COLOR ATLAS & SYNOPSIS OF PEDIATRIC DERMATOLOGY

Kay Shou-Mei Kane, MD
Assistant Professor of Dermatology
Harvard Medical School
Clinical Associate of Dermatology
Children's Hospital
Boston, Massachusetts
Clinical Associate of Dermatology
Mt. Auburn Hospital
Boston, Massachusetts

Vinod E. Nambudiri, MD, MBA
Attending Physician, Internal Medicine
Grand Strand Regional Medical Center
Myrtle Beach, South Carolina
Associate Physician, Department of Dermatology
Brigham and Women's Hospital
Boston, Massachusetts

Alexander J. Stratigos, MD
Professor of Dermatology—Venereology
University of Athens School of Medicine
Andreas Syngros Hospital for Skin and Venereal Diseases
Athens, Greece

COLOR ATLAS & SYNOPSIS OF PEDIATRIC DERMATOLOGY

THIRD EDITION

Kay Shou-Mei Kane, MD

Vinod E. Nambudiri, MD, MBA

Alexander J. Stratigos, MD

New York   Chicago   San Francisco   Athens   London   Madrid
Mexico City   Milan   New Delhi   Singapore   Sydney   Toronto

Color Atlas & Synopsis of Pediatric Dermatology, Third Edition

2 3 4 5 6 7 8 9   DSS   21 20 19 18

ISBN   978-0-07-184394-2
MHID   0-07-184394-9

This book was set in Minion Pro by Aptara, Inc.
The editors were Karen G. Edmonson and Robert Pancotti.
The production supervisor was Catherine H. Saggese.
Project management was provided by Nomeeta Devi, Aptara, Inc.
The text designer was Alan Barnett; the cover designer was Dreamit, Inc.
RR Donnelley was the printer and binder.

Library of Congress Cataloging-in-Publication Data

Names: Kane, Kay Shou-Mei, author. | Nambudiri, Vinod E., author. |
    Stratigos, Alexander J., author.
Title: Color atlas & synopsis of pediatric dermatology / Kay Shou-Mei Kane,
    Vinod E. Nambudiri, Alexander J. Stratigos.
Other titles: Color atlas and synopsis of pediatric dermatology
Description: Third edition. | New York : McGraw-Hill Education, [2016] |
    Preceded by Color atlas & synopsis of pediatric dermatology / Kay
    Shou-Mei Kane ... [et al.]. 2nd ed. c2009. | Includes bibliographical
references and index.
Identifiers: LCCN 2015041709| ISBN 9780071843942 (pbk.) | ISBN 0071843949
Subjects: | MESH: Infant–Atlases. | Skin Diseases–Atlases. |
    Adolescent–Atlases. | Child–Atlases.
Classification: LCC RJ511 | NLM WS 17 | DDC 618.92/5–dc23 LC record
available at http://lccn.loc.gov/2015041709

McGraw-Hill Education books are available at special quantity discounts to use as premiums and sales promotions or for use in corporate training programs. To contact a representative, please visit the Contact Us pages at www.mhprofessional.com.

Once again to my wonderful family: David, Michaela, and Cassandra.
And to the readers who have purchased all three editions of this book.
Kay S. Kane

To my wife Navya and my son Abhinav for their love,
To my family and friends for their support,
To my teachers and mentors for their guidance,
And to my patients for their inspiration.
Vinod E. Nambudiri

To my wife Natassa and my sons Yannis and Aristomenis for their love and
unlimited support,
To my teachers for their mentorship and guidance,
And to my patients with endless gratitude.
Alexander J. Stratigos

CONTENTS

SECTION 17

SECTION 18

SECTION 19

SECTION 20

PREFACE

The third edition of the *Color Atlas & Synopsis of Pediatric Dermatology* builds upon its predecessors with new photographs plus up-to-date management and treatment recommendations for pediatric skin diseases. The book is written primarily for primary care specialists, residents, and medical students with the hopes of providing an easy-to-read, image-rich resource to aid in the in-office diagnosis and treatment of pediatric skin disorders.

The authors have made every attempt to provide accurate information regarding the disease entities and the therapies approved for pediatric usage at the time of publication. However, in this world of ever-changing medicine, it is recommended that the reader confirm information contained herein with other sources.

ACKNOWLEDGMENTS

"Practicing dermatologists are like the woodwind section of the orchestra—small in number . . . when they play they must play well."
Thomas B. Fitzpatrick, MD

I would like to thank my colleagues who have supported me throughout the years: Richard Allen Johnson, MD, Stephen Gellis, MD, Marilyn Liang, MD, Jennifer Huang, MD, Elena Hawryluk, MD, Jeffrey Dover, MD, Kenneth Arndt, MD, Thomas Rohrer, MD, Robin Travers, MD, Tania Phillips, MD, Brooke Sikora, MD, Jeffrey Sobell, MD, Katrina Dy, MD, Joyce Hennessy, RN, Maria Benoit, RN, Janet Weaver, RN, Karol Timmons, RN, Lisa Fitzgerald, Maria Alfeo, Maureen Teehan, Andrea DiGiulio, Beth Hartigan, Lenore Rosen, Diane Lysak, Jenna Mazzaferro, Micaela Berger, Shannon Patti, and Laura Mateo. From the previous editions we will always be indebted to Peter Lio, MD, Howard Baden, MD, Jennifer Ryder, MD, Karen Wiss, MD, and Lisa Cohen, MD. And finally, a shout-out to the Buckingham, Browne & Nichols Parents' Association Executive Board, without whom this book would have been completed five years earlier.

Kay S. Kane

COLOR ATLAS & SYNOPSIS OF PEDIATRIC DERMATOLOGY

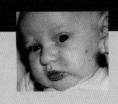
CUTANEOUS FINDINGS IN THE NEWBORN

PHYSIOLOGIC SKIN FINDINGS IN THE NEWBORN

VERNIX CASEOSA

Vernix, derived from the same root as *varnish*, is the whitish-gray covering on newborn skin and is composed of degenerated fetal epidermis and sebaceous secretions.

EPIDEMIOLOGY

AGE Newborns.
GENDER M = F.
PREVALENCE Seen in all infants.

PATHOPHYSIOLOGY

The vernix caseosa is thought to play a protective role for the newborn skin with both water-barrier and antimicrobial properties.

PHYSICAL EXAMINATION

Skin Findings

TYPE OF LESION Adherent cheesy material which dries and desquamates after birth (Fig. 1-1).
COLOR Gray-to-white.
DISTRIBUTION Generalized.

DIFFERENTIAL DIAGNOSIS

The vernix caseosa is generally very distinctive but must be differentiated from other membranous coverings such as collodion baby and harlequin fetus. Both of these are much thicker, more rigid, and more dry.

COURSE AND PROGNOSIS

In an otherwise healthy newborn, the vernix caseosa will fall off in 1 to 2 weeks.

TREATMENT

No treatment is necessary. Much of the vernix caseosa is usually wiped from the skin at birth. The rest of the vernix is shed over the first few weeks of life.

Current newborn skin care recommendations are as follows:

1. Full immersion baths are not recommended until the umbilical stump is fully healed and detached.
2. At birth, blood and meconium can be gently removed with warm water and cotton balls.
3. Umbilical cord care and/or circumcision varies from hospital to hospital. Several methods include simply maintaining a dry cord environment, local application of alcohol (alcohol wipes), topical antibiotic (bacitracin, Polysporin, or neosporin), or silver sulfadiazine cream (Silvadene) to the area(s) with each diaper change. The umbilical cord typically falls off in 7 to 14 days.
4. Until the umbilical and/or circumcision sites are healed, spot cleaning the baby with cotton balls and warm water is recommended. After the open sites have healed, the baby can be gently immersed in lukewarm water and rinsed from head to toe.
5. Avoiding perfumed soaps and bubble baths is best. Fragrance-free, soap-free cleansers are the least irritating. Such cleansers should be used only on dirty areas and rinsed off immediately.
6. After bathing, newborn skin should be patted dry (not rubbed). The vernix caseosa may still be present and adherent for several weeks. Topical moisturizers are usually not recommended.

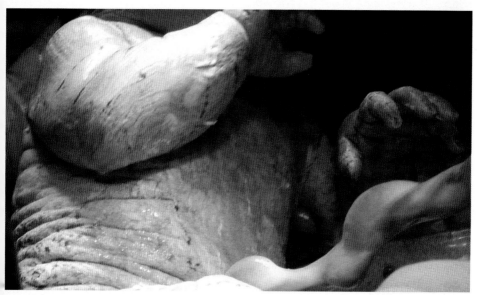

FIGURE 1-1 Vernix caseosa White, cheesy vernix caseosa on a newborn baby, just a few seconds old. (Used with permission from Dr. Mark Waltzman.)

CUTIS MARMORATA

A physiologic red–blue reticulated mottling of the skin of newborn infants. It is seen as an immature physiologic response to cold with resultant dilatation of capillaries and small venules. Skin findings usually disappear with rewarming and the phenomenon resolves as the child gets older.

 INSIGHT While cutis marmorata is essentially always normal, its analog in adults, livedo reticularis, can be associated with connective tissue disease and vasculopathies.

EPIDEMIOLOGY

AGE Onset during first 2 to 4 weeks of life; associated with cold exposure.
GENDER M = F.
PREVALENCE More prevalent in premature infants.

PATHOPHYSIOLOGY

Thought to be owing to the immaturity of the autonomic nervous system of newborns. Physiologically normal and resolves as child gets older.

HISTORY

Reticulated mottling of the skin resolves with warming.

PHYSICAL EXAMINATION

Skin Findings

TYPE Reticulated mottling (Fig. 1-2).

COLOR Reddish-blue.
DISTRIBUTION Diffuse, symmetric involvement of the trunk and extremities.

DIFFERENTIAL DIAGNOSIS

Cutis marmorata is benign and self-limited. It can be confused with cutis marmorata telangiectatica congenita (CMTC), a more severe condition that can also present as reticulated vascular changes at birth which do not ameliorate with warming the infant. CMTC is a rare, chronic, relapsing, severe form of vascular disease that can lead to permanent scarring skin changes.

COURSE AND PROGNOSIS

Recurrence is unusual after 1 month of age. Persistence beyond neonatal period is a possible marker for trisomy 18, Down syndrome, Cornelia de Lange syndrome, hypothyroidism, or CMTC and children with such persistent presentations should be evaluated for additional workup.

TREATMENT AND PREVENTION

Usually self-resolving.

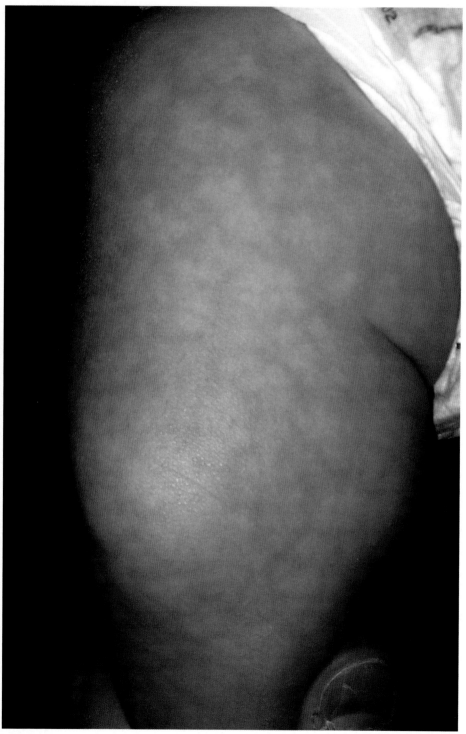

FIGURE 1-2 Cutis marmorata Reticulated, vascular mottling on the leg of a healthy newborn which resolves quickly with warming.

NEONATAL HAIR LOSS

Neonatal hair at birth is actively growing in the anagen phase, but within the first few days of life converts to telogen (the rest period before shedding hair). Consequently, there is normally significant hair shedding during the first 3 to 4 months of life.

 INSIGHT Parents may complain that "back to sleep" is the cause of hair loss in their child; the sleep position only accentuates the normal loss and is not the cause.

SYNONYM Telogen effluvium of the newborn.

EPIDEMIOLOGY

AGE Newborns, can be seen at 3 to 4 months of age.
GENDER M = F.
PREVALENCE Affects all infants to some degree.

PATHOPHYSIOLOGY

There are three stages in the hair life cycle:

1. Anagen (the active growing phase that typically lasts from 2 to 6 years).
2. Catagen (a short-partial degeneration phase that lasts from 10 to 14 days).
3. Telogen (resting and shedding phase that lasts from 3 to 4 months).

At any given time in a normal scalp, approximately 89% of the hair are in anagen phase, 1% are in catagen phase, and 10% are in telogen phase. Neonatal hair loss occurs because most of the anagen hair at birth simultaneously converts to telogen phase in the first few days of life, resulting in whole-scalp shedding of the birth hair in 3 to 4 months.

HISTORY

During the first 3 to 6 months of life, there will be physiologic shedding of the newborn hair.

In some cases, the growth of new hair balances the shedding hair and the process is almost undetectable.

PHYSICAL EXAMINATION

Skin Findings

TYPE OF LESION Nonscarring alopecia (Fig. 1-3).
DISTRIBUTION Diffuse involving the entire scalp.

DIFFERENTIAL DIAGNOSIS

Neonatal hair loss is a normal physiologic process that is diagnosed clinically by history and physical examination. The alopecia may be accentuated on the occipital scalp because of friction and pressure from sleeping on the back. If associated with significant crusting, scale, or inflammation, other causes of hair loss should be excluded such as seborrheic dermatitis (cradle cap) and tinea capitis.

COURSE AND PROGNOSIS

In an otherwise healthy newborn, the hair loss self-resolves by 6 to 12 months of age.

TREATMENT

No treatment is necessary. The parents should be reassured that neonatal hair loss is a normal physiologic process and that the hair will grow back by 6 to 12 months of age without treatment. If hair regrowth does not occur or is irregular, structural disorders of the hair shaft, vitamin deficiencies, mineral deficiencies, and other processes such as alopecia areata should be ruled out.

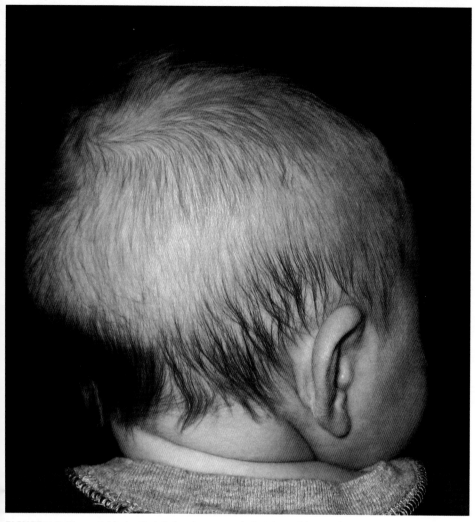

FIGURE 1-3 Neonatal hair Occipital and vertex scalp hair loss of the newborn hair in a healthy 4-month-old baby.

MISCELLANEOUS CUTANEOUS DISORDERS OF THE NEWBORN

MILIARIA, NEWBORN

Miliaria is a common neonatal dermatosis resulting from sweat retention caused by incomplete differentiation of the epidermis and its appendages. Obstruction and rupture of epidermal sweat ducts is manifested by a vesicular eruption.

 INSIGHT In older children and adults, miliaria rubra is the most common form, usually seen in areas of moist occlusion, such as on the back of a bedridden patient with fever.

SYNONYMS Prickly heat, heat rash.

EPIDEMIOLOGY

AGE Newborn.
GENDER M = F.
INCIDENCE Greatest in the first few weeks of life.
PREVALENCE Virtually, all infants develop miliaria. More common in warmer climates with greater proclivity for sweating.
ETIOLOGY Immature appendages and keratin plugging of eccrine duct lead to vesicular eruption.

PATHOPHYSIOLOGY

Incomplete differentiation of the epidermis and its appendages at birth leads to keratinous plugging of eccrine ducts and subsequent leakage of eccrine sweat into the surrounding tissue. Staphylococci on the skin may play a role in the occlusion process as well.

PHYSICAL EXAMINATION

Skin Findings
Miliaria Crystallina (Sudamina)

TYPE Superficial pinpoint clear vesicles (Fig. 1-4). No surrounding inflammation.
COLOR Skin-colored, pink.
DISTRIBUTION Generalized in crops.
SITES OF PREDILECTION Intertriginous areas, commonly neck and axillae, or clothing-covered truncal areas.

Miliaria Rubra (Prickly Heat, Heat Rash)

TYPE Pinpoint papules/vesicles.
COLOR Erythematous.
SITES OF PREDILECTION Covered parts of the skin, forehead, upper trunk, volar aspects of the arms, and body folds.

DIFFERENTIAL DIAGNOSIS

The diagnosis of miliaria is made based on observation of characteristic lesions. Vesicles may be ruptured with a fine needle, yielding clear, entrapped sweat; infectious organisms are NOT present. Miliaria rubra—and particularly miliaria pustulosa (comprising pustular lesions)—requires close inspection to ascertain its nonfollicular nature to distinguish it from folliculitis. Miliaria can also be confused with candidiasis and acne.

LABORATORY EXAMINATIONS

In miliaria crystallina, vesicles are often found superficially in the stratum corneum and serial sectioning demonstrates direct communication with ruptured sweat ducts. Miliaria rubra histologically demonstrates degrees of spongiosis and vesicle formation within the epidermal sweat duct.

MANAGEMENT

PREVENTION Avoid excessive heat and humidity. Lightweight and/or absorbent clothing, cool baths, and air conditioning help prevent sweat retention.
TREATMENT Preventative measures only for newborns; in older patients, cool moist dressings, antibacterial cleansers, and cream-based emollients may speed healing.

FIGURE 1-4 Miliaria Superficial, clear, pinpoint vesicles of miliaria crystallina on the back of an infant.

MILIA

Multiple 1- to 2-mm milky-white/yellow superficial tiny cysts seen over the forehead, cheeks, and nose of infants. They may be present in the oral cavity (Epstein's pearls).

 INSIGHT So-called secondary milia (milia after trauma to the skin) can be seen in patients with blistering disorders such as epidermolysis bullosa.

EPIDEMIOLOGY

AGE All ages, especially newborns.
GENDER M = F.
PREVALENCE Up to 40% of infants have milia on the skin, up to 85% of infants have the intraoral counterpart (Epstein's pearls) on the palate.
ETIOLOGY May be related to trauma to the skin surface during delivery.

PATHOPHYSIOLOGY

Milia and Epstein's pearls are caused by the cystic retention of keratin in the superficial epidermis.

PHYSICAL EXAMINATION

Skin Findings

TYPE Few to numerous pinpoint white papules (Fig. 1-5).
SIZE 1 to 2 mm.
COLOR Yellow to pearly white.
DISTRIBUTION Forehead, nose, cheeks, gingiva, midline palate (Epstein's pearls), rarely on the penis, and at sites of trauma.

DIFFERENTIAL DIAGNOSIS

Milia must be differentiated from molluscum contagiosum and sebaceous hyperplasia.

Molluscum contagiosum does not typically appear in the immediate neonatal period and is characterized by dome-shaped papules with central umbilication. Sebaceous hyperplasia is usually more yellow than white in color and, on close inspection, is found to be composed of tiny aggregates of micropapules with central umbilication. Epstein's pearls can be differentiated from intraoral mucinous cysts by their typical midline palate location and spontaneous resolution.

LABORATORY EXAMINATIONS

DERMATOPATHOLOGY Superficial, tiny epithelial cysts containing keratin and developing in connection with the pilosebaceous follicle.

COURSE AND PROGNOSIS

Milia and Epstein's pearls should spontaneously exfoliate during the first few weeks of life. Unusually, persistent milia or widespread milia can be seen in conjunction with more severe developmental problems, namely, oral-facial-digital syndrome, steatocystoma multiplex, and hereditary trichodysplasia.

TREATMENT AND PREVENTION

No treatment is necessary. Cosmetically, lesions may be incised and expressed. For long-standing or persistent lesions in older children, topical retinoids may be another useful treatment option.

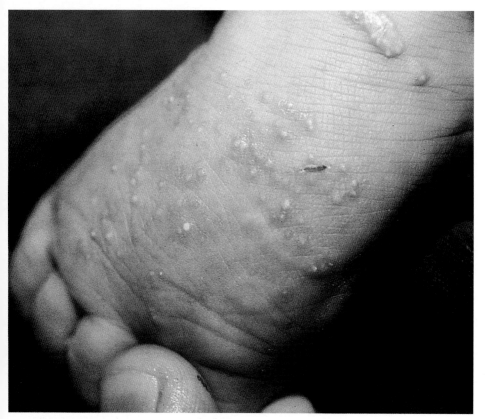

FIGURE 1-5 Milia Numerous pinpoint, white papules on the foot of a premature infant.

ACNE NEONATORUM

Acne neonatorum is a benign, self-limited, acneiform eruption that develops within the first 30 days of life.

INSIGHT

In severe cases that do not resolve, evaluation for underlying androgen excess is warranted.

SYNONYMS Transient cephalic neonatal pustulosis, neonatal cephalic pustulosis.

EPIDEMIOLOGY

AGE Rare at birth, peaks between the age of 2 and 4 weeks of life.
GENDER M = F.
PREVALENCE Up to 50% of infants.

PATHOPHYSIOLOGY

Some, perhaps most, of these cases are thought to be related to *Malassezia* yeasts on the skin. Transient increases in circulatory androgens may also contribute to neonatal acne.

HISTORY

Multiple discrete papules develop between the age of 2 and 4 weeks of life, evolve into pustules, and spontaneously resolve.

PHYSICAL EXAMINATION

Skin Findings

TYPE Inflammatory papules and pustules; comedones are rare (Fig. 1-6).

COLOR Erythematous.
DISTRIBUTION Face, scalp >> chest, back, and groin.

DIFFERENTIAL DIAGNOSIS

Erythema toxicum, candidiasis, and staphylococcal infection can be considered.

LABORATORY EXAMINATIONS

DERMATOPATHOLOGY Increased number of sebaceous glands and keratin-plugged pilosebaceous orifices lead to rupturing and neutrophilic or granulomatous inflammation.

COURSE AND PROGNOSIS

Neonatal acne may persist up to 8 months of age. There is some suggestion that infants with extensive neonatal acne may experience severe acne as adults, though data are conflicting.

TREATMENT AND PREVENTION

Neonatal acne typically resolves spontaneously. For severe involvement, 2% ketoconazole cream, 2.5% benzoyl peroxide gel applied twice daily, or a mild 1% hydrocortisone cream may be used.

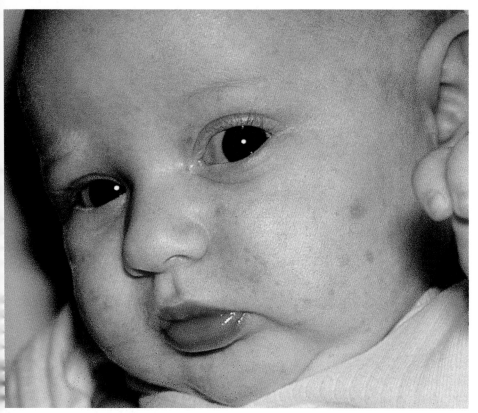

FIGURE 1-6 Acne neonatorum Acneiform lesions on the cheek of an infant.

ERYTHEMA TOXICUM NEONATORUM

Benign transient, blotchy erythema with central vesiculation is seen in newborns.

EPIDEMIOLOGY

AGE Newborns.
GENDER M = F.
PREVALENCE Reports range from 4.5% to 70% of term infants. Less common in premature infants. May be slightly more common in infants delivered via cesarean section or from multiparous births.

PATHOPHYSIOLOGY

The cause of erythema toxicum is unknown. The eosinophil response is suggestive of a hypersensitivity reaction, but specific allergens have not been identified.

HISTORY

Macular erythema with central vesicles and pustules appear between 24 and 48 hours of life.

PHYSICAL EXAMINATION

Skin Findings

TYPE Blotchy erythematous macules 2 to 3 cm in diameter with a central 1- to 4-mm central papule, vesicle, or pustule (Fig. 1-7).
COLOR Erythematous.
DISTRIBUTION Chest, back, face, and proximal extremities, sparing the palms and soles.

DIAGNOSIS AND DIFFERENTIAL DIAGNOSIS

DIAGNOSIS Wright stain of a vesicle will reveal a predominance of eosinophils. Gram stain will be negative for bacteria.
DIFFERENTIAL DIAGNOSIS Erythema toxicum must be differentiated from miliaria rubra and transient neonatal pustular melanosis. The lesions of erythema toxicum are usually larger than those of miliaria rubra and have wider erythematous halos surrounding them. Transient neonatal pustular melanosis has a predominance of neutrophils rather than eosinophils in the vesicles and typically heals with residual pigmentation. Bacterial and fungal culture of erythema toxicum lesions will be negative differentiating it from neonatal bacterial infections and congenital candidiasis. More worrisome considerations include herpes infection and Langerhans cell histiocytosis. These entities may require virologic testing and skin biopsy for definitive diagnosis and must not be overlooked.

LABORATORY EXAMINATIONS

WRIGHT STAIN A smear of a vesicle with Wright stain reveals numerous eosinophils.
GRAM STAIN Negative.
DERMATOPATHOLOGY Intraepidermal vesicle filled with eosinophils.
HEMATOLOGIC EXAMINATION Peripheral eosinophilia of up to 20% may be seen in some cases.

COURSE AND PROGNOSIS

Lesions may occur from birth to the 10th day of life and individual lesions clear spontaneously within 5 days. All lesions resolve by 2 weeks.

TREATMENT

No treatment is necessary.

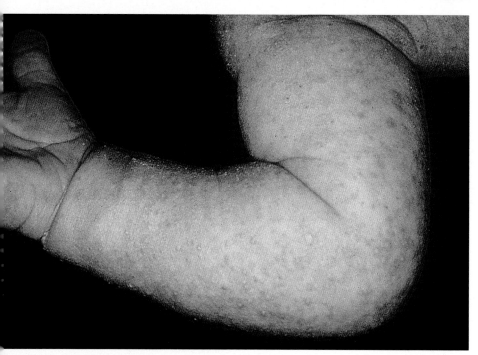

FIGURE 1-7 Erythema toxicum neonatorum Erythematous macules with central vesicles scattered diffusely over the arm of a newborn. A smear of the vesicle contents would show a predominance of eosinophils.

TRANSIENT NEONATAL PUSTULAR MELANOSIS

A benign and self-limited condition characterized by blotchy erythema and superficial vesicopustules of the newborn that heal with residual pigmentation.

 INSIGHT Many times, particularly in postterm infants, no pustules or vesicles remain at birth and only pigmented macules are found.

EPIDEMIOLOGY

AGE Newborns.
GENDER M = F.
RACE More common in black infants.
PREVALENCE 0.2% to 4% of newborns.

PATHOPHYSIOLOGY

The pathophysiology is unknown.

HISTORY

Idiopathic, superficial, sterile vesicles and pustules that are present at birth rupture in 24 to 48 hours and heal with pigmented macules that slowly fade over several months.

PHYSICAL EXAMINATION

Skin Findings

TYPE Tiny vesicles, pustules (Fig. 1-8), or ruptured lesions with a collarette of scale. There is generally minimal or no surrounding erythema.
COLOR Hyperpigmented macules may develop at the site of resolving vesicles and pustules.

DISTRIBUTION Clusters on face, trunk, and proximal extremities, rarely palms and soles may be involved.

DIAGNOSIS AND DIFFERENTIAL DIAGNOSIS

DIAGNOSIS Wright stain of a vesicle will reveal a predominance of neutrophils. Gram stain will be negative for bacteria.
DIFFERENTIAL DIAGNOSIS Includes erythema toxicum neonatorum, staphylococcal and other bacterial infections, candidiasis, herpes, and miliaria.

LABORATORY EXAMINATIONS

WRIGHT STAIN A smear of a vesicle with Wright stain reveals numerous neutrophils and an occasional eosinophil.
GRAM STAIN Negative.
DERMATOPATHOLOGY Vesicular lesions show intraepidermal vesicles filled with neutrophils. Macular hyperpigmented lesions show mild hyperkeratosis and basilar hyperpigmentation.

COURSE AND PROGNOSIS

The vesicles and pustules usually disappear by 5 days of age and the pigmented macules fade over 3 to 6 months.

TREATMENT

No treatment is necessary.

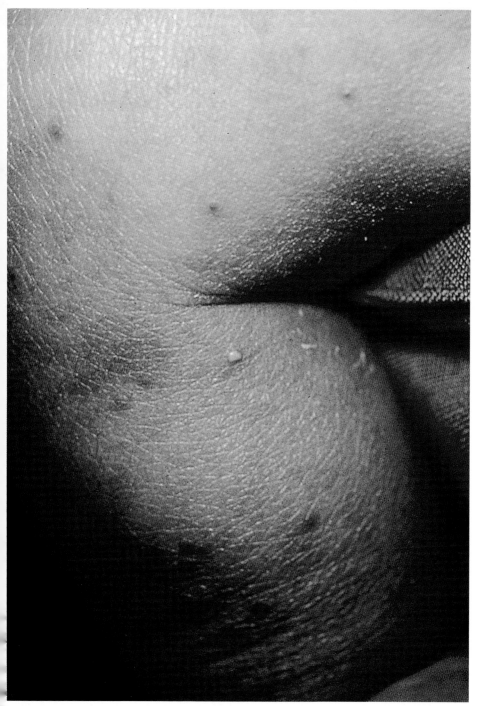

FIGURE 1-8 Transient neonatal pustular melanosis Vesicles and pustules scattered diffusely on the leg of an infant. Note the hyperpigmented areas at sites of resolved lesions. A smear of the vesicle contents would reveal a predominance of neutrophils.

ACROPUSTULOSIS OF INFANCY

A benign vesicular and pustular pruritic eruption that begins in infancy and often has a waxing and waning course with recurrences every few months over the first years of life. Children with a prior exposure to scabies may be at a higher risk.

EPIDEMIOLOGY

AGE Usually starts in first year of life; resolves over 2 years.
GENDER Male = Female.
RACE No clear racial predilection; Black race reported as having a higher incidence in some studies.
PREVALENCE Uncommon.

PATHOPHYSIOLOGY

The exact pathophysiology of infantile acropustulosis is not known. One postulated mechanism is a persistent localized allergic hypersensitivity or inflammatory response to a foreign antigen. Reports suggest an increased prevalence of the eruption in children with a prior history of scabies, but no conclusive pathophysiologic link has been demonstrated. Other etiologic theories include an atypical infectious cause.

HISTORY

Lesions typically present during the first year of life. The skin eruption consists of crops of erythematous macules that evolve into vesicles and pustules predominantly on the palms and soles, as well as the dorsal hands and feet. The eruption is pruritic and infants may exhibit discomfort and irritability associated with the eruption. The lesions may spontaneously heal after 1 to 2 weeks and return periodically.

PHYSICAL EXAMINATION

Skin Findings

TYPE Vesicles, pustules.
COLOR Pink to whitish; tan brown residual hyperpigmentation after resolution (Fig. 1-9).
DISTRIBUTION Palms, soles > dorsal feet, dorsal hands, extremities.

DIAGNOSIS AND DIFFERENTIAL DIAGNOSIS

DIAGNOSIS Clinical history and physical findings with vesicles and pustules confined to the feet and hands are sufficient to make the diagnosis. Skin scrapings of vesicles should be performed to rule out scabies infestation. Gram stain and KOH preparations should be negative in acropustulosis.
DIFFERENTIAL DIAGNOSIS The differential diagnosis includes scabies, atopic dermatitis, pustular psoriasis, contact dermatitis, impetigo, and transient neonatal pustular melanosis.

LABORATORY EXAMINATIONS

GRAM STAIN Negative.
KOH PREP Negative.
SCABIES (MINERAL OIL) PREP Negative.
DERMATOPATHOLOGY Subcorneal pustules filled with neutrophils and eosinophils.

COURSE AND PROGNOSIS

The vesicles and pustules usually resolve within 2 weeks, but recurrent eruptions may persist for up to 2 years. Lesions may heal with postinflammatory hyperpigmentation that gradually fades over 3 to 6 months.

TREATMENT

The eruption is generally self-limited. Treatment with topical corticosteroids has been reported to lead to symptomatic improvement. If pruritus is strongly associated with the eruption, oral antihistamines such as hydroxyzine or diphenhydramine at bedtime may be useful for symptomatic relief. Refractory cases have been reported to respond to oral erythromycin (40 mg/kg/d) and dapsone (1–2 mg/kg/d), presumably for their anti-inflammatory effects.

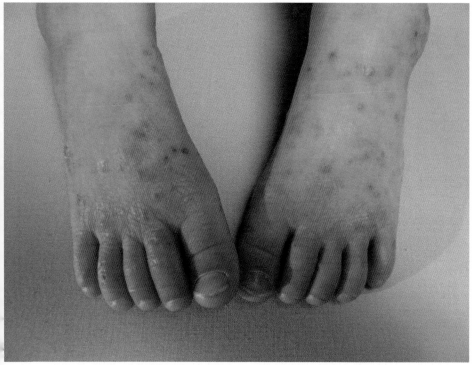

FIGURE 1-9 Acropustulosis of infancy Erythematous vesicles and pustules on the bilateral dorsal feet. Scattered areas of hyperpigmentation from prior eruptions are present.

NEONATAL LUPUS ERYTHEMATOSUS

Neonatal lupus erythematosus (NLE) is an uncommon autoimmune disease caused by the transplacental antibodies from mother to fetus. The skin lesions are usually nonscarring and similar to those of subacute cutaneous lupus erythematosus (SCLE) in adults. Rarely, however, skin atrophy can result. The lesions may be accompanied by cardiac conduction defects, hepatobiliary diseases, or hematologic disturbances.

INSIGHT

If a newborn is thought to have "widespread ringworm," neonatal lupus must be considered.

EPIDEMIOLOGY

AGE Skin lesions may be present at birth or may appear within the first few months of life. Lesions typically last several weeks to months, but typically resolve by 6 months of age. Heart block appears typically during gestation (at about 18 weeks of gestational age, but may occur later) and is generally irreversible.

GENDER M = F.

INCIDENCE Unknown. One estimate, based on the incidence of congenital heart block with NLE being the most frequent etiology, approximates the incidence of NLE to be near 1:20,000 births. NLE with cutaneous involvement occurs in up to 10% to 20% of mothers with SLE and anti-Ro antibodies.

ETIOLOGY AND TRANSMISSION Maternal autoantibodies cross the placenta during pregnancy and are thought to produce both the cutaneous and systemic findings of NLE. Many mothers of neonatal lupus patients have no symptoms of connective tissue disease.

PATHOPHYSIOLOGY

Mothers of babies with NLE possess autoantibodies (95% of cases possess anti-Ro/SSA, others may have anti-La/SSb or anti-U_1RNP antibodies). These IgG autoantibodies pass through the placenta from mother to fetus and can be found in the neonate's serum. It is felt that these autoantibodies are implicated in the development of cutaneous and systemic findings of NLE. The skin lesions are temporary and begin to resolve at or before the time that maternal autoantibodies are cleared from the child's system (typically at 6 months of age). Conduction defects may be caused by anti-Ro/SSA-mediated interference of specific cardiac serotoninergic receptors.

PHYSICAL EXAMINATION

About half of the NLE cases exhibit skin disease while fewer exhibit congenital heart block. Approximately 10% have both skin disease and heart block.

Skin Findings

TYPE Scaly plaques, epidermal atrophy. Generally, no scarring or follicular plugging.

COLOR Pink, erythematous. May be hypopigmented.

SHAPE Round, elliptical, or annular.

DISTRIBUTION Frequently on face and scalp. Lesions may be concentrated in the periorbital and malar areas. Widespread involvement may occur (Fig. 1-10).

General Findings

Typically, disease presents with complete heart block that begins during gestation. Occasionally, lesser degrees of conduction abnormality are present. Fibrosis of the AV node (in rare instances, the SA node) may lead to bradycardia. NLE typically presents with isolated heart block and no associated cardiac anomalies. Other findings include liver disease, thrombocytopenia, and leukopenia.

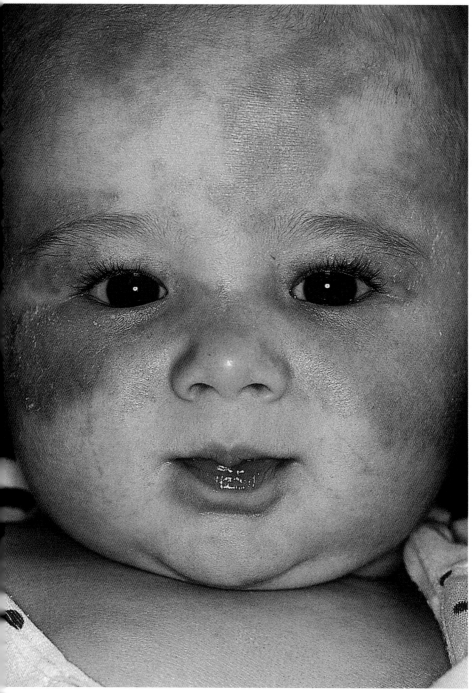

FIGURE 1-10 Neonatal lupus erythematous Erythematous, annular plaques on the face of a healthy 5-week-old baby. Skin lesions resolved after 6 months.

DIFFERENTIAL DIAGNOSIS

The skin findings of the newborn may be confused with other scaly, erythematous plaques such as seborrhea, eczema, psoriasis, or tinea. Heart block may be detected during routine obstetrical examination and confirmed by fetal ultrasound. Finally, the diagnosis can be confirmed by serologic studies.

LABORATORY EXAMINATIONS

HISTOPATHOLOGY Biopsy of lesional skin reveals findings similar to that of SCLE lesions. There is vacuolar basal cell degeneration in the epidermis and a sparse mononuclear cell infiltrate in the superficial dermis. Immunofluorescence studies demonstrate a granular deposition pattern of IgG in the dermoepidermal junction with variable C3 and IgM deposition. **SEROLOGY** Sera of mother and baby should be tested for autoantibodies. Ninety-five percent of cases are owing to anti-Ro/SSA antibodies. Anti-La/SSB antibodies may also be present but almost never without the presence of anti-Ro/SSA antibodies. Anti-U_1RNP autoantibodies account for the NLE cases that do not have anti-Ro/SSA antibodies present. **OTHER** Obstetrical detection of slowed fetal heart rate or ultrasound documentation of heart block may be found as early as 16 weeks of gestational age.

COURSE AND PROGNOSIS

Infants with NLE who survive the neonatal period have a good prognosis and rarely go on to develop autoimmune disease. The estimated mortality rate is 10%, with deaths being secondary to intractable heart failure during the neonatal period. Mothers with babies, who develop NLE do not have an increased rate of spontaneous abortion but often develop autoimmune disease, on an average, 5 years after delivery. The risk of NLE in future pregnancies is approximately 25% for mothers who have had one child with NLE.

Skin Findings

The cutaneous lesions of NLE in the neonate are benign and transient, usually lasting weeks to months and regress by the age of 6 months, occasionally with residual postinflammatory hypopigmentation or atrophy that gradually improves.

General Findings

Despite complete heart block and a subsequent slowed heart rate, babies with cardiac involvement of NLE tend to be well compensated. Half of them do not require any treatment, and the other half need pacemakers. Approximately 10% do not respond despite pacemaker placement likely because of coexistent myocardial disease, and die of intractable heart failure.

MANAGEMENT

During Gestation

Testing for autoantibodies during pregnancy is appropriate for women with anti-Ro/SSA autoantibody symptomatology: Sjögren's syndrome, SCLE, SLE, arthralgias, dry eyes, dry mouth, or photosensitivity. Women with previous births with heart block or other signs/symptoms suggestive of NLE should also be tested. It is important to keep in mind that 50% of women with babies with NLE are asymptomatic at delivery and conversely, most women with anti-Ro/SSA antibodies will have normal babies. It is estimated that only 1% to 2% of women with anti-Ro/SSA autoantibodies will have a baby with NLE demonstrating cardiac involvement. Risk factors that increase these percentages include a previous baby with NLE and mothers with the diagnosis of SLE. Screening tests should include fluorescent antibody tests for anti-Ro/SSA, anti-La/SSB, and anti-U$_1$RNP autoantibodies.

Obstetrical screening for a slowed fetal heart rate is also important and if heart block is con-firmed, the fetus should be monitored carefully for the development of hydrops fetalis. The delivery room should be equipped to manage a newborn with possible heart failure. The use of systemic steroids or plasmapheresis during gestation has been utilized in life-threatening circumstances. Data suggest the use of antimalarials such as hydroxychloroquine by a mother with anti-Ro antibodies during pregnancy can reduce the risk of developing NLE or the severity of the disease in newborns.

Neonatal Period

SKIN FINDINGS Skin disease is generally benign and self-limited. Supportive care includes strict sun protection and topical steroids for more severe cutaneous involvement. Systemic treatment is not indicated.

GENERAL FINDINGS Treatment of heart disease is not always indicated. For those children with heart failure because of a slowed heart rate, pacemaker implantation is the treatment of choice.

APLASIA CUTIS CONGENITA

Aplasia cutis congenita is a congenital defect of the scalp characterized by localized loss of the epidermis, dermis, and sometimes, subcutaneous tissue.

EPIDEMIOLOGY

AGE Present at birth.
GENDER M = F.
INCIDENCE Unclear; one estimate is 1 in 10,000 births.
ETIOLOGY Unknown for most cases; whereas, some are related to genetic syndromes, fetus papyraceous, and teratogens.
GENETICS Most cases are sporadic, some familial cases are reported.

PATHOPHYSIOLOGY

The exact mechanism of this disorder is not known. It is hypothesized that aplasia cutis congenita results from incomplete neural tube closure or an embryonic arrest of skin development. Mutations in cell cycle signaling pathways are postulated to be associated with the genetic forms of the disease.

HISTORY

Aplasia cutis congenita presents as an asymptomatic ulceration of the scalp at birth that heals with scarring. Lesions from earlier in gestation may present as membrane-like scars at birth.

PHYSICAL EXAMINATION

Skin Findings

TYPE OF LESION Ulceration that is replaced with scar tissue (Fig. 1-11). In the scar, no hair or appendages are present. A ring of long hair around the lesion (hair collar sign) may be present.
SIZE 1 to 3 cm, may be larger.
SHAPE Round, oval, or stellate.
NUMBER Solitary lesion (70% of cases), two lesions (20% of cases), three or more lesions (10% of cases).
COLOR Pink to red healing to white–gray.
DISTRIBUTION Scalp vertex, midline (50% of cases) or adjacent areas (30%). Can also rarely be seen on the face, trunk, or extremities.

General Findings

Typically, aplasia cutis congenita is an isolated skin finding. In rare instances, it may be seen with other developmental abnormalities such as skeletal, cardiac, neurologic, or vascular malformations.

DIFFERENTIAL DIAGNOSIS

The diagnosis of aplasia cutis congenita is made by history and physical examination. It should be differentiated from scalp electrode monitors, forceps, or other iatrogenic birth injuries as well as neonatal herpes simplex virus infection. Parental history regarding any similar congenital lesions should be elicited.

LABORATORY EXAMINATIONS

DERMATOPATHOLOGY Skin biopsy reveals an absence of the epidermis and appendageal structures. There is a decrease in dermal elastic tissue, and, in some deep cases, a loss of all skin layers and subcutaneous tissues.

COURSE AND PROGNOSIS

The prognosis of cutis aplasia congenita as an isolated finding is good. The ulceration typically heals with scarring in a few weeks. The scarred area will persist as an asymptomatic lesion for life.

TREATMENT

Localized care of the ulcerated area at birth includes the following:

1. Gentle cleansing of the area with warm water and cotton balls.
2. A thin layer of topical antibiotic ointment (Bactroban, bacitracin, Polysporin, or neosporin) to prevent secondary infection.
3. Protective coverings to prevent further trauma to the area. The area will heal with scarring and, as the child grows, the scar usually becomes inconspicuous and covered with surrounding hair.

In instances of aplasia cutis congenita associated with a hair collar sign, evaluation for underlying associated CNS anomalies should be considered.

Long-term management options for aplasia cutis congenita are:

1. No treatment. The scarred area should be examined annually for any changes since scarred areas do have a higher risk of neoplastic transformation.
2. Surgical correction of the area by excision or hair transplant.

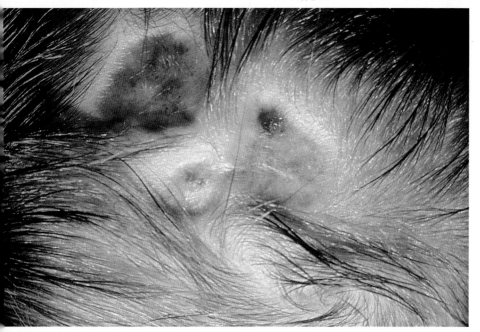

FIGURE 1-11 Aplasia cutis congenita Three localized areas of scarring alopecia on the vertex of the scalp. These areas began as ulcerated lesions at birth and are otherwise asymptomatic.

HETEROTOPIC NEURAL NODULES

Heterotopic neural nodules refer to a group of malformations that includes ectopic leptomeningeal or brain tissue in the dermis and subcutis. These lesions are present on the scalp at birth and may communicate directly with the CNS.

 INSIGHT Thick, dark hair forming a ring around a scalp lesion is known as the "hair collar sign" and suggests underlying CNS malformations or ectopic neural tissue in the scalp.

SYNONYMS Primary cutaneous meningioma, atretic meningocele or encephalocele, heterotopic neural rest, cutaneous ectopic brain.

EPIDEMIOLOGY

AGE Present at birth.
GENDER M = F.
INCIDENCE Rare.
ETIOLOGY Unknown.

PATHOPHYSIOLOGY

Herniation of neural tissue during development with subsequent severing is thought to be the cause of most of these lesions. "Rests" are collections of surviving embryonic cells that appear to have been misdirected during development and may explain some types of these malformations. The neural tissue can be composed of leptomeningeal tissues, neurons, or glial cells.

HISTORY

Heterotopic neural nodules present on the scalp at birth or shortly after and persist. They may become secondarily infected and some may swell with crying or Valsalva maneuvers.

PHYSICAL EXAMINATION

Skin Findings

TYPE OF LESION Papule, plaque, or cyst, without scalp hair (Fig. 1-12). Likely to have surrounding area of thick, coarse hair (hair collar sign). May also have associated capillary stain. More than one lesion may be present.
SIZE 2 to 4 cm.
SHAPE Round.

NUMBER Solitary lesion.
COLOR Skin-colored, erythematous, or bluish.
DISTRIBUTION Parietal and occipital scalp, almost always near midline.

General Findings

Typically, heterotopic neural nodules are an isolated skin finding. However, because there may be connection with the brain, infection can be transmitted in a retrograde fashion from the skin.

DIFFERENTIAL DIAGNOSIS

The diagnosis is generally made by history and physical examination. Radiologic imaging is essential to evaluate for intracranial connection. Dermoid cyst, meningocele, encephalocele, nevus, lipoma, aplasia cutis congenita, and vascular neoplasms must be considered in the differential diagnosis.

LABORATORY EXAMINATIONS

DERMATOPATHOLOGY Skin biopsy reveals thin central epidermis with dermal collagen surrounded by cystic spaces with meningothelial cells. Thickened hair follicles may be seen at the periphery associated with large apocrine and sebaceous glands.
IMAGING Computed tomography (CT) scan or magnetic resonance imaging (MRI) may reveal intracranial extension.

COURSE AND PROGNOSIS

The prognosis of heterotopic neural nodules is good. With surgery, future risk of retrograde infection can be eliminated.

TREATMENT

Identification of the lesion as a heterotopic neural nodule and involving a neurosurgeon or plastic surgeon with experience in the area is paramount. Imaging is essential prior to surgery or manipulation of any sort. Complete excision is curative.

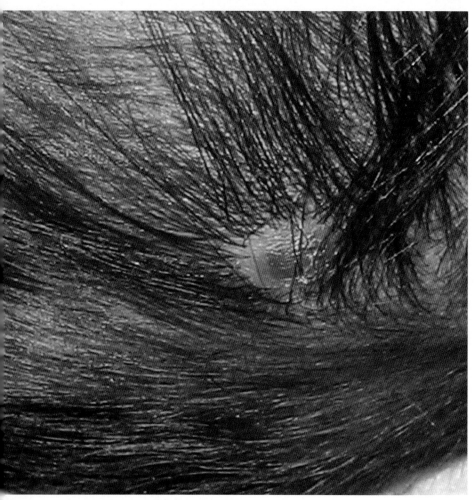

FIGURE 1-12 Heterotopic neural nodule Slightly erythematous, cystic papule with surrounding hair collar sign.

ACCESSORY TRAGUS

Accessory tragi result when a branchial arch or cleft fails to fuse or close properly. Defects occur unilaterally or bilaterally and may have accompanying facial anomalies.

SYNONYM Preauricular skin tag.

EPIDEMIOLOGY

AGE Newborn.
GENDER M = F.
INCIDENCE 4 in 1,000.
ETIOLOGY May be related to an underlying genetic anomaly.

PATHOPHYSIOLOGY

Accessory tragi are caused by first or second branchial arch fusion abnormality during embryonic development.

HISTORY

Noted at birth and persists asymptomatically for life. Usually, it is an isolated, congenital defect. Rarely, there may be other associated branchial arch abnormalities or other genetic syndromes present. The presence of preauricular tags is associated with urinary tract abnormalities such as vesicoureteral reflux. Accessory tragi are a feature of Goldenhar syndrome, Treacher Collins, and VACTERL association, among others.

PHYSICAL EXAMINATION

Skin Findings

TYPE Small, pedunculated papule (Fig. 1-13). Usually single; occasionally multiple.

COLOR Skin color, tan to brown.
SIZE 1 to 7 mm.
SHAPE Pedunculated, round to oval lesions.
SITES OF PREDILECTION Preauricular area.

DIFFERENTIAL DIAGNOSIS

Differential diagnosis includes epidermal inclusion cyst, fibroma, adnexal tumor, or lipoma.

LABORATORY EXAMINATIONS

DERMATOPATHOLOGY Skin biopsy or removal would show a loose fibrous stroma with overlying thinned epidermis and numerous vellus hairs. Cartilage is frequently present.

COURSE AND PROGNOSIS

Accessory tragi are typically asymptomatic but persist for life, occasionally becoming inflamed.

MANAGEMENT

Solitary, uncomplicated lesions may be tied off shortly after birth but otherwise can be excised during childhood for cosmetic purposes. Screening urinary tract ultrasonography is recommended by some authors given the potential for systemic associations.

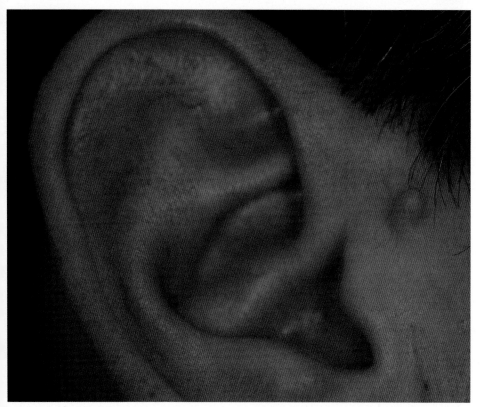

FIGURE 1-13 Accessory tragus Asymptomatic skin-colored papule in the preauricular region of an otherwise healthy person.

BRANCHIAL CLEFT CYST

An epithelial cyst on the lateral neck caused by an incomplete obliteration of the branchial clefts during embryologic development.

INSIGHT

Branchial cleft cysts are the most common etiology of congenital neck masses.

SYNONYMS Branchial cyst, branchial sinus.

EPIDEMIOLOGY

AGE Newborn.
GENDER M = F.
PREVALENCE Unknown.
ETIOLOGY Arises from failure of involution of the second or third branchial clefts. Remnants of the cleft membrane form cysts or sinuses.
GENETICS Most are sporadic but case reports of autosomal dominant inheritance patterns exist.

PATHOPHYSIOLOGY

Branchial cleft cysts are nonregressed remnants of the embryonic second and third branchial clefts. Similar lesions, thyroglossal ducts, and/or sinuses, can be seen more near the midline of the neck.

HISTORY

ONSET Lesions are evident at birth or appear in early childhood as cystic swellings in the neck, deep to the sternocleidomastoid muscle. Occasionally, they can become infected and painful.

PHYSICAL EXAMINATION

Skin Findings

TYPE Fluctuant papule or nodule. Open draining sinus or pit may be seen on the skin surface.

COLOR Skin-colored.
SIZE 2 to 10 mm.
DISTRIBUTION Unilateral or bilateral swellings in the neck, deep to the sternocleidomastoid muscle (Fig. 1-14).

DIFFERENTIAL DIAGNOSIS

Branchial cleft cysts can be confused with other nodular lesions on the neck such as lymph nodes or epidermal or pilar cysts. The location and presence at birth can help distinguish them from other neck lesions.

LABORATORY EXAMINATIONS

DERMATOPATHOLOGY On skin biopsy, the cyst will have a stratified squamous epithelial lining.

COURSE AND PROGNOSIS

Cysts often form sinuses or fistulae, draining mucus internally to the pharynx and/or externally through the skin of the neck along the anterior edge of the sternomastoid muscle. Cysts and associated sinuses may also become infected.

MANAGEMENT

These lesions are benign, however, they can be symptomatic with recurrent infections and swelling. Symptomatic lesions can be surgically excised.

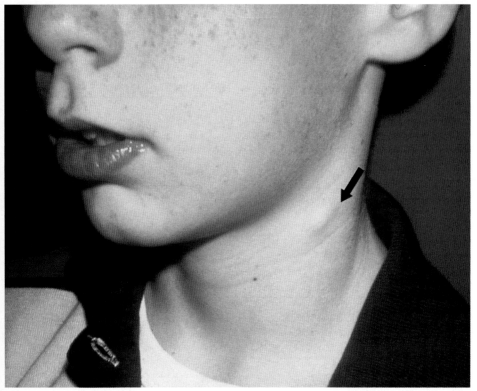

FIGURE 1-14 Branchial cleft cyst An asymptomatic, unilateral cystic swelling on the neck present since birth.

ACCESSORY NIPPLE

An additional nipple appearing anywhere along an imaginary line drawn from the midaxilla to the inguinal area. Nipples may appear unilaterally or bilaterally and with or without areolae.

SYNONYMS Supernumerary nipple, polythelia.

EPIDEMIOLOGY

AGE Newborn.
GENDER M = F, with some studies reporting a slight male predominance.
PREVALENCE Common.
ETIOLOGY Developmental defect with persistence of the embryonic milkline.

PATHOPHYSIOLOGY

Accessory nipples represent persistent, fetal, embryonic milkline lesions.

HISTORY

Lesions are present at birth, asymptomatic, and persist for life.

PHYSICAL EXAMINATION

Skin Findings

TYPE Papule with or without surrounding areola.
COLOR Pink to brown.
SIZE Usually smaller than normal anatomically placed nipples.
SHAPE Often round to oval in shape.
DISTRIBUTION Chest, abdomen >> thigh, vulva.
SITES OF PREDILECTION Along a line from the midaxillae to the inguinal area (Fig. 1-15).

DIFFERENTIAL DIAGNOSIS

When occurring without an areola, the nipple may be misdiagnosed as a congenital nevus.

LABORATORY EXAMINATIONS

DERMATOPATHOLOGY Skin biopsy would reveal histologic findings of a normal nipple (lactation ducts and glands).

DIAGNOSIS

The diagnosis of an accessory nipple can be made clinically, especially if it is present along the anterior milkline. Other ectopically placed lesions may need a biopsy and histologic confirmation.

COURSE AND PROGNOSIS

Accessory nipples are present at birth and persist asymptomatically for life. Changes in appearance may be noted due to hormonal surges during puberty. Malignant degeneration is rare.

MANAGEMENT

Accessory nipples do not need treatment but should be monitored, since those with associated breast tissue can have the same malignant potential as normal breast tissue. Surgical removal can be performed for diagnostic, cosmetic, or therapeutic purposes.

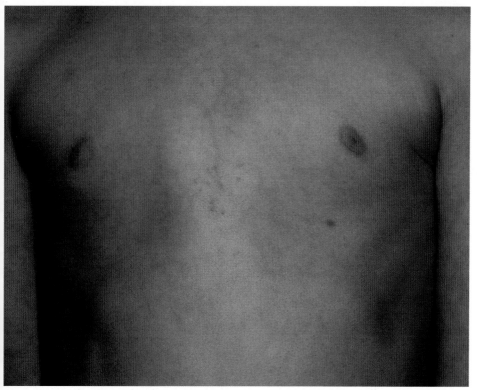

FIGURE 1-15 Accessory nipple Asymptomatic, symmetric brown papule since birth along the milkline on the chest.

CONGENITAL INFECTIONS OF THE NEWBORN

NEONATAL HERPES SIMPLEX VIRUS INFECTION

Neonatal herpes simplex infection is a potentially fatal disease. Neonatal herpes has a broad clinical spectrum and may be categorized into three patterns: localized infection confined to the skin, eyes, or mouth; CNS disease; and disseminated disease.

INSIGHT Many infants with CNS and disseminated neonatal herpes do not develop cutaneous lesions.

EPIDEMIOLOGY

AGE Neonatal herpes can present up to 4 weeks of age. Disseminated disease often presents during the first week of life, while localized infection typically presents later. CNS infection presents between 14 and 21 days of life.
GENDER M = F.
PREVALENCE Approximately 1:3,000 to 1:10,000 live births. Correlates with population prevalence of new genital HSV.
ETIOLOGY Approximately 75% result from herpes simplex virus-2 (HSV-2) infection, 25% result from herpes simplex virus-1 (HSV-1) infection.
TRANSMISSION Herpes virus is most commonly inoculated onto the baby's mucous membranes during its passage through the birth canal; however, ascending infection and transmission in the perinatal period from the mouth or hands of caregivers may occur.

PATHOPHYSIOLOGY

Herpes virus inoculation occurs mucocutaneously; systemic infection can ensue with disease limited to the brain or diffuse hematogenous dissemination.

HISTORY

Pregnant women with recurrent genital herpes are at very low risk of transmitting HSV to their babies (<5%) because of anti-HSV antibodies, which pass through the placenta and convey immunity to the baby. The majority of cases occur in asymptomatic mothers with primary genital herpes infection making it very difficult to predict those at risk.

PHYSICAL EXAMINATION

Skin Findings

TYPE OF LESION Skin lesions begin as 2- to 8-mm macules or papules that progress to single or grouped vesicles that then rupture

leaving an erosion or ulcer, which crusts over and heals (Fig. 1-16).
COLOR Pink to erythematous.
SHAPE Round to oval.
DISTRIBUTION Oral lesions are most frequently located on the tongue, palate, gingiva, lips, and buccal mucosa. Ocular lesions appear as erosions on the conjunctiva and cornea. Skin lesions occur at sites of inoculation; infant monitoring scalp electrodes may produce enough skin trauma to allow invasion by the herpes virus. At birth in vertex deliveries, the scalp is a common site for the development of initial herpetic lesions and conversely, in breech deliveries, the buttocks and perianal area frequently manifest the first lesions. The vesicles may become generalized in the disseminated pattern of the disease.

General Findings

Early in the infection, infants typically present with nonspecific symptoms such as lethargy, poor feeding, and fever. CNS involvement is manifested by isolated encephalitis with frequent seizures that are nonfocal in nature. Eye involvement is seen in 10% to 20% of these patients and is noted characteristically between 2 days and 2 weeks of life. Disseminated infection presents with irritability, respiratory distress, jaundice, and seizures from viral infection of the brain, lungs, liver, and adrenal glands.

DIFFERENTIAL DIAGNOSIS

The diagnosis of neonatal herpes is made by history and clinical presentation and confirmed by detection of the herpes virus. The differential diagnosis includes other blistering diseases of the newborn such as congenital varicella, bullous impetigo, pemphigus vulgaris, and other causes of neonatal sepsis.

LABORATORY EXAMINATIONS

TZANCK PREPARATION Cells scraped from the base of vesicular lesions are positive for multinucleated giant cells in 60% of culture-proven HSV.
HISTOPATHOLOGY Intraepidermal vesicles produced by ballooning degeneration. Inclusion bodies (eosinophilic structures with a surrounding

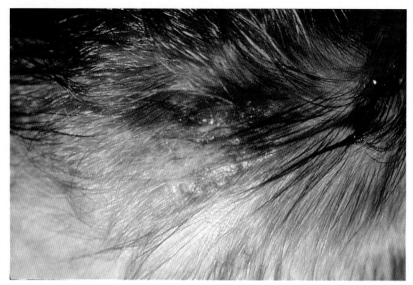

FIGURE 1-16 Congenital herpes simplex virus, localized Grouped vesicles on an erythematous base on the scalp of a newborn.

clear halo) are frequently seen in the center of enlarged, round nuclei of balloon cells.

DIRECT IMMUNOFLUORESCENCE Cells scraped from the base of vesicular lesions can be tested for the presence of herpes virus infection using HSV-1 or HSV-2 specific monoclonal antibodies. Sensitivity and specificity correlate highly with tissue culture results.

SEROLOGY Antibody measurement in the baby is of little value because the seropositivity rate for HSV-2 among all women of childbearing age exceeds 20%.

CULTURE HSV may be cultured within 2 to 5 days from infected samples of skin, throat, conjunctiva, cerebrospinal fluid, blood, urine, and stool.

POLYMERASE CHAIN REACTION Herpes simplex DNA can be detected in the CSF using the polymerase chain reaction, an extremely sensitive technique that is frequently used for CSF evaluation.

COURSE AND PROGNOSIS

Morbidity and mortality of neonatal herpes is strongly associated with disease classification. Additionally, HSV-2 neonatal disease has been associated with worse clinical outcomes.

LOCALIZED INFECTION Treated infants with cutaneous infection have virtually a 100% survival rate, although some will suffer a cutaneous relapse in the first year of life. Approximately 10% will manifest herpetic lesions in the oropharynx. Up to 40% will have persistent ocular pathology, although this is seen most frequently in children suffering from severe neurologic residua (see below).

CNS INFECTION Untreated cases have a mortality rate of 50% and treated cases have a mortality rate of 15% to 30%. HSV-2 causes significantly worse encephalitis as compared to HSV-1. Many of these cases sustain permanent neurologic impairment.

DISSEMINATED These neonates frequently progress to cardiovascular compromise, coagulopathy, and, in the absence of therapy, about 80% of cases result in death. With antiviral therapy, the mortality rate is reduced to approximately 25%.

MANAGEMENT

In light of the varied clinical manifestations of neonatal herpetic infections and the severe consequences of untreated disease, immediate institution of antiviral chemotherapy has been recommended for any infant presenting with signs of severe, unidentified infection in the first month of life, even in the absence of any characteristic skin findings.

Antiviral therapy of IV acyclovir 60 mg/kg divided into three equal doses and administered every 8 hours for 14 days if limited disease, 21 days if disseminated or involving CNS. If ocular involvement is present, addition of topical 1% trifluridine or 3% vidarabine drops can be instituted. Infants with CNS or disseminated disease that have been treated successfully may require long-term suppressive antiviral therapy to prevent subclinical CNS recurrences.

CONGENITAL VARICELLA ZOSTER VIRUS

The majority of infants exposed to varicella zoster virus (VZV) infection during pregnancy are asymptomatic and normal. There are two exceptions: congenital VZV syndrome and neonatal varicella.

Congenital VZV Syndrome Occurs if a mother is infected in the first 20 weeks of pregnancy and transplacental infection of fetus occurs before maternal immunity can protect the infant. Though only a small percentage of infants born to mothers with VZV infection before 20 weeks will ultimately be affected, this acquired infection leads to severe fetal sequelae and mortality in up to 30% of affected infants.

Neonatal Varicella Occurs if the mother is infected with VZV within 3 weeks of delivery. Since the infant is born before maternal antibodies have been generated, the infant has no immunity and will have a severe infection in the first 12 days of life with pneumonitis, hepatitis, meningoencephalitis, and up to a 20% mortality.

EPIDEMIOLOGY

AGE Newborn.
GENDER M = F.
INCIDENCE Both congenital VZV and neonatal VZV are very rare.
ETIOLOGY VZV.
TRANSMISSION Varicella causes maternal viremia, which can cause transplacental infection; ascending infection from the birth canal and transmission in the perinatal period may also occur.

PHYSICAL EXAMINATION

Skin Findings

Congenital VZV Syndrome

TYPE Cicatricial scars, skin loss, limb contractures.
DISTRIBUTION Sometimes in a dermatomal pattern.
GENERAL FINDINGS Low-birth-weight, eye defects, encephalomyelitis, hypoplastic limbs, microcephaly, pneumonitis.

Neonatal Varicella

TYPE Monomorphic progression from macule, papules, vesicles to crust (Fig. 1-17).
COLOR Erythematous.
DISTRIBUTION Generalized.
GENERAL FINDINGS Pneumonitis, hepatitis, and meningoencephalitis.

DIFFERENTIAL DIAGNOSIS

Congenital HSV, other TORCH [toxoplasmosis, other (syphilis), rubella, cytomegalovirus (CMV), HSV] infections, sepsis.

LABORATORY EXAMINATIONS

Direct immunofluorescence (DFA), polymerase chain reaction, or skin biopsy of cutaneous lesions can demonstrate VZV. Cultures of tissue or CSF have not been shown to reliably grow VZV in infants with congenital VZV syndrome. IgG and IgM antibodies to VZV can be demonstrated in the mother's sera to determine either previous immunity or active infection to confirm the findings and VZV-specific IgG antibodies in the baby that persist older than 7 months of life (by which point any maternal antibodies should have disappeared) may confirm the findings.

DIAGNOSIS

Based on history or maternal infection, clinical appearance of the newborn, and laboratory findings.

COURSE AND PROGNOSIS

Infants in utero of mothers with VZV are generally protected by the transplacental-acquired antibodies generated during maternal VZV infection. Thus, most infants are unaffected and are born normal even though they may develop unusual manifestations of attenuated immunity later in life such as herpes zoster at an early age. Such children are immunocompetent, but had an utero primary VZV infection (chicken pox) and an attenuated immune response since maternal antibodies were present to help fight the infection. Infants born to mothers who develop varicella from 5 days prior to delivery to 2 days postpartum are at highest risk for a fatal course because of insufficient time for maternal antibody acquisition.

Congenital VZV syndrome has up to a 30% mortality rate but long-term outcome can be good for surviving patients.

Herpes zoster (shingles) in a pregnant woman is generally thought to have minimal risk for sequelae for the fetus.

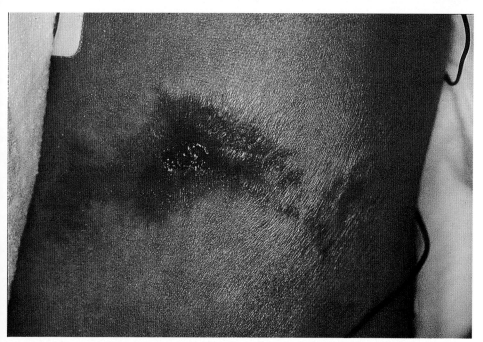

FIGURE 1-17 Congenital varicella zoster virus infection T5 dermatomal erythematous plaque on the right side of a newborn's body. (Image used with permission from Dr. Karen Wiss.)

MANAGEMENT

Those pregnant women who have been exposed to varicella should have a VZV-IgG level measured if they do not have a history of varicella infection or vaccination. For those with negative histories or serologies, varicella zoster immune globulin (VZIG) is indicated at any point during pregnancy.

Administration of acyclovir should be given at the first clinical sign of VZV infection. For VZV infections between 5 days before and 2-day postpartum, mothers should be given acyclovir and an attempt to delay the delivery may be made. The neonates should be given VZIG and systemic acyclovir immediately upon delivery and should be isolated and observed for 2 weeks.

BLUEBERRY MUFFIN BABY

The "blueberry muffin baby" is so named because of the baby's clinical presentation, with disseminated red–blue papules and nodules representing islands of extramedullary hematopoiesis. The blueberry muffin baby can be seen following in utero infections with toxoplasmosis, varicella, CMV, human immunodeficiency virus (HIV), and rubella.

EPIDEMIOLOGY

AGE Newborn.
GENDER M = F.
INCIDENCE Rare.
ETIOLOGY Maternal infection during pregnancy and transplacental infection with toxoplasmosis, varicella, CMV, HIV, or rubella.

PHYSICAL EXAMINATION

Skin Findings

TYPE Purpuric macules, papules, and nodules (Fig. 1-18).
COLOR Bluish-red to purple.
SIZE 2 to 8 mm in diameter.
SHAPE Circular to oval.
PALPATION Infiltrated, larger lesions are palpable 1 to 2 mm above the skin's surface.
DISTRIBUTION Generalized.

General Findings

TOXOPLASMOSIS Lymphadenopathy, hepatosplenomegaly, hydrocephaly, microcephaly, cataracts, pneumonitis, chorioretinitis, convulsions.
VARICELLA See "Congenital Varicella Zoster Virus."
CMV Jaundice, hepatosplenomegaly, anemia, thrombocytopenia, respiratory distress, convulsions, and chorioretinitis.
HIV Hepatosplenomegaly, other opportunistic infections.
RUBELLA Cataracts, deafness, growth retardation, hepatosplenomegaly, cardiac defects, and meningoencephalitis.

DIFFERENTIAL DIAGNOSIS

The differential diagnosis of a blueberry muffin baby is typically the infectious causes of extramedullary dermal hematopoiesis: toxoplasmosis, varicella, CMV, HIV, and rubella. The diagnosis is typically made by maternal history and detection of one of the above-named infectious agents.

LABORATORY EXAMINATIONS

DERMATOPATHOLOGY Blueberry muffin lesions show aggregates of large nucleated and non-nucleated erythrocytes.

Toxoplasmosis

DNA Detection of parasite DNA in amniotic fluid or fetal blood.
SEROLOGY Higher infant antitoxoplasma IgM than maternal IgM is diagnostic of congenital infection.
WRIGHT OR GIEMSA STAIN CSF or lymph node, spleen, or liver demonstrating *Toxoplasma gondii*.
SKULL FILMS Diffuse, punctate, comma-shaped, intracranial calcifications.

CMV

CULTURE Urine, liver, CSF, gastric washing, and pharynx will show characteristic large cells with intranuclear and cytoplasmic inclusions.
HEAD CT SCAN Intracranial calcifications may be present.

Rubella

SEROLOGY Elevated anti-rubella IgM in infant or persistent anti-rubella IgG in infants older than 6 months. Fourfold or greater increase in acute and convalescent sera is also diagnostic.
CULTURE Virus can be isolated from nasopharynx, urine, CSF, skin, stool, or eyes.

COURSE AND PROGNOSIS

TOXOPLASMOSIS Infected infants may be stillborn, premature, or full term. At birth, they may present with malaise, fever, rash, lymphadenopathy, hepatosplenomegaly, convulsions, and chorioretinitis, though most are asymptomatic. Overall prognosis is poor, especially with infants that have liver and bone marrow involvement.
CMV Affected infants may have sensorineural hearing loss, mental retardation, learning disabilities, and seizures. Poor prognosis, especially with intracranial calcifications or hydrocephalus.
RUBELLA Rubella acquired during the first trimester may lead to low-birth-weight, microcephaly, mental retardation, cataracts, deafness, and heart abnormalities. Rubella acquired during second or third trimester can lead to hepatosplenomegaly, pneumonitis, myocarditis, encephalitis, osteomyelitis, or retinopathy.

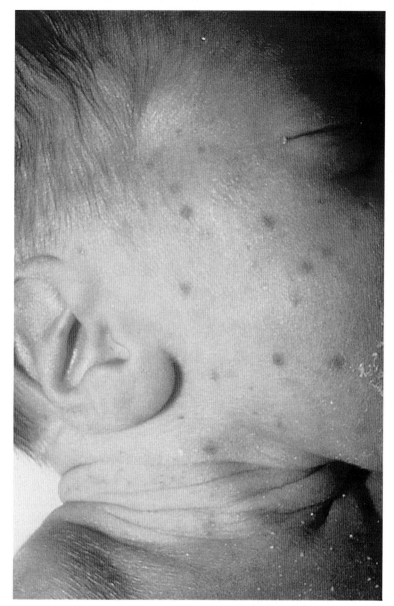

FIGURE 1-18 Blueberry muffin baby Scattered red–blue papules and nodules on the face of a newborn. The lesions represent sites of extramedullary hematopoiesis.

MANAGEMENT

TOXOPLASMOSIS 30+ days of sulfadiazine (150–200 mg/kg/d divided qid) plus pyrimethamine (1–2 mg/kg/d divided bid). Infants with chorioretinitis or high CSF protein levels may need systemic steroids.

CMV Ganciclovir can be used to treat retinitis and organ involvement.

RUBELLA Immune globulin administered to exposed pregnant mother within 22 hours of onset can prevent/reduce fetal infection. Neonatal rubella requires ophthalmologic and supportive care. However, infected infants can shed the virus for up to a year.

CONGENITAL SYPHILIS

A prenatal spirochetal infection with characteristic early and late signs and symptoms. Clinical manifestations of early congenital syphilis (first several months of life) include anemia, fever, wasting, hepatosplenomegaly, lymphadenopathy, rhinitis (snuffles), mucocutaneous lesions (including rhagades: radial fissures and furrows around the mouth), and pseudoparalysis. Symptoms of late congenital syphilis, which appears after 2 years of age, include interstitial keratitis, Hutchinson teeth (notched central incisors), and eighth nerve deafness; these three compose the Hutchinson triad. Frontal bossing, mulberry molars, saddle nose deformity, Clutton joints (painless knee swelling), and anterior bowing of the shins are also features of late congenital syphilis.

SYNONYM Prenatal syphilis.

EPIDEMIOLOGY

AGE Bimodal; within first months of life and after the age of 2.
GENDER M = F.
INCIDENCE Incidence had dropped to insignificant levels in 1959, but since then has been increasing.
ETIOLOGY Spirochete *Treponema pallidum* crosses the placenta to infect the fetus.

HISTORY

Neonates with syphilis are often born without signs of disease at time of birth. Clinical manifestations in the first month of life are common. Skin findings include macules, papules, papulosquamous, and vesicobullous lesions. Widespread desquamation can occur (Fig. 1-19). Mucocutaneous involvement of mouth and lips is common. Systemically, there is lymphadenopathy, hepatosplenomegaly, and pseudoparalysis.

PHYSICAL EXAMINATION

EARLY CONGENITAL SYPHILIS Signs and symptoms appearing in first 2 months of life.

Skin Findings

Noted in one-third to one-half of affected infants. Skin lesions are infectious.
TYPE Macules, papules, or papulosquamous lesions on body. Patches on mucous membranes; raised verrucous plaques on anogenital or oral membranes.
COLOR Bright pink to erythematous; fades to copper-colored or brownish.
SIZE AND SHAPE Large, round, or oval.
DISTRIBUTION Generalized or localized to any area.
SITES OF PREDILECTION Face, dorsal surface of trunk and legs, diaper area, palms, and soles.

General Findings

Hepatomegaly, lymphadenopathy (especially epitrochlear), splenomegaly, jaundice, anemia, thrombocytopenia, osteochondritis, and meningitis. "Barber-pole umbilical cord" with spiral red, white, and black discoloration of necrotizing umbilical cord.
LATE CONGENITAL SYPHILIS Signs and symptoms appearing after 2 years of age.

Skin Findings

Hypersensitivity-type reaction or scars and deformities related to infection. Skin lesions no longer infectious.

General Findings

Hutchinson triad: (1) interstitial keratitis, (2) Hutchinson teeth, (3) eighth nerve deafness; dental changes (mulberry molars or bony gums that progress to necrotic ulcers), Higoumenakis sign (unilateral, thickened inner one-third of clavicle), arthritis, Parrot lines (radial scars after rhagades heal), and eye changes (choroiditis, retinitis, and optic atrophy).

DIFFERENTIAL DIAGNOSIS

The diagnosis of congenital syphilis can be made based on clinical suspicion and confirmed by positive dark-field microscopy or fluorescent antibody tests of the umbilical cord, placenta or skin lesions, by radiologic bony changes, and positive serology for syphilis. A serologic titer in the newborn at least fourfold higher than the mother is diagnostic of congenital syphilis.

LABORATORY EXAMINATIONS

DARK-FIELD MICROSCOPY Of the umbilical cord, skin lesions, or mucous membranes for *T. pallidum*.
RADIOLOGIC STUDIES For bone abnormalities: widening of the epiphyseal line with increased density of the shafts.

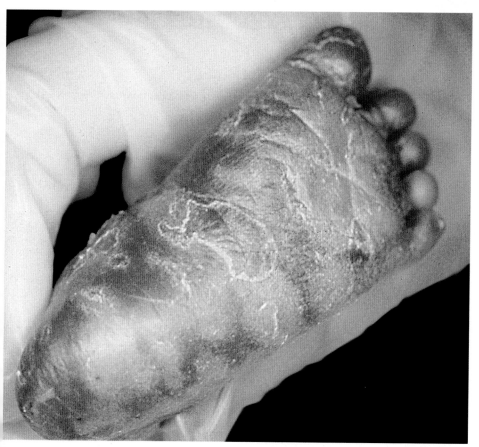

FIGURE 1-19 Neonatal syphilis Copper-colored macules and diffuse desquamation on the plantar surface of a newborn with secondary syphilis.

PLACENTAL CHANGES Include focal villositis, endovascular and perivascular proliferation in villous vessels, and relative immaturity of villi.

COURSE AND PROGNOSIS

Relative to time during pregnancy of maternal spirochetemia and subsequent fetal inoculation. Up to 4 months of gestation, spontaneous abortion is common. Infection after 4 months of gestation may result in stillborn or fatally ill neonate. Prognosis with contracted disease is dependent on early and proper diagnosis and adequate treatment.

MANAGEMENT

Treatment of disease without CNS involvement:

1. Aqueous crystalline penicillin G: 100,000–150,000 units/kg IM or 50,000 units/kg IV q8–12h × 14 days. Infants older than 4 weeks may require higher doses.

2. Procaine penicillin G: 50,000 units/kg IM q24h × 10–14 days.
3. Benzathine penicillin G: 50,000 units/kg IM × 1 dose.

Treatment with CNS involvement:

1. Crystalline penicillin G: 30,000–50,000 units/kg divided bid–tid × 3 weeks. Again, older infants may require higher doses.
2. Procaine penicillin G: 50,000 units/kg qid × 3 weeks.

CONGENITAL CUTANEOUS CANDIDIASIS

An intrauterine contracted infection that presents at the time of birth as erythematous or generalized eczematous, scaly skin.

SYNONYM Moniliasis.

EPIDEMIOLOGY

AGE Birth.
GENDER M = F.
ETIOLOGY Candida organisms, most commonly *Candida albicans,* existing in the microflora of the mouth, GI and vaginal tracts of the mother. Infants harbor *C. albicans* in the mouth or GI tract and recurrently on the skin.
OTHER FEATURES Endocrine disorders, genetic disorders (Down syndrome, acrodermatitis enteropathica, chronic mucocutaneous candidiasis, chronic granulomatous disease) and immune disorder or systemic antibiotics can predispose an individual to candidiasis.

HISTORY

ONSET Present at birth or shortly thereafter.
REVIEW OF SYMPTOMS Usually no constitutional symptoms.

PHYSICAL EXAMINATION

Skin Findings

TYPE Erythema, papules, pustules to exfoliative lesions (Fig. 1-20).
COLOR Red or white.
SIZE 1 to 2 mm.
DISTRIBUTION Head, neck, trunk, and extremities. Occasional nail, palm, and sole involvement. Spares diaper area.

SITES OF PREDILECTION Intertriginous areas, posterior aspect of trunk and extensor surfaces of extremities.

DIFFERENTIAL DIAGNOSIS

The diagnosis of cutaneous candidiasis is based on clinical suspicion and confirmed by demonstration of candidal organisms. Clinical presentation is similar to erythema toxicum, transient neonatal pustular melanosis, bacterial folliculitis, bullous impetigo, congenital herpes, congenital varicella, congenital syphilis, or acne neonatorum. The course of congenital candidiasis can be progressive, but benign and without constitutional symptoms.

LABORATORY EXAMINATIONS

Direct microscopic examination of pustules and culture from the cutaneous lesions yield yeast forms.

COURSE AND PROGNOSIS

Congenital candidiasis clears spontaneously after several weeks.

MANAGEMENT

Systemic (50,000–100,000 units qid) and topical nystatin hasten resolution of lesions in 3 to 10 days. In more severe cases, fluconazole (3–6 mg/kg po qd) may be needed.

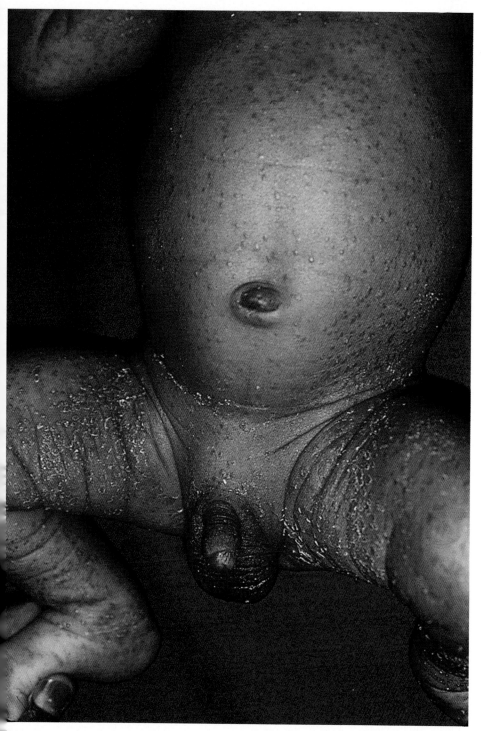

FIGURE 1-20 Congenital candidiasis Diffuse erythematous papules, pustules and exfoliation on a newborn with congenital candidiasis.

ABNORMALITIES OF SUBCUTANEOUS TISSUE

SUBCUTANEOUS FAT NECROSIS

A benign, self-limited panniculitis in which subcutaneous fat is injured and becomes inflamed, presenting as a firm, erythematous nodule or plaque in an otherwise healthy newborn.

INSIGHT

Frequently, these children are the product of long, difficult labor and delivery.

EPIDEMIOLOGY

AGE First several weeks of life.
GENDER M = F.
PREVALENCE Rare.
ETIOLOGY Cold injury, trauma at delivery, asphyxia, ischemia, and other neonatal stressors may initiate the disease.

PATHOPHYSIOLOGY

The fat of neonates contains more saturated fatty acids, which have a higher melting point than adult fatty acids. Once the temperature of the skin drops below the melting point of the fat, crystallization occurs with subsequent necrosis and granulomatous inflammatory response. This feature may play a role in enhancing physical or metabolic trauma leading to necrosis. The exact pathophysiology is still debated.

HISTORY

Asymptomatic single or multiple red nodules or plaques that begin within the first 2 weeks of life and resolve spontaneously over several weeks.

PHYSICAL EXAMINATION

Skin Findings

TYPE OF LESION Sharply demarcated indurated nodules coalescing into larger plaques, occasionally ulcerated (Fig. 1-21).
COLOR Reddish to purple.
PALPATION Firm to palpation.
DISTRIBUTION Cheeks, buttocks, back, arms, or thighs.

General Findings

Infrequently, hypercalcemia can present with irritability, vomiting, weight loss, and failure to thrive.

DIFFERENTIAL DIAGNOSIS

Subcutaneous fat necrosis must be differentiated from bacterial cellulitis, sclerema neonatorum, and congenital tumors such as a sarcoma. Babies with subcutaneous fat necrosis generally appear healthy, are afebrile, and feed vigorously, which are helpful in eliminating cellulitis and sclerema neonatorum from the differential.

LABORATORY EXAMINATIONS

DERMATOPATHOLOGY Foci of fat necrosis often with needle-shaped clefts surrounded by granulomatous inflammation. Areas of calcification may be present.
LABORATORY EXAMINATION OF BLOOD Hypercalcemia may be found infrequently, usually around the time of resolution of the skin lesions. Hypoglycemia, thrombocytopenia, and hypertriglyceridemia may also occur.

COURSE AND PROGNOSIS

Lesions evolve slowly over weeks-to-months from red nodules, to bruise-like discoloration, to a hard subcutaneous mass that usually resolves without atrophy or scarring. In the case of hypercalcemia left untreated, seizures, cardiac arrhythmias, renal failure, and death may result.

MANAGEMENT

No treatment is necessary for these self-resolving lesions in general. Fluctuant lesions may be aspirated for comfort and to minimize overlying epidermal necrosis.

The calcium level should be monitored at least biweekly in these infants as the skin lesions resolve, since hypercalcemia must be treated aggressively.

The lesions tend to heal with subcutaneous atrophy consistent with the evolution of other disorders of the subcutaneous fat.

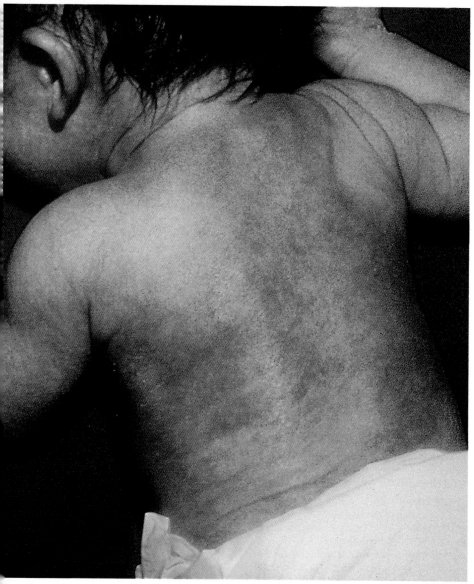

FIGURE 1-21 Subcutaneous fat necrosis Confluent erythematous, well-demarcated subcutaneous nodules of fat on the back of a newborn.

SCLEREMA NEONATORUM

A diffuse skin hardening seen in severely ill newborns with multiple etiologies.

EPIDEMIOLOGY

AGE Newborns, premature infants are more susceptible.
GENDER Sclerema occurs slightly more frequently in males.
INCIDENCE Rare.
ETIOLOGY Sclerema can result from a number of physiologic insults and is a nonspecific sign of poor prognostic outcome rather than a primary disease. In 25% of affected infants, the mother is severely ill at the time of delivery.

PATHOPHYSIOLOGY

The fat of neonates contains more saturated fatty acids, which have a higher melting point than adult fatty acids. Once the temperature of the skin drops below the melting point of the fat, crystallization occurs. Vascular collapse, hypothermia, and metabolic derangements seen in severe illness may induce crystallization.

HISTORY

Onset typically in first week of life in severely ill infants with sepsis, hypoglycemia, hypothermia, or severe metabolic abnormalities.

PHYSICAL EXAMINATION

Skin Findings

TYPE OF LESION Diffuse wood-like hardening and thickening of the skin (Fig. 1-22).
COLOR Yellow–white mottled appearance.
PALPATION Stony, hard, and cool.
DISTRIBUTION Symmetrical, beginning on the legs and progressing upward to involve the buttocks and trunk.

General Findings

Infant is severely ill with an underlying medical condition such as sepsis, cardiac or respiratory problems, hypothermia, or metabolic abnormalities. Infants are weak, lethargic, and feed poorly.

DIFFERENTIAL DIAGNOSIS

Clinically, the diffuse skin thickening and hardening are characteristic of sclerema. These skin changes are similar morphologically to scleroderma which is not seen in this context. Sclerema neonatorum may be confused with subcutaneous fat necrosis of the newborn. Several distinguishing features include: (1) appearance of the infant: in sclerema neonatorum, the infant appears extremely ill; in subcutaneous fat necrosis, the infant appears remarkably well; (2) distribution of the lesions: in sclerema neonatorum, the sclerosis is diffuse and in subcutaneous fat necrosis, the lesions are localized; (3) morphology of the lesions: in subcutaneous fat necrosis, there is often significant erythema of the nodules, which may be mobile, while sclerema tends to be more pale and bound down.

LABORATORY EXAMINATIONS

DERMATOPATHOLOGY Edema and thickening of fibrous septa surrounding fat lobules, occasionally with needle-like clefts within fat cells; usually less necrosis than seen in subcutaneous fat necrosis of the newborn.

COURSE AND PROGNOSIS

The prognosis of sclerema neonatorum is poor. By the time the skin is diffusely hardened, the infant is usually very ill with high morbidity and mortality.

TREATMENT AND PREVENTION

Careful neonatal monitoring of premature infants with precise temperature control, appropriate antibiotic therapy, and correction of metabolic abnormalities, possibly with repeated exchange transfusions, IVIG, or systemic corticosteroids may arrest and reverse the process.

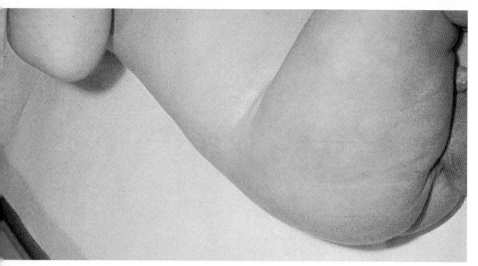

FIGURE 1-22 Sclerema neonatorum Diffuse wood-like hardening of the thigh in a sick newborn infant.

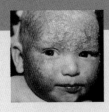

ECZEMATOUS DERMATITIS

ATOPIC DERMATITIS

Atopic dermatitis is a chronic disorder characterized by xerosis, pruritus, scaly erythematous patches, and thickening of the skin with enhancement of normal skin markings (lichenification). It is frequently associated with a personal or family history of hay fever, asthma, or allergic rhinitis. It can be divided into three phases based on the age of the individual: infantile, childhood, and adolescent.

INSIGHT Although many patients and families will insist on "finding the cause," experience and studies confirm that specific allergen identification and avoidance or dietary modification is less helpful than focusing on skin treatment and maintaining healthy skin barrier function.

EPIDEMIOLOGY

AGE Onset usually from age 2 to 12 months, and almost all cases by age 5 years. Nearly 80% of cases will resolve by adulthood.
GENDER M = F.
INCIDENCE Common and thought to be increasing.
HEREDITARY PREDISPOSITION More than two-thirds have personal or family history of allergic rhinitis, hay fever, or asthma. Many children with atopic dermatitis develop asthma and/or hay fever later in life.
PREVALENCE 10% to 15% of the childhood population with significant regional variability. Up to 11% of the US pediatric population affected.

PATHOPHYSIOLOGY

The cause of atopic dermatitis is unknown; however, multiple factors are known to play a role in the development of atopic dermatitis. Certain genetic factors (such as filaggrin gene abnormalities) may lead to xerosis while others may result in immune dysregulation. Factors such as stress, climate, infections, irritants, and allergens seem to play a role in many patients as well. For the vast majority of patients, there is no one "trigger" or "cause," but rather an unfortunate collection of constituents that all

can worsen the disease. A central tenet in the pathophysiology of atopic dermatitis is believed to be the interplay between epidermal disruption and inflammation mediated by T-cells and Langerhans cells.

HISTORY

Atopic dermatitis is sometimes called "the itch that rashes." Dry skin and pruritus are found in essentially all patients. Scratching the skin leads to the characteristic eczematous changes and a vicious itch-scratch cycle. Itching may be aggravated by cold weather, frequent bathing (particularly with hot water), wool, detergent, soap, and stress. The disease can wax and wane unpredictably, however, which probably contributes to the numerous misattributions of causes and remedies.

PHYSICAL EXAMINATION

Skin Findings

TYPE Patches and plaques with scale, crust, and lichenification. Lesions usually confluent and ill defined.
COLOR Erythematous.

Special Clinical Features

Atopic children may demonstrate increased palmar markings, periorbital atopic pleats (Dennie–Morgan lines), keratosis pilaris, or white dermatographism. They also can develop widespread herpetic, wart, molluscum, or tinea infections because of their impaired skin barrier function.

DIFFERENTIAL DIAGNOSIS

Atopic dermatitis can be confused with seborrheic dermatitis, contact dermatitis, psoriasis, or scabies. Several metabolic disorders may manifest eczematous dermatitis and should be considered, including acrodermatitis enteropathica and phenylketonuria. Some disorders of immunity may also include atopic dermatitis, such as Wiskott–Aldrich syndrome, X-linked agammaglobulinemia, and hyper-IgE syndrome (Job syndrome).

DERMATOPATHOLOGY

Acute lesions show intraepidermal intercellular edema (spongiosis) with occasional vesicle formation and a dermal infiltrate comprised largely of lymphocytes with few eosinophils. Chronic lesions show acanthosis, hyperkeratosis, and spongiosis.

LABORATORY EXAMINATION

Laboratory studies are not needed to make the diagnosis of atopic dermatitis. Patients may have an increased IgE and/or eosinophilia. Radioallergosorbent testing (RAST) is frequently positive for multiple antigens but direct applicability to the dermatitis is exceedingly rare.

COURSE AND PROGNOSIS

Conflicting data and great individual variability preclude definitive prognostication. However, the majority of patients significantly improve by school age with a minority requiring lifelong management. A significant portion of affected children will develop asthma or hay fever later in life.

MANAGEMENT

Because atopic dermatitis cannot be cured, the goal is to keep the condition under control and maintain the quality of life for the patient and the family. A four-pronged approach can be helpful in maximizing treatment, addressing each major aspect of atopic dermatitis, summarized in Figure 2-1: the treatment tetrahedron.

MOISTURIZATION

Improving moisturization is universally helpful and is the foundation of treatment for atopic dermatitis. The best moisturizer is the one that the patient will use. While greasier ointment preparations are better, such as hydrated petrolatum, Aquaphor, or Eucerin, low compliance limits the use in some patients. Less greasy creams such as CeraVe, Cetaphil, and Aveeno can still be highly effective and used more frequently throughout the day.

The "soak and seal" technique is highly effective in locking in moisture and consists of the following:

1. Bathing in lukewarm water for approximately 15 minutes daily.
2. Using a mild nonsoap cleanser such as Dove, Aveeno, or Cetaphil.
3. Patting the skin dry lightly with a towel to remove most of the water.
4. While still moist, applying the moisturizer liberally.

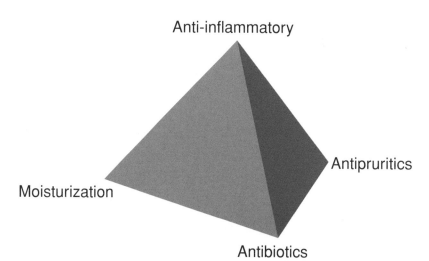

FIGURE 2-1 Atopic dermatitis treatment tetrahedron The four main treatment categories.

Anti-Inflammatory Agents

For the mildest cases, improved moisturization can often suffice. However, for more significant disease, anti-inflammatory agents are necessary. Systemic corticosteroids are generally best avoided; while incredibly effective in the short term, the rebound effect can be devastating and can create systemic corticosteroid dependence that is extremely difficult to manage.

While topical corticosteroids are the traditional cornerstone of treatment for atopic dermatitis, the topical calcineurin inhibitors tacrolimus and pimecrolimus have an important defined role in the management of this disease.

TOPICAL CORTICOSTEROIDS The most frequent reason for treatment failure is using a potency that is too low for the body site and severity. Fear of side effects from corticosteroids is very common and not necessarily without good reason, but must be tempered by the knowledge that proper use minimizes such adverse effects while providing true relief from the disease. In general, ointments are preferred but as with moisturizers, compliance may dictate use of a cream despite the fact that these can be more drying and even irritating in some cases.

a. Low-potency steroids (e.g., hydrocortisone 2.5% or desonide 0.05%) may be used for mild disease or on sensitive skin areas such as the face, axillae, or groin twice daily, no more than 2 weeks per month.
b. Mid-potency steroids (e.g., triamcinolone 0.1% and fluticasone propionate 0.005% ointment) may be used on the body or extremities twice daily, no more than 2 weeks per month.
c. High-potency steroids (e.g., fluocinonide 0.05% and clobetasol propionate 0.05% ointment) are reserved for older children on severely affected areas twice daily, no more than 2 weeks per month.

Patients need to be cautioned about steroid side effects. Continuous or overzealous use may cause thinning of the skin, stretch marks (striae), telangiectasia, and significant systemic absorption. Infants are at greater risk for increased absorption because of their increased body surface area-to-weight ratio. Topical steroids applied near the eye area may lead to cataracts and glaucoma.

TOPICAL CALCINEURIN INHIBITORS Tacrolimus has been used as a systemic treatment for transplant rejection and is an approved topical preparation for atopic dermatitis. Tacrolimus and the related chemical pimecrolimus are important additions to the armamentarium as they are not corticosteroids and do not share the same side effects. However, they are very expensive and have a shorter history of safety data than corticosteroids. The FDA has issued a black box warning for these medications highlighting a possible association with skin cancer and lymphoma, prompting concern from clinicians and patients alike. While more than 15 years of clinical practice has yielded minimal data suggesting a significant increase in long-term adverse effects from the use of topical calcineurin inhibitors in the management of atopic dermatitis or other cutaneous conditions, ongoing surveillance is warranted. These medications are probably best used as steroid-sparing agents in patients with moderate-to-severe atopic dermatitis who would be at significant risk from steroid side effects. Side effects reported include burning and itching in some patients, which tend to resolve as the skin improves.

Antibiotics

Topical or oral antibiotics may be needed if the skin becomes secondarily infected, a very common scenario in atopic dermatitis. However, systemic antibiotics are not indicated in the absence of infection; use in this context may unnecessarily promote antibiotic resistance.

Open and moist areas, which may weep or become crusted, vesiculation and frank pustules frequently indicate bacterial infection in patients with severe disease. Topical mupirocin is generally the antibiotic of choice because of its efficacy against *Staphylococcus* and the relatively rare rate of contact allergy. It may be applied thrice daily to such impetiginized areas for 7 to 14 days. Bacitracin and neomycin are frequent contact dermatitis sensitizers and should be avoided. Daily bleach baths—adding a half cup of bleach to a full bathtub, achieving a very dilute bleach solution—can also be helpful for decolonization of skin flora that may contribute to secondary infection.

In more widespread infection, oral antibiotics may be used for 7 to 10 days. In patients with recurrent infections a longer maintenance course of antibiotics may be considered. Commonly prescribed antibiotics include empiric cephalexin (25–50 mg/kg/d divided qid, not to exceed 4 g/d) and dicloxacillin (25–50 mg/kg/d divided qid, not to exceed 2 g/d), though obtaining skin culture with sensitivities can be very helpful in guiding antibiotic therapy, especially in patients with recurrent infections.

Antipruritics

This corner of the tetrahedron is least populated with good options and, perhaps as a result of this, most frequently ignored. However, there is still a role for antipruritic treatments.

ANTIHISTAMINES These oral medications are unfortunately not very effective at controlling the itch of atopic dermatitis. They continue to be useful at bedtime as the side effect of drowsiness is often effective at improving sleep. In rare instances, a paradoxical hyperactivity may be seen. The most commonly prescribed antihistamines are hydroxyzine (2 mg/kg/d divided tid or qid) and diphenhydramine (1–2 mg/kg tid, not to exceed 300 mg/d). Topical antihistamines are not recommended because of the relatively high risk of developing allergic contact dermatitis and limited efficacy in controlling atopic dermatitis-associated itch.

ANESTHETICS Topical pramoxine (available as 1% cream and in combination creams) can be helpful at alleviating itch very quickly by literally inhibiting the nerves, which convey the sensation.

COOLING PREPARATIONS Topical preparations of menthol, camphor, and calamine may all be helpful, especially in combination form. Aveeno Anti-Itch cream (regular strength), Sarna Sensitive Skin lotion, and Eucerin Itch-Relief Moisturizing spray all contain combinations of these ingredients and can be helpful for acute pruritus. Encouraging patients to apply the antipruritic preparations instead of scratching can be extremely helpful. In all patients, but especially in children younger than 2 years, camphor use should be carefully limited as camphor toxicity can occur.

INFANTILE ATOPIC DERMATITIS

Frequently appearing on the face, this common problem is often extremely worrisome to new parents. Many of these patients have atopic diseases in the family. Milk-protein allergy is frequently blamed, but the high rate of improvement with time alone makes this observation very suspect.

EPIDEMIOLOGY

AGE Symptoms appear between age 2 and 6 months and the majority clear by age 2 to 3 years.

PHYSICAL EXAMINATION

Skin Lesions

TYPE Patches and erosions with scaling, exudation with wet crusts, and fissures.

COLOR Erythematous pink to red.

DISTRIBUTION Begins on face (cheeks, forehead, and scalp) and then spreads to body, usually sparing diaper area (Fig. 2-2).

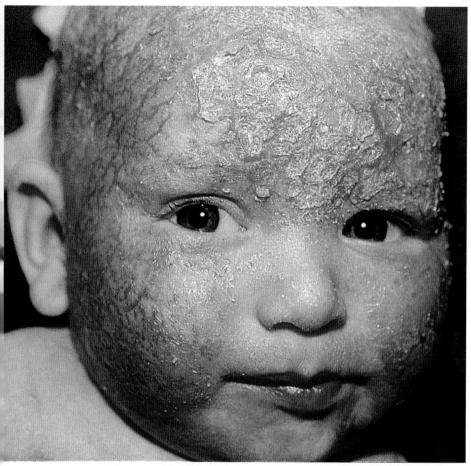

FIGURE 2-2 Infantile atopic dermatitis Erythematous, scaling exudative patches predominantly on the face of a 6-month-old child.

CHILDHOOD-TYPE ATOPIC DERMATITIS

EPIDEMIOLOGY

AGE Typically follows infantile atopic dermatitis and is seen from age 4 to 10 years.

PHYSICAL EXAMINATION

Skin Lesions

TYPE Papules coalescing into lichenified plaques with erosions and crusts (Figs. 2-3 and 2-4).

DISTRIBUTION Wrists, ankles, antecubital, and popliteal fossae.

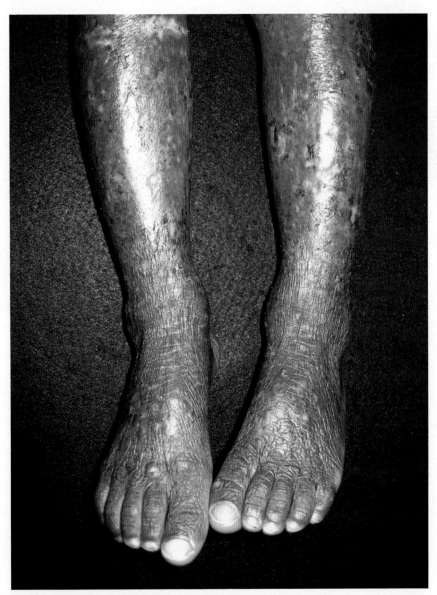

FIGURE 2-3 **Atopic dermatitis, childhood-type** Ill-defined lichenified papules and plaques with excoriations and dyspigmentation on the legs of a child.

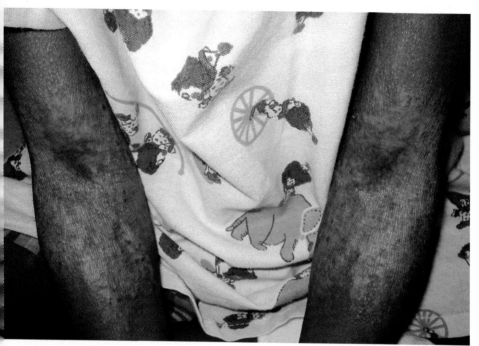

FIGURE 2-4 Atopic dermatitis, childhood-type Lichenification and erythematous patches in the antecubital fossae of a child.

ADOLESCENT-TYPE ATOPIC DERMATITIS

EPIDEMIOLOGY

AGE Begins at age 12 years and continues into adulthood.

PHYSICAL EXAMINATION

Skin Lesions

TYPE Papules coalescing into lichenified plaques.
DISTRIBUTION Flexor folds (Fig. 2-5), face, neck, upper back, hands, and feet.

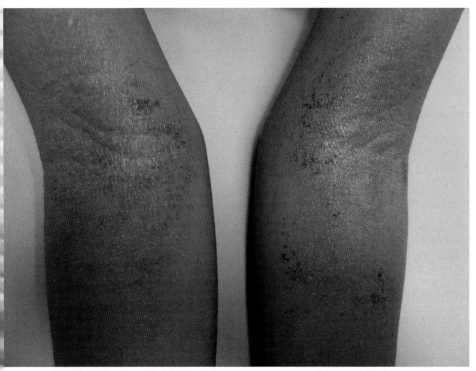

FIGURE 2-5 Atopic dermatitis, adolescent-type Erythematous, lichenified plaques on the antecubital fossae of an adolescent.

STRIAE DISTENSAE

Atrophic, scar-like lesions that may be seen from topical or systemic corticosteroid use. While they do not cause significant morbidity, numerous striae can be disfiguring and are difficult to reverse.

SYNONYM Stretch marks.

EPIDEMIOLOGY

AGE Persons of all ages may be affected; seen more commonly in adolescents and adults.
GENDER F > M.
INCIDENCE Common.

PATHOPHYSIOLOGY

Damage to the connective tissue (collagen and elastin) due to mechanical stretching, particularly in genetically susceptible individuals, causes permanent breakage and alteration of elastic fibers. During the adolescent growth spurt striae frequently develop on the back and arms; during pregnancy they are frequently found on the abdomen. Topical or systemic corticosteroids (endogenous or exogenous) facilitate striae while topical retinoids mitigate against their formation.

HISTORY

DURATION OF LESION(S) Years. The lesions often start as deep red–blue plaques and over time become more white in color and thinner.

PHYSICAL EXAMINATION

Skin Lesions

TYPE Atrophic linear plaques with fine wrinkling of the epidermis.

SIZE 1 to 10 cm.
COLOR Erythematous in younger lesions to hypopigmented in older lesions.
SHAPE Linear.
DISTRIBUTION Frequently on the lower back, upper arms, and abdomen, but may occur anywhere topical steroids are applied (Fig. 2-6).

DIFFERENTIAL DIAGNOSIS

Striae secondary to rapid growth or weight gain must be distinguished from endogenous or exogenous Cushing syndrome associated with excess corticosteroid exposure.

MANAGEMENT

Cautious use of topical and corticosteroids with frequent breaks from the medication can minimize the risk of striae. Avoiding high-potency steroids to more delicate skin such as that of the face, axillae, or groin is also helpful. Concurrent use of tretinoin cream or gel has been shown to prevent the formation of striae and improve the appearance even after their development. Pulsed dye laser is helpful for decreasing the erythema and various forms of laser treatment may increase the collagen in the lesions.

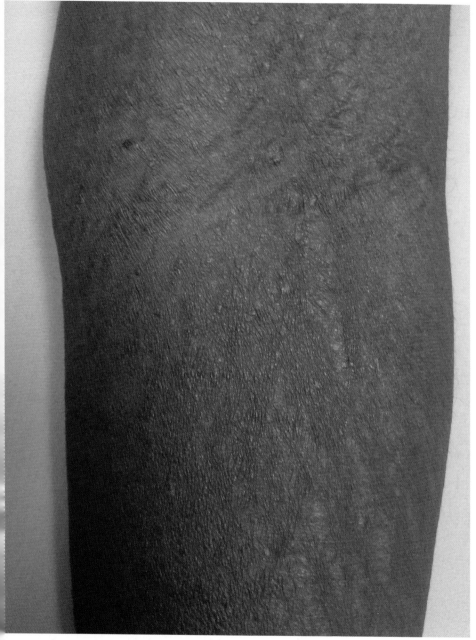

FIGURE 2-6 Striae distensae Atrophic linear striae secondary to overuse of topical corticosteroids.

LICHEN SIMPLEX CHRONICUS

Lichen simplex chronicus (LSC) is a localized, well-circumscribed area of lichenification (thickened skin with enhanced skin markings) resulting from repeated rubbing, itching, or scratching of the skin. It is frequently seen in individuals with atopic dermatitis, seborrheic dermatitis, contact dermatitis, or psoriasis.

EPIDEMIOLOGY

AGE Rarely seen in young children. Occurs in adolescents and adults.
GENDER F > M.
INCIDENCE Common.

PATHOPHYSIOLOGY

A response to physical trauma resulting in epidermal hyperplasia and acanthosis. The skin becomes highly sensitive to touch, probably related to proliferation of nerves in the epidermis. This leads to an itch-scratch cycle that is difficult to stop.

HISTORY

DURATION OF LESION(S) Weeks to months or years.

PHYSICAL EXAMINATION

Skin Lesions

TYPE Well-defined plaque of lichenification (Figs. 2-7 and 2-8); at times with scale or excoriations.
SIZE 5 to 15 cm.
COLOR Usually hyperpigmented but occasionally hypopigmented.
SHAPE Round, oval, linear (following path of scratching).
DISTRIBUTION Easily reached areas such as neck, wrists, ankles, pretibial area, thighs, vulva, scrotum, and perianal area. Spares difficult-to-reach areas such as upper central back.

DIFFERENTIAL DIAGNOSIS

LSC can be confused with tinea corporis, psoriasis, contact, or atopic dermatitis.

LABORATORY EXAMINATIONS

DERMATOPATHOLOGY Hyperkeratosis, acanthosis, and elongated and broad rete ridges. Spongiosis is infrequent and vesiculation is absent. In the dermis, there is a chronic inflammatory infiltrate with fibrosis.

MANAGEMENT

Topical corticosteroids or calcineurin inhibitors (i.e., tacrolimus or pimecrolimus) will decrease pruritus. Occlusive dressings or wraps such as the Unna boot (gauze impregnated with zinc oxide and calamine) can also prevent scratching. Flurandrenolide, a mid-potency steroid, is available as a tape, which can be very useful for covering an area of LSC. It should be used sparingly as steroids under occlusion are much more potent.

The side effects of prolonged or potent topical steroids should be reviewed. Continued use of topical steroids can lead to thinning of the skin, stretch marks, and accentuation of the blood vessels in the skin. For small localized areas of LSC, intralesional corticosteroids are often highly effective.

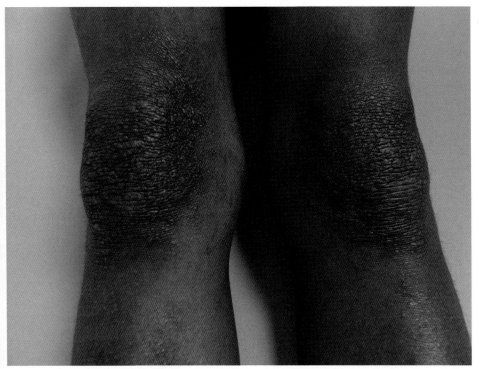

FIGURE 2-7 Lichen simplex chronicus Excoriated, lichenified plaque with accentuated skin lines caused by repeated scratching of the area.

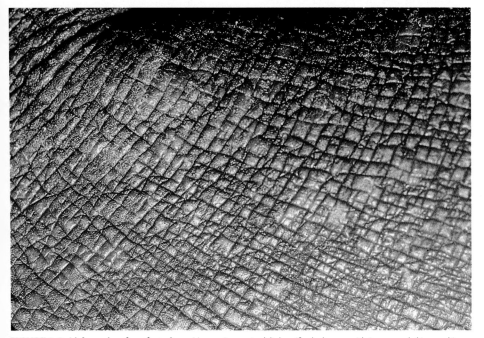

FIGURE 2-8 Lichen simplex chronicus Hyperpigmented, lichenified plaque with increased skin markings caused by repeated rubbing of the area.

PRURIGO NODULARIS

Prurigo nodularis (PN) is characterized by multiple lichenified intensely pruritic papules on the extremities. It is more frequently seen in individuals with a history of atopic dermatitis or allergies.

 INSIGHT Simply asking the patient to demonstrate how he or she scratches, picks, or rubs will frequently confirm the diagnosis as the patient gladly obliges.

SYNONYM Nodular prurigo.

EPIDEMIOLOGY

AGE Rarely seen in young children. Occurs in adolescents and adults.
GENDER M = F.
INCIDENCE Rare.

PATHOPHYSIOLOGY

Although the pathophysiology is uncertain, PN may begin as a response to an insect bite or an area of dermatitis that is scratched, picked, or rubbed. As with LSC, the trauma results in skin thickening, hyperkeratosis, and increased size (and, some studies suggest, responsiveness) of nerve fibers in the skin. Hepatic or renal dysfunction may be an associated factor in some cases, though the relationship may be simply as an underlying cause of pruritus.

HISTORY

DURATION OF LESION(S) Months to years.

PHYSICAL EXAMINATION

Skin Lesions

TYPE Papules and nodules (Fig. 2-9); at times with scale or excoriation.
SIZE 3 to 20 mm.

COLOR Usually hyperpigmented but occasionally hypopigmented.
SHAPE Round, dome-shaped.
DISTRIBUTION From several lesions in a localized area to hundreds of widespread nodules, frequently on the legs and arms.

DIFFERENTIAL DIAGNOSIS

Papular urticaria (insect bites), transepidermal elimination disorders (perforating dermatoses), bacterial or deep fungal infection of the skin including atypical mycobacteria, and some tumors can mimic this condition.

LABORATORY EXAMINATIONS

Skin biopsy can be helpful in confirming the diagnosis and eliminating infectious or neoplastic etiologies. Complete blood count, liver function tests, and chemistries are useful for evaluating the underlying hepatic or renal dysfunction.

MANAGEMENT

Topical corticosteroids or calcineurin inhibitors (i.e., tacrolimus or pimecrolimus) may decrease pruritus but frequently are ineffective. Occlusive dressings or wraps such as the Unna boot (gauze impregnated with zinc oxide and calamine) help prevent picking. Flurandrenolide, a mid-potency steroid, is available as a tape, which can be very useful for covering an individual lesion. Intralesional corticosteroids are often effective but difficult when the lesions are widespread. Phototherapy with ultraviolet B can be effective for some patients. Discussion of avoiding the picking or scratching behavior is important as well.

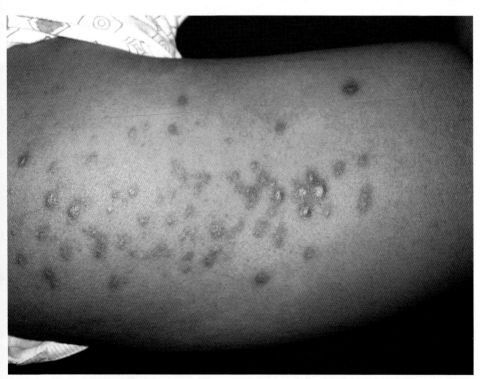

FIGURE 2-9 Prurigo nodularis Multiple dyspigmented nodules on the arm.

DYSHIDROTIC ECZEMATOUS DERMATITIS

Dyshidrotic eczema is a special vesicular type of hand and foot eczema. It is an acute, chronic, or recurrent dermatosis of the fingers, palms, and soles characterized by a sudden onset of deep-seated pruritic, clear, "tapioca-like" vesicles; later, scaling, fissures, lichenification, and occasionally, secondary bacterial infection may occur.

SYNONYM Pompholyx (from the Greek for *bubble*).

EPIDEMIOLOGY

AGE 12 to 40 years old.
GENDER M = F.

PATHOPHYSIOLOGY

The etiology is unclear and likely multifactorial. Approximately half the patients have an atopic background. Emotional stress is sometimes a precipitating factor. Hyperhidrosis may or may not be present. External contactants may play a role in some cases.

HISTORY

DURATION OF LESIONS Several days.
SKIN SYMPTOMS Pruritus and painful fissures that may be incapacitating. Summer exacerbations are not infrequent.

PHYSICAL EXAMINATION

Skin Lesions

Type

a. *Early* Vesicles, usually small (1 mm), deep-seated, appear like "tapioca" in clusters (Fig. 2-10), occasionally bullae, especially on the feet.
b. *Late* Scaling, lichenification, painful fissures, and erosions (Fig. 2-11).

ARRANGEMENT Vesicles grouped in clusters.
DISTRIBUTION Hands and feet with sites of predilection bilaterally on the sides of fingers, palms, and soles.
NAILS Dystrophic changes (transverse ridging, pitting, and thickening) may occur.
OTHER Hyperhidrosis is present in some patients.

DIFFERENTIAL DIAGNOSIS

Pompholyx can mimic a vesicular reaction to active dermatophytosis on the feet, an "id"

(autoeczematization) reaction to inflammation or infection elsewhere, pustular psoriasis, or an acute contact dermatitis.

DERMATOPATHOLOGY

Intraepidermal vesicles with balloon cells and sparse inflammation.

COURSE AND PROGNOSIS

Recurrent attacks with intervals of weeks to months with spontaneous remissions in 2 to 3 weeks.

MANAGEMENT

1. Dry skin care with minimization of hand washing and wet-work, mild soap-free cleansers for washing, followed by ointments (e.g., hydrated petrolatum).
2. For the active vesicular stage (early): Burrow's wet dressings, commonly available as Domeboro Astringent Solution Powder Packets q6h for 15 minutes; large bullae may be drained but not unroofed.
3. For the more chronic eczematous stage (late): High-potency topical corticosteroid ointments are successful in some patients; rarely, a short course of systemic corticosteroids may be used, though the disease may rebound severely after cessation.
4. Bacterial infection may be present and topical (mupirocin ointment tid to open or crusted areas) or oral antibiotics (e.g., cephalexin 25–50 mg/kg/d divided qid, not to exceed 4 g/d for 7 days) may be helpful.
5. PUVA (oral or topical as "soaks" in psoralen with controlled ultraviolet A light treatment) is successful in older patients if given over prolonged periods of time, especially in severe cases.

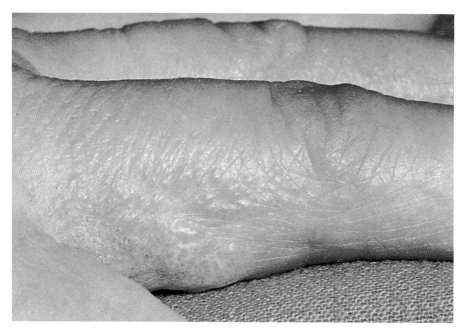

FIGURE 2-10 Atopic dermatitis, dyshidrotic type Tapioca-like, deep-seated vesicles on the sides of the fingers. (Reproduced with permission from IM Freedberg et al., *Dermatology in General Medicine.* 5th ed. New York: McGraw-Hill; 1999.)

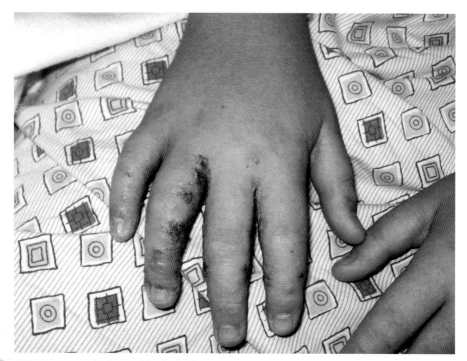

FIGURE 2-11 Atopic dermatitis, dyshidrotic type Fissuring, scaling, and eroded patches after widespread vesiculation in a severe case.

NUMMULAR ECZEMA

Nummular eczema is a chronic, pruritic, inflammatory dermatitis occurring in the form of coin-shaped plaques. It is seen in individuals with dry skin and/or atopic dermatitis.

 INSIGHT Nummular eczema may be very refractory to treatment; oftentimes a much more potent corticosteroid must be used to these areas than for routine atopic dermatitis.

SYNONYMS Discoid eczema; nummular dermatitis.

EPIDEMIOLOGY

AGE Any age. Seen more commonly in older children and adolescents.
GENDER M = F.
INCIDENCE Common.
ETIOLOGY Unclear. Exacerbated by winter, excessive bathing, irritants.

PATHOPHYSIOLOGY

Unclear. A common eczematous reaction pattern, frequently occurring in atopic patients.

HISTORY

DURATION OF LESIONS Weeks, with remissions and recurrences.
SKIN SYMPTOMS Pruritus, may be mild or severe.

PHYSICAL EXAMINATION

Skin Lesions

TYPE Closely grouped, small vesicles and papules that coalesce into lichenified plaques, often 3 to 5 cm.
COLOR Deeply erythematous to hyperpigmented.

SHAPE Round or coin-shaped (Fig. 2-12), hence the adjective nummular (from Latin *nummularis*, "like a coin").
DISTRIBUTION Extensor surfaces of hands, arms, legs.

DIFFERENTIAL DIAGNOSIS

Nummular dermatitis must be distinguished from tinea corporis, contact dermatitis, and psoriasis. Early on, the round shape may also be mistaken for an annular lesion, such as that of granuloma annulare or erythema annulare centrifugum.

LABORATORY EXAMINATIONS

POTASSIUM HYDROXIDE EXAMINATION Scrapings negative for fungal elements excludes tinea corporis.
DERMATOPATHOLOGY Subacute inflammation with acanthosis, intraepidermal vesicles, and spongiosis in the epidermis.

COURSE AND PROGNOSIS

Remissions with treatment but frequent recurrences unless the skin is kept moisturized.

MANAGEMENT

1. Dry skin care consisting of mild soap-free cleansers for washing, followed by frequent moisturization with CeraVe, Aveeno, or hydrated petrolatum.
2. Topical corticosteroids can be applied for a limited time to the more moderate to severely affected areas.

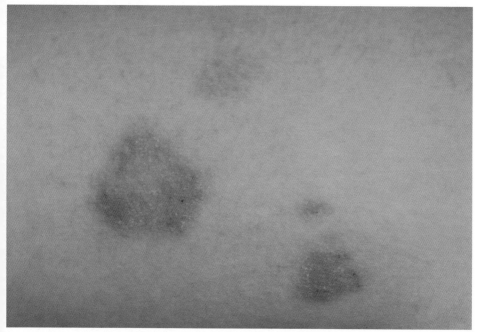

FIGURE 2-12 Nummular eczema Lichenified coin-shaped plaques on the arm.

CONTACT DERMATITIS

There are two types of contact dermatitis:
1. Allergic contact: caused by sensitization of the skin to a topical allergen with type IV hypersensitivity.
2. Irritant contact: caused by mechanical or chemical injury to the skin without specific immunity.
Both reactions are characterized by pruritus, stinging, or burning of the skin and an eczematous rash.

EPIDEMIOLOGY

AGE Irritant dermatitis may occur at any age, whereas allergic contact dermatitis is unusual in <1 year of age given time needed to expose and sensitize skin to allergen.
GENDER M = F.
INCIDENCE May affect 20% of the pediatric population.
ETIOLOGY Exposure to an antigen that has previously caused sensitization in the case of allergic contact (see Table 2-1). A primary irritant that produces inflammation via injury in the case of irritant contact.

TABLE 2-1 Common Contact Allergens in Children

Nickel

Cobalt
Gold

Cocamidopropyl betaine
Balsam of Peru

Thimerosal
Neomycin

Bacitracin
Benzalkonium chloride

Disperse blue dye
Carba mix

Cinnamic aldehyde
Formaldehyde

Fragrance Mix

Adapted from Jacob SE, Yang A, Herro E, Zhang C. Contact allergens in a pediatric population. *J Clin Aesthet Dermatol.* 2010; 3(10): 29–35.

PATHOPHYSIOLOGY

Allergic contact dermatitis is the classic example of type IV hypersensitivity reaction (delayed type) caused by sensitized lymphocytes (T cells) after contact with antigen. The tissue damage results from cytotoxicity by T cells and from release of lymphokines.

Irritant contact dermatitis is caused by immediate physical damage to an area of skin and subsequent inflammatory response.

HISTORY

DURATION OF LESION(S) Acute contact: days, weeks; chronic contact: months, years.
SKIN SYMPTOMS Pruritus, often severe. Extensive lesions may be painful.

PHYSICAL EXAMINATION

Skin Findings

Type
a. *Acute* Inflammatory papules and vesicles coalescing into plaques (Fig. 2-13A,B).
b. *Subacute* Patches of mild erythema showing small, dry scales, or superficial desquamation, sometimes associated with small, red, pointed or rounded, firm papules.
c. *Chronic* Patches of lichenified (thickening of the epidermis with enhancement of the skin markings) firm, rounded or flat-topped papules, excoriations, and pigmentation (Fig. 2-14).

ARRANGEMENT Well-demarcated patterns suggestive of an external cause or "outside job." Plant allergic contact dermatitis often results in linear lesions.
DISTRIBUTION In exposed areas that come into contact with irritant or allergen.

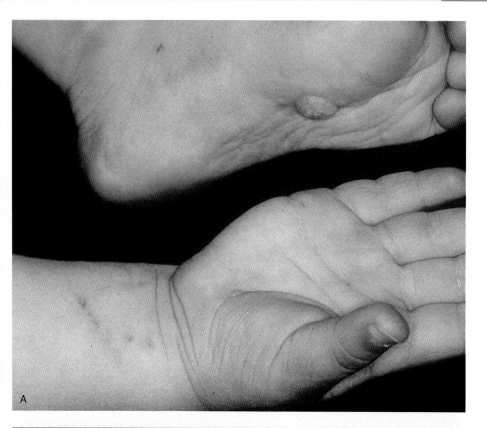

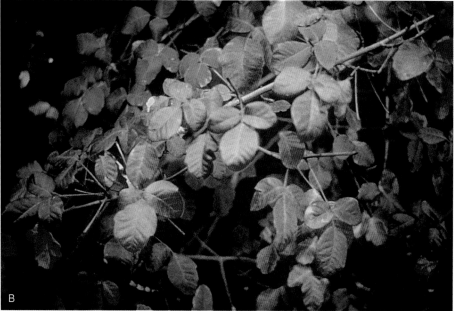

FIGURE 2-13 Allergic contact dermatitis, acute **(A)** linear arrangement of vesicles on wrist and bulla on the foot of a child exposed to poison ivy. **B:** Plant: poison ivy with characteristic shiny red, three-leaf configuration.

LABORATORY EXAMINATIONS

DERMATOPATHOLOGY Inflammation with intraepidermal intercellular edema (spongiosis) and monocyte and histiocyte infiltration in the dermis suggest allergic contact dermatitis, whereas more superficial vesicles containing polymorphonuclear leukocytes suggest a primary irritant dermatitis. In chronic contact dermatitis, there is lichenification (hyperkeratosis, acanthosis, elongation of rete ridges, and elongation and broadening of papillae).

PATCH TESTING Numerous allergens may be specifically tested in suspected allergic contact dermatitis. Standardized mixtures of the allergens are placed against the skin for 24 to 48 hours and then removed looking for reactions at each site.

MANAGEMENT

Prompt identification and removal of the offending agent is critical.

ACUTE Domeboro Astringent Solution soaks 15 minutes 4 times per day may be helpful. High-potency topical corticosteroids can be very helpful for localized reactions. For more widespread reactions and those involving very sensitive skin such as the face or genitals, a short course of systemic corticosteroids may provide relief. It is important to taper systemic steroids slowly (over several weeks) as rebound is common if the taper is performed too quickly.

SUBACUTE AND CHRONIC Short courses of potent topical corticosteroid preparations (such as clobetasol ointment) may be used sparingly bid for up to 2 weeks along with aggressive moisturization and avoidance of scratching and rubbing.

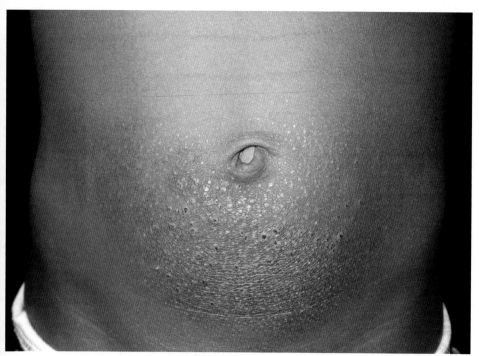

FIGURE 2-14 Allergic contact dermatitis, chronic lichenified papules grouped near the umbilicus in a child with nickel allergy from his belt buckle and button.

SEBORRHEIC DERMATITIS

Seborrheic dermatitis is a recurrent, waxing and waning dermatosis, which occurs on the areas of the skin in which the sebaceous glands are most active, such as the face and scalp, and in the diaper area.

SYNONYMS Cradle cap; seborrhea.

EPIDEMIOLOGY

AGE Infancy (within the first 10 weeks) and adolescence (puberty).
GENDER More common in males.
INCIDENCE 2% to 5% of the population.
ETIOLOGY Unknown. *Malassezia furfur* yeast, a normal skin constituent, is highly associated with seborrheic dermatitis.

PATHOPHYSIOLOGY

Malassezia does not appear to be present in higher numbers in these patients, thus an abnormal immune response is postulated.

HISTORY

DURATION OF LESIONS Gradual onset, commonly in infancy.
SKIN SYMPTOMS Typically asymptomatic or mildly pruritic.

PHYSICAL EXAMINATION

Skin Lesions

TYPE Patches with yellowish often greasy scale which can be very thick and adherent.
COLOR Erythematous.
ARRANGEMENT Scattered, discrete patches on the face and chest (Fig. 2-15); diffuse involvement of scalp and diaper area.
DISTRIBUTION Scalp, face, chest, and diaper area.

DIFFERENTIAL DIAGNOSIS

Differential includes dermatophytosis, candidiasis, and atopic dermatitis. There is an overlap seen in some patients with psoriasis, the so-called "sebopsoriasis."

DERMATOPATHOLOGY

Focal parakeratosis, with few pyknotic neutrophils, moderate acanthosis, spongiosis (intercellular edema) and nonspecific inflammation of the dermis.

COURSE AND PROGNOSIS

Infantile seborrhea usually is asymptomatic and clears spontaneously within months. Childhood and adolescent seborrheic dermatitis can clear spontaneously but may have a recurrent course.

TREATMENT

SCALP (CRADLE CAP) Removal of the thick scale with mineral oil and fine tooth comb lifting off of scale can provide symptomatic and cosmetic relief. For older children, shampoos containing selenium sulfide, zinc pyrithione, tar, or ketoconazole used intermittently 2 to 3 times a week can control the eruption. It is important to instruct the patient or parent to lather the shampoo and let it sit on the scalp for 5 minutes before rinsing.
FACE AND DIAPER AREA Creams containing ketoconazole are helpful and safe; these may be used bid on a regular basis for prevention. Low-potency topical steroid preparations (e.g., 2.5% hydrocortisone cream or fluticasone cream) may be used bid sparingly for 2 to 3 days for acute flares.

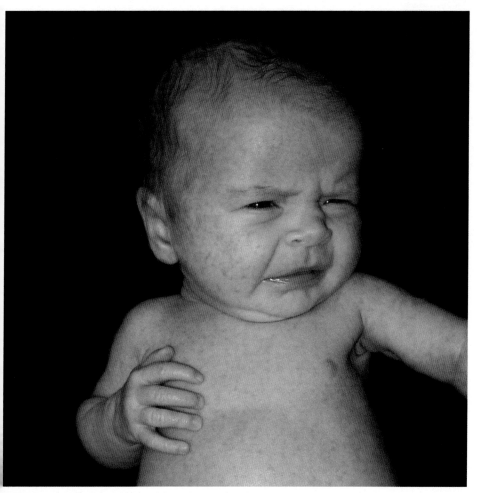

FIGURE 2-15 Seborrheic dermatitis Widespread erythematous patches on the face and chest; yellowish adherent scale on the scalp.

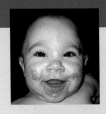

DIAPER DERMATITIS AND RASHES IN THE DIAPER AREA

DIAPER DERMATITIS

Diaper dermatitis generally refers to the irritant contact dermatitis that may result from multiple factors in the area: macerated skin (softened by being wet), rubbing and wiping, and possibly the presence of ammonia in urine and proteases and lipases in stool—all of which cause skin irritation and breakdown. It can become complicated by secondary bacterial or yeast infections as well.

INSIGHT The so-called "Greek method" of washing the soiled diaper area under a running tap of warm water rather than using abrasive wipes is said to prevent diaper dermatitis.

SYNONYMS Diaper rash, nappy rash.

EPIDEMIOLOGY

AGE Most babies develop some form of diaper dermatitis during their diaper-wearing years. The peak incidence is between ages 9 and 12 months.

GENDER M = F.

PREVALENCE At any one point in time, up to one-third of infants may have diaper dermatitis. The prevalence of severe diaper dermatitis (defined as erythema with ulcerations, oozing papules, and pustules) is 5%.

ETIOLOGY Excessive hydration of the skin and frictional injury lead to a compromised skin barrier, compounded by irritation from ammonia, feces, cleansing products, fragrances, and possible superinfection with *Candida albicans* or bacteria.

SEASON Reportedly highest during winter months, perhaps due to less frequent diaper changing.

PATHOPHYSIOLOGY

The warm moist environment inside the diaper and frictional damage decrease the protective barrier function of the skin in the diaper area. Additional predisposing factors such as seborrhea, atopic dermatitis, and systemic disease—as well as activating factors such as allergens (in detergents, rubbers, and plastic), primary irritants (ammonia from urine and feces), and infection (by yeast or bacteria)—lead to a rash in the diaper area. Diarrheal illnesses may acutely worsen diaper dermatitis given the frequent wet diapers with fecal material and propensity for maceration.

PHYSICAL EXAMINATION

Skin Findings

TYPE OF LESION Ranges from macular erythema (Fig. 3-1) to papules, plaques, vesicles, erosions, and rarely ulcerated nodules.

COLOR Ranges from mild erythema to diffuse beefy redness.

PALPATION Ranges from nonindurated to prominently elevated lesions.

DISTRIBUTION Diaper area, convex surfaces involved, folds spared. Severe cases may involve folds and have characteristic C. *albicans* satellite pustules if superinfected.

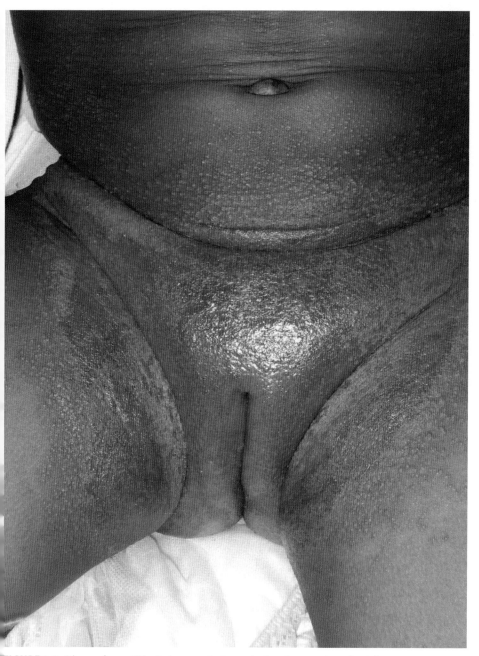

FIGURE 3-1 Diaper dermatitis Red, macerated areas in the diaper region of an infant.

DIFFERENTIAL DIAGNOSIS

DIAGNOSIS The diagnosis of diaper dermatitis may be made clinically, although refractory response to conventional treatments should raise the suspicion of less common rashes in the diaper area.

DIFFERENTIAL DIAGNOSIS Diaper dermatitis must be differentiated from psoriasis, granuloma gluteale infantum (likely a foreign body reaction, typically to baby powder, or topical steroids), primary candidiasis (perianal or intertriginous involvement with satellite lesions), perianal streptococcal infection, seborrheic dermatitis, acrodermatitis enteropathica (AE; caused by zinc deficiency), and Langerhans cell histiocytosis (LCH).

COURSE AND PROGNOSIS

Most episodes of diaper dermatitis are self-limited with a duration of 3 days or less. Severe cases of diaper dermatitis are usually caused by chronic irritants or secondary infection with candida or bacteria.

MANAGEMENT

The following help minimize rashes in the diaper area:

1. Keeping the diaper area clean and dry with gentle cleansing of the area (cotton balls dipped in warm water or nondetergent cleanser) and frequent diaper changes promptly after defecation and urination.
2. Remove any irritating agent or allergen from the diaper environment; hypoallergenic or cloth diapers may be less irritating. Similarly, fragrance-free, alcohol-free, or hypoallergenic wipes should be used sparingly to avoid contributing to further irritation.

3. Exposing the skin to air periodically will help keep it dry.
4. Protective creams and ointments such as zinc oxide (Desitin, Triple Paste), petrolatum (Hydrolatum, Vaseline), mineral oils, baby oils, lanolin, or vitamins A and D (A&D ointment) may protect the skin from moisture and help heal the infant's skin. These can be applied as a thick layer to the involved area with each diaper change, and may also be used as prophylaxis against future irritation by creating a barrier between the skin and urinary or fecal material.
5. For severe inflammation, mild topical steroids (2.5% hydrocortisone ointment) may be used sparingly. Since the diaper area is always under occlusion the steroid effects will be augmented in the already very sensitive baby skin of the groin area.

6. Cutaneous candidiasis requires topical antifungal treatment with nystatin or clotrimazole creams. Avoid anticandidal preparations that are mixed with cortisone to prevent steroid side effects in the occluded diaper area.
7. Bacterial infections may be treated with topical mupirocin; caution is advised with bacitracin and neomycin preparations as the incidence of allergic contact dermatitis is very high. Oral antibiotics may be indicated in severe cases.
8. Powders (talc, baby powder, cornstarch, magnesium stearate, zinc stearate, and baking soda) can be used to absorb moisture and reduce friction but should be applied carefully and sparingly so accidental inhalation does not occur.

RASHES IN THE DIAPER AREA

PSORIASIS IN DIAPER AREA

Psoriasis can first manifest itself as a recalcitrant diaper rash, and should be considered if conventional diaper rash remedies are not effective. Other stigmata of early psoriasis include seborrhea, nail pitting, and intergluteal erythema. A family history of psoriasis can also suggest this diagnosis.

EPIDEMIOLOGY

AGE Any age, typically seen first in the diaper area of children younger than 2 years.
GENDER F > M.
INCIDENCE Uncommon.
ETIOLOGY Unclear.
GENETICS Possible autosomal dominant inheritance with incomplete penetrance. Associated with HLA Cw6 (strongest association with early-onset or childhood psoriasis), as well as HLA B13, HLA B17, and HLA B57.

PATHOPHYSIOLOGY

In normal skin, the cells mature, shed, and are replaced every 3 to 4 weeks. In psoriasis, there is shortening of the cell cycle to 3 to 4 days. This leads to increased epidermal cell turnover with decreased shedding and, hence, the accumulation of dead cells as layers of silvery-white scale. However, psoriasis in the diaper area may not show the characteristic silvery-white scale given the constant dampness of the local environment.

PHYSICAL EXAMINATION

Skin Findings

TYPE Scattered erythematous papules, may coalesce into a well-delineated erythematous plaque. May demonstrate maceration in the diaper region.
COLOR Dark-red plaques, silvery mica-like scale variably present.
SIZE Pinpoint to several centimeters.
DISTRIBUTION Anogenital area; may also involve intergluteal cleft, umbilicus, behind or inside the ears, scalp, extremities (Fig. 3-2). Involvement of the inguinal folds may help distinguish from irritant diaper dermatitis.
NAILS May have pinpoint pits indicative of psoriasis.

DIFFERENTIAL DIAGNOSIS

The well-delineated bright-red plaque and silvery mica-like scale is characteristic of psoriasis. Removal of the scale may result in punctate bleeding (Auspitz sign). Macerated plaques without scale may be mistaken for irritant diaper dermatitis or allergic contact dermatitis.

LABORATORY EXAMINATIONS

DERMATOPATHOLOGY Epidermal thickening with edema of dermal papillae, thinning of suprapapillary area.

COURSE AND PROGNOSIS

Chronic course with remissions and exacerbations, very unpredictable. Some children progress to mild disease with intermittent exacerbations. Other children have a more severe course with recurrent flares, and 5% develop an associated arthritis.

MANAGEMENT

Psoriasis in the diaper area can be both refractory and/or recurrent.

1. Emollients such as petrolatum, moisturizers, or diaper creams can help minimize flares and reduce itching.
2. Allowing the diaper area to be exposed to air for short periods can also help reduce the chafing that can exacerbate psoriasis (Koebner phenomenon).
3. Sunlight exposure is thought to help psoriasis, but sunburns should be avoided.
4. Topical tar preparations are anti-inflammatory and can be used in the bath water (Cutar or Polytar) or in creams (MG217 or Elta tar creams). Prolonged use of these agents is not recommended.
5. More severe cases may require short courses of mild topical steroids (hydrocortisone 2.5%, desonide 0.05% cream or ointment). It is important to use steroid in the diaper area sparingly since the occlusive diaper increases the steroid potency as well as the risk of steroid side effects such as skin thinning and striae.

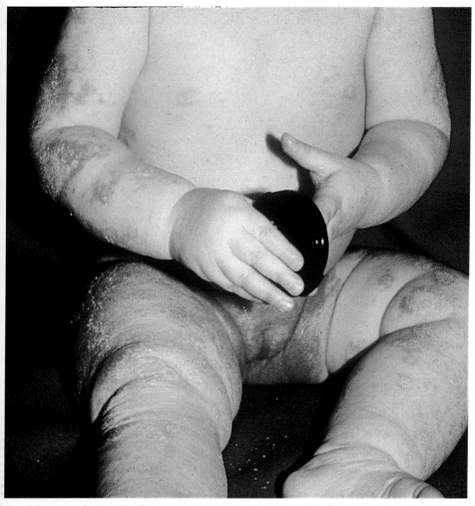

FIGURE 3-2 Psoriasis in the diaper area Well-delineated bright-red erythematous plaques in the diaper area and on the extremities of a child.

CANDIDAL INFECTION

Commonly overlooked, *Candida* diaper dermatitis should be suspected whenever a diaper rash fails to respond to conventional treatment, especially following a course of systemic antibiotic therapy. The infection is propagated by the chronic occlusive state of diapers worn during infancy.

SYNONYM Monilial diaper dermatitis.

EPIDEMIOLOGY

AGE Any diaper-wearing stage (approximately infancy to 3 years of age).
GENDER M = F.
INCIDENCE Common.
ETIOLOGY *C. albicans* organisms are harbored in the lower intestinal tract of the infant. Upon defecation, infected feces introduce yeast into area. The moist occlusive diaper environment favors candidal overgrowth and leads to a rash.

PATHOPHYSIOLOGY

C. albicans in mouth or GI tract of infant can proliferate in moist diaper environment. Predisposing factors such as systemic antibiotics can also contribute to *Candida* overgrowth.

HISTORY

Candidal overgrowth is seen most frequently following systemic antibiotic therapy. Lesions appear first in the perianal area and then spread to perineum and inguinal creases. The diaper rash may occur in conjunction with oral thrush. Pre-existing maceration in the diaper area can also predispose to superinfection by candidal species.

PHYSICAL EXAMINATION

Skin Findings

TYPE Erythema with fragile satellite pustules (Fig. 3-3). Rash involving perineum is sharply demarcated with elevated rim and variable scaling along the border. Pinpoint satellite vesicopustules often present.
COLOR Beefy red erythematous base.
DISTRIBUTION Genitocrural area, buttocks, lower abdomen, and inner aspects of the thighs, does not spare folds.

DIAGNOSIS AND DIFFERENTIAL DIAGNOSIS

DIAGNOSIS Observation of beefy red rash with vesicopustular satellite lesions is diagnostic. Scrapings and cultures can be confirmatory.
DIFFERENTIAL DIAGNOSIS Primary candidal infection in the diaper area has characteristic satellite papules and pustules that are virtually diagnostic. It may be confused with other recalcitrant rashes in the diaper area such as psoriasis, AE, or histiocytosis X. Most commonly, it can be seen in conjunction with other diaper rashes as a secondary infection.

LABORATORY EXAMINATIONS

Microscopic examination of skin scrapings with potassium hydroxide, Gram stain, or periodic acid-Schiff stain demonstrate budding yeasts and hyphae or pseudohyphae. Lesions may be cultured on Sabouraud's or Nickerson's media. White mucoid colonies grow within 48 to 72 hours.

COURSE AND PROGNOSIS

Rash progresses until *Candida* is treated. Area may become eroded and painful.

MANAGEMENT

1. Topical nystatin (Mycostatin) or clotrimazole (Lotrimin) creams tid to area will clear rash. Care should be taken to avoid anticandidal preparations that are mixed with coticosteroids (Lotrisone, Vytone) since these may be too strong and result in unwanted steroid side effects on the occluded diaper area against baby skin.
2. Oral nystatin suspension (nystatin swish and swallow, 1–3 mL po qid) can be applied to the affected mouth areas to treat oral thrush or gastrointestinal candidal overgrowth. This will also reduce chances of candidal recurrence in the diaper area.

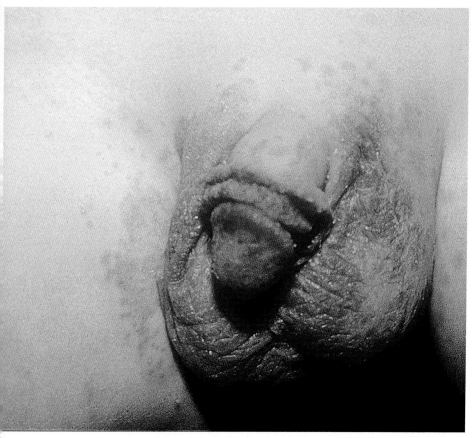

FIGURE 3-3 **Primary candidal infection in the diaper area** Beefy red plaque in the diaper area surrounded by characteristic satellite pustules.

ACRODERMATITIS ENTEROPATHICA

AE is a hereditary or acquired clinical syndrome caused by zinc deficiency. It is characterized by an acral, vesiculobullous eczematous dermatitis characteristically distributed on the face, hands, feet, and anogenital area.

 INSIGHT If acrodermatitis enteropathica is suspected, an alkaline phosphatase level can be helpful; this zinc-dependent enzyme is often low in such patients.

EPIDEMIOLOGY

Age

HEREDITARY In infants given bovine milk: days to few weeks after birth. In breastfed infants: soon after weaning.

ACQUIRED Older children and adults with illness that depletes zinc supply or chronic malnutrition.

GENDER M = F.

ETIOLOGY Hereditary or acquired deficiency in zinc.

HEREDITARY Autosomal recessively inherited disorder in zinc absorption secondary to abnormal zinc-uptake transporter proteins encoded by the *SLC39A4* gene. Zinc in human milk appears to be more bioavailable to infants than zinc from bovine milk, resulting in breastfed infants not displaying signs or symptoms until weaning.

ACQUIRED Long-term zinc deficiency can be seen in patients with parenteral nutrition lacking zinc, such as in bowel bypass syndrome, Crohn's disease, HIV, cystic fibrosis, alcoholism, vegetarian diets, essential fatty acid deficiencies, and other syndromes.

PATHOPHYSIOLOGY

Low serum zinc levels in infancy or childhood lead to AE. The basic defect is a GI malabsorption of zinc. Hereditary AE is due to abnormal zinc-uptake protein. Acquired AE can be seen with any systemic disease with GI malabsorption of zinc. The major function of zinc is to be incorporated into enzymes, and there are more than 200 zinc-dependent metalloenzymes in the body.

HISTORY

Review of systems may include diarrhea, weight loss, listlessness, and behavioral changes (irritability, crying, and restlessness).

PHYSICAL EXAMINATION

Skin Findings

TYPE OF LESION Eczematous or psoriasiform plaques may progress to vesiculobullae or erosions that crust and become dry (Fig. 3-4A and B).

COLOR Erythematous base.

DISTRIBUTION Perioral and symmetrically located on buttocks, extensor surfaces (elbows and knees), and acral areas (fingers and toes).

General Findings

Diarrhea, cachexia, alopecia, nail dystrophy, glossitis, stomatitis, hypogeusia (decreased sense of taste), photophobia, drooling, and growth retardation. Hypogonadism in males (more evident in adolescence). Emotional disturbances.

LABORATORY EXAMINATIONS

Low serum zinc (<50 µg/dL) or alkaline phosphatase levels. "Zebra striped" light banding of hair can be seen with polarized light microscopy. However, zinc levels may fluctuate with stress or infection.

DIFFERENTIAL DIAGNOSIS

The differential diagnosis includes other bullous diseases (such as linear IgA chronic bullous disease of childhood and bullous impetigo), psoriasis, LCH, and candidal infection. Refractory diaper dermatitis associated with periorificial and acral findings should lead the clinician to suspect AE.

COURSE AND PROGNOSIS

If unrecognized, AE has a relentlessly progressive course leading to infection and disability. Once recognized and treated, AE manifestations are quickly corrected and reversed.

TREATMENT

1. Topical zinc creams (Desitin, A&D ointment, zinc oxide paste, and Triple Paste) can begin to improve the rash.
2. Dietary supplement of zinc gluconate, acetate, or sulfate (3 mg/d of elemental zinc, divided bid/tid) is usually curative. The recommended daily allowance (RDA) of elemental zinc is up to 3 mg/d for children up to age 3 years.
3. In severe cases, $ZnCl_2$ may be administered intravenously.

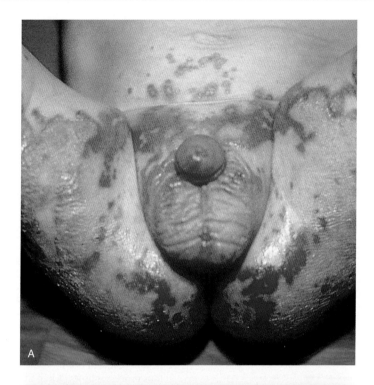

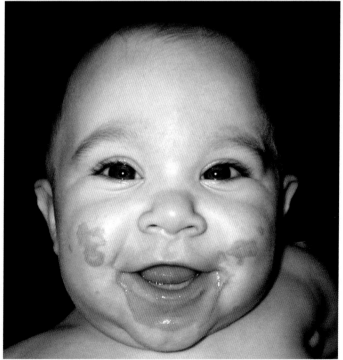

FIGURE 3-4 Acrodermatitis enteropathica A: Refractory erythematous, scaly macerated plaque in the diaper area. **B:** Erythematous and eroded plaques in the perioral region.

GRANULOMA GLUTEALE INFANTUM

Granuloma gluteale infantum is a benign rash in the diaper area characterized by reddish-purple granulomatous nodules. The disorder represents a cutaneous response to a foreign body (talc or zirconium), topical steroids, infection *(candida)*, or inflammation.

SYNONYMS Kaposi sarcoma–like granuloma; granuloma intertriginosum infantum; vegetating bromidism.

EPIDEMIOLOGY

AGE Any diaper-wearing age, typically from birth to 3 years.
GENDER M > F.
INCIDENCE Rare.
ETIOLOGY Initiating inflammatory process with maceration and secondary infection leads to a granulomatous response.

PATHOPHYSIOLOGY

Lesions believed to be a unique, benign granulomatous response to a foreign body, inflammation, maceration, and/or secondary infection.

HISTORY

Lesions appear in the diaper area several months after treatment of inciting factors. The rash symptoms can range from being asymptomatic to very painful.

PHYSICAL EXAMINATION

Skin Findings

TYPE Granulomatous papules and nodules (Fig. 3-5).
COLOR Reddish-purple.
SIZE 0.5 to 4.0 cm in diameter.
DISTRIBUTION Groin, buttocks, lower aspect of abdomen, penis, rarely intertriginous areas of axillae, and/or neck.

DIFFERENTIAL DIAGNOSIS

The papular and nodular lesions of granuloma gluteale infantum can appear very worrisome despite their benign nature because similar lesions can also be seen in sarcomas and lymphomas. Similar lesions may be found in Kaposi sarcoma, tuberculosis, syphilis, and deep fungal infections. The diagnosis of granuloma gluteale infantum is often made clinically and can be confirmed by skin biopsy.

LABORATORY EXAMINATIONS

LIGHT AND ELECTRON MICROSCOPY Hyperplastic epidermis with inflammatory cells (mostly neutrophils), a parakeratotic stratum corneum, and a dense inflammatory infiltrate throughout the depth of the cutis with hemorrhage, neutrophils, lymphocytes, histiocytes, plasma cells, eosinophils, newly formed capillaries, and giant cells. Lesions of granuloma gluteale infantum lack the masses of patchy accumulations of lymphoma cells seen in lymphomatous disorders. Granuloma gluteale infantum may be differentiated from more severe granulomatous processes by its lack of fibrous proliferative features, spindle cell formations, and mitoses.

COURSE AND PROGNOSIS

Benign. Lesions resolve completely and spontaneously several months after treatment of the primary inciting inflammatory process and/or infection.

MANAGEMENT

Treatment begins with the identification and elimination of the primary inciting inflammatory process and/or infection.
For the nodular lesions:

1. If topical steroids are being used, discontinuation often leads to resolution of the nodules
2. Conversely, if topical steroids are not being used, a short 2-week trial of topical, intralesional, or impregnated steroid tape (Cordran tape) may hasten resolution of these nodules Close follow-up is necessary because steroid may worsen the condition.

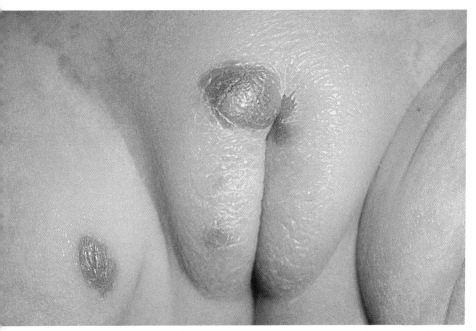

FIGURE 3-5 Granuloma gluteale infantum Nodular granulomatous response in the diaper area to topical steroids.

LANGERHANS CELL HISTIOCYTOSIS IN THE DIAPER AREA

LCH is a rare proliferative disorder of the Langerhans cell (a histiocyte that migrates throughout the skin as an antigen-presenting cell). Although the disease is rare, it frequently presents in infancy as a rash in the diaper area. LCH should be considered if a diaper rash is particularly recalcitrant to usual remedies, especially if systemic symptoms are present.

INSIGHT In refractory diaper dermatitis with petechiae or purpura, Langerhans cell histiocytosis must be excluded.

SYNONYM Histiocytosis X, Langerhans cell granulomatosis, type II histiocytosis, LCH.

EPIDEMIOLOGY

AGE Usually in the first year of life. Can be seen up to 3 years of age.
GENDER M > F in children.
INCIDENCE Extremely rare, 1 per 5 million children annually.
ETIOLOGY Unclear.
GENETICS Possibly autosomal recessive with reduced penetrance.

PATHOPHYSIOLOGY

Unclear. Several proposed mechanisms include a disturbance of intracellular lipid metabolism, a reactive histiocytic response to infection, or a neoplastic process. Some cases may be hereditary. All theories somehow implicate the development of a Langerhans cell–like histiocyte as a primary component.

PHYSICAL EXAMINATION

Skin Findings

TYPE Begins as erythema and scale and progresses to purpuric papules, nodules, or vesicles (Fig. 3-6).
COLOR Reddish-brown or purple.
SIZE Pinpoint to 1 cm.
DISTRIBUTION Inguinal and perineal areas, axilla, behind ears, and scalp, can be on the trunk.

General Findings

Decreased immunity can lead to increased susceptibility to infections. Severe forms of the disease can have cell infiltrates of the bone, lung, liver, and lymph nodes.

LABORATORY EXAMINATIONS

DERMATOPATHOLOGY Skin biopsy will reveal characteristic Langerhans cells, which are diagnostic of a histiocyte proliferative disorder. Langerhans cells can be identified with positive S-100 and CD1a stains. Electron microscopy demonstrates racquet-shaped Birbeck granules in the cytoplasm of the histiocytes.

DIFFERENTIAL DIAGNOSIS

The initial presentation of LCH is similar to seborrhea, with an erythematous scaly rash that becomes more extensive cutaneously and can have associated systemic disease. A skin biopsy is usually needed to confirm the diagnosis.

COURSE AND PROGNOSIS

LCH constitutes a spectrum of disease. The highest mortality rate (38–54%) is seen in the most severe form: Letterer–Siwe disease (associated with fever, anemia, thrombocytopenia, lymphadenopathy, hepatosplenomegaly, and skeletal tumors). Less severe clinical courses are seen with Hand–Schuller–Christian disease (associated with osteolytic defects, diabetes mellitus, and exophthalmos). Eosinophilic granuloma (associated with osteolytic defects and spontaneous fractures) and Hashimoto–Pritzker disease (aka congenital self-healing reticulohistiocytosis; a benign, self-limited entity with skin lesions only) represent the mildest forms. See Section 19 for additional discussion of these entities.

MANAGEMENT

The diagnosis of LCH is important to recognize when an ill infant presents with a refractory or recurrent diaper rash. The diagnosis should be entertained and confirmed by skin biopsy at an early age. For localized skin disease, topical corticosteroids, topical antibiotics, PUVA (for older children), and topical nitrogen mustard may be used. For noncutaneous lesions, more supportive and aggressive therapies may be needed (see Section 19, "Skin Signs of Reticulo endothelial Disease" for more details).

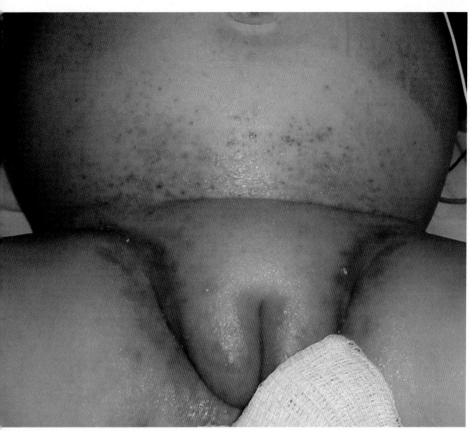

FIGURE 3-6 Langerhans cell histiocytosis in the diaper area Refractory diaper rash with scattered erythematous papules and a petechial component. Skin biopsy revealed Langerhans cells, which confirmed the diagnosis.

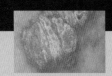

DISORDERS OF
EPIDERMAL PROLIFERATION

PSORIASIS

Psoriasis is a hereditary disorder of skin characterized by chronic scaling papules and plaques in a characteristic distribution, largely at sites of repeated minor trauma. The HLA types most frequently associated with psoriasis are HLA-Cw6, -B13, -B17, -Bw16, -B37, and -DR7.

INSIGHT It can be difficult to distinguish between atopic dermatitis and psoriasis in infancy. If family history and cutaneous findings are not helpful, one hint is atopic dermatitis usually spares the diaper area and psoriasis favors that location.

EPIDEMIOLOGY

AGE 10% have onset of lesions before age 10, and up to 33% have onset by age 20 years.
GENDER Slight predominance F > M.
PREVALENCE 2% of the world's population. United States and Canada: 4% to 5% of the population.
RACE Low incidence in Asians, Africans, African Americans, American Indians, and Japanese relative to Caucasians.
OTHER FEATURES Multifactorial inheritance. Minor trauma is a predisposing factor (45% of patients) in eliciting lesions (Koebner's phenomenon). Infection (particularly streptococcal) also plays a role. Many episodes of psoriasis—and particularly guttate psoriasis—follow sore throats or upper respiratory infections. Stress, cold weather, hypocalcemia, and lack of sunlight exposure aggravate the condition. Certain drugs (lithium, interferon, β-blockers, alcohol, antimalarials, corticosteroid withdrawal, and paradoxically anti-TNFα biologics) can also precipitate psoriasis.

PATHOPHYSIOLOGY

Psoriasis is likely a polygenic disease caused by the inappropriate activation of T cells (the adaptive immune system) as well as abnormal keratinocyte proliferation (the innate immune system). A predominantly T_H1 inflammatory milieu underlies the chronic inflammation

of psoriasis. Several cytokines including interferon-α, TNF-α, interleukin 23, and interleukin 17 are known to play critical roles in the initiation and prolongation of the inflammation in psoriasis that drives T-cell recruitment and increased keratinocyte proliferation.

HISTORY

ONSET OF LESIONS Usually slowly over the course of months but may be sudden as in acute guttate psoriasis and generalized pustular psoriasis (von Zumbusch).
SKIN SYMPTOMS Pruritus is reasonably common, especially in scalp and anogenital psoriasis.
CONSTITUTIONAL SYMPTOMS In 5% of cases, psoriasis can be associated with arthritis, fever, and/or an "acute illness" syndrome (weakness, chills, fever) with generalized erythroderma.

PHYSICAL EXAMINATION

Skin Findings

TYPE Well-delineated, erythematous, thickened plaques with a characteristic silvery-white scale (Fig. 4-1A). Removal of scale results in the appearance of miniscule blood droplets (Auspitz sign).
COLOR Salmon pink to red.
SIZE Can range from pinpoint 1-mm papules to large 20- to 30-cm plaques.
SHAPE Round, oval, polycyclic, or annular. Lesions may take on sharply geometric shapes when arising in sites of trauma or repeated pressure (Koebner's phenomenon).
DISTRIBUTION Localized (e.g., elbows), regional (e.g., scalp), generalized (e.g., guttate psoriasis or erythroderma). Often symmetrically distributed over the body.
SITES OF PREDILECTION Favors elbows (Fig. 4-1B) knees, facial region, scalp, and intertriginous areas (axillae, inguinal folds, intergluteal cleft).

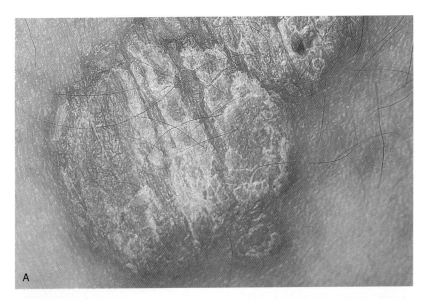

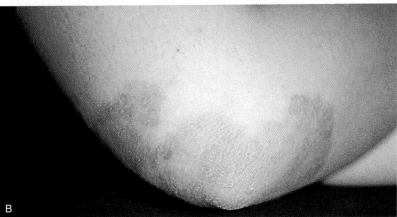

FIGURE 4-1 Psoriasis vulgaris A: Well-delineated erythematous plaques with a silvery-white scale characteristic of psoriasis. **B:** Well-delineated erythematous plaque located on the elbow of a child with psoriasis. *(continued)*

OTHER Scalp involvement is common (Fig. 4-1C), with predilection for the occiput. Hair loss (alopecia) is not a common feature even with severe scalp involvement. Fingernails and toenails are sometimes involved. Nail changes include pitting, subungual hyperkeratosis, onycholysis, and yellow spots under the nail plate "oil spot" (Fig. 4-1D).

General Findings

Psoriatic arthritis is rare before age 40 and occurs in 5% to 30% of the patients with skin findings. Arthritis may be mono- and symmetric oligoarthritis of the DIPs and PIPs, arthritis exclusively of the DIPs, rheumatoid arthritis-like in medium-sized joints (PIP, MCP, wrists, ankles, and elbows), arthritis mutilans with severe joint destruction or spondylitis, and sacroiliitis. Children with psoriasis are more likely to be obese.

DIFFERENTIAL DIAGNOSIS

Psoriasis may be confused with seborrheic dermatitis. The two entities may be indistinguishable and often an overlap, so-called sebopsoriasis presentation can be seen. Psoriasis must also be distinguished from atopic dermatitis, lichen simplex chronicus, pityriasis rosea, tinea corporis, contact dermatitis, psoriasiform drug eruptions (such as from β-blockers, gold, and methyldopa), and cutaneous T-cell lymphoma.

LABORATORY EXAMINATIONS

DERMATOPATHOLOGY Skin biopsy reveals (1) epidermal hyperplasia with thinning of the suprapapillary plates and elongation of the rete ridges; (2) increased mitosis of keratinocytes, fibroblasts, and endothelial cells; (3) parakeratotic hyperkeratosis (nuclei retained in the stratum corneum); and (4) inflammatory cells in the dermis (usually lymphocytes and monocytes) and in the epidermis (polymorphonuclear cells), forming microabscesses of Munro in the stratum corneum.

THROAT CULTURE Throat culture for β-hemolytic streptococcus is indicated in cases of guttate psoriasis or in cases that are precipitated by a sore throat. If positive, antibiotic may be needed to clear the infection, which in some cases may speed resolution of the psoriasis.

COURSE AND PROGNOSIS

Psoriasis typically has a chronic course with numerous remissions and exacerbations. Some children progress to mild disease with intermittent asymptomatic flares. Other children have a more severe course with recurrent extensive flares, and 5% may develop an associated arthritis in adulthood.

MANAGEMENT

The treatment of psoriasis depends upon the extent and severity of the disease, as well as the site involved. While not usually as itchy as atopic dermatitis, many patients complain of pruritus. Patients should be instructed never to rub or scratch the areas since trauma can precipitate psoriatic plaques (Koebner's phenomenon).

1. Emollients such as petrolatum, mineral oil, Vaseline, or moisturizers (CeraVe, Eucerin, Moisturel, and Aquaphor creams) should be used to keep the skin well hydrated.
2. Judicious ambient sunlight exposure helps psoriasis, and children should be encouraged to cautiously expose the affected areas to the sun for short periods of 15 to 20 minutes during the day. Sunscreen should be used, and sunburning should be avoided.
3. Baths are helpful in soothing the pruritus and removing the scale. They should be lukewarm and limited to 10 minutes in duration. For some, it may be helpful to add bath oil, salt, or tar (Balnetar bath oil) to the water to soften scale and soothe dry skin.
4. Tar preparations can be suggested to reduce the skin inflammation. Bath emulsions, creams (Elta tar), and ointments (MG217) can be used twice daily, but are not recommended for prolonged periods of time.
5. Topical steroid creams are effective if used in appropriate strengths:
   a. Low-potency steroids (desonide 0.05%, 1% or 2.5% hydrocortisone) can be used on the face and groin area, no more than bid × 2 weeks per month.
   b. Medium-potency steroids (mometasone 0.1%, fluticasone 0.05%, triamcinolone 0.1%) can be used on the extremities or body no more than bid × 2 weeks per month.
   c. High-potency steroids (clobetasol 0.05%, diflorasone 0.05%, betamethasone dipropionate 0.05%) should be reserved for older children/adults on severely affected areas bid for no more than 2 weeks.
6. Oral antibiotics may be effective, especially in guttate psoriasis flares precipitated by *Streptococcus* pharyngitis. Certain antibiotics also possess anti-inflammatory properties and can help if there are signs of secondary infection—open moist areas that weep or become crusted. Some commonly prescribed antibiotics include penicillin VK (25–50 mg/kg/d divided qid, not to exceed 3 g/d), cephalexin (25–50 mg/kg/d divided qid, not to exceed 4 g/d), dicloxacillin (25–50 mg/kg/d divided qid, not to exceed 2 g/d), and erythromycin (30–50 mg/kg/d divided qid, not to exceed 2 g/d).
7. Steroid-sparing topical creams include the following:
   a. Vitamin D analogs (calcipotriene 0.005%) typically used bid to affected areas. Calcipotriene may also be used in conjunction with topical steroids. A commonly used maintenance schedule recommends calcipotriene applied bid to affected areas Monday through Friday and a topical steroid applied bid Saturday and Sunday.
   b. Retinoids (tazarotene 0.1% cream or gel) can be used to decrease epidermal proliferation and is applied qhs to affected areas. The retinoids typically help reduce the psoriatic scale, but often are too irritating for use in younger children.
   c. Anthralins (Drithocreme, Dritho-Scalp) have an antiproliferative effect and can be used qid to affected areas, but often are too irritating for use in younger children.

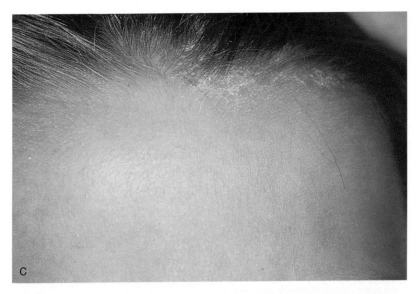

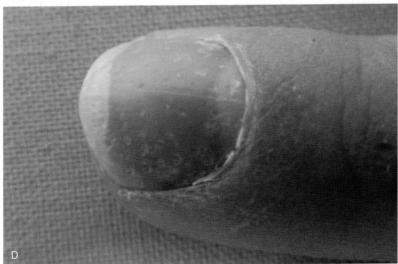

FIGURE 4-1 *(Continued)* **Psoriasis vulgaris, scalp, and nail findings C:** Diffuse erythema and scale in the scalp of a child with psoriasis. Hair loss is minimal. **D:** Pinpoint pits, distal onycholysis, and yellowish discoloration (so-called oil-spot) seen in the fingernails of a child with psoriasis.

8. For the scalp, tar (T/Gel, DHS) selenium sulfide (Selsun), zinc pyrithione (Head & Shoulders), salicylic acid (T/Sal), or ketoconazole (Nizoral) shampoos used two or three times per week can help reduce scaling. Topical steroid solutions (fluocinolone 0.01% scalp solution) can be applied qam sparingly to the affected areas to help decrease erythema and itching.
9. Phototherapy with UVB, narrow band UVB, or PUVA (psoralen with UVA) works well, but increases the lifetime risk of skin cancer, and is usually not recommended for children.
10. Systemic agents including methotrexate, cyclosporine, systemic retinoids (acitretin), and systemic biologic agents (etanercept, infliximab, adalimumab, ustekinumab) are reserved for severe, refractory cases or those with significant associated arthritis and warrant careful prescreening and close blood monitoring.

PSORIASIS VULGARIS, GUTTATE TYPE

Guttate psoriasis is an acute flare of multiple generalized small psoriatic plaques that often follows streptococcal pharyngitis. This form is relatively rare (2% of all psoriasis cases), but commonly seen in children and often clears. Guttate psoriasis may be more chronic, especially in adults, and may be unrelated to streptococcal infection.

PHYSICAL EXAMINATION

Skin Lesions

TYPE Papules 2 mm to 1 cm.
COLOR Salmon pink.
SHAPE Guttate, "spots that resemble drops" (Fig. 4-2).
ARRANGEMENT Scattered discrete lesions.
DISTRIBUTION Generalized, usually sparing the palms and soles and concentrating on the trunk, less on the face, scalp, and nails.

DIFFERENTIAL DIAGNOSIS

Guttate psoriasis needs to be differentiated from pityriasis rosea, viral exanthem, psoriasiform drug eruption, and secondary syphilis.

LABORATORY EXAMINATION

SEROLOGIC An increased antistreptolysin O, anti-DNase B, or streptozyme titer in those patients with antecedent streptococcal infection.

THROAT CULTURE May be positive for β-hemolytic *Streptococcus pyogenes* (Group A β-hemolytic streptococcus).

COURSE AND PROGNOSIS

Often, but not always, this type of psoriasis spontaneously disappears in a few weeks. Resolution may be expedited in some individuals with antibiotic treatment.

MANAGEMENT

The resolution of lesions can be accelerated by judicious exposure to sunlight. For persistent lesions, treatment is same as for generalized plaque psoriasis. Penicillin VK (25–50 mg/kg/d divided qid, not to exceed 3 g/d) if group A β-hemolytic *Streptococcus* is cultured from throat.

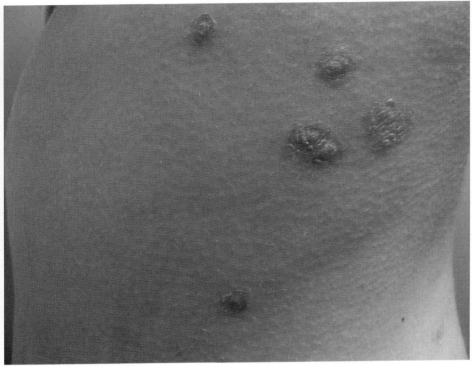

FIGURE 4-2 Psoriasis vulgaris, guttate type Erythematous scaly papules on the trunk of an adolescent.

PALMOPLANTAR PUSTULOSIS

Palmoplantar pustulosis is a rare, relapsing eruption limited to the palms and the soles characterized by numerous sterile yellow, deep-seated pustules that evolve into crusts and scales. It is believed by some to be a localized variant of pustular psoriasis.

PHYSICAL EXAMINATION

Skin Lesions

TYPE Pustules that evolve into crusts and scaling.
COLOR Dusky red base, yellow pustules.
SIZE 2 to 5 mm.
DISTRIBUTION Localized to palms (Fig. 4-3A) and soles (Fig. 4-3B).

DIFFERENTIAL DIAGNOSIS

Palmoplantar pustulosis needs to be differentiated from tinea manuum, tinea pedis, dyshidrotic eczema, and contact dermatitis.

LABORATORY EXAMINATION

DERMATOPATHOLOGY Skin biopsy reveals edema and exocytosis of mononuclear cells forming a vesicle. Later, neutrophils form a pustule.

COURSE AND PROGNOSIS

Palmoplantar pustulosis can recur for years and is difficult to treat. Infrequently, psoriasis vulgaris may develop elsewhere. Pustulosis of the palms and soles can very rarely be associated with sterile inflammatory bone lesions (chronic recurrent multifocal osteomyelitis, pustulotic arthroosteitis, and SAPHO syndrome: *s*ynovitis, *a*cne, *p*ustulosis, *h*yperostosis, and *o*steitis). Some hereditary cases have been associated with a mutation in the IL36RN gene encoding the interleukin-36 receptor antagonist protein.

MANAGEMENT

The resolution of lesions can be accelerated by judicious exposure to sunlight. Steroids under occlusion at night can hasten resolution. Systemic treatments such as methotrexate, cyclosporine, retinoids, or biologic agents are often necessary to achieve disease control.

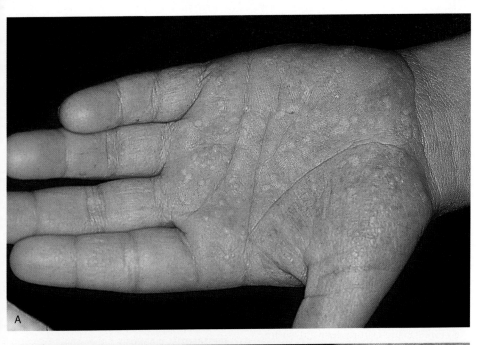

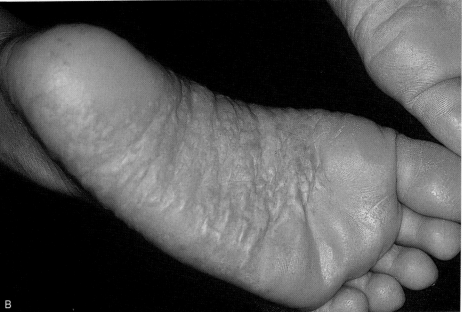

FIGURE 4-3 Palmoplantar pustulosis, palms, and soles A: Deep-seated yellow vesicles on the palms which progress to crusts and scales. **B:** The soles of the same individual with similar deep-seated pustular lesions.

PSORIASIS VULGARIS, ERYTHRODERMIC

Erythrodermic psoriasis is a serious, often life-threatening condition in patients with psoriasis, characterized by full-body redness (erythroderma) and scaling. A pre-existing dermatosis can be identified in 50% of patients and psoriasis is the second most common cause of erythroderma after atopic dermatitis.

 INSIGHT Erythroderma is one of the true dermatologic emergencies. An etiology should be sought quickly and supportive care initiated immediately.

SYNONYMS Dermatitis exfoliativa, erythroderma of Wilson–Brocq.

EPIDEMIOLOGY

AGE Any age.
GENDER M > F.
INCIDENCE Rare.
ETIOLOGY In childhood, erythroderma is more likely owing to pre-existing dermatitis such as atopic dermatitis or psoriasis.
CLASSIFICATION Acute phase with generalized scaly erythema and fever, lymphadenopathy. Chronic form characterized by nail dystrophy but no loss of scalp and body hair (compared to other forms of erythroderma, e.g., drugs, mycosis fungoides).

HISTORY

DURATION OF LESIONS Acute onset of systemic symptoms and red swollen patches and plaques that evolve into a widespread exfoliative erythema in the setting of previous psoriasis.
SKIN SYMPTOMS Generalized pruritus.
GENERALIZED SYMPTOMS Chills, malaise, fatigue, anorexia, weight loss.

PHYSICAL EXAMINATION

Skin Findings

TYPE OF LESIONS Confluent diffuse erythema covered by laminated scales. Skin becomes dull, scarlet, swollen, with areas of oozing (Fig. 4-4). Desquamation usually occurs after a few days. The palms and soles are covered by thick scales and have deep fissures. Secondary infections by bacteria can develop.
COLOR Bright red.
ARRANGEMENT Confluent.

DISTRIBUTION Generalized.
HAIR Normal.
NAILS Onycholysis, shedding of nails with dystrophy.

General Findings

Generalized lymphadenopathy.

DIAGNOSIS AND DIFFERENTIAL DIAGNOSIS

DIAGNOSIS Clinical diagnosis of psoriatic erythroderma is not always easy, especially in the absence of previous history of psoriasis. Cutaneous signs of psoriasis are helpful, such as pitting of the nails, psoriasiform plaques on the scalp, or intergluteal erythema.
DIFFERENTIAL DIAGNOSIS Other causes of erythroderma include pityriasis rubra pilaris (PRP), seborrheic dermatitis (erythroderma desquamativa), drug hypersensitivity, atopic dermatitis, cutaneous T-cell lymphoma, lichen planus, pemphigus foliaceous, epidermolytic hyperkeratosis (EHK), and acute graft-versus-host disease.

LABORATORY EXAMINATIONS

HEMATOLOGY Elevated sedimentation rate.
CHEMISTRY Low serum albumin and increased γ-globulins. Young children may be especially prone to dehydration from increased insensible transepidermal water losses and present with hypernatremia. Hypocalcemia may also be seen in erythrodermic states.
MICROBIOLOGY Blood cultures will be negative (usually obtained to rule out infection in the setting of high fever).
DERMATOPATHOLOGY Psoriasiform dermatitis with elongated and thickened ridges, marked parakeratosis, absent granular layer, intra- and intercellular edema, epidermal invasion by leukocytes, and a dermal perivascular inflammatory infiltrate.

COURSE AND PROGNOSIS

Variable. Can be very prolonged and recurrent.

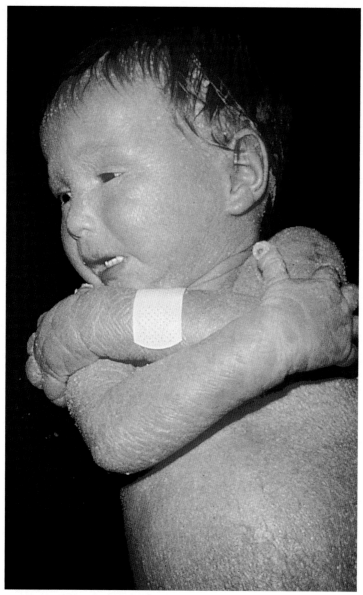

FIGURE 4-4 Psoriasis vulgaris: erythrodermic Entire skin surface is dull-red in color with diffuse swelling and oozing.

MANAGEMENT

Supportive care often requiring hospitalization is necessary to maintain fluid–electrolyte homeostasis and body temperature. Skin biopsy should be performed if the cause of the erythroderma is not known (no known predisposition to psoriasis). Topical treatments include emollients and steroids under occlusive wraps. Systemic steroids, retinoids, or immunosuppressives (methotrexate or cyclosporin) may be necessary. In older children, phototherapy with UVB, narrow band UVB, or PUVA may be helpful.

PITYRIASIS AMIANTACEA

Pityriasis amiantacea ("asbestos like") refers to the condition of large, adherent flakes of thick scale that coat the scalp and hair. It may be associated with hair loss which is generally not permanent.

SYNONYM Tinea amiantacea.

EPIDEMIOLOGY

AGE Typically school age children and adolescents.
GENDER F > M.
INCIDENCE Uncommon.
ETIOLOGY Often a manifestation of other underlying skin disease with scalp involvement such as psoriasis, seborrheic dermatitis, or atopic dermatitis.
RACE All races.

HISTORY

DURATION OF LESIONS Individuals present with chronic scalp flaking associated with bound-down areas of thick, adherent scales. The shiny appearance of the heaped-up scales gives rise to the name "amiantacea," resembling the appearance of asbestos.
SKIN SYMPTOMS Associated symptoms may include pruritus, tingling, or burning of the scalp. The chronicity of the lesions may be associated with patchy or diffuse alopecia.

PHYSICAL EXAMINATION

TYPE Erythematous plaques with adherent, thick yellowish scale (Fig. 4-5).
COLOR Yellow to white or gray.
ARRANGEMENT Individual plaques or confluent, diffuse involvement.
DISTRIBUTION May be localized or present throughout the scalp and the scale may be adherent to the hair.

GENERAL FINDINGS May be associated with other signs of underlying skin disease (e.g., plaques of psoriasis on the body).

DIFFERENTIAL DIAGNOSIS

Pityriasis amiantacea is generally thought to be a subset of scalp psoriasis or seborrheic dermatitis; it needs to be differentiated from tinea capitis. No pathogenic organisms are present in pityriasis amiantacea.

COURSE AND PROGNOSIS

Pityriasis amiantacea is chronic, remitting, and difficult to treat.

MANAGEMENT

Topical tar (T/Gel) selenium sulfide (Selsun), zinc pyrithione (Head & Shoulders), or ketoconazole, salicylic acid (T/Sal, Sebulex) shampoos used 2 or 3 times per week can help reduce scaling.

Often the adherent scale can be difficult to remove, especially in individuals with long hair. In such cases, warm towel wraps to loosen the scale, and fine tooth combing may be helpful.

Topical steroid solutions (fluocinolone 0.01% or fluocinonide 0.05%) can be applied sparingly to the affected areas to help decrease erythema and itching, but then should be tapered to avoid adverse effects.

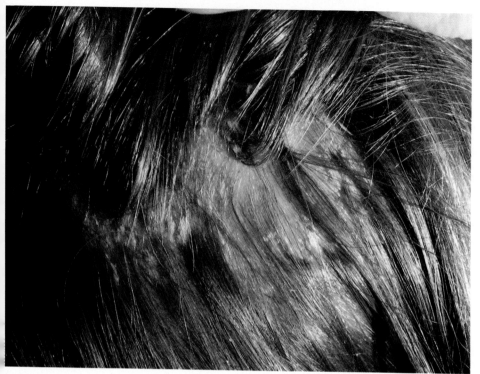

FIGURE 4-5 Pityriasis amiantacea Erythematous patches on the scalp with resultant adherent scale in the hair.

ICHTHYOSIFORM DERMATOSES AND ERYTHROKERATODERMAS

The ichthyosiform dermatoses and erythroker-atodermas are disorders of cornification. The ichthyoses are a group of hereditary disorders, characterized by generalized scaling of the skin. The erythrokeratodermas are a group of inherited conditions characterized by erythema and hyperkeratosis, with no scale. The clinical severity for all these disorders varies from very mild and asymptomatic to life-threatening.

INHERITANCE

ICHTHYOSIS VULGARIS (IV): Autosomal dominant. Mutation in the *FLG* gene encoding filaggrin.
X-LINKED ICHTHYOSIS (XLI): Recessive X-linked, only expressed in males. Mutation in *STS* gene encoding steroid sulfatase.
BULLOUS CONGENITAL ICHTHYOSIFORM ERYTHRODERMA [Also known as epidermolytic hyperkeratosis (EHK)]: Autosomal domi-nant. Mutation in genes encoding keratin 1 or keratin 10.
CONGENITAL ICHTHYOSIFORM ERYTHRODERMA: Autosomal recessive. Multiple genes; most common mutation in *TGM1* encoding kerati-nocyte transglutaminase.
LAMELLAR ICHTHYOSIS (LI): Autosomal recessive. Multiple genes; most common mutation in *TGM1* encoding keratinocyte transglutaminase.

PATHOPHYSIOLOGY

In IV and XLI, the formation of thickened stra-tum corneum is caused by increased adhesive-ness of the stratum corneum cells and/or failure of normal cell–cell separation. EHK shows increased epidermal cell turnover with vacuol-ization because of intracellular edema. LI shows increased germinative cell hyperplasia and increased transit rate through the epidermis.

HISTORY

All types of ichthyosis tend to be worse during the dry, cold winter months and improve dur-ing the hot, humid summer. Patients living in tropical climates may remain symptom free, but may experience symptomatic appearance or worsening on moving to a more temperate climate.

DIAGNOSIS

Usually, the diagnosis can be made based on clinical findings.

MANAGEMENT

HYDRATION OF STRATUM CORNEUM Pliability of stratum corneum is a function of its water content. Hydration is best accomplished by immersion in bath followed by the application of petrolatum (petroleum jelly, hydrated petrolatum, or Aquaphor).

KERATOLYTIC AGENTS Propylene glycol with lactic acid (Epilyt) is effective without occlusion. Combinations of salicylic acid and propylene glycol (Keralyt) can be used alone or under plastic occlusion. α-Hydroxy acids such as lactic acid bind water or control scaling. Urea-containing preparations (2–20%) (Aquacare, Carmol) help to bind water in the stratum corneum. Lac-hydrin contains buffered lactic acid and is a mild keratolytic.

SYSTEMIC RETINOIDS Retinoids such as isotretinoin and acitretin are reserved for severe cases of LI, but careful monitoring for toxicity is required. Severe cases may require intermittent therapy over long periods of time. Continuous long-term use in children is contraindicated.

COLLODION BABY

Ichthyosis in the newborn often presents as a collodion baby (Fig. 4-6). It is not a distinct disorder, but can be the first presentation of several (usually autosomal recessive) ichthyoses. At birth, the collodion baby is encased in a clear, parchment-like membrane, which may impair respiration and sucking. When the membrane is shed 2 to 3 weeks later, the infant may have difficulties with thermal regulation and an increased susceptibility to infections. After healing the skin will appear normal. Sixty to seventy percent of these babies will go on to develop some form of ichthyosis later in life.

INSIGHT

20% of collodion babies will go on to have totally normal skin.

SYNONYMS Self-healing collodion fetus, desquamation of the newborn, ichthyosis congenita, lamellar exfoliation of the newborn.

EPIDEMIOLOGY

AGE Newborn.
GENDER M = F.
INCIDENCE Rare.
ETIOLOGY Unclear.

PATHOPHYSIOLOGY

Collodion membranes can be seen in various forms of ichthyoses, but the mechanism behind the formation of the membrane is not clear. In the case of LI, transglutaminase-1 deficiency leads to abnormal cornification which causes the membrane, but in other ichthyoses, the pathogenesis is unclear.

HISTORY

ONSET Membrane is present at birth.
DURATION OF LESIONS Desquamation of the membrane is usually complete by 2 to 3 weeks of life.

PHYSICAL EXAMINATION

Skin Findings

TYPE Transparent, parchment-like membrane encasing the newborn.
COLOR Skin-colored.
DISTRIBUTION Membrane covers the entire body surface.

General Findings

Collodion babies are often premature with an increased morbidity and mortality. If the membrane is thin, it can spontaneously resolve leaving normal or dry skin in the newborn. If the membrane is thick, it can impair respiration, sucking, and the infant's mobility. The stiffness of the membrane can also cause an ectropion, eclabion, and hypoplasia of the nose and ear cartilage. In severe cases, when the membrane sheds, the infant can experience temperature and fluid–electrolyte instability.

LABORATORY EXAMINATION

DERMATOPATHOLOGY Skin biopsy shows a thickened stratum corneum, but the collodion membrane is generally not diagnostic of the underlying ichthyotic condition. Deferring skin biopsy until the membrane is shed may be preferable.

DIFFERENTIAL DIAGNOSIS

Clinical findings are diagnostic. A collodion baby needs to be clinically differentiated from a harlequin fetus, a more severe frequently lethal condition. The skin in a harlequin baby has a thickened stratum corneum with deep cracks and fissures (Fig. 4-6).

COURSE AND PROGNOSIS

The collodion membrane breaks up and peels during the first 2 weeks of life predisposing the infant to difficulties in thermal regulation and an increased risk of infection. The final appearance of the skin depends on the etiology of the condition. The collodion baby may be the initial presentation of LI or congenital ichthyosiform erythroderma. In rare instances, the collodion baby progresses to Sjogren–Larsson syndrome, trichothiodystrophy, infantile Gaucher disease, or Netherton syndrome.

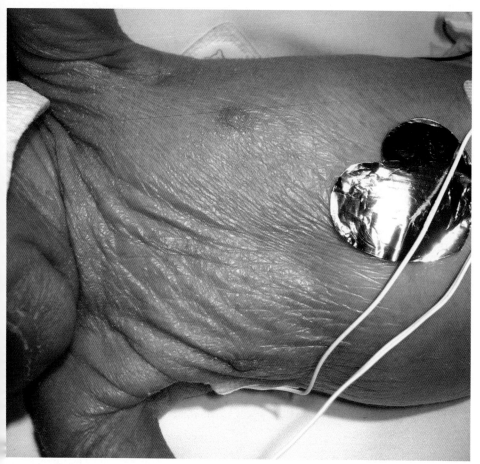

FIGURE 4-6 Collodion baby at birth A baby soon after birth with a clear parchment-like membrane covering the entire skin.

MANAGEMENT

The management of the collodion baby is primarily supportive. Collodion babies require hospitalization and incubation at birth. The infant should be kept in a high-humidity incubator to maximize membrane hydration. Wet compresses and lubricants or emollients can also increase skin pliability. Clear fluids or IV hydration may be needed until the infant's ability to eat has been ascertained. Respiratory efforts may also need external support. As the membrane begins to shed 2 to 3 weeks later, the infant should be frequently monitored for temperature and electrolyte instability. Throughout the shedding process, careful monitoring for skin and lung infections is also recommended.

HARLEQUIN FETUS

A harlequin baby is very rare, severe form of congenital ichthyosis with thickened stratum corneum that cracks and fissures shortly after birth. The condition is associated with premature delivery and poor fetal outcome.

SYNONYMS Harlequin fetus, harlequin ichthyosis, ichthyosis congenita gravior.

EPIDEMIOLOGY

AGE Newborn.
GENDER M = F.
INCIDENCE Fewer than 100 case reports.
GENETICS Autosomal recessive mutation in *ABCA12* gene.

PATHOPHYSIOLOGY

The abnormally thickened stratum corneum is thought to be caused by a defect in *ABCA12* which encodes a keratinocyte lipid transporter protein, leads to defective lamellar body formation and secretion in the skin.

HISTORY

ONSET Thickened skin is present at birth and cracks forming large adherent plates of skin separated by deep fissures.
SKIN SYMPTOMS Skin is rigid and thick.

PHYSICAL EXAMINATION

Skin Findings

TYPE Polygonal/triangular/diamond-shaped plaques because of skin fissuring.
COLOR Gray/yellow cracked skin forming plaques, deep red fissures.
DISTRIBUTION Whole body is involved with a marked ectropion (turning out of the eyelids), eclabium (fish-mouth deformity), distorted flat ears, and sometimes microcephaly (Fig. 4-7).

General Findings

Most infants are stillborn or die in the neonatal period. Newborns exhibit poor feeding and difficulties with temperature and electrolyte

regulation. The rigidity of the skin impairs movement and respiration. The large fissures in the skin can lead to infection and sepsis.

DIFFERENTIAL DIAGNOSIS

The clinical presentation of a harlequin fetus is diagnostic. It should be differentiated from the less severe form of congenital ichthyosis (collodion baby).

LABORATORY EXAMINATIONS

HISTOPATHOLOGY Skin biopsy reveals a characteristic thick and compact orthokeratotic stratum corneum, absent granular layer, plugged sweat ducts, and sebaceous follicles filled with hyperkeratotic debris. Hair follicles have a characteristic marked accumulation of keratin material around the hair shaft, which can be used to diagnose the condition prenatally.
ULTRASTRUCTURAL FINDINGS Abnormal or missing lamellar bodies in the granular layer, absent lipid lamellae, and/or lipid inclusions in the stratum corneum.

COURSE AND PROGNOSIS

The course and prognosis for a harlequin fetus is very poor. Most infants die early because of prematurity, infection, or thermal or electrolyte imbalance.

MANAGEMENT

Intensive supportive measures are necessary to provide adequate nutrition, manage body temperature, monitor fluid and electrolyte balance, and prevent infections in the perinatal period. Systemic retinoids such as isotretinoin and acitretin may increase survival, but the harlequin skin is permanent and the resultant quality of life is poor.

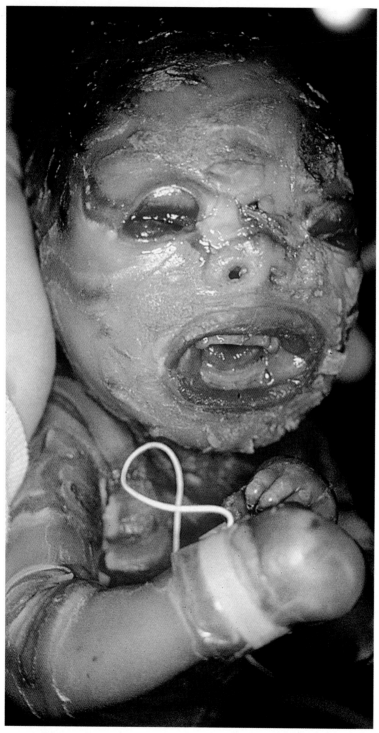

FIGURE 4-7 Harlequin fetus Newborn with rigid skin, marked ectropion, fish-mouth deformity, and distorted flat ears.

ICHTHYOSIS VULGARIS

IV is characterized by mild, generalized hyperkeratosis with xerosis (dry skin) most pronounced on the lower legs. It is frequently associated with atopy.

INSIGHT The pretibial area usually shows prominent scaling; many of these patients also have keratosis pilaris.

SYNONYMS Ichthyosis simplex, autosomal dominant ichthyosis.

EPIDEMIOLOGY

AGE OF ONSET Childhood.
GENDER M = F.
MODE OF INHERITANCE Autosomal dominant, variable clinical presentation.
INCIDENCE Common, 1/250 people. More common in Caucasians, Asians.
ETIOLOGY Decreased or absent profilaggrin leads to decreased keratohyalin granules and an abnormal granular layer of the epidermis.

HISTORY

Very commonly associated with atopy (atopic dermatitis, allergies, hay fever, asthma). Xerosis and pruritus worse in winter months. Hyperkeratosis and less commonly xerosis are of cosmetic concern to many patients.

PHYSICAL EXAMINATION

Skin Findings

TYPE Xerosis (dry skin) with fine powdery scale (Fig. 4-8). Increased accentuation of the palmar and plantar skin markings.
COLOR Normal skin color, white powdery scale.
DISTRIBUTION Diffuse involvement, accentuated on the shins, arms, and back, but sparing the body folds (axillae, antecubital, and popliteal fossae); face is also usually spared.

General Findings

IV may be seen with other signs of atopy: atopic dermatitis, asthma, allergies, hay fever, and keratosis pilaris (KP).

DIFFERENTIAL DIAGNOSIS

IV needs to be differentiated from xerosis, XLI, LI, and drug-induced ichthyoses.

LABORATORY EXAMINATIONS

DERMATOPATHOLOGY Mild orthokeratotic hyperkeratosis with a thickened stratum corneum and a reduced or absent granular layer.
ELECTRON MICROSCOPY May demonstrate abnormal or decreased keratohyalin granules.

COURSE AND PROGNOSIS

May show improvement in the summer and in adulthood.

MANAGEMENT

1. Emollients such as petrolatum, mineral oil, Vaseline, or moisturizers (Lubriderm, Eucerin, Moisturel, and Aquaphor creams) should be used to keep the skin well hydrated.
2. Ceramide-containing creams seem particularly effective (CeraVe).
3. Moisturizing cleansers can be helpful (Dove, CeraVe).
4. Keratolytic agents containing urea (Carmol), α-hydroxy (Aquaglycolic), lactic acid (AmLactin, Lac-hydrin), and salicylic acids can be used bid to the affected areas to help exfoliate the diffuse scale, but should be avoided in young children because the stinging sensation is usually not well tolerated. The face and groin areas should also be avoided.

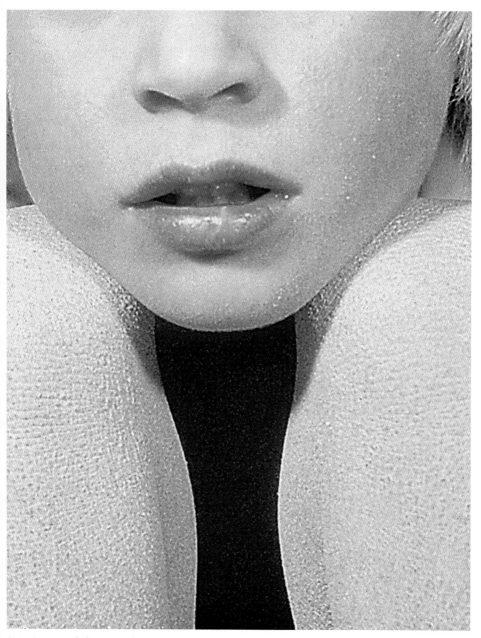

FIGURE 4-8 Ichthyosis vulgaris Fine powdery scale on the shins of a child with ichthyosis vulgaris. The face is spared.

X-LINKED ICHTHYOSIS

XLI occurs in males and is characterized by prominent dirty brown scales occurring on the neck, trunk, and extensor surfaces with onset soon after birth. Female carriers may exhibit mild skin findings.

 INSIGHT Because of placental sulfatase deficiency, the delivery of these patients may be complicated by failure of initiation and/or progression of labor. Female carriers may also show low levels of serum estriol on maternal serum screening.

SYNONYMS Ichthyosis nigricans, steroid sulfatase deficiency.

EPIDEMIOLOGY

AGE OF ONSET Usually appears in the first 3 to 12 months of life.
GENDER Males only. Female carriers may exhibit partial abnormalities.
INCIDENCE 1 in 2,000 to 9,500 males.
MODE OF INHERITANCE X-linked recessive. Prenatal diagnosis is possible.
GENETIC DEFECT Reduced or absent steroid sulfatase caused by the deletion of *STS* gene on chromosome Xp22.32.

PATHOPHYSIOLOGY

XLI is caused by a deficiency or absence of steroid sulfatase. Impaired hydrolysis of cholesterol sulfate and DHEAS leads to an increased accumulation of cholesterol-3-sulfate in the epidermis. This, in turn, leads to increased cellular adhesion and clinically apparent hyperkeratosis.

HISTORY

In addition to the discomfort caused by xerosis, the dirty brown scales on the neck, ears, scalp, and arms are a major cosmetic disfigurement, causing the patient to appear "dirty" all the time.

PHYSICAL EXAMINATION

Skin Findings

TYPE Large firmly adherent scales separated by zones of normal-appearing skin gives the area a cracked appearance (Fig. 4-9).

COLOR Scales are light to dark brown.
SHAPE Fish-scale pattern.
DISTRIBUTION Lateral neck, back, upper arms, chest, and abdomen; prominent scalp scaling may occur. Palms, soles, and face are spared.

General Findings

During the second or third decades, deep corneal opacities develop in 10% to 50% of affected males and some female carriers for XLI. In women pregnant with an affected male fetus, the decreased estrogen levels can cause the cervix not to dilate during labor, necessitating C-section. Affected males have an increased risk of cryptorchidism, putting them at higher risk for testicular cancer and hypogonadism.

DIFFERENTIAL DIAGNOSIS

XLI needs to be differentiated from xerosis, IV, LI, and drug-induced ichthyoses.

LABORATORY EXAMINATIONS

DERMATOPATHOLOGY Skin biopsy will show hyperkeratosis with a moderately increased stratum corneum and a granular layer present in contrast to IV.
LABORATORY FINDINGS High levels of cholesterol sulfate can be measured in the serum, stratum corneum, nails, placenta, or amniotic fluid. A biochemical assay for steroid sulfatase activity can also be performed. In pregnant women with an affected fetus, decreased estrogen or nonhydrolyzed sulfated steroids in the urine can be detected. Finally, a Southern blot, FISH, or PCR assay can be used to detect the exact genetic defect.

COURSE AND PROGNOSIS

XLI is chronic and persistent but may wax and wane with the seasonal variation in humidity. It does not improve with age. The skin findings do not cause physical limitations, but can be cosmetically distressing.

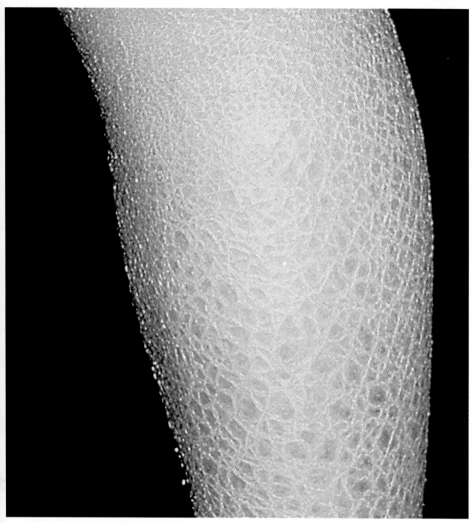

FIGURE 4-9 X-linked ichthyosis More pronounced fish-scale pattern on the leg of a child with X-linked ichthyosis. The diffuse brown scale gives the child a "dirty" appearance.

MANAGEMENT

1. Emollients such as propylene glycol, petrolatum, mineral oil, Vaseline, or moisturizers (Lubriderm, Eucerin, Moisturel, and Aquaphor creams) should be used to keep the skin well hydrated.
2. Keratolytic agents such as Epilyt, Keralyt, Lac-Hydrin, and Carmol can be used bid to the affected areas to help exfoliate the diffuse scale, but should be avoided in young children because the stinging sensation is usually not well tolerated. The face and groin areas should also be avoided.
3. Topical retinoids such as tazarotene may be helpful, but may be too irritating in young children.

BULLOUS CONGENITAL ICHTHYOSIFORM ERYTHRODERMA

Bullous congenital ichthyosiform erythroderma is a chronic disfiguring disorder that initially presents with blistering and erosions. Gradually, the skin changes to a more diffuse, hyperkeratotic, almost verrucous appearance.

SYNONYMS EHK, bullous ichthyosis, bullous congenital ichthyosiform erythroderma of Brocq.

EPIDEMIOLOGY

ONSET The disease is present at or shortly after birth.
GENDER M = F.
PREVALENCE One in 200,000 to 300,000.
ETIOLOGY Genetic mutation of keratin 1, 10 (or keratin 2e in ichthyosis bullosa of Siemens).
INHERITANCE The disease has an autosomal dominant inheritance, but 50% of patients exhibit new mutations.

PATHOPHYSIOLOGY

Mutations in keratins 1 and 10 localized on chromosome 12q11–q13 and 17q12–q21, respectively. The genetic mutations affect keratin alignment, oligomerization, and filament assembly resulting in a weakened cellular skeleton and skin blistering.

HISTORY

The major complaint early in life is blistering, which is painful and can cause widespread denudation. Later, the hyperkeratosis becomes disfiguring and malodorous.

PHYSICAL EXAMINATION

Skin Findings

TYPE Early flaccid blisters (Fig. 4-10A) can lead to peeling, erosions, and large denuded areas. Later, there is erythematous hyperkeratosis with verrucous plaques (Fig. 4-10B).
COLOR Early, skin is erythematous. Later, thick scales are dark brown.
DISTRIBUTION All surfaces of the body can be involved, and flexural areas are accentuated. Many patients have palmar and plantar involvement (keratoderma).

General Findings

Hair, nails, and teeth are usually normal.

DIFFERENTIAL DIAGNOSIS

Bullous congenital ichthyosiform erythroderma at birth needs to be differentiated from other blistering disorders such as epidermolysis bullosa, staphylococcal-scalded skin syndrome, toxic epidermal necrolysis, and bullous impetigo. The clinical appearance of the later verrucous form may be confused with LI but the pathology is usually diagnostic.

LABORATORY EXAMINATIONS

DERMATOPATHOLOGY Skin biopsy reveals dense orthokeratotic hyperkeratosis and keratinocytes show intracellular vacuolization with keratin intermediate filament clumping described as "epidermolytic hyperkeratosis."
ELECTRON MICROSCOPY Reveals clumping of keratin intermediate filaments.
OTHER Genetic screening for keratin 1 and 10 defects can be used prenatally.

COURSE AND PROGNOSIS

The blistering ceases during the second decade, but hyperkeratosis persists for life. Later, the hyperkeratosis is a problem because of the disfigurement, malodor from secondary infection, and discomfort from limitation of motion. Severe scalp involvement can lead to hair loss.

MANAGEMENT

Early in the blistering stage of the disease, supportive care is needed to prevent infection, dehydration, fluid/electrolyte imbalances, and temperature fluctuations. Once denuded, lubricants and careful handing is necessary.
The following are helpful in the later verrucous form:

1. Regular lukewarm soaking baths can be useful to help remove the accumulated scale. The addition of bath salts or bath oils may help exfoliate the thickened scale.
2. Keratolytic agents with urea (Carmol), salicylic acid (Salex), and α-hydroxy acids (Aquaglycolic) can be used to help exfoliate the diffuse scale, but should be avoided in young children because the stinging sensation is usually not well tolerated. The face and groin areas should also be avoided.
3. Systemic retinoids such as isotretinoin and acitretin are useful in controlling the hyperkeratosis, but they may cause flares of the blistering. The side effects of the drugs on bones and tendons are a concern and long-term use is generally not recommended.

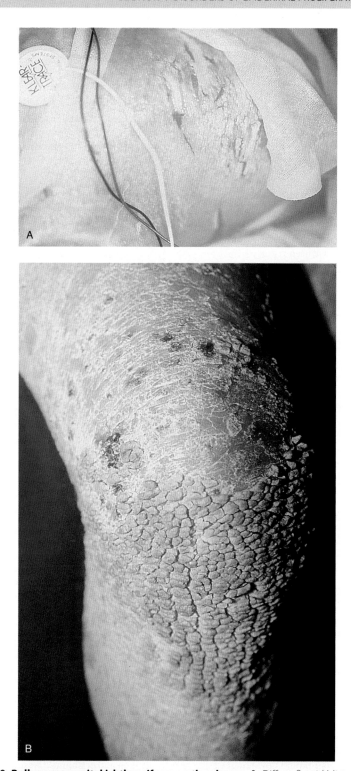

FIGURE 4-10 Bullous congenital ichthyosiform erythroderma A: Diffuse flaccid blistering of the skin and erythroderma at birth. **B:** Extensive verrucous plaques on the knee of a child.

LAMELLAR ICHTHYOSIS

LI often presents at birth with the infant encased in a collodion membrane (see "Collodion Baby," Fig. 4-6), which is soon shed with subsequent formation of large, coarse scales in a generalized distribution.

SYNONYMS Nonbullous, congenital, ichthyosiform erythroderma, nonerythrodermic AR LI.

EPIDEMIOLOGY

AGE OF ONSET A collodion baby at birth is usually the initial presentation (Fig. 4-6). In some cases, the disease is not evident until 3 months of age.
GENDER M = F.
INCIDENCE One in 200,000 to 300,000.
MODE OF INHERITANCE Most families exhibit an autosomal recessive inheritance. Autosomal dominant cases have been reported.

PATHOPHYSIOLOGY

Mutation of transglutaminase-1 (chromosome 14q11.2) has been found in a number of patients, but at least two other genetic loci (on chromosomes 2q33–q35 and 19p12–q12) have been identified. Transglutaminase-1 helps cross-link the structural proteins (involucrin, loricrin, keratin intermediate filaments) in the upper epidermis; malfunction leads to abnormal skin cornification and desquamation.

HISTORY

LI typically presents at birth as a collodion baby. After 2 to 3 weeks, the collodion membrane is shed and replaced by large scales. During exercise and hot weather, hyperthermia may occur because of a decreased ability to sweat. Fissuring of stratum corneum may result in excess water loss and dehydration. Young children have increased nutritional requirements because of excessive shedding of stratum corneum. Fissures on hands and feet are painful.

PHYSICAL EXAMINATION

Skin Lesions

TYPE At birth, infant typically presents with a collodion membrane which is shed in 2 to 3 weeks. Subsequently, large parchment-like scales develop over the entire body (Fig. 4-11A). Scales are large and very thick. Fissuring of hands and feet is common.
DISTRIBUTION Generalized. Hyperkeratosis around joints may be verrucous (Fig. 4-11B). Patients may have ectropion (eyelids are turned outward) and eclabium (lips turned outward).
HAIR AND NAILS Hair bound down by scales; frequent infections result in scarring alopecia. Nails show ridges and grooves.

General Findings

Tightness of facial skin leads to ectropion, eclabium, and hypoplasia of the nose and ear cartilage. Hyperkeratosis results in obstruction of eccrine sweat glands with resultant impairment of sweating and risk of overheating. Scale accumulation in the ear canal can lead to occlusion and infection.

LABORATORY EXAMINATIONS

DERMATOPATHOLOGY Skin biopsy shows dense hyperkeratosis, patchy parakeratosis, increased granular layer (in contrast to IV), acanthosis, and papillomatosis.
OTHER Tranglutaminase-1 activity of the keratinocytes can be measured and will be low in LI patients with transglutaminase-1 mutations. Genetic testing for the transglutaminase-1 gene mutation can be performed for prenatal diagnosis.

DIFFERENTIAL DIAGNOSIS

At birth, the collodion baby presentation can precede a number of ichthyotic disorders and the differential is long (see "Collodion Baby"). Later in life, the dark plate-like scale is clinically diagnostic.

COURSE AND PROGNOSIS

For LI, the collodion membrane present at birth is shed. However, plate-like, diffuse scales persist throughout life and there is no improvement with age.

MANAGEMENT

Patients with LI should avoid situations that may lead to overheating. Their skin appearance can be improved with:

1. Topical calcipotriene has anecdotally been shown to be somewhat helpful.
2. Topical retinoids (tazarotene) can increase skin turnover with reported success.
3. Topical lactic acid and propylene glycol have also shown some improvement in decreasing scale.
4. Systemic retinoids such as isotretinoin and acitretin are useful in controlling the hyperkeratosis and clinical improvement of the ectropion and eclabium. The side effects of the retinoids on bones and tendons are a concern and long-term use is not recommended.

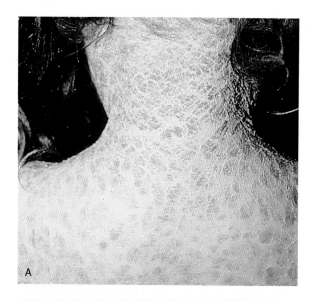

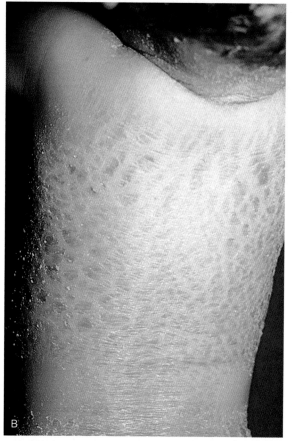

FIGURE 4-11 Lamellar ichthyosis A: Generalized plate-like scales on the posterior neck of a child with lamellar ichthyosis. **B:** Large plate-like scales on the back of the same child.

KERATOSIS PILARIS

KP is a common benign skin condition characterized by follicular-based hyperkeratosis with mild erythema. It is most prominent on the lateral upper arms and thighs, but can also be seen on the cheeks of children. It is commonly seen in individuals with a personal or family history of atopy.

EPIDEMIOLOGY

AGE Appears in early childhood.
GENDER M = F.
INCIDENCE Common.
ETIOLOGY Excessive keratinization within hair follicles.
GENETICS Autosomal dominant inheritance. Potential associated with chromosome 18p deletion.
SEASON Worse during cold seasons.

PHYSICAL EXAMINATION

Skin Findings

TYPE OF LESION Discrete follicular papules often with superimposed keratotic plug (Fig. 4-12A). Variable background erythema.
COLOR Red or brown.
DISTRIBUTION Lesions are prominent on the outer aspects of upper arms and thighs, sometimes on the cheeks of children.
PALPATION Skin has a rough texture reminiscent of gooseflesh or plucked chicken skin.

General Findings

Often associated with other signs of atopy: atopic dermatitis, asthma, allergies, hay fever, or IV.

DIFFERENTIAL DIAGNOSIS

The diagnosis of KP is made clinically. KP is common, but there are rare KP-like variants:

1. Ulerythema ophryogenes (KP rubra atrophicans faciei). X-linked condition notable for widespread KP that begins with follicular-based keratotic papules on the lateral eyebrows that resolve with depressed pits and alopecia.
2. KP rubra faciei. Similar to ulerythema ophryogenes, except that the lesions begin on the cheeks and temples (Fig. 4-12B).

3. Atrophoderma vermiculata (folliculitis ulerythema reticulata). Characterized by symmetric atrophic pits on the cheeks, forehead, and eyebrows.
4. Keratosis follicularis spinulosa decalvans. A variant of KP occurring on the scalp with loss of hair secondary to follicular scarring.

LABORATORY EXAMINATIONS

DERMATOPATHOLOGY Skin biopsy reveals follicular hyperkeratosis and a sparse inflammatory infiltrate in the dermis.

COURSE AND PROGNOSIS

KP is benign but persistent and chronic. Occasionally, it subsides after the age of 20 years. Patients are most distressed by its rough texture and cosmetic appearance.

MANAGEMENT

1. Emollients such as petrolatum, mineral oil, Vaseline, or moisturizers (CeraVe, Eucerin, Moisturel, and Aquaphor creams) should be used to keep the skin well hydrated.
2. Keratolytic agents such as Epilyt, Keralyt, Lac-Hydrin, and Carmol may be used bid to the affected areas to help exfoliate the diffuse scale, but should be avoided in young children because the stinging sensation is usually not well tolerated. The face and groin areas should also be avoided.
3. Topical steroid creams can be used intermittently to decrease the erythematous appearance of the rash:
   a. Low-potency steroids (2.5% hydrocortisone) can be used on the face or body no more than 2 weeks per month.
   b. Medium-potency steroids (triamcinolone 0.1%) can be used on the extremities or body no more than 2 weeks per month.

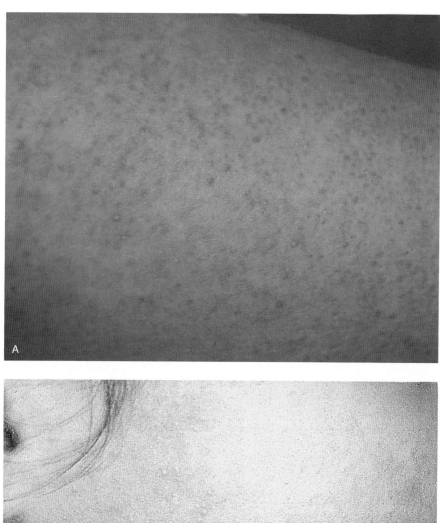

FIGURE 4-12 Keratosis pilaris A: Erythematous follicular-based papules with keratosis plugs on the chin of an adolescent. **Keratosis rubra faciei B:** Follicular-based erythematous papules on the cheek of child.

PITYRIASIS RUBRA PILARIS

PRP is a chronic disease characterized by follicular papules, orange to pink scaly plaques, and a palmo-plantar keratoderma.

EPIDEMIOLOGY

AGE Two peaks: before the age of 20 years, and after the age of 60 years.

CLASSIFICATION PRP presenting in childhood may be either familial or acquired. Childhood PRP can be classified as either classical juvenile onset, circumscribed juvenile onset, or atypical juvenile onset forms.

GENDER M = F.

INCIDENCE Uncommon.

INHERITANCE Nearly all cases are acquired. Some reports of autosomal dominant or autosomal recessive inheritance. Autosomal dominant familial forms associated with mutations in the *CARD14* gene have been reported.

PATHOPHYSIOLOGY

Genetic abnormal cornification of unclear pathogenesis. Possible mechanisms hypothesized include abnormal vitamin A metabolism, physical (UV exposure, infections), superantigens, or autoimmune triggers.

HISTORY

SKIN SYMPTOMS Mild-to-moderate pruritus or burning sensation. Pain in areas of fissured skin.

PHYSICAL EXAMINATION

Skin Findings

TYPE Follicular hyperkeratosis on an erythematous base. Ranges from scale and erythema of the face, scalp, and ears (often the initial presentation) to punctate papules on the body coalescing into large plaques with characteristic "islands of normal skin" (Fig. 4-13).

COLOR Reddish-brown papules, orange and salmon-colored plaques.

DISTRIBUTION In some children: focally on the elbows and knees, in other children and adults: generalized form with plaques on the trunk and extremities. Punctate keratoses (resembling a "nutmeg grater") on the dorsal aspects of first and second phalanges, hands, wrists, knees, ankles, feet, sides of neck, and trunk.

General Findings

Thickened hyperkeratotic palms and soles (forming "sandal"-like thickened skin). Nail dystrophy (thickening, opacification, subungual hyperkeratosis; pitting not common).

Disease can rarely progress into an exfoliative erythroderma associated with fever, chill, malaise, and diarrhea.

DIFFERENTIAL DIAGNOSIS

The differential diagnosis for PRP includes psoriasis, seborrheic dermatitis, lichen planus, atopic dermatitis, and viral exanthem. Clinically, the classic "islands of spared normal skin" differentiate PRP from all other dermatoses.

LABORATORY EXAMINATIONS

DERMATOPATHOLOGY Skin biopsy reveals irregular "checkerboard pattern" hyperkeratosis with alternating vertical and horizontal parakeratosis of the stratum corneum, follicular plugging, a mononuclear cell infiltrate in the dermis, and focal acantholytic dyskeratotic cells or acantholysis within the epidermis.

COURSE AND PROGNOSIS

Childhood PRP has a persistent course characterized by spontaneous remissions and exacerbations.

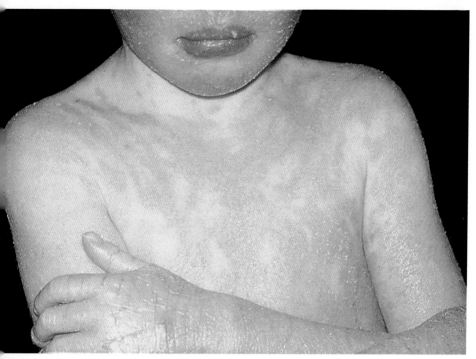

FIGURE 4-13 Pityriasis rubra pilaris Diffuse salmon-colored plaques with characteristic islands of sparing on the chest of a child.

MANAGEMENT

1. Emollients such as petrolatum, mineral oil, Vaseline, or moisturizers (CeraVe, Eucerin, Moisturel, and Aquaphor creams) should be used to keep the skin well hydrated.

2. Keratolytic agents such as Epilyt, Keralyt, Lac-Hydrin, and Carmol can be used bid to the affected areas to help exfoliate the diffuse scale, but should be avoided in young children because the stinging sensation is usually not well tolerated. The face and groin areas should also be avoided.

3. Topical steroids creams can be used intermittently to decrease the erythematous appearance of the rash:

   a. Low-potency steroids (2.5% hydrocortisone) can be used on the face or body no more than 2 weeks per month.

   b. Medium-potency steroids (triamcinolone 0.1%) can be used on the extremities or body no more than 2 weeks per month.

   c. High-potency steroids (clobetasol 0.05%, diflorasone 0.05%, betamethasone dipropionate 0.05%) should be reserved for older children/adults on severely affected areas bid for no more than 2 weeks.

4. Less toxic regimens are recommended for the childhood form of PRP, but in severe refractory cases oral retinoids (isotretinoin, acitretin), systemic steroids, and/or methotrexate may be necessary. Phototherapy with ultraviolet-A or ultraviolet-B radiation has also been reported helpful in some cases. Recent experience with biologic agents suggests some improvement in patients with PRP treated with TNF-α inhibitors.

DARIER DISEASE

Vernix, derived from the same root as *varnish*, is the whitish-gray covering on newborn skin and is composed of degenerated fetal epidermis and sebaceous secretions.

SYNONYMS Keratosis follicularis, Darier-White disease.

EPIDEMIOLOGY

AGE 70% of patients have disease onset between 6 and 20 years.
GENDER M = F.
INCIDENCE One in 55,000 to 100,000.
GENETICS Autosomal dominant disease with complete penetrance, but varying clinical severity. Genetic mutation localized to the *ATP2A2* gene on chromosome 12q23–24.
SEASON Exacerbation during summer months/sun exposure (photo-Koebner's phenomenon).

PATHOPHYSIOLOGY

The disease has been localized to the *ATP2A2* gene on chromosome 12q23–24. The defective gene leads to abnormal functioning of an endoplasmic reticulum Ca^{2+} ATPase (SERCA2) resulting in abnormal intracellular Ca^{2+} signaling. The inadequate Ca^{2+} stores impair correct protein synthesis of molecules necessary for good cell-to-cell adhesion. This causes acantholysis (loss of suprabasilar cellular adhesion) and apoptosis (increased cellular death).

PHYSICAL EXAMINATION

Skin Lesions

TYPE Small keratotic crusted papules and plaques with greasy scale coalescing into warty plaques (Fig. 4-14A).
COLOR Skin-colored to yellow-brown or red.
PALPATION Rough.
DISTRIBUTION Follicular distribution on face, scalp, chest. Intertriginous lesions (axillae, groin) are common.
SITES OF PREDILECTION Seborrheic areas (trunk scalp, face, neck) are sites of predilection. Keratotic papules on dorsal surface of hands and feet and punctate lesions on palms/soles.
NAIL FINDINGS Red, gray, or white longitudinal streaks with V-shaped notch at the distal end and subungual hyperkeratosis (Fig. 4-14B).
MUCOUS MEMBRANES White painless cobblestone papules coalescing into plaques.

Oropharynx (palate, gingiva, mucosa, and tongue), larynx, or anorectal mucosa may be involved.

General Findings

Skin lesions are malodorous and patients have an increased susceptibility to infections. Rarely, mental deficiency, schizophrenia, epilepsy, small stature reported.

DIFFERENTIAL DIAGNOSIS

Darier disease may be confused with seborrheic dermatitis, transient acantholytic dermatosis, pemphigus foliaceous, and Hailey–Hailey disease. These can be differentiated clinically or histopathologically.

LABORATORY EXAMINATIONS

DERMATOPATHOLOGY Skin biopsy shows suprabasal acantholysis and dyskeratotic cells because of apoptosis. Hyperkeratosis is present and can be quite thick. Darier disease has characteristic findings:

1. Corps ronds (acantholytic keratinocytes with partially fragmented nuclei surrounded by clear cytoplasm and a ring of collapsed keratin bundles) in the Malpighian layer.
2. Corp grains (oval cells with bright eosinophilic cytoplasm of collapsed keratin bundles and shrunken nuclear remnants) in the stratum corneum.

ELECTRON MICROSCOPY Ultrastructurally, skin lesion demonstrate a loss of desmosomes and detachment of the keratin filaments from the desmosomes.

COURSE AND PROGNOSIS

Darier disease persists throughout life, but doe have periods of exacerbation and partial remission. The most distressing aspects of the condition are the odor, disfigurement, and pruritus. Up to 50% have oral involvement. Patients report worsening of the skin symptoms in the summer months and aggravation by sun exposure, heat, sweat, and humidity. Additionally, individuals are more susceptible to infections with bacteria, yeast, or fungus.

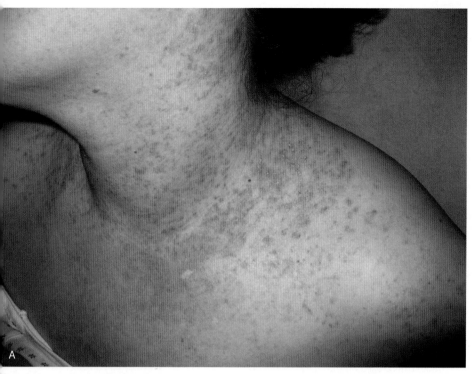

FIGURE 4-14 Darier disease A: Keratotic, crusted papules with scale on the neck. *(continued)*

MANAGEMENT

1. Lightweight clothing and sun protecting help prevent exacerbations of Darier disease, which can be triggered by heat, sun, or sweating.
2. Antimicrobial cleansers (Panoxyl, Hibiclens) can be used to decrease malodorous bacterial colonization. Secondary bacterial infections can be treated with oral antibiotics (cephalexin 25–50 mg/kg/d divided qid, not to exceed 4 g/d, dicloxacillin 25–50 mg/kg/d divided qid, not to exceed 2 g/d, and erythromycin 30–50 mg/kg/d divided qid, not to exceed 2 g/d).
3. Keratolytic agents such as Epilyt, Keralyt, Lac-Hydrin, and Carmol can be used to reduce scaling and irritation, but should be used cautiously in young children because stinging may not be tolerated. The face and groin areas should also be avoided.
4. Topical retinoid creams may also be helpful (tretinoin, tazarotene, adapalene) but are limited by their irritating side effects.
5. Topical steroid creams can be used intermittently but are often not effective:
   a. Low-potency steroids (2.5% hydrocortisone) can be used on the face or body no more than 2 weeks per month.
   b. Medium-potency steroids (triamcinolone 0.1%) can be used on the extremities or body no more than 2 weeks per month.
   c. High-potency steroids (clobetasol 0.05%, diflorasone 0.05%, betamethasone dipropionate 0.05%) should be reserved for older children/adults on severely affected areas bid for no more than 2 weeks.
6. Patients need to be cautioned about topical steroid side effects. Continued use can cause thinning of the skin, striae formation, and systemic absorption, especially in younger children and infants. Steroids used around the eye area for prolonged periods can lead to glaucoma and/or cataract formation.
7. Systemic retinoids such as isotretinoin and acitretin are effective at smoothing the keratotic surface; however, long-term use of these agents is not recommended.
8. In severe refractory cases of disfiguring disease, reports of cyclosporine dermabrasion, CO_2, erbium:YAG laser resurfacing, and photodynamic therapy have yielded some clinical success in individual cases.

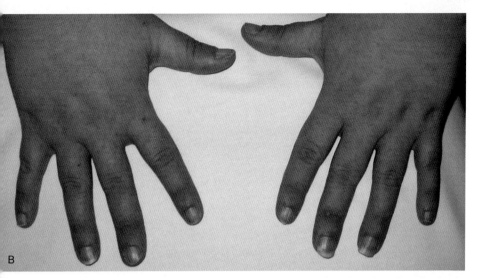

B

FIGURE 4-14 *(Continued)* **B:** Nails with red, white longitudinal streaks with V-shaped notch at the distal end and subungual hyperkeratosis.

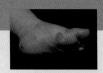

PRIMARY BULLOUS DERMATOSES

EPIDERMOLYSIS BULLOSA

Epidermolysis bullosa (EB) defines a group of rare inherited mechanobullous skin disorders that are characterized by skin fragility and bullae formation. There are three major categorizations of the disease: epidermolysis bullosa simplex (EBS), junctional epidermolysis bullosa (JEB), and dystrophic epidermolysis bullosa (DEB) with over 20 different phenotypes representing mutations in the genes of at least 18 structural proteins of the skin (in the epidermis, dermal–epidermal junction, or upper papillary dermis).

INSIGHT Melanocytic nevi in children with recurrent blistering disorders may appear clinically atypical (large and dark with irregular borders) while having reassuring histological patterns.

CLASSIFICATION

Inherited EB can be classified based on phenotype and genotype, subdividing EB into types and subtypes as follows:

1. Epidermolysis bullosa simplex (EBS, with intraepidermal bullae)

    Major subtypes:
    EBS, localized (also known as EBS, Weber–Cockayne).
    EBS, generalized intermediate (also known as EBS, Koebner).
    EBS, generalized severe (also known as EBS, Dowling-Meara).
    EBS with muscular dystrophy.
    Minor subtypes:
    EBS with mottled pigmentation.
    Autosomal recessive EBS.
    EBS, Ogna.
    EBS with pyloric atresia.
    EBS superficialis/suprabasal EBS.

2. Junctional epidermolysis bullosa (JEB, with bullae cleavage plane at lamina lucida)

    Major subtypes:
    JEB, generalized severe (also known as JEB, Herlitz).
    JEB, generalized intermediate (also known as JEB, non-Herlitz).
    JEB with pyloric atresia.
    Minor subtypes:
    JEB inversa.
    JEB localized.
    JEB laryngo-onycho-cutaneous syndrome.

3. Dystrophic epidermolysis bullosa (DEB, with bullae cleavage plane below lamina densa)

    Major subtypes:
    Dominant (D) DEB.
    Recessive (R) DEB, generalized severe (also known as RDEB, Hallopeau–Siemens).
    RDEB, generalized intermediate (also known as RDEB non-Hallopeau–Siemens).
    Minor subtypes:
    DDEB, pretibial.
    DDEB pruriginosa.
    RDEB inversa.
    RDEB centripetalis.
    DEB, transient bullous dermolysis of the newborn.
    DEB, autosomal, dominant/autosomal, recessive heterozygote.

EPIDERMOLYSIS BULLOSA SIMPLEX

EBS is typically an autosomal dominantly inherited, typically nonscarring, blistering disorder which results from cleavage within or above the basal cell layer of the epidermis.

There are three major subtypes of EBS which have a mutation in the genes coding for keratin 5 or keratin 14 which are found in the basal keratinocyte, and a fourth major subtype associated with muscular dystrophy which arises from mutations in the gene encoding the protein plectin:

Major subtypes:
   EBS, localized (also known as EBS, Weber–Cockayne).
   EBS, generalized intermediate (also known as EBS, Koebner).
   EBS, generalized severe (also known as EBS, Dowling-Meara).
   EBS with muscular dystrophy.

There are more rare autosomal recessive generalized EBS forms with a variety of causative mutations:

Minor subtypes:
   EBS with mottled pigmentation—mutation in keratin 5.
   Autosomal recessive EBS—mutation in keratin 5 or 14.
   EBS, Ogna—mutation in plectin.
   EBS with pyloric atresia—mutation in plectin.
   EBS superficialis (unknown genetic defect, intraepidermal blister just beneath the granular layer, may be a clinical variant of another form of EB).

SYNONYM Epidermolytic EB.

EPIDEMIOLOGY

AGE
   Major subtypes:
   EBS, localized (Weber–Cockayne): Blisters may appear in first 2 years of life. It can also begin in adolescence.
   EBS, generalized intermediate (Koebner): Bullae at birth, at areas of friction; improves in adolescence.
   EBS, generalized severe (Dowling-Meara): Bullae at birth; widespread, severe, and extensive spontaneous blisters; improves in adolescence.

EBS with muscular dystrophy: Bullae at birth.

INCIDENCE 10 per 1 million live births. EBS, localized (Weber–Cockayne) variant is most common, estimated at 1/50,000 live births.
GENDER M = F.
ETIOLOGY Mutations in genes encoding keratins 5 or 14, or mutations in gene encoding plectin. See Table 5-1.
GENETICS Autosomal dominant in inheritance, rarely can be autosomal recessively inherited. See Table 5-1.
PRECIPITATING FACTORS Bullae are mechanically induced by friction and can be exacerbated by warm temperatures, running, prolonged walking, and other sources of trauma.

TABLE 5-1 Epidermolysis Bullosa Simplex: Disease Type With Gene Defect and Inheritance Pattern

Disease Type	Gene	Inheritance
Epidermolysis Bullosa Simplex		
EBS, localized (Weber–Cockayne)	Keratin 5, Keratin 14	AD
EBS, generalized intermediate (Kobner)	Keratin 5, Keratin 14	AD
EBS, generalized severe (Dowling-Meara)	Keratin 5, Keratin 14	AD
EBS with muscular dystrophy	Plectin	AD
EBS with pyloric atresia	Plectin	AR
EBS with mottled pigmentation	Keratin 5	AD
EBS, autosomal recessive	Keratin 5, Keratin 14	AR
EBS, Ogna type	Plectin	AD
EBS superficialis	Unknown	AD

PATHOPHYSIOLOGY

Mutations in the genes encoding keratin 5 (chromosome 12q) or 14 (chromosome 17q) or plectin (chromosome 8q) cause abnormal keratinocyte tonofilaments or hemidesmosomes in the basal cell layer of the skin. Trauma leads to intraepidermal cleavage at the level of the basal cell layer with resultant blister formation.

HISTORY

Healthy infants are born with seemingly fragile skin. Blisters form in areas of greatest friction, but blistering tendency usually improves with age.

PHYSICAL EXAMINATION

Skin Findings

Type and Distribution

Major subtypes:
EBS, localized (Weber–Cockayne): flaccid bullae on hands and feet (Fig. 5-1).
EBS, generalized intermediate (Koebner): generalized bullae with milia formation on healing areas. Little to no mucosal involvement, 20% with nail dystrophy.
EBS, generalized severe (Dowling-Meara): widespread bullae with arcuate, herpetiform grouping, palmoplantar keratoderma.
EBS with muscular dystrophy: localized bullae.
Minor subtypes:
EBS with mottled pigmentation: bullae associated with reticulate hyperpigmented macules.
Autosomal recessive EBS: may be either local or generalized bullae, often presenting shortly after birth.
EBS, Ogna: similar phenotype to EBS, localized (Weber–Cockayne) with additional clinical feature of perilesional bruising and hemorrhagic bullae.
EBS with pyloric atresia: severe with bullae at birth; poor prognosis often with death in infancy.
EBS superficialis: superficial peeling often without blisters (split just beneath the granular layer).

LABORATORY EXAMINATION

DERMATOPATHOLOGY Light microscopy reveals an intraepidermal split consistent with basal cell cytolysis, but this is not diagnostic.
TRANSMISSION ELECTRON MICROSCOPY AND IMMUNOFLUORESCENCE ANTIGENIC MAPPING More sensitive technique demonstrating the cleavage through the basal layer and basal cell cytolysis. In EBS, generalized severe (Dowling-Meara), EM will show clumping of tonofilaments in addition to basal cell cytolysis. Immunofluorescence staining shows the BP antigen, laminin, and collagen IV to be located beneath the level of cleavage. Immunofluorescent antigenic mapping with monoclonal antibodies can demonstrate absent keratins 5 or 14 or plectin.
MOLECULAR TESTING Can be performed based on keratin gene mutations and/or abnormal production of keratins 5 or 14 or plectin.

DIFFERENTIAL DIAGNOSIS

If family history is noncontributory, clinical bullae formation in an otherwise seemingly healthy newborn should lead one to suspect mechanobullous disorders. The differential diagnosis includes other genodermatoses with blisters (bullous congenital ichthyosiform erythroderma), autoimmune bullous diseases (linear IgA, pemphigoid, pemphigus), infections (herpes, staphylococcal scalded skin, bullous impetigo), benign entities (suction blister, friction blister), or rarely signs of child abuse or neglect (scalding, thermal injury).

COURSE AND PROGNOSIS

Most common forms of EBS improve with age, and blister formation can be limited by decreasing traumatic activities. Of the common subtypes, EBS, generalized severe (Dowling-Meara) variant can be extensive enough to cause significant morbidity and mortality, and EBS associated with muscular dystrophy may have a varied phenotype with progressive muscular wasting in severe forms.

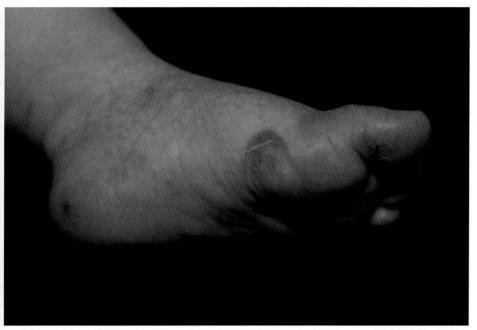

FIGURE 5-1 Epidermolysis bullosa simplex Localized flaccid bullae on the foot of an infant.

MANAGEMENT

The treatment of EBS is palliative:

1. Bullae formation can be minimized by limiting traumatic activities; using soft, well-fitted shoes; and avoiding warm temperatures.
2. When blisters occur, extension may be avoided by careful aseptic aspiration of the blister fluid with a sterile pin or needle. The roofs of the blisters may be carefully trimmed with sterile scissors. Then the lesion can be dressed with a hydrocolloid dressing or petrolatum-impregnated gauze that will not stick to the healing blister site.
3. Daily baths, gentle cleansers (Aquanil or Cetaphil liquid cleansers), and bandaging can help reduce chance of secondary infection and will also help healing of the blistered area.
4. Topical emollients (Vaseline petroleum jelly, hydrated petrolatum, or Aquaphor healing ointment) can reduce friction in the healing area.
5. Topical antibiotics (mupirocin) may be used if evidence of bacterial secondary infection is present (yellow exudate, purulence, crusting).
6. A water mattress with fleece covering may be necessary to reduce pressure and friction to limit extensive blistering.
7. Widespread denudation of the skin requires hospitalization with IV fluids, IV antibiotics if appropriate, and burn unit wound care.
8. Tissue-cultured derived artificial skin dressings are expensive, but may be helpful in nonhealing sites.
9. Genetic counseling to the family is important and prenatal testing should be offered if available. At present, there is no gene therapy available.
10. An international epidermolysis registry (www.debra.org) has been established and can be used as a support and informational system for families who have children with EB.

JUNCTIONAL EPIDERMOLYSIS BULLOSA

JEB is a rare autosomal recessively inherited mechanobullous disease that leads to cleavage within the lamina lucida layer (at the junction of the epidermis and dermis) of the skin.

JEB subtypes have inherited mutations in the anchoring filaments (laminin 332) or hemidesmosomes [bullous pemphigoid antigen 2 (also known as type XVII collagen) or α_6- and β_4-integrins]:
Several subtypes have been described:

1. JEB, generalized severe (also known as JEB, Herlitz type, letalis)
2. JEB, generalized intermediate (also known as non-Herlitz type, mitis)
3. JEB with pyloric atresia (mutations of α_6- and β_4-integrin)

EPIDEMIOLOGY

AGE Onset of blisters at birth or early infancy (Fig. 5-2A).
GENDER M = F.
INCIDENCE 2 per 1 million live births.
ETIOLOGY Mutation in the gene that codes for laminin 332, type XVII collagen (also known as bullous pemphigoid antigen 2), or α_6- and β_4-integrin. See Table 5-2.
GENETICS Autosomal recessive.

PATHOPHYSIOLOGY

Abnormal hemidesmosome formation leads to skin fragility at the lamina lucida level of the basement membrane. Molecular defects identified include abnormalities in hemidesmosome components: laminin 332, type VII collagen, or α_6- and β_4-integrin.

HISTORY

Blistering onset occurs during infancy for all types of JEB. The spectrum of disease (depending on subtype) can range from mild blistering tendencies to severe widespread blistering with a poor prognosis (JEB, generalized severe or Herlitz variant). Mucosal/esophageal/laryngeal blistering and scarring can lead to death in infancy.

PHYSICAL EXAMINATION

Skin Findings

Type and Distribution

1. JEB, generalized severe (Herlitz type, letalis): Extensive bullae formation (Fig. 5-2B), which heals with excessive granulation tissue periorifically (Fig. 5-2C), around the neck, and in the axillae. Nails may have paronychial inflammation, teeth may be dysplastic.
2. JEB, generalized intermediate (non-Herlitz type, mitis): Serosanguineous blisters, atrophic scarring, dystrophic or absent nails, mild mucous membrane involvement.

General Findings

1. JEB, generalized severe (Herlitz type, letalis): Laryngeal involvement leads to 50% mortality within first 2 years of life. Survivors have severe growth retardation and anemia.
2. JEB, generalized intermediate (non-Herlitz type, mitis): Scarring alopecia.
3. All JEB types have dental enamel hypoplasia leading to caries and tooth loss.

LABORATORY EXAMINATIONS

DERMATOPATHOLOGY Light microscopy reveals a subepidermal cleavage.

TABLE 5-2 Junctional Epidermolysis Bullosa: Disease Type With Gene Defect and Inheritance Pattern

Disease Type	Gene	Inheritance
Junctional Epidermolysis Bullosa		
JEB, generalized severe (Herlitz)	Laminin 332	AR
JEB, generalized intermediate (non-Herlitz)	Laminin 332, Collagen 17A1	AR
JEB with pyloric atresia	Integrin β_4, Integrin α_6	AR
JEB, localized	Collagen 17A1	AR
JEB inversa	Laminin 332	AR
JEB, laryngo-onycho-cutaneous syndrome	Laminin 332	AR

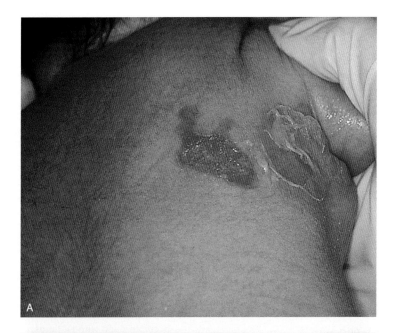

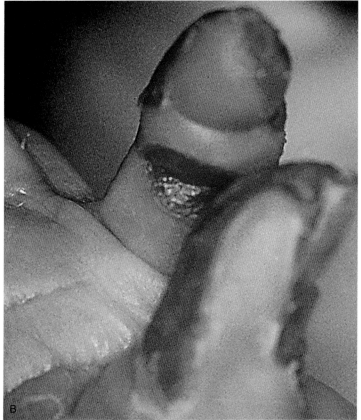

FIGURE 5-2 **A: Junctional epidermolysis bullosa in a newborn** Blister formation noted at areas of mild friction on the right chest wall of an otherwise healthy 7-day-old infant. **B: Junctional epidermolysis bullosa in a 1-month-old infant** Same child 4 weeks later with severe blistering of the distal fingertips. *(continued)*

TRANSMISSION ELECTRON MICROSCOPY AND IMMU-NOFLUORESCENCE ANTIGENIC MAPPING EM will show abnormal or absent hemidesmosomes and/or subbasal dense plates as well as a split in the lamina lucida. Immunofluorescence staining can demonstrate abnormal or absent laminin 5 (laminin 332), type XVII collagen, and/or α_6- and β_4-integrin.

DIFFERENTIAL DIAGNOSIS

Family history is usually helpful, but if non-contributory, blister formation tendencies in the newborn could implicate a mechanobul-lous disease. The differential diagnosis includes other genodermatoses with blisters (bullous congenital ichthyosiform erythroderma), autoimmune bullous diseases (linear IgA, pemphigoid, pemphigus), infections (herpes, staphylococcal scalded skin, bullous impetigo), benign entities (suction blister, friction blister), or rarely signs of child abuse or neglect (scald-ing, thermal injury).

COURSE AND PROGNOSIS

1. JEB, generalized severe (Herlitz type, letalis): Severe blistering at birth and laryngeal lesions lead to a 50% mortality before age 2. Pyloric atresia can also be seen. Patients who survive heal with atrophic changes of the skin. Attempts at laminin 5 (laminin 332) replacement and gene therapy are in progress but have not been successfully performed to date.
2. JEB, generalized intermediate (non-Herlitz type, mitis): Affected patients have normal growth and lifespan.

MANAGEMENT

The treatment of JEB is palliative:

1. Bullae formation can be minimized by limiting traumatic activities; using soft, well-fitted shoes; and avoiding warm temperatures.
2. When blisters occur, extensive blisters may be avoided by careful aseptic aspiration of the blister fluid with a sterile pin or needle. The roofs of the blisters may be carefully trimmed with sterile scissors. Then the lesion can be dressed with a hydrocolloid dressing or petrolatum-impregnated gauze that will not stick to the healing blister site.
3. Daily baths, gentle cleansers (Aquanil or Cetaphil liquid cleansers), and bandag-ing can help reduce chance of secondary infection and will also help healing of the blistered area.
4. Topical emollients (Vaseline petroleum jelly, hydrated petrolatum, or Aquaphor healing ointment) can reduce friction on the healing area.
5. Topical antibiotics (mupirocin) can be used if evidence of bacterial secondary infection is present (yellow exudate, purulence, crusting).
6. A water mattress with fleece covering may be necessary to reduce pressure and friction to limit extensive blistering.
7. Widespread denudation of the skin requires hospitalization with IV fluids, IV antibiotics if appropriate, and burn unit wound care.
8. Watching for respiratory or GI involve-ment is important. Soft foods and liquid diets may help symptomatically. Ultimately, corrective surgical intervention may be necessary.
9. For severe disease systemic steroids, hyperbaric chambers, laminin replacement, and other therapeutic attempts have been reported, with limited success.
10. Tissue-cultured derived artificial skin dress-ings are expensive, but may be helpful in nonhealing sites.
11. Genetic counseling to the family is impor-tant and prenatal testing should be offered if available. At present, there is no gene therapy available, though clinical trials are investigating this approach.
12. An international epidermolysis registry (www.debra.org) has been established and can be used as a support and informational system for families who have children with EB.

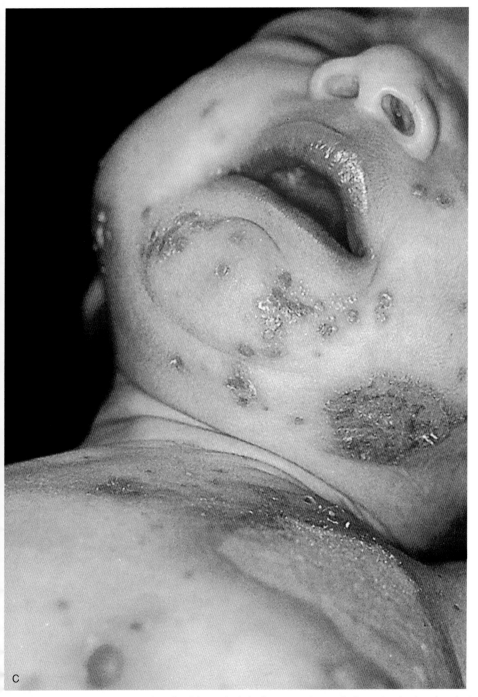

C

FIGURE 5-2 *(Continued)* **C: Junctional epidermolysis bullosa, age 1 month** Severe perioral, oral, and GI involvement. The infant was subsequently hospitalized and despite burn unit supportive measures, eventually passed away because of sepsis.

DYSTROPHIC EPIDERMOLYSIS BULLOSA

DEB is a deeper mechanobullous disease caused by a mutation in the collagen VII gene. This results in a defective anchoring fibril in the sublamina densa of the skin and leads clinically to subepidermal blisters which scar.

The subtypes of DEB are based on inheritance patterns:

1. Dominant DEB, generalized (AD inherited)
2. Recessive DEB, generalized severe (also known as Hallopeau–Siemens, AR inherited)
3. Recessive DEB, generalized intermediate (AR inherited)

SYNONYMS Dermolytic bullous dermatosis, dysplastic EB.

EPIDEMIOLOGY

AGE Blistering in both forms appears at birth.
GENDER M = F.
INCIDENCE Recessive DEB: 3 in 1 million live births, Dominant DEB: 2 in 1 million live births.
ETIOLOGY Mutation in genes encoding for collagen type VII.
GENETICS Autosomal dominant and autosomal recessive forms. See Table 5-3.

PATHOPHYSIOLOGY

In dominant DEB, the genetic defect leads to abnormal collagen VII resulting in impaired anchoring fibrils in the lamina densa. In recessive DEB, the genetic defect leads to severe defects in type VII collagen leading to undetectable anchoring fibrils in the lamina densa. Both DEB forms result in a split in the dermal–epidermal junction which clinically results in deep blisters that can heal with scarring, fusion, and flexion deformities.

HISTORY

Blistering onset at infancy (Fig. 5-3A), then:

1. Dominant DEB: Intermittent blistering episodes noted at birth or shortly thereafter that improve with age. Mild hair and teeth involvement.

2. Recessive DEB: Widespread dystrophy and scarring leading to incapacity and nail and mucous membrane involvement leading to poor growth and poor development.

PHYSICAL EXAMINATION

Skin Findings

Type and Distribution

1. Dominant DEB: Bullae on dorsal aspect of extremities result in either hypertrophic (Cockayne-Touraine variant) or atrophic (Pacini variant) scars and milia. Mucous membrane involvement in 20%; 80% have thickened nails. Hair and teeth abnormalities are typically mild if present.

2. Recessive DEB: In the generalized severe form (Hallopeau–Siemens variant), there is widespread dystrophic scarring, severe involvement of the mucous membranes, and severe nail dystrophy. Bullae heal with atrophic scarring and milia resulting in mitten deformities of the hands and feet, extremities become contracted with scars (Fig. 5-3B). Recurrent scarring can lead to the development of aggressive life-threatening squamous cell carcinomas with metastases. In the more mild generalized intermediate, blistering is less severe.

General Findings

1. Dominant DEB: Generally healthy and of normal stature.

TABLE 5-3 Dystrophic Epidermolysis Bullosa: Disease Type With Gene Defect and Inheritance Pattern

Disease Type	Gene	Inheritance
Dystrophic Epidermolysis Bullosa		
DDEB	Collagen 7A1	AD
RDEB, generalized severe	Collagen 7A1	AR
RDEB, generalized intermediate	Collagen 7A1	AR

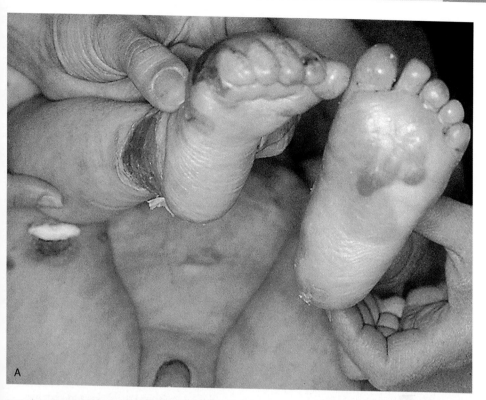

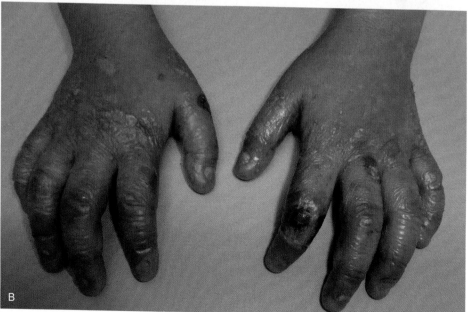

FIGURE 5-3 A: Recessive dystrophic epidermolysis bullosa in a newborn. Bullae occur at areas of minimal trauma at or near birth. **B:** Recessive dystrophic epidermolysis bullosa in a child. Scarring of the hands in a child with RDEB.

2. Recessive DEB: In the generalized severe form (Hallopeau–Siemens variant), progressive deformity of the extremities leads to increasing incapacity. Eye involvement leads to blepharitis, symblepharon, conjunctivitis, keratitis, and corneal opacities. Laryngeal and pharyngeal involvement leads to hoarseness and aphonia (inability to speak). Esophageal strictures and intestinal disease can lead to malabsorption and failure to thrive. Renal involvement can lead to ureteral reflux, hydronephrosis, glomerulonephritis, and renal failure. Teeth are malformed and susceptible to caries. Scalp and body hair is sparse or absent. In the generalized intermediate form, internal involvement is typically less pronounced.

LABORATORY EXAMINATIONS

DERMATOPATHOLOGY Light microscopy reveals a split at the dermal–epidermal junction. TRANSMISSION ELECTRON MICROSCOPY AND IMMUNOFLUORESCENCE ANTIGENIC MAPPING EM will show abnormal or absent anchoring fibrils and a split at the sublamina densa level. Immunofluorescence staining can demonstrate abnormal (DDEB or generalized intermediate RDEB) or absent collagen VII (usually in generalized severe RDEB).

DIFFERENTIAL DIAGNOSIS

Family history is usually helpful, but if noncontributory, blister formation tendencies in the newborn could implicate a mechanobullous disease. The differential diagnosis includes other genodermatoses with blisters (bullous congenital ichthyosiform erythroderma), autoimmune bullous diseases (linear IgA, pemphigoid, pemphigus), infections (herpes, staphylococcal scalded skin, bullous impetigo), benign entities (suction blister, friction blister), or rarely signs of child abuse or neglect (scalding, thermal injury).

COURSE AND PROGNOSIS

1. Dominant DEB: After blisters at birth, intermittent episodes of less severe blistering occur, but lifespan and growth/development are normal. The blistering episodes are worse than EBS, but milder than recessive DEB.
2. Recessive DEB: In individuals with the generalized severe variant Hallopeau–Siemens, the extensive blistering may result in scarring, fusion, and flexion deformities that are functionally incapacitating. Recessive DEB blistering may result in death secondary to sepsis, fluid loss, or malnutrition. Surviving patients are chronically susceptible to infection and repeated blistering leads to further and further disabilities. These patients tend to have difficulties with laryngeal complications, esophageal strictures, and scarring of the anal area, and have a predisposition to basal cell and squamous cell carcinomas in the scarred skin areas. In the generalized intermediate variant, life expectancy is normal and there is little to no increased risk of carcinoma formation.

MANAGEMENT

The treatment of DEB is palliative:

1. Bullae formation can be minimized by limiting traumatic activities; using soft, well-fitted shoes; and avoiding warm temperatures.
2. When blisters occur, extensive blisters may be avoided by careful aseptic aspiration of the blister fluid with a sterile pin or needle. The roofs of the blisters may be carefully trimmed with sterile scissors. Then the lesion can be dressed with a hydrocolloid dressing or petrolatum-impregnated gauze that will not stick to the healing blister site.
3. Daily baths, gentle cleansers (Aquanil or Cetaphil liquid cleansers), and bandaging can help reduce chance of secondary infection and will also help healing of the blistered area.
4. Topical emollients (Vaseline petroleum jelly, hydrated petrolatum, or Aquaphor healing ointment) can reduce friction on the healing area.
5. Topical antibiotics (mupirocin) can be used if evidence of bacterial superinfection is present (yellow exudate, purulence, crusting).
6. A water mattress with fleece covering may be necessary to reduce pressure and friction to limit extensive blistering.
7. Widespread denudation of the skin requires hospitalization with IV fluids, IV antibiotics if appropriate, and burn unit wound care.
8. Tissue-cultured derived artificial skin dressings are expensive, but may be helpful in nonhealing sites.
9. Genetic counseling to the family is important and prenatal testing should be offered if available. At present, there is no gene therapy available, though clinical trials are investigating this approach.
10. Oral and GI complications lead to aphonia and aphasia. A liquid or soft food diet may help symptoms. Aggressive oral, dental, and nutritional care should be given. Ultimately, surgical intervention may be needed.
11. Occupational and physical therapy for the fusion and flexion deformities is recommended, and repeated plastic surgical reconstruction may be needed to prolong functional use of the hands and feet.
12. Other reported treatments include systemic steroids, phenytoin, tetracycline, thalidomide, and tacrolimus, which all have anecdotal limited success.
13. Genetic counseling to the family is important and prenatal testing should be offered if available.
14. An international epidermolysis registry (www.debra.org) has been established and can be used as a support and informational system for families who have children with EB.

OTHER

LINEAR IGA BULLOUS DISEASE OF CHILDHOOD

Linear IgA bullous disease of childhood is a rare, benign, self-limited bullous eruption thought to be caused by IgA autoantibodies targeting antigens at the basement membrane zone of the skin.

SYNONYMS Chronic bullous disease of childhood, benign chronic bullous dermatitis of childhood, childhood linear IgA dermatitis herpetiformis, linear IgA disease of childhood.

EPIDEMIOLOGY

AGE Mostly preschool children (mean age 4.5 years).
GENDER Possible slight female predominance, F:M = 3:2.
INCIDENCE One in 250,000.
ETIOLOGY IgA autoantibodies to antigens in the basement membrane zone.

PATHOPHYSIOLOGY

Circulating IgA autoantibodies target a 97 kDa protein in the basement membrane zone, leading to cleavage of the skin at that level and blister formation. Reports of GI disease (gluten-sensitive enteropathy, ulcerative colitis), autoimmune diseases (lupus, dermatomyositis), malignancies (lymphoma, leukemia), infection (zoster), or medications (vancomycin, penicillins cephalosporins, NSAIDs) are postulated possible triggers for linear IgA disease of childhood.

HISTORY

DURATION OF LESIONS Several months to 3 years.
SKIN SYMPTOMS Mild-to-severe pruritus.
REVIEW OF SYSTEMS Negative.

PHYSICAL EXAMINATION

Skin Findings

TYPE Large tense bullae, central crusting (Fig. 5-4A).
COLOR Annular erythema, clear or hemorrhagic bullae on erythematous base.
SIZE Bullae 1 to 2 cm.
ARRANGEMENT Annular or rosette configuration like "a string of pearls" (Fig. 5-4B).

DISTRIBUTION Widespread.
SITES OF PREDILECTION Face (especially perioral area) (Fig. 5-4C), scalp, lower abdomen, buttock, perineum, thighs, dorsa of feet.

DIFFERENTIAL DIAGNOSIS

Linear IgA bullous disease of childhood needs to be distinguished from other blistering diseases such as other genodermatoses with blisters (bullous congenital ichthyosiform erythroderma), autoimmune bullous diseases (pemphigoid, pemphigus), or infections (herpes, staphylococcal scalded skin, bullous impetigo). A thorough medication history should be taken to exclude drug-induced linear IgA bullous dermatosis or a bullous drug hypersensitivity.

LABORATORY EXAMINATIONS

DERMATOPATHOLOGY Subepidermal blister with dermal papillary edema, neutrophils (newer lesions), and occasionally eosinophils (older lesions).
IMMUNOELECTRON MICROSCOPY Reveals linear deposits of IgA in the basement membrane zone. Indirect immunofluorescence may detect circulating IgA autoantibodies against antigens in the lamina lucida and sublamina densa. Some individuals will also have circulating IgG autoantibodies against target antigens as well, though their clinical significance is uncertain.

COURSE AND PROGNOSIS

Most cases of linear IgA bullous disease of childhood are self-limited. Affected children have disease-free remissions and then spontaneously clear within 2 to 4 years, typically before puberty. Only a small subset of patients experience episodic recurrences that persist into adulthood.

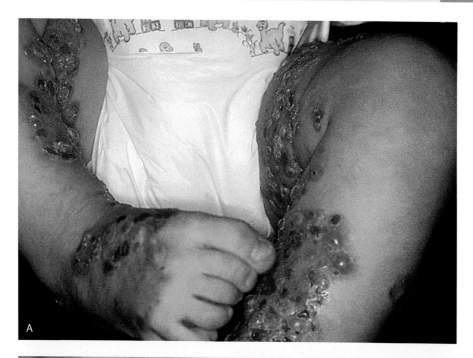

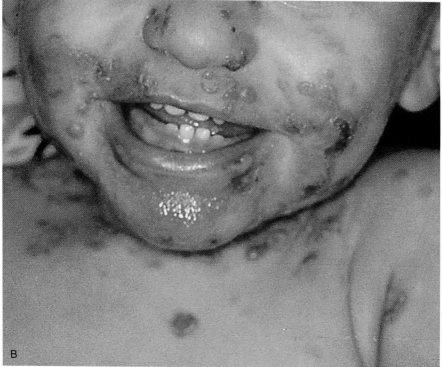

FIGURE 5-4 Linear IgA bullous disease of childhood A: Legs of a 13-month-old infant with characteristic annular plaques and "string of pearls" bullae configuration. **B:** Perioral blistering on the face of the same infant. *(continued)*

MANAGEMENT

Treatment of linear IgA chronic bullous diseases is directed at reducing the frequency and severity of outbreaks. Two first-line agents for the disease include sulfapyridine and dapsone.

1. Dapsone (1–2 mg/kg/d, not to exceed 100 mg/d) is effective at treating linear IgA bullous dermatosis in childhood. All individuals should be screened for glucose-6-phosphate dehydrogenase (G6PD) deficiency prior to starting treatment as well as a baseline complete blood count (CBC) and liver function tests (LFTs). Once the existing lesions have improved after initiation of treatment (usually in a matter of days), the dosage may be tapered to the least amount required to keep the skin under control. Side effects of dapsone include hemolysis, methemoglobinemia, nausea, vomiting, headache, tachycardia, psychoses, fever, dermatitis, liver necrosis, lymphadenitis, and neuropathy. Monthly blood work with specific monitoring of the CBC for hemolysis as well as a regular urinalysis is recommended.

2. The disease is also very responsive to sulfapyridine (100–200 mg/kg/d divided qid, not to exceed 4 g/d). Once the existing lesions have improved, the dosage may be tapered to the least amount needed to keep the skin under control (usually less than 0.5 g po qid). Signs of sulfapyridine toxicity include nausea, vomiting, headache, fever, leukopenia, agranulocytosis, hemolytic anemia, serum sickness, hepatitis, dermatitis, and renal crystalluria. As with initiation of dapsone, a screening test for G6PD deficiency should be performed, and pretreatment as well as monthly blood work should be followed.

3. Reports of improvement have been seen with oral tetracycline, erythromycin, or dicloxacillin.

4. Patients who fail to respond to sulfonamides alone may improve with the addition of systemic steroids.

5. Mycophenolate mofetil, azathioprine, IVIG, and cyclosporine may be tried in refractory cases.

6. Medications may be required anywhere from several months to 3 years until the disease remits.

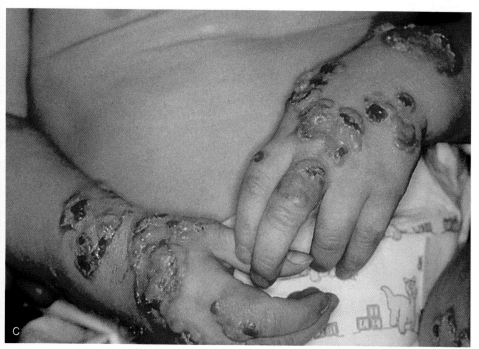

FIGURE 5-4 *(Continued)* **C:** Large tense bullae with central crusting on the hands of the same infant.

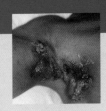

DISORDERS OF THE SEBACEOUS AND APOCRINE GLANDS

ACNE VULGARIS

Acne vulgaris is the most common skin disorder in adolescents. It is a multifactorial disease characterized by chronic inflammation of the pilosebaceous units of certain areas (most commonly the face and trunk) that manifests as comedones, papules, nodules, cysts, or papulopustules. Resolving lesions are often but not always followed by scars.

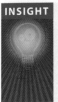

INSIGHT Neonatal acne (presenting between the age of 2 weeks and 3 months of life) is common and self-limited; it has been associated with inflammation in response to *Malassezia* overgrowth. Infantile acne (presenting between 3 and 6 months of age) may foreshadow more severe acne later in life.

EPIDEMIOLOGY

AGE Typically begins at puberty.
GENDER M > F, and males tend to be more severely affected.
PREVALENCE Approximately 85% of 12- to 24-year-old patients have some form of acne. Forty to fifty million people in the United States have acne annually.
DRUGS Systemic corticosteroids, iodides, bromides, anticonvulsants (phenytoin and trimethadione), antidepressants (lithium), and epidermal growth factor receptor (EGFR) inhibitors can exacerbate acne in susceptible patients.
GENETIC ASPECTS Family history may be a predictor of acne severity. Additionally, individuals with an XXY karyotype are at increased risk for severe acne. Acne may rarely be a component of syndromes such as SAPHO (synovitis, acne, pustulosis, hyperostosis, osteitis) and PAPA (pyogenic arthritis, pyoderma gangrenosum, acne).
OTHER FACTORS Emotional stress, lack of sleep, and menses can cause exacerbations. Pressure or rubbing of skin can cause local outbreaks (acne mechanica). Androgen excess can also lead to severe refractory cases.

PATHOPHYSIOLOGY

The lesions of acne (comedones) are the result of genetics (increased number and size of sebaceous glands), mechanical factors (accumulation of sloughed corneocytes leading to pilosebaceous unit blockage), hormones (androgens), bacteria (*Propionibacterium acnes*), and the inflammatory response in the pilosebaceous unit. Androgens stimulate sebaceous glands to produce larger amounts of sebum; bacteria contain lipase that converts lipids into fatty acids. Both excess sebum and fatty acids cause the corneocytes to block the pilosebaceous unit and comedones are formed. If the comedo is open to the skin surface, the oxidized keratin and lipid debris, along with corneocyte melanin, protrudes and darkens in color (blackheads). Closed comedones may break under the skin and the contents (sebum, lipid, fatty acids, keratin) enter the dermis, provoking inflammation (papules, pustules, nodules). Rupture plus intense inflammation may lead to scarring.

HISTORY

DURATION OF LESIONS Weeks to months.
SEASON Worse in fall and winter.
SYMPTOMS Itching or pain in lesions (especially nodulocystic type). Rarely, systemic symptoms such as fever may be associated with extreme presentations of acne fulminans.

PHYSICAL EXAMINATION

Skin Lesions

TYPE

Comedones: open comedones are "blackheads," closed comedones are "whiteheads" (Fig. 6-1A).

Papules with or without inflammation, pustules (Fig. 6-1B).

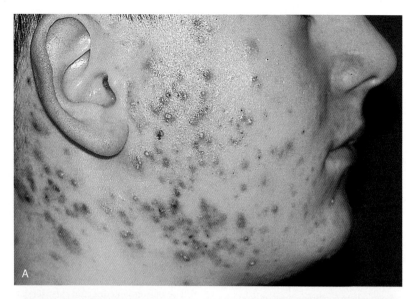

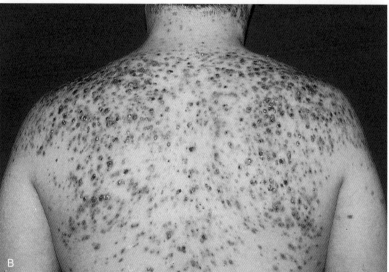

FIGURE 6-1 Acne vulgaris A: Scattered inflammatory papules and pustules on the cheek of an adolescent. **B:** Scattered inflammatory papules, pustules, and nodules on the back of the same individual. *(continued)*

Nodules, noduloulcerative lesions, 2 to 5 cm in diameter.

Postinflammatory hyperpigmentation (more common in darker skin types).

Scars. Atrophic depressed (often pitted), box-car, ice-pick, rolling, or hypertrophic (keloid) scars (Fig. 6-1C).

SHAPE Round; nodules may coalesce to form linear plaques.

ARRANGEMENT Isolated single lesion (e.g., nodule) or scattered discrete lesions (papules, cysts, nodules).

SITES OF PREDILECTION Face, chest, back, shoulders.

DIFFERENTIAL DIAGNOSIS

Acne has many morphologies and thus has a large differential including milia, miliaria, candidal infections, pustulosis, sebaceous hyperplasia, appendageal tumors, folliculitis, keratosis pilaris, and rosacea. Persistent lesions may mimic facial growths associated with genetic syndromes such as adenoma sebaceum of tuberous sclerosis.

COURSE AND PROGNOSIS

Acne may have a mild self-limited course or a protracted recurrent course that may persist into adulthood.

LABORATORY STUDIES

Persistent acne may be a result of XYY chromosomal genotype or endocrine disorders such as polycystic ovarian syndrome, hyperandrogenism, hypercortisolism, or precocious puberty. Patients suspected of hyperandrogenism should have screening tests including serum levels of total and free testosterone (to detect ovarian excess androgen), didehydroepiandrosterone sulfate (DHEAS, detects excess adrenal androgen), and 17-hydroxyprogesterone (detects adrenal excess androgen). Patients suspected of hypercortisolism should have an AM serum cortisol checked.

MANAGEMENT

Patients and parents should be educated on factors that may aggravate acne:

1. Repeated pressure, leaning, touching, or scrubbing acne-prone areas.
2. Occlusive garments such as headbands, chin-straps, helmets, and hats.
3. Oil and grease in moisturizers, face creams, makeup, or hair products.
4. Greasy air–filled environments such as fast-food kitchens.
5. Squeezing or popping pimples can lead to scarring.
6. Certain medications taken for other problems [e.g., oral contraceptives (OCPs), lithium, hydantoin, topical, and systemic steroids].
7. Emotional stress.
8. Hormonal changes with menses.
9. Foods typically do not play a major role, but some people find specific foods trigger their acne and are helped by avoiding them.

MILD ACNE

1. Topical antibiotics such as clindamycin or erythromycin help decrease bacterial load and inflammation.
2. Topical benzoyl peroxide also suppresses *P. acnes* and microbial resistance has not been reported. Topical benzoyl peroxide and topical antibiotics have synergistic effects when used in combination and help reduce bacterial resistance when combined.
3. Topical salicylic acid or α-hydroxy acid preparations can help slough the outer layer of skin preventing follicular blockage.
4. Topical retinoids (tretinoin, adapalene, tazarotene) are effective, but require detailed instructions and gradual increases in concentration. Retinoids help the skin turn over more rapidly to decrease follicular blockage and rupture.
5. Topical sulfur is antimicrobial and keratolytic.
6. Use of noncomedogenic cleansers and cosmetics should be encouraged in individuals who are acne-prone once clear to minimize recurrences.

MODERATE TO SEVERE ACNE

1. Oral antibiotics such as tetracycline (25–50 mg/kg/d divided bid, not to exceed 3 g/d), erythromycin (30–50 mg/kg/d divided bid, not to exceed 2 g/d), doxycycline (5 mg/kg/d divided qid–bid, not to exceed 200 mg/d), or minocycline (2 mg/kg/d, not to exceed 200 mg/d) are probably the most effective and can be tapered to lower doses once the acne is under good control. Minocycline, tetracycline, and doxycycline should only be used in children older than 8 years because of potential permanent staining of growing teeth. Erythromycin can increase theophylline and digoxin levels and should be used with caution in patients taking these medications. All oral antibiotics may also theoretically interfere with the efficacy of OCPs through alteration of gut flora and backup contraceptive methods should be used.
2. In certain females, acne is quite responsive to hormonal influences and can be controlled with OCPs. Three OCPs are currently FDA-approved for the treatment of acne:
   (1) A triphasic OCP with norgestimate (progestin)-ethinyl estradiol 35 μg (Estrostep).
   (2) Graduated ethinyl estradiol (20–35 μg) with norethindrone acetate (Ortho-tri-cyclin).

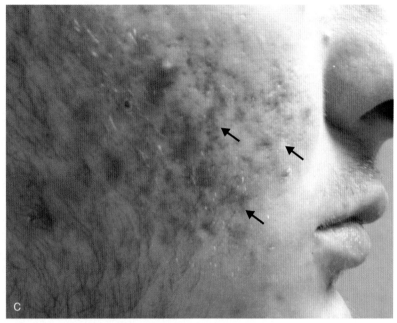

FIGURE 6-1 *(Continued)* **Acne vulgaris scarring C:** Atrophic depressed scars *(arrows)* on the cheek of an adolescent with acne.

(3) 20 µg of ethinyl estradiol with 3 mg drospirenone (Yaz or Yasmin).

In Europe and Canada, 2-mg cyproterone (a progestational antiandrogen) with ethinyl estradiol (35 or 50 µg) is available (Diane-35) and highly effective.

3. Oral spironolactone blocks androgen receptors and 5α-reductase. Doses of 50 to 100 mg daily can reduce sebum production and improve acne. Patients taking spironolactone should be cautioned regarding hyperkalemia and hypotension side effects.

4. Oral 13-*cis*-retinoic acid (isotretinoin) is highly effective for cystic acne. As retinoids are teratogenic, it is necessary that female patients be on two forms of birth control at least 1 month prior to beginning treatment, throughout treatment, and for 1 month after treatment is discontinued. Furthermore, a patient must have a negative serum pregnancy test within the 2 weeks prior to beginning treatment. Prescribers, patients, and pharmacies must all comply with the national isotretinoin registry program (see below). Dosage: 0.5 to 2 mg/kg/d with meals for a 15- to 20-week course, which is usually adequate. Approximately 30% of patients require a second course. Careful

monitoring of the blood is necessary during therapy, especially in patients with elevated blood triglycerides before therapy is begun. Currently, isotretinoin use is regulated in the United States by the iPLEDGE program which requires prescriber, patient, and pharmacist to sign off electronically on a monthly basis during treatment.

Common side effects of isotretinoin include xerosis, dry oral and nasal mucosa, xerophthalmia, myalgias, and skeletal hyperostoses. Serious side effects include idiopathic intracranial hypertension (pseudotumor cerebri), depression, suicidal ideation, and teratogenicity. The concomitant use of isotretinoin and tetracyclines increases the risk of pseudotumor cerebri and should be avoided.

5. Incising and expressing comedones can improve cosmetic appearance transiently.

6. Intralesional steroids for deep and inflamed lesions can quickly help them resolve.

7. Cosmetic camouflage can reduce the prominence of bothersome acne lesions.

8. Acne scarring can be treated with dermabrasion, laser resurfacing, chemical peels, filler substances, or punch grafting.

INFANTILE ACNE

Infantile acne is acne that appears when the infant is 3 to 4 months or older. Unlike neonatal acne, which is short-lived and self-resolving, infantile acne can be more long-standing, refractory to treatment, and predictive of a more severe resurgence of acne at puberty.

EPIDEMIOLOGY

AGE Onset age 3–4 months to 24 months. Rarely onset up to age 8 years (prior to adrenarche).
GENDER M > F.
GENETICS More common in children with a family history of acne.

PHYSICAL EXAMINATION

Skin Findings

TYPE Comedones (closed and open), papules, pustules, and occasional cystic nodules (Fig. 6-2).
DISTRIBUTION Face.

COURSE AND PROGNOSIS

Infantile acne has a variable course. In some individuals, it clears spontaneously after a few weeks without long-term sequelae. In others, especially cases with earlier onset and a family history of acne, the course is more protracted and severe with likely resurgence at puberty. Persistent severe infantile acne should be worked up for an endocrine abnormality, and an elevated level (>0.5 µg) of 17-ketosteroids in a 24-hour urine collection is suggestive of gonadal and adrenal hyperactivity.

MANAGEMENT

Infant skin is usually very sensitive, and mild cases of infantile acne can be managed with gentle cleansing. More severe cases may require topical medications, but they should be used sparingly and in low doses to the affected areas qid–bid to avoid overdrying and irritating the skin. Topical medications include the following:

1. Topical antibiotics such as clindamycin or erythromycin help decrease bacterial load and inflammation.
2. Topical benzoyl peroxide also suppresses P. acnes with no risk of resistance.
3. Topical sulfur is antimicrobial and keratolytic.
4. Topical salicylic acid, hydroxy acid preparations, or retinoids are effective, but may be too irritating in this age group.

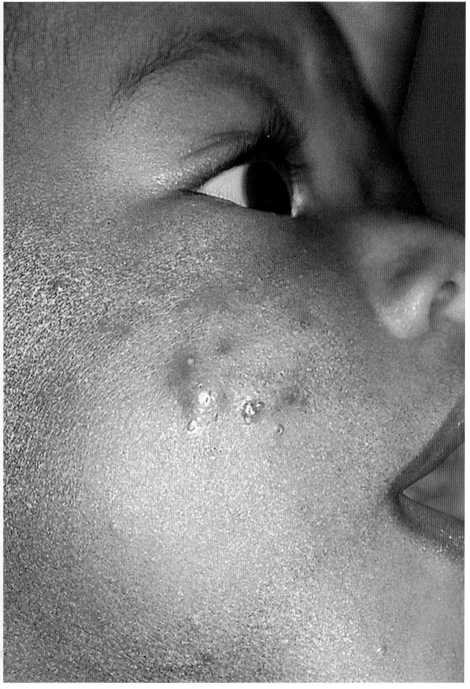

FIGURE 6-2 Infantile acne Scattered inflammatory papules and pustules on the cheek of a 5-month-old child.

PERIORIFICIAL DERMATITIS

Periorificial dermatitis is an acne-like eruption on the perioral, periocular, or rarely anogenital skin characterized by discrete erythematous papules that often coalesce, forming inflammatory plaques.

INSIGHT Unlike acne, periorificial dermatitis lacks true comedones (blackheads and whiteheads) and can be thus differentiated.

EPIDEMIOLOGY

AGE Any age. Seen in both young children and adults, from 15 to 40 years old.
GENDER F > M.
ETIOLOGY Unknown.
OTHER FACTORS May be precipitated or markedly aggravated by potent topical (fluorinated) corticosteroids, inhaled or nebulized corticosteroids, topical calcineurin inhibitors, and/or cosmetics.

HISTORY

DURATION OF LESIONS Weeks to months.
SKIN SYMPTOMS Occasional itching or burning.

PHYSICAL EXAMINATION

Skin Lesions

TYPE Initial lesions are erythematous papules. Confluent plaques may appear eczematous with erythema and scale (Fig. 6-3).
COLOR Pink to red.
SIZE 1- to 2-mm papules coalescing into larger plaques.
ARRANGEMENT Papules are irregularly grouped.
DISTRIBUTION Initial lesions usually around mouth and nasolabial folds, rarely in the periocular or anogenital area.

DIFFERENTIAL DIAGNOSIS

The diagnosis of periorificial dermatitis is made clinically and needs to be differentiated from contact dermatitis, atopic dermatitis, seborrheic dermatitis, rosacea, acne vulgaris, and sarcoidosis.

COURSE AND PROGNOSIS

Appearance of lesions is usually subacute over weeks to months. Periorificial dermatitis is, at times, misdiagnosed as an eczematous or seborrheic dermatitis and treated with a fluorinated corticosteroid preparation, which worsens the condition. Untreated, periorificial dermatitis fluctuates in activity over months to years. With treatment for several months, mild recurrences can occur but clear easily.

MANAGEMENT

Treatment should begin by eliminating any topical agents that may be aggravating or precipitating the condition, such as fluorinated corticosteroids, toothpaste with fluoride, or cosmetics. Often, just by eliminating the offending agent, the rash will clear. More refractory cases may require topical medications sparingly to the affected areas:

1. Topical antibiotics such as clindamycin, erythromycin, or metronidazole can help decrease inflammation.
2. Topical benzoyl peroxide is antimicrobial.
3. Topical sulfur preparations are antimicrobial and keratolytic.
4. Topical salicylic acid, hydroxy acid, or retinoids can help but must be used sparingly to avoid irritation.
5. Many cases require a course of oral antibiotics such as a macrolide or tetracycline. Tetracyclines should only be used in children older than 8 years because of potential permanent staining of growing teeth.

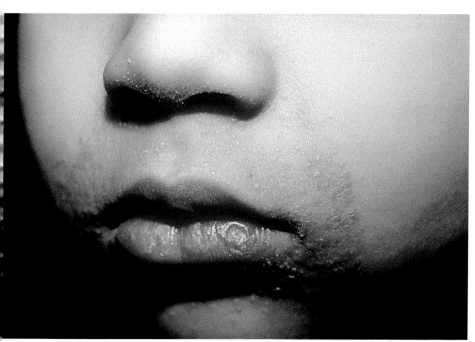

FIGURE 6-3 Perioral dermatitis Scattered inflammatory papules, erythema, and scale in a child who has been applying topical steroids to the area.

HIDRADENITIS SUPPURATIVA

Hidradenitis suppurativa is a chronic disease of apocrine gland–bearing skin (typically the axillae, inguinal folds, and anogenital region) that results in recurrent suppurative nodules (boils), draining sinus tracts, and cribriform scarring of the involved areas.

 INSIGHT Incision and drainage of these lesions is almost completely unhelpful save for temporary pain and pressure relief; they tend to refill immediately upon healing.

SYNONYMS Apocrinitis, hidradenitis axillaris, acne inversa, Verneuil's disease, pyoderma fistulans sinifica.

EPIDEMIOLOGY

AGE Develops at or soon after puberty.
GENDER F:M = 3:1.
RACE Affects blacks more than whites.
INCIDENCE Affects up to 1% of the population.
ETIOLOGY Predisposing factors: obesity, genetic predisposition to acne, occlusion of the follicular infundibulum, follicular rupture, and secondary bacterial infection.

PATHOPHYSIOLOGY

Sequence of changes: (1) keratinous plugging of the apocrine duct, (2) dilatation of apocrine duct and hair follicle, (3) severe inflammatory changes limited to a simple apocrine gland, (4) bacterial growth in dilated duct, (5) ruptured duct/gland results in extension of inflammation/infection, (6) extension of suppuration/tissue destruction, and (7) ulceration and fibrosis, sinus tract formation.

HISTORY

Intermittent pain, abscess formation in axilla(e), and/or inguinal area. The area under the breast may also be affected, and associated severe cystic acne of the face, chest, and back is also seen. The "follicular occlusion tetrad" labels the common association of hidradenitis suppurtiva with acne conglobata, dissecting cellulitis of the scalp, and pilonidal sinus. Other associated syndromes with hidradenitis include PASH (pyoderma gangrenosum, acne, suppurative hidradenitis) or PAPASH (pyogenic arthritis, pyoderma gangrenosum, acne, suppurative hidradenitis).

PHYSICAL EXAMINATION

Skin Findings

TYPE OF LESION Inflammatory nodule or abscess that drains purulent or seropurulent material. Eventually, sinus tracts form and result in fibrosis and "bridge," hypertrophic, and keloidal scars (Fig. 6-4). Multiple nodules are usually present. The so-called bridge lesions have the appearance of a sinus tract with double-ended comedones.
SIZE 0.5- to 1.5-cm nodules.
COLOR Erythematous nodules.
PALPATION Lesions moderately to exquisitely tender. Pus may be expressed from abscesses.
DISTRIBUTION OF LESIONS Axillae, under breasts, inguinal folds, anogenital areas.

General Findings

Often associated with obesity. Associated with severe cystic acne of the face (acne conglobata), chest, or back.

DIFFERENTIAL DIAGNOSIS

The diagnosis of hidradenitis suppurativa is made clinically by the characteristic distribution of the rash and by the resultant cribriform scarring. Early disease may be confused with furunculosis, lymphadenitis, ruptured trichilemmal cysts, cat scratch disease, or tularemia. Late disease can resemble lymphogranuloma venereum, donovanosis, scrofuloderma, actinomycosis, or the sinus tracts and fistulae associated with ulcerative colitis and regional enteritis.

LABORATORY EXAMINATIONS

BACTERIOLOGY *Staphylococcus aureus* or streptococci are organisms that commonly secondarily infect skin lesions; usually cultures of the lesions or pus reveal polymicrobial normal skin flora.
DERMATOPATHOLOGY Early: keratin occlusion of apocrine duct and hair follicle, ductal/tubular dilatation, and inflammatory changes. Late: abscesses followed by destruction of apocrine/eccrine/pilosebaceous apparatus, fibrosis, and scarring.

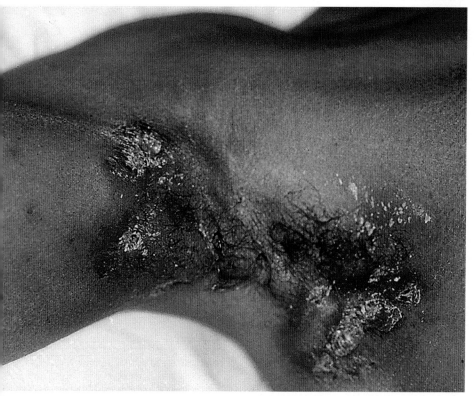

FIGURE 6-4 Hidradenitis suppurativa Axillae with inflammatory cysts, sinus tract formation, and keloids.

COURSE AND PROGNOSIS

Spectrum of disease is very broad. Many patients have mild involvement. The disease sometimes undergoes a spontaneous remission with age (more than 35 years). In some individuals, the course can be relentlessly progressive, with marked morbidity related to chronic pain, draining sinuses, and scarring. Pain control and exuberant drainage requiring hospitalization are not uncommon.

TREATMENT

1. Weight reduction and methods of decreasing friction and moisture are helpful. Loose clothing/undergarments, absorbent powders can help provide symptomatic relief.
2. Antibacterial soaps and topical clindamycin has been useful to reduce *S. aureus* carriage and secondary infection.
3. Intralesional triamcinolone (3–5 mg/mL) into early inflammatory lesions can hasten resolution and decrease pain.
4. Systemic steroids, systemic antibiotics, cyproterone acetate, ethinyl estradiol, isotretinoin, acitretin, finasteride, cyclosporine, TNF-α inhibitors and TNF inhibition in combination with botulinum toxin have been used in refractory severe cases with limited success.
5. With extensive, chronic disease, complete excision or CO_2 laser ablation of involved axillary tissue or inguinal area may be required.

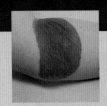

DISORDERS OF MELANOCYTES

ACQUIRED MELANOCYTIC NEVI

Acquired melanocytic nevocellular nevi are small (<1 cm), benign, well-circumscribed, pigmented lesions comprised of groups of melanocytes or melanocytic nevus cells.
They can be classified into three groups:

1. Junctional nevi (cells grouped at the dermal–epidermal junction, above the basement membrane).
2. Dermal nevi (cells grouped in the dermis).
3. Compound nevi (combination of histologic features of junctional and dermal).

Clinical overlap exists among all three types.

INSIGHT Only some 30% of melanomas arise from pre-existing nevi; thus prophylactically removing all the nevi on a person is neither warranted nor protective.

SYNONYMS Pigmented nevi, nevocellular nevus, moles.

EPIDEMIOLOGY

AGE Nevi appear after 6 to 12 months of age, peak during the third decade, and then slowly disappear.
INCIDENCE Common. By age 25, most Caucasians will have 20 to 40 moles.
GENDER M = F.
RACE Caucasians have more total body nevi than darker skin types. Asians and blacks have more nevi on atypical locations (palms, soles, nail beds, and conjunctivae) than whites.

GENETICS Increased number of nevi tend to cluster in families. Increased clinically atypical nevi may be more prevalent in families with melanoma.

HISTORY

DURATION OF LESIONS Commonly called *moles*, lesions appear after the age of 6 to 12 months and reach a maximum number between ages 20 and 29. By age 60, many moles fade and/or disappear.
SKIN SYMPTOMS Nevocellular nevi are asymptomatic. If a mole is symptomatic, it should be evaluated and/or removed.

DIFFERENTIAL DIAGNOSIS

Melanocytic nevi need to be differentiated from seborrheic keratoses, dermatofibromas, neurofibromas, fibroepithelial polyps, basal cell carcinomas, and melanomas.

MANAGEMENT

Indications for removal of acquired melanocytic nevi are the following:

1. *Asymmetry in shape.* One-half is different from the other.
2. *Border.* Irregular borders are present.
3. *Color.* Color is or becomes variegated. Shades of gray, black, white are worrisome.
4. *Diameter.* Greater than 6 mm (may be congenital mole, but should be evaluated).
5. *Evolution:* If the lesion is growing rapidly, distinct from other nevi or a child's overall growth pattern.
6. *Symptoms.* Lesion begins to persistently itch, hurt, or bleed.
7. *Site.* If the lesion is repeatedly traumatized in any given location (e.g., waistline, neck) or if the lesion is in a high-risk/difficult-to-monitor site such as the mucous membranes or anogenital area, it may warrant removal.

These criteria are based on anatomic sites at risk for change of acquired nevi to malignant melanoma *or* on changes in individual lesions (color, border) that indicate the development of a focus of cells with *dysplasia,* the precursor of malignant melanoma. Dysplastic nevi are *usually* >6 mm, and darker, with a variegation of color (tan, brown), and irregular borders. Approximately one-third of melanomas are associated with precursor nevi, and an increased number of nevi increases the melanoma risk.

Melanocytic nevi, if treated, should always be excised for histologic diagnosis and for definitive treatment. Destruction by electrocautery, laser, or other means is not recommended.

JUNCTIONAL NEVUS

PHYSICAL EXAMINATION

Skin Lesions

TYPE Macule.
SIZE Less than 1 cm.
COLOR Uniform tan, brown, or dark brown.
SHAPE Round or oval with smooth regular borders (Fig. 7-1).
ARRANGEMENT Scattered discrete lesions.
DISTRIBUTION Random.

SITES OF PREDILECTION Trunk, upper extremities, face, lower extremities; may be located on palms, soles, and genitalia.

DERMATOPATHOLOGY

HISTOLOGY In junctional nevi, the cells and/or nest of nevus cells are located in the lower epidermis.
DERMOSCOPY Uniform pigment network thinning out toward the periphery of the lesion.

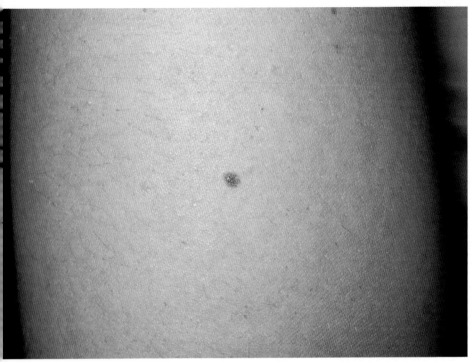

FIGURE 7-1 Junctional nevus Brown macule with regular borders and uniform pigment.

DERMAL NEVUS

SYNONYM Intradermal nevus.

PHYSICAL EXAMINATION

Skin Lesions

TYPE Elevated papule, nodule, polypoid, or papillomatous lesion.
COLOR Skin-colored, tan, or brown.
SHAPE Round, dome-shaped (Fig. 7-2).
DISTRIBUTION More common on the face and neck, but can occur on the trunk or extremities.
OTHER FEATURES Coarse hairs may be present within the lesion. Dermal nevi usually appear in late adolescence, 20s, and 30s.

DIFFERENTIAL DIAGNOSIS

Dermal nevi may be mistaken for other nevi such as junctional nevi, and on the face, from basal cell carcinoma.

DERMATOPATHOLOGY

HISTOLOGY Dermal nevi have nevus cells and/or nests in the dermis.
DERMOSCOPY Focal globules and white structure-less areas.

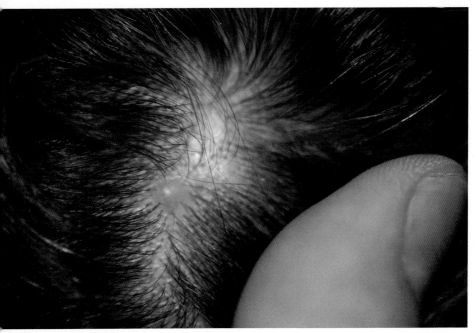

FIGURE 7-2 Dermal nevus Raised brown dome-shaped papule with regular borders and uniform pigment on the scalp of an adolescent.

COMPOUND NEVUS

PHYSICAL EXAMINATION

Skin Lesions

TYPE Macule or slightly elevated papule, or nodule (Fig. 7-3).
COLOR Tan, brown, or dark brown.
SHAPE Round.
DISTRIBUTION Any site.
OTHER FEATURES In late childhood, compound nevi can increase in darkness and become more elevated.

DERMATOPATHOLOGY

HISTOLOGY In compound nevi, nevus cells and/or nests are seen in both the epidermis and dermis.
DERMOSCOPY Globular ovoid pattern sometimes in a cobblestone pattern, structureless brown or hypopigmented areas with reticulated periphery, or mixed pattern.

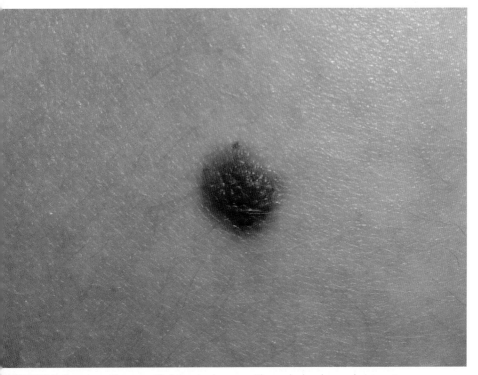

FIGURE 7-3 Compound nevus Slightly raised nevus with regular borders and pigment.

CONGENITAL NEVOMELANOCYTIC NEVUS

Congenital melanocytic nevi (CMN) are pigmented lesions of the skin usually present at birth. CMN may be of any size from very small to very large. CMN are benign neoplasms comprising cells called *nevomelanocytes,* which are derived from melanoblasts.

SYNONYMS Giant pigmented nevus, congenital nevomelanocytic nevus, garment nevus, bathing-trunk nevus, and giant hairy nevus.

EPIDEMIOLOGY

AGE Present at birth (congenital). Rarely, a CMN becomes visible after birth ("tardive"), usually within the first 3 to 12 months of life.
GENDER M = F.
RACE All races.
INCIDENCE Small CMN: 0.5% to 2.5% of the population. Large/giant CMN: 0.005% of the population.
ETIOLOGY Likely multifactorial. Rare familial cases have been reported.

PATHOPHYSIOLOGY

CMN are derived from neural crest-derived melanoblasts embryologically migrating to form the nevus after 10 weeks in utero but before the sixth month of gestation. It is unclear what causes these melanoblasts to migrate differently from other melanoblasts when forming nevi in the skin. CMN have shown an increase in mutations in the gene *NRAS,* suggesting a possible contributor to their etiology.

HISTORY

Congenital nevi are present at or soon after birth. They begin as pale brown to tan macules, which become darker and more elevated during adolescence. Most of them are benign and grow proportionally with the child and are asymptomatic for life. As the child grows older, the lesions develop coarse terminal hairs and may become more verrucous in appearance.

PHYSICAL EXAMINATION

Skin Lesions

TYPE Well-circumscribed macules, slightly raised papules or plaques with or without coarse terminal hairs.
BORDERS Sharply demarcated, regular contours.
SURFACE May or may not have altered skin surface ("pebbly," mammillated, rugose, cerebriform, bulbous, tuberous, or lobular).

COLOR Light or dark brown. May exhibit a "halo" phenomenon with a peripheral rim of depigmentation over time.
SIZE Small CMN: <1.5 cm; medium CMN: 1.5 to 20 cm (Fig. 7-4); large/giant CMN: >20 cm. CMN >9 cm on the scalp or >6 cm on the trunk in newborns qualify as large/giant CMN based on an expected adult size of >20 cm.
SHAPE Oval or round, symmetric. Large/giant plaques may have a geographic appearance.
DISTRIBUTION Isolated, discrete lesions on any site.

DIFFERENTIAL DIAGNOSIS

Without a good birth history, small CMN are often confused with common acquired nevomelanocytic nevi. A CMN can also be confused with a dysplastic nevus, Mongolian spot, nevus of Ota, congenital blue nevus, nevus spilus, Becker's nevus, neurofibroma, smooth muscle hamartoma, pigmented epidermal nevus, or café au lait macule (CALM).

LABORATORY EXAMINATIONS

HISTOPATHOLOGY In congenital nevi, the nevomelanocytes occur as well-ordered clusters in the epidermis, and in the dermis as sheets, nests, or cords. Unlike the common acquired nevomelanocytic nevus, the nevomelanocytes in CMN tend to occur in the skin appendages (eccrine ducts, hair follicles, and sebaceous glands), in nerve fascicles and/or arrectores pilorum muscles, blood vessels (especially veins), and lymphatic vessels, and extend into the lower two-thirds of the reticular dermis and deeper.
DERMOSCOPY Reticular, globular, reticular-globular, diffuse brown or multicomponent pigment pattern.

COURSE AND PROGNOSIS

By definition CMN appear at birth but varieties of CMN may arise during infancy (so-called tardive CMN). The lifetime risk for development of melanoma in small or medium CMN is low. Patients with large/giant CMN have been estimated to have a lifetime risk of 4.5% to 6.3% for developing melanoma within the CMN, though estimates vary widely both below and above this range.

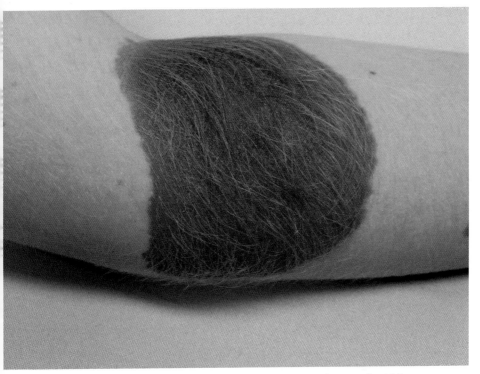

FIGURE 7-4 Congenital nevus A medium-sized congenital nevus on the arm of a child.

Neurocutaneous melanosis is a rare condition associated with large/giant CMNs, or multiple >3 cm smaller CMNs. Histologically, melanosis may be seen at the base of the brain, ventral surfaces of the pons, medulla, upper cervical, or lumbosacral spinal cord. It may be asymptomatic, or cause seizures, focal neurologic deficits or obstructive hydrocephalus. The latter symptomatic form carries a worse prognosis.

MANAGEMENT

Small (<1.5 cm) and medium (1.5–20 cm) benign-appearing congenital nevi can be safely monitored clinically. Their risk of malignant transformation is too low to warrant removal, thus patients should be instructed about signs of malignant transformation and regular skin examinations should suffice:

1. *Changes in shape.* One-half is different from the other.
2. *Irregular or fuzzy borders.* Irregular borders are present.
3. *Color variegation.* Shades of gray, black, white are worrisome.
4. *Symptoms.* Lesion begins to persistently itch, hurt, or bleed.

Large/giant CMN (>20 cm) are clinically difficult to manage since the risk of malignant transformation is present at birth, plus they are logistically more difficult to remove. It is important to follow these lesions clinically with measurements and/or photographs. Complete surgical removal of the lesion is difficult and often requires multiple-staged surgeries with tissue expansion, skin grafting, and/or artificial skin replacement.

An MRI to screen for neurocutaneous melanosis should be considered in neonates with large posterior axial lesions or multiple satellite nevi. Asymptomatic neurocutaneous melanosis can be monitored with repeat scans. Symptomatic neurocutaneous melanosis carries such a poor prognosis that surgical removal of the large CMN is typically not pursued.

Dermabrasion, laser removal, cryosurgery, electrocautery, or curettage of congenital nevi of any size is currently *not* recommended.

ATYPICAL "DYSPLASTIC" MELANOCYTIC NEVUS

Atypical "dysplastic nevi" are acquired nevi with a clinically atypical appearance: asymmetry, irregular borders, and/or color variation. Histologically, they may exhibit architecturally or cytologically atypical cells, the significance of which is controversial.

SYNONYMS Clark's nevus, B-K mole.

EPIDEMIOLOGY

AGE May appear at any age.
GENDER M = F.
RACE White = black.
INCIDENCE Estimated 5% of the population.
ETIOLOGY Familial tendency.
GENETICS Autosomal dominant.

PATHOPHYSIOLOGY

Genetic loci (especially *CDKN2A* located at 9p21) have been implicated in familial cases of dysplastic nevi/melanoma. Immunosuppression is also associated with an increased risk of dysplastic nevi.

HISTORY

Dysplastic nevi typically appear later in childhood (puberty) than benign nevi. They most frequently involve the trunk and show a predilection for covered areas of the body (scalp, breasts in females, and bathing trunk in males), and are more numerous in sun-exposed areas.
SKIN SYMPTOMS Typically asymptomatic. Itching or bleeding may be indicators of malignant change.

PHYSICAL EXAMINATION

Skin Findings

TYPE Macules, papules, or poorly circumscribed nodules.
SIZE 6 to 15 mm.
COLOR Asymmetrically brown, tan, pink, or variegated (Fig. 7-5).
SHAPE Round to oval with irregular or angulated borders.

DISTRIBUTION Back > chest > extremities. Predilection for covered areas (scalp, breasts in females, and bathing trunk in males).

DIFFERENTIAL DIAGNOSIS

Dysplastic nevi can be confused with acquired nevomelanocytic nevi, small congenital nevi, melanoma, Spitz nevi, seborrheic keratoses, solar lentigines, and other pigmented lesions.

LABORATORY EXAMINATIONS

DERMATOPATHOLOGY The histologic criteria for a dysplastic nevus include the following:

1. Architectural disorder with asymmetry of the lesion.
2. Intraepidermal melanocytes in a single file or nests beyond the dermal component.
3. Lentiginous hyperplasia with elongation of the rete ridges (may be "bridging").
4. ± Fibrotic changes around the rete ridges.
5. ± Vascular changes.
6. ± Inflammation.

COURSE AND PROGNOSIS

Clinically, it seems atypical nevi are an intermediate on the continuum between normal common nevi and melanoma. The majority of atypical nevi are clinically stable and *not* inevitable precursors to melanoma. A rare few do progress to melanoma, especially in patients with numerous atypical nevi or a family history of melanoma. Thus these patients should self-check for changes in their moles and routinely have their skin checked by a physician.

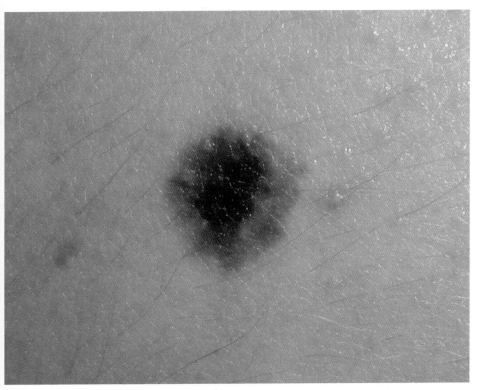

FIGURE 7-5 Dysplastic nevus Nevus with irregular borders and several shades of pigment.

MANAGEMENT

Patients with atypical nevi should have regular skin examinations with excision and histologic evaluation of any changing or worrisome lesions. These patients should also be educated and instructed on worrisome signs in moles:

1. *Asymmetry in shape.* One-half is different from the other.
2. *Border.* Irregular borders are present.
3. *Color.* Color is or becomes variegated. Shades of gray, black, white are worrisome.
4. *Diameter.* Greater than 6 mm (may be congenital mole, but should be evaluated).
5. *Evolution:* If the lesion is growing rapidly, distinct from other nevi or a child's overall growth pattern.
6. *Symptoms.* Lesion begins to persistently itch, hurt, or bleed. If a skin lesion is constantly trau-

matized in any given location (e.g., waistline, neck) or if lesion is in a high-risk/difficult-to-monitor site such as the mucous membranes or anogenital area, it may warrant removal.

It may be harder for patients to follow these general guidelines given the atypical presentation of their dysplastic nevi at baseline, thus routine skin examinations (± photos) with a physician are recommended. Physicians will be looking for lesions that "stand out" or differ from the patient's other baseline nevi. It is not recommended to remove all clinically atypical nevi; rather, close follow-up and removal of changing or worrisome nevi is indicated. Additionally, first-degree relatives of patients with melanoma or atypical nevi should have regular skin checks, and counseling regarding sun avoidance and protection.

BLUE NEVUS

A blue nevus is an acquired, benign, small, dark blue to blue–black, sharply defined papule or nodule of melanin-producing dermal melanocytes.

SYNONYMS Blue neuronevus, dermal melano-cytoma, common blue nevus, blue nevus of Jadassohn–Tieche.

EPIDEMIOLOGY

AGE May appear at any age; up to 25% are present at birth.
GENDER F > M, 2:1.
RARE VARIANTS Cellular blue nevus, combined blue nevus–nevomelanocytic nevus, plaque-type blue nevi.

PATHOPHYSIOLOGY

A blue nevus arises from ectopic dermal mela-nocytes. It is thought that melanocytes migrate away from the dermis during the second half of embryogenesis, and that blue nevi represent arrested embryonal migration of the melano-cytes. They appear blue because of the Tyndall's phenomenon refracting light from the deeper location of the nevus cells. Mutations in the gene *GNAQ*, encoding a membrane G-protein with GTPase activity, have been found in a majority of blue nevi.

HISTORY

Blue nevi are benign growths that appear during childhood and adolescence, remain stable in size, and persist for life. In contrast, cellular blue nevi are generally >1 cm in size and have a low but distinct danger of malignant transfor-mation. Rarely, multiple blue nevi have been associated with the Carney complex, with find-ings including lentigines, and both cutaneous and internal myxomas.

PHYSICAL EXAMINATION

Skin Lesions

TYPE Macule or dome-shaped papule.
SIZE 2 to 10 mm.
COLOR Blue, blue–gray, blue–black (Fig. 7-6). Occasionally has target-like pattern of pigmen-tation.

SHAPE Usually round to oval.
DISTRIBUTION Dorsa of the hands and feet (50%), scalp or the face (34%), or buttocks (6%).

DIFFERENTIAL DIAGNOSIS

The diagnosis of a blue nevus is usually made on clinical findings. Although worrisome in color, blue nevi can be diagnosed by their normal skin markings. The diagnosis can be confirmed by excision and histologic examina-tion. The differential diagnosis includes a radia-tion tattoo, traumatic tattoo (e.g., pencil lead tip), dermatofibroma, glomus tumor, primary or metastatic melanoma, venous lake, angio-keratoma, sclerosing hemangioma, apocrine hidrocystoma, and a pigmented spindle cell (Spitz) nevus.

DERMATOPATHOLOGY

HISTOLOGY Skin biopsy reveals spindle-shaped melanocytes grouped in bundles in the middle and lower third of the dermis.
DERMOSCOPY Homogenous blue–gray or blue–black pigmentation.

COURSE AND PROGNOSIS

Common blue nevi appear and persist throughout life. They may flatten and fade in color over time. Malignant degeneration is rare.

MANAGEMENT

Common blue nevi smaller than 10 mm in diameter and stable for many years usually do not need excision. Those larger than 10 mm are more likely to be the cellular blue nevus vari-ant, which does have a low risk of malignant degeneration, and for which surgical removal is recommended. The sudden appearance or change of an apparent blue nevus also warrants surgical excision.

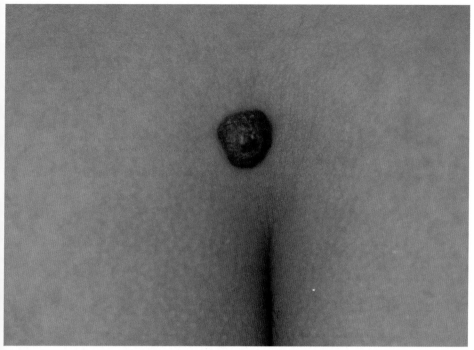

FIGURE 7-6 Blue nevus Blue–black 6-mm lesion on the buttock of a child.

HALO NEVUS

A halo nevus is a nevus (usually compound or dermal nevus) that becomes surrounded by a halo of depigmentation. The nevus then typically undergoes spontaneous involution and regression followed by repigmentation of the depigmented area.

SYNONYMS Sutton's nevus, leukoderma acquisitum centrifugum, perinevoid vitiligo.

EPIDEMIOLOGY

AGE Typically in patients <20 years. Age range: first through fifth decades.
GENDER M = F.
INCIDENCE <1% of patients under age 20 years.
FAMILY HISTORY Halo nevi occur in siblings and in persons with a family history of vitiligo.
ASSOCIATED DISORDERS 20% of patients with halo nevi have vitiligo. Most of them also have dysplastic nevi.
HALO DEPIGMENTATION AROUND OTHER LESIONS Typically halo nevi are compound or dermal nevi at the outset. However, halos have also been reported with blue nevi, congenital nevi, Spitz nevi, and melanomas.

PATHOPHYSIOLOGY

The triggering mechanism for halo nevi is unclear. It is thought perhaps a halo nevus represents a cell-mediated and/or humoral autoimmune response against nonspecifically altered nevomelanocytes. This results in cross-reactivity to distant nevomelanocytes (supported by the clinical observation that 20% of patients with halo nevi also exhibit vitiligo).

HISTORY

Three Stages

1. Development (in months) of halo around pre-existing nevus.
2. Disappearance (months to years) of nevus.
3. Repigmentation (months to years) of halo.

PHYSICAL EXAMINATION

Skin Lesions

TYPE Nevus: papular. Halo: macular.
SIZE Nevus: 3 to 10 mm. Halo: 1 to 5 mm beyond the nevus periphery (Fig. 7-7).
SHAPE Round to oval.
COLOR Nevus: pink, brown. Halo: initial erythema followed by depigmented white.
NUMBER 25% to 50% of patients have two or more halo nevi.

ARRANGEMENT Scattered discrete lesions (1 to 90 lesions).
DISTRIBUTION Trunk (especially the back).

LABORATORY EXAMINATIONS

DERMATOPATHOLOGY Dermal or compound nevus surrounded by lymphocytic infiltrate (lymphocytes and histiocytes) around and between nevus cells. In the halo areas, there is a decrease or absence of melanin and melanocytes (as shown by electron microscopy or immunohistochemistry).
DERMOSCOPY Symmetric, white structure-less area surrounding the nevus.
WOOD'S LAMP Examination of the clinical lesion with a Wood's lamp will accentuate the areas of depigmentation.

DIFFERENTIAL DIAGNOSIS

Halo nevi are clinically distinctive, and characterized by a nonworrisome junctional, dermal, or compound central nevus. In rare instances, halos of depigmentation can be seen around congenital nevi, atypical nevi, blue nevi, Spitz nevi, primary or metastatic melanoma, dermatofibromas, warts, or molluscum.

COURSE AND PROGNOSIS

The majority of halo lesions undergo spontaneous resolution, with subsequent clearing of the depigmented areas. In a few cases, the halo nevi persist or the nevus regresses, yet the depigmentation persists. Finally, in very rare instances (in adults), multiple halo nevi may be a precursor or sign of melanoma.

MANAGEMENT

Halo lesions undergo spontaneous resolution and the central regressing nevus need not be removed. The central nevus and complete skin should routinely be evaluated for clinical criteria of malignancy (variegation of pigment and irregular borders) as a halo can rarely be associated with melanoma (ocular or cutaneous). Worrisome or atypical lesions should be excised and sent for histologic evaluation.

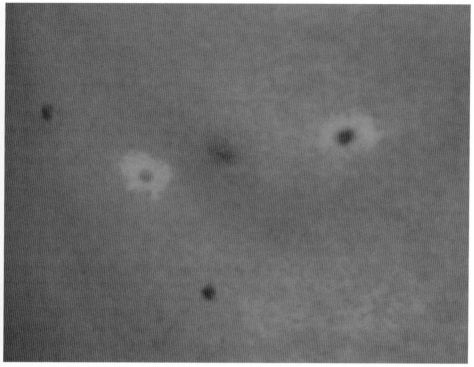

FIGURE 7-7 Halo nevus Scattered red–brown nevi, two with a depigmented halo.

NEVUS SPILUS

A nevus spilus is a flat brown macule dotted with superimposed smaller dark brown-to-black nevi (junctional nevi, compound nevi, Spitz nevi, blue nevi) that develop over time.

SYNONYMS Speckled lentiginous nevus, spotty nevus, spotted grouped pigmented nevus, nevus-on-nevus, zosteriform lentiginous nevus.

EPIDEMIOLOGY

AGE Macular component usually present at birth, but can appear later in life.
INCIDENCE Present in fewer than 2/1,000 newborns, found in 2% of the adult population.
GENDER M = F.

PATHOPHYSIOLOGY

The pathogenesis of a nevus spilus is unclear, but may represent a localized change in neural crest melanoblasts leading to the simultaneous or subsequent development of multiple different types of nevi; nevus spilus may be a variant of CMN. Genetic and environmental factors may play a role.

HISTORY

The macular component of a nevus spilus is usually present at birth, but can be acquired. Gradually more and more nevi appear superimposed on the congenital macule giving the nevus a "speckled" appearance. The entire lesion is typically asymptomatic and persists for life, growing proportionately with the child. Rarely, the nevi within the nevus spilus can become atypical. Nevus spilus may also rarely be associated with underlying muscle weakness or excessive sweating (hyperhidrosis), termed "speckled lentiginous nevus syndrome."

PHYSICAL EXAMINATION

Skin Findings

TYPE Background: macular. Superimposed nevi: small macules or papules (Fig. 7-8).
COLOR Background: light brown. Superimposed nevi: brown, blue, or dark brown–black.
SIZE AND SHAPE Background: 1 to 20 cm. Superimposed nevi: 1 to 6 mm.
SITES OF PREDILECTION Torso and extremities.
ARRANGEMENT May have a blaschkoid, segmental, or zosteriform configuration.

DIFFERENTIAL DIAGNOSIS

A nevus spilus can be confused with a CALM, Becker's nevus, compound nevus, congenital nevus, and/or junctional nevus.

LABORATORY EXAMINATIONS

DERMATOPATHOLOGY Background: epidermal hyperpigmentation with macromelanosomes or lentiginous melanocytic hyperplasia. Superimposed nevi: histologic changes of a congenital, junctional, compound, blue, Spitz, or atypical nevus.

DIFFERENTIAL DIAGNOSIS

A nevus spilus can be confused with a CALM or with agminated nevi (the latter has no background lesion).

COURSE AND PROGNOSIS

Nevus spilus rarely develop into malignant melanoma, and often persist throughout life asymptomatic and unchanging.

MANAGEMENT

Because nevus spilus does have nevus areas within it, its nevi should be monitored clinically for signs of worrisome changes, which include the following:

1. *Asymmetry in shape.* One-half is different from the other.
2. *Border.* Irregular borders are present.
3. *Color.* Color is or becomes variegated. Shades of gray, black, white are worrisome.
4. *Symptoms.* Lesion begins to persistently itch, hurt, or bleed.
5. *Evolution*: If the lesion is growing rapidly, distinct from other nevi or a child's overall growth pattern.

The lesions of nevus spilus tend to be several centimeters in diameter, thus prophylactic surgical excision is not recommended nor warranted. Routine clinical examination with biopsies and histologic evaluation of any worrisome central nevi is the current recommended approach.

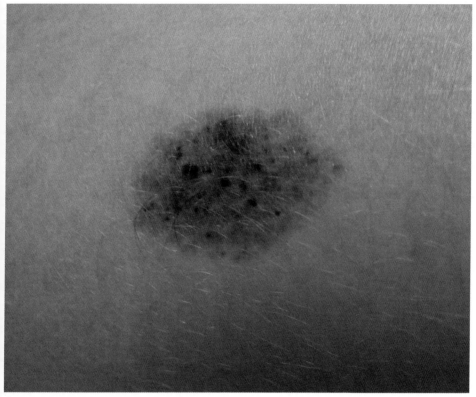

FIGURE 7-8 Nevus spilus Large tan macule dotted with numerous superimposed small dark nevi.

SPITZ (SPINDLE AND EPITHELIOID CELL) NEVUS

A Spitz nevus is a benign small red–brown, dome-shaped papule or nodule that appears suddenly (typically on the face) in a child. Despite the benign nature of the lesion, the histology is misleadingly worrisome, with spindle and epithelioid cells, some of which are atypical in appearance, resembling a melanoma.

 INSIGHT An experienced dermatopathologist is critical when evaluating Spitz nevi since histologically they can look very worrisome and be mistaken for melanoma with dire consequences for the child.

SYNONYMS Spitz tumor, benign juvenile melanoma, epithelioid cell–spindle cell nevus, Spitz juvenile melanoma.

EPIDEMIOLOGY

AGE One-third appear before age 10 years, one-third between ages 10 and 20 years. Rarely seen at birth. Rare in persons >40 years.
GENDER M = F.
INCIDENCE 1.4:100,000 in Australia.

PATHOPHYSIOLOGY

The pathogenesis of a Spitz nevus is unclear. The increased incidence in children, during pregnancy, and during puberty suggests developmental and hormonal influences.

HISTORY

Spitz nevi typically appear suddenly, rapidly grow, and then plateau. They can remain stable for years. They are typically asymptomatic and may persist for life or develop into a dermal nevus.

PHYSICAL EXAMINATION

Skin Findings

TYPE Papule or nodule.
COLOR Pink, tan to red–brown color (Fig. 7-9).
SIZE 2 mm to 2 cm (average diameter: 8 mm)
SHAPE Round, dome-shaped.
DISTRIBUTION Up to 42% found on the head and neck of children/adolescents. May have an agminated or grouped arrangement with multiple lesions clustered together.

DIAGNOSIS AND DIFFERENTIAL DIAGNOSIS

The diagnosis of a Spitz nevus is usually made clinically. The differential diagnosis includes a dermal nevus, pyogenic granuloma, hemangioma, molluscum contagiosum, dermatofibroma, mastocytoma, juvenile xanthogranuloma, and nodular melanoma.

LABORATORY EXAMINATIONS

DERMATOPATHOLOGY Skin biopsy shows large nests of epithelioid and spindle cells with abundant cytoplasm and occasional mitotic figures. The nests extend into the dermis in a characteristic "raining down" pattern. There are also coalescent eosinophilic globules (Kamino bodies) present in the basal layer in 80% of biopsies.

COURSE AND PROGNOSIS

Spitz nevi appear suddenly and enlarge rapidly. They then plateau and persist for years, some may morphologically change into a dermal nevus. Spitz nevi are benign but there are case reports of "metastatic Spitz nevi" in which nevus cells are found in local lymph nodes (the significance of which is unclear) and rare instances of Spitz progression to melanoma.

MANAGEMENT

Because Spitz nevi are benign, in cases with a classic appearance and clinical history, no treatment is needed. However, the rapid onset and growth of the lesion is often worrisome to clinicians and the lesions are often removed by excisional biopsy. Once excised, good dermatopathologic examination is needed to distinguish the Spitz nevi from melanoma. Several consultative opinions may be necessary to rule out melanoma in borderline or atypical Spitz lesions. If atypical features are noted on the pathology, close regular follow-up with a dermatologist may be warranted for periodic skin examinations and surveillance.

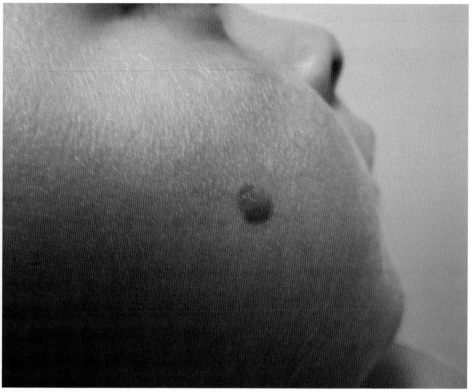

FIGURE 7-9 Spitz nevus A red–brown dome-shaped papule on a child's face.

EPIDERMAL MELANOCYTIC DISORDERS

EPHELIDES

Ephelides (freckles) are light brown macules that occur on sun-exposed skin most frequently observed in light-skinned individuals.

SYNONYM Freckles.

EPIDEMIOLOGY

AGE Not present at birth. Usually appear before age 3 with sun exposure.
GENDER M = F.
SEASON Increase in size, number, and degree of pigmentation during summer. Decrease in winter.
ETIOLOGY Related to sun exposure. Maybe autosomal dominantly inherited. Linked with light skin color and red or blond hair.

PATHOPHYSIOLOGY

Sun exposure stimulates the melanocytes to focally produce more melanin, and the more fully melanized melanosomes are transported from the melanocytes to the keratinocytes. Ephelides also demonstrate larger melanocytes compared to normal uninvolved skin.

PHYSICAL EXAMINATION

Skin Findings

GENETICS Ephelides have been associated with variants in the melanocortin 1 receptor (MC1R) gene
TYPE 1- to 5-mm macules.
COLOR Light brown to brown.
SHAPE Round to stellate.
DISTRIBUTION Sun-exposed skin: nose, cheeks (Fig. 7-10), chest, shoulders, arms, and upper back.

LABORATORY EXAMINATIONS

DERMATOPATHOLOGY Normal number of melanocytes but increased melanin content in the basal keratinocytes.
WOOD'S LAMP May accentuate and reveal more freckling.

DIFFERENTIAL DIAGNOSIS

The diagnosis of ephelides is made clinically. Ephelides (freckles) differ from lentigines in that ephelides are only in sun-exposed areas and eventually fade with time, whereas lentigines can be found on any site and persist despite sun avoidance. Small macular nevi may also be mistaken for ephelides, but tend to be darker and persist similar to lentigines.

COURSE AND PROGNOSIS

Mild sun-induced ephelides are benign [unless associated with xeroderma pigmentosum (XP)] and tend to disappear with age. Severe sunburn-induced freckles (from a blistering sunburn) are typically more stellate in shape and permanent. When extensive ephelides are seen in persons with dark hair, XP or a heterozygous carrier for XP should be considered.

MANAGEMENT

Ephelides are benign, fade with time, and do not require treatment. However, they are a marker for increased sun susceptibility coupled with past UV damage. Thus freckled individuals should have regular skin examinations and be counseled regarding avoidance of sun exposure and good sunscreen application.

Cosmetically, ephelides can be masked by cover-up makeup, and eventually lighten with time and sun avoidance. For faster results, ephelides can be lightened with α-hydroxy acid, salicylic acid, azelaic acid, hydroquinone, tretinoin, liquid nitrogen, or laser. Care must be taken in these approaches not to worsen the cosmetic outcome with subsequent dyspigmentation or depigmentation of uninvolved skin.

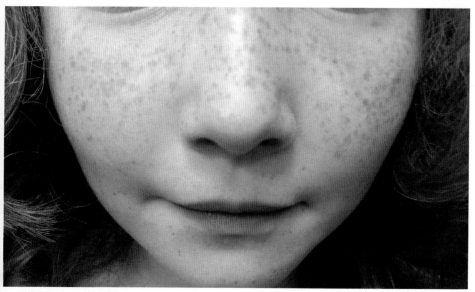

FIGURE 7-10 Ephelides Scattered brown freckles on the cheeks of a child with red hair.

LENTIGO SIMPLEX AND LENTIGINES-ASSOCIATED SYNDROMES

A lentigo simplex is a well-circumscribed brown macular lesion with increased numbers of melanocytes (which distinguishes it from ephelides) without any predilection for sun-exposed areas (differing from adult solar lentigines). There are also several syndromes characterized by lentiginosis (Table 7-1).

EPIDEMIOLOGY

AGE Can be present at or near birth, increase during adolescence, and persist for life. May also be a marker for a lentiginosis syndrome (Table 7-1).
GENDER M = F.
RACE All equally.

PATHOPHYSIOLOGY

An increased number of melanocytes produce more melanin resulting in hyperpigmented macules. The cause is unknown, but may be from a genetic alteration of the neuroectoderm.

PHYSICAL EXAMINATION

Skin Findings

TYPE Macules to patches (Fig. 7-11).
SIZE <5 mm.
COLOR Tan, light brown, dark brown, or black.
SHAPE Round or oval.
NUMBER Maybe solitary or numerous.
DISTRIBUTION Can be found on any cutaneous surface including palms, soles, and mucous membranes. Genital lentigines are not uncommon.

DIFFERENTIAL DIAGNOSIS

The diagnosis of lentigines is made by clinical examination. Simple lentigines can be difficult to distinguish from ephelides, junctional nevi, solar lentigines, or macular seborrheic keratoses. Lentigines differ from ephelides (freckles) in that while ephelides eventually fade, lentigines persist for life.

LABORATORY EXAMINATIONS

DERMATOPATHOLOGY Increased number of melanocytes along the dermal–epidermal junction and elongation of the rete ridges.
ELECTRON MICROSCOPY Melanin macroglobules found in the melanocytes, keratinocytes, and melanophages.
WOOD'S LAMP May accentuate and reveal more lentigines.
DERMOSCOPY Light brown structure-less or reticular pattern.

COURSE AND PROGNOSIS

Lentigines, as an isolated finding, are benign and asymptomatic. Typically, the pigmented macules are present at or near birth, increase in number during puberty, and persist for life (but may fade slightly in adulthood). The presence of multiple lentigines may be a marker of a more systemic lentiginosis syndrome.

MANAGEMENT

Lentigines are benign and do not require treatment.

Cosmetically, lentigines can be masked by cover-up makeup, and eventually lighten with time. For faster results, lentigines can be lightened with α-hydroxy acids, salicylic acid, azelaic acid, hydroquinone, tretinoin, liquid nitrogen, or laser. Care must be taken in these approaches not to worsen the cosmetic outcome with subsequent dyspigmentation.

Lesions on acral skin or mucous membranes should be monitored for clinical atypia because they can rarely progress to lentigo maligna. Although commonly restricted to the cutaneous surface only, patients with generalized lentiginosis should be monitored for systemic disease.

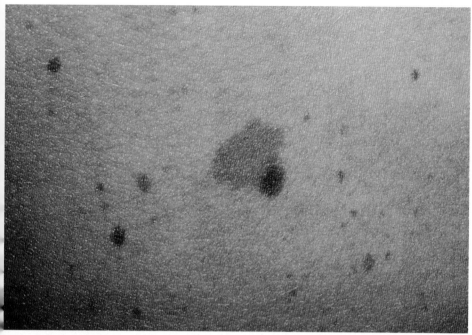

FIGURE 7-11 Lentigines Scattered brown macular spots on the back of a child with multiple lentigines (LEOPARD) syndrome.

TABLE 7-1 Lentiginous Syndromes

Disorder	Synonyms	Age	Etiology	Cutaneous Findings	Associated Features
Eruptive lentiginosis		Adolescents and young adults		Widespread occurrence of several hundred lentigines over months to years	
Segmental lentiginosis				Lentigines confined to one side of the body	Dermatomal type: benign. Nondermatomal type: may be associated with CNS abnormality or neurofibromatosis.
Nevus spilus	Nevoid lentigo; speckled lentiginous nevus	Infancy or childhood		Macular café au lait background with overlying 1–3 mm more deeply pigmented spots	Typically benign. Rare malignant transformation into melanomas have been reported.
PUVA lentigines			PUVA treatments	Disseminated hyperpigmented macules	Occur in 10–40% of PUVA patients; more prevalent in those treated for >5 years
Inherited patterned lentiginosis		Infancy or early childhood	AD inherited	Lentiginosis of face, lips, extremities, buttocks, and palmoplantar surfaces	
Multiple lentigines syndrome	LEOPARD syndrome	Infancy and evolve until adulthood	AD inherited, mutation in *PTPN11* gene	Multiple lentigines especially on upper trunk and neck. Mucosal surfaces spared. Café noir macules—similar to CALM but with darker pigmentation closer to lentigines.	L = Lentigines E = EKG abnormalities O = Ocular hypertelorism P = Pulmonary stenosis A = Abnormal genitalia R = Retardation of growth D = Deafness
LAMB and NAME syndromes	Carney complex, Syndrome myxoma	Childhood	AD inherited, mapped to gene *PRKAR1A*, 17q24	Multiple lentigines; ephelides, blue nevi, mucocutaneous myxoma. Also at risk for psammomatous schwannomas and adrenocortical disease, and testicular tumors.	L = Lentigines A = Atrial myxoma M = Mucocutaneous myxoma B = Blue nevi N = Nevi A = Atrial myxoma M = Mucocutaneous myxoma E = Ephelides

Peutz–Jeghers syndrome	Infancy and early childhood	AD inherited, mutation in the *STK11* gene, 19p13	Brown–black macules around mouth, lips, buccal mucosa, hands, and feet	Jejunal polyposis, increased risk of GI and non-GI malignancies
Cronkhite–Canada syndrome	Onset typically in adulthood		Diffuse brown macules on face and extremities. Alopecia and dystrophic nail changes	GI polyposis, diarrhea
Bannayan–Riley–Ruvalcaba syndrome; Macrocephaly, multiple lipomas, hemangioma syndrome	Onset in childhood	AD inherited, mutation in *PTEN* gene	Penile lentigines, vascular malformations, cutaneous lipomas, CALM	Macrocephaly, intestinal hamartomas
Sotos syndrome		Sporadic; *NSD1* or *NFIX* gene mutations	Lentigines of the penile shaft and glans penis	Macrocephaly, acromegaly, unusual facies, skeletal abnormalities
Centrofacial neurodysraphic lentiginosis	Lentiginosis centrofacial	Lesions appear at age 1–10	AD inherited	Closely clustered lentigines on the nose and infraorbital areas; mucous membranes spared	Status dysraphicus, neuropsychiatric disorder, epilepsy, increased risk of mental retardation

PEUTZ–JEGHERS SYNDROME

Peutz–Jeghers syndrome is a rare autosomal dominantly inherited disorder characterized by familial polyposis and lentigines on the lips and oral mucous membranes. Polyps in the GI tract may occur, with abdominal symptoms manifesting in childhood or early adulthood.

EPIDEMIOLOGY

AGE Lentigines appear in infancy and early childhood. GI polyps appear in late childhood, before age 30.
GENDER M = F.
GENETICS Autosomal dominant with 100% penetrance and variable expressivity; >40% of cases are due to spontaneous mutations.
ETIOLOGY Mutation in the *STK11* gene.

HISTORY

The lentigines can be congenital or may develop during infancy and early childhood. The pigmented macules may disappear over time on the lips, but the pigmentation of the mouth does not disappear and is therefore the *sine qua non* for the diagnosis. The lentigines occur in some patients who have never had abdominal symptoms.
SYSTEMS REVIEW Abdominal pain can present anytime between ages 10 and 30. GI bleeding, melena, hematemesis, and anemia may also occur. The small bowel is most often affected, but large bowel, stomach, and esophageal polyps may also occur.

PHYSICAL EXAMINATION

Skin Findings

TYPE Macule.
COLOR Dark brown or black.
SIZE 2 to 5 mm. Lentigines on the face are smaller than those on the palms and soles and in the mouth.
SHAPE OF INDIVIDUAL LESION Round or oval.
ARRANGEMENT OF MULTIPLE LESIONS Closely set clusters of lesions.
DISTRIBUTION OF LESIONS Intraoral lentigines are the *sine qua non* of Peutz–Jeghers syndrome; the lesions are dark brown, black, or bluish-black. They are irregularly distributed on the gums, buccal mucosa, and hard palate (Fig. 7-12). Lentigines also occur on the lips, around the mouth, nose, palms, soles, hands, and nails.
NAILS May have longitudinal melanonychia (pigmented streaks or diffuse involvement of the nail bed).

GI TRACT Polyps, which may lead to abdominal pain, GI bleeding, intussusception, and obstruction.
OTHER ORGAN SYSTEMS Long-term slight increased risk of pancreatic cancer, ovarian/testicular tumors.

LABORATORY EXAMINATIONS

DERMATOPATHOLOGY On skin biopsy, there is increased melanin in the melanocytes and basal cells.
ELECTRON MICROSCOPY Numerous melanosomes with melanocytes and keratinocytes.
PATHOLOGY OF GI POLYPS Hamartomas, with mixture of glands and smooth muscle.
HEMATOLOGIC Anemia from blood loss may be present.
GASTROENTEROLOGY Stool examinations may reveal occult bleeding.
RADIOLOGIC STUDIES Imaging of the GI tract is important in patients with the clinical presentation of multiple lentigines of the type noted earlier.

DIFFERENTIAL DIAGNOSIS

In Peutz–Jeghers syndrome the mucosal pigmentation (intraorally) is the constant feature that remains throughout life. The differential diagnosis for mucosal hyperpigmentation includes normal mucosal pigmentation in darker skin types, amalgam tattoos, and staining from zidovudine therapy. The lentigines of Peutz–Jeghers can be differentiated from ephelides by being much darker and occurring in areas not exposed to sunlight (e.g., palms, soles). Also, the lentigines are not widely distributed as in the multiple lentigines syndrome (LEOPARD syndrome); they do not occur on the trunk or proximal extremities, but are localized to the central areas of the face, palms and soles, and dorsa of the hands.

COURSE AND PROGNOSIS

There is a normal life expectancy. Symptomatic GI polyps are the most difficult aspect of this syndrome and may require multiple polypectomies to relieve the symptoms. There is also an increased risk of developing gastrointestinal and pancreatic carcinoma.

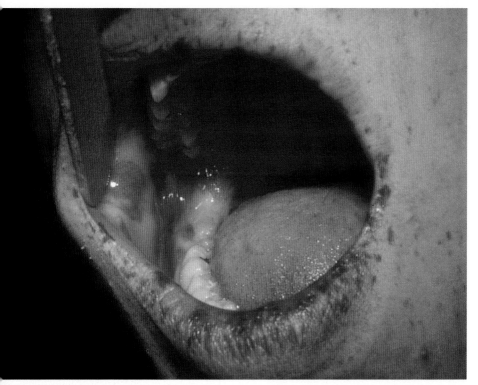

FIGURE 7-12 Peutz–Jeghers syndrome Scattered dark brown macules on the lips and buccal mucosa of a child with Peutz–Jeghers syndrome. The pigmented macules on the lips may fade with time, but the intraoral pigmentation persists for life.

MANAGEMENT

SKIN Lentigines are benign and do not require treatment. Cosmetically, lentigines can be masked by cover-up makeup, and eventually lighten with time. For faster results, lentigines can be lightened with α-hydroxy acids, salicylic acid, azelaic acid, hydroquinone, tretinoin, liquid nitrogen, or laser. Care must be taken in these approaches not to worsen the cosmetic outcome with subsequent dyspigmentation.

OTHER It is recommended that patients with Peutz–Jeghers syndrome have the following:

1. Hematocrit checked every 6 months for anemia.
2. Stool examination annually looking for occult blood.
3. Routine examinations with a gastroenterologist and appropriate GI studies (for patients >10 years old, small bowel follow-through examinations, upper endoscopies, and colonoscopies every 2 years).
4. Surgical polypectomies for symptomatic or large (>1.5 cm) GI polyps.

MULTIPLE LENTIGINES SYNDROME

The multiple lentigines syndrome is a multiorgan genodermatosis commonly referred to by its mnemonic: LEOPARD syndrome. Its principal visible manifestation is generalized lentigines (dark brown macules).

The seven features in the mnemonic are the following:

L (lentigines)
E (EKG abnormalities)
O (ocular hypertelorism)
P (pulmonary stenosis)
A (abnormal genitalia)
R (retardation of growth or dwarfism)
D (deafness).

SYNONYMS Multiple lentigines syndrome, cardiocutaneous syndrome, hypertrophic obstructive cardiomyopathy and lentiginosis, lentiginosis profusa syndrome, progressive cardiomyopathic lentiginosis.

EPIDEMIOLOGY

AGE Lentigines usually present at birth. Extracutaneous features do not appear until puberty. Mean age of diagnosis: 14 years.
GENDER M > F.
INCIDENCE Rare.
GENETICS Autosomal dominant inheritance with variable expressivity.
ETIOLOGY Mutation in *PTPN11* gene which encodes a protein-tyrosine phosphatase.

HISTORY

The lentigines are often congenital and increase in number, size, and darkness around puberty. They then begin to fade slowly throughout adulthood. Extracutaneous features are usually not manifested until puberty and include pulmonary stenosis, obstructive cardiomyopathy, atrial septal defects, primary pulmonary hypertension, pectus deformities, kyphoscoliosis, hypospadias, cryptorchidism, mental retardation, and sensorineural hearing loss. Cardiac abnormalities result in the greatest morbidity associated with the syndrome.

PHYSICAL EXAMINATION

Skin Findings

TYPE Numerous (generally hundreds to thousands) well-demarcated macules.
SIZE 1 to 5 mm.
COLOR Tan, brown, or black.
SHAPE Round or oval.
DISTRIBUTION Lentigines are concentrated on the face (Fig. 7-13A), neck, and upper trunk

(Fig. 7-13B) but may also involve the arms, palms, soles, and genitalia. Mucous membranes are spared.

General Findings

SKELETAL Growth retardation (<25th percentile), hypertelorism, pectus deformities, kyphoscoliosis, and winged scapulae.
CARDIOPULMONARY Includes pulmonary stenosis and conduction defects.
GENITOURINARY Gonad hypoplasia, renal agenesis.
NEUROLOGIC Sensorineural deafness, abnormal EEG, slowed peripheral nerve conduction.

LABORATORY EXAMINATIONS

DERMATOPATHOLOGY There is increased number of melanocytes in the basal layer.
ELECTRON MICROSCOPY Increased number/size of melanosomes in the keratinocytes.

DIFFERENTIAL DIAGNOSIS

Other lentiginous syndromes such as Peutz–Jeghers should be considered. The multiple lentigines syndrome typically has facial lentigines with sparing of the mucous membranes, whereas Peutz–Jeghers syndrome has marked intraoral involvement. Other syndromes with lentigines and their features are listed in Table 7-1.

COURSE AND PROGNOSIS

The skeletal, cardiac, and endocrine abnormalities are the most problematic. The lentigines are only of cosmetic concern and can get darker, larger, and more numerous with age.

MANAGEMENT

Lentigines are benign and do not require treatment. Cosmetically, lentigines can be masked by cover-up makeup, and eventually lighten

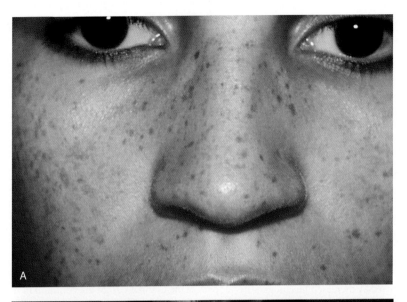

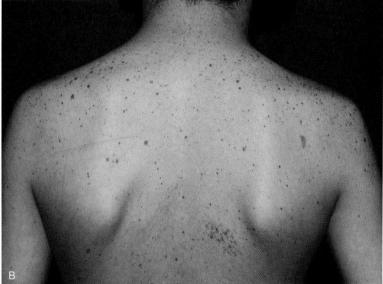

FIGURE 7-13 Multiple lentigines syndrome A: Scattered brown macules on the face of an individual with the multiple lentigines syndrome. **B:** Scattered brown macules on the back of an individual with multiple lentigines syndrome.

with time. For faster results, lentigines can be lightened with α-hydroxy acids, salicylic acid, azelaic acid, hydroquinone, tretinoin, liquid nitrogen, or laser. Care must be taken in these approaches not to worsen the cosmetic outcome with subsequent dyspigmentation.

The skeletal, cardiac, and endocrine abnormalities are the most problematic for LEOPARD patients. Although the extracutaneous fea-

tures are usually not manifested until puberty, LEOPARD patients need to be monitored and managed for pulmonary stenosis, obstructive cardiomyopathy, atrial septal defects, primary pulmonary hypertension, pectus deformities, kyphoscoliosis, hypospadias, cryptorchidism, mental retardation, and sensorineural hearing loss. Cardiac abnormalities result in the greatest morbidity associated with the syndrome.

CAFE AU LAIT MACULES AND ASSOCIATED SYNDROMES

CALM are large, round, well-circumscribed, light brown patches that range in size from 1 to 5 cm. One to three CALM are seen in 10% to 28% of normal individuals, but more than three CALM may be a marker for several syndromes such as neurofibromatosis (Table 7-2).

EPIDEMIOLOGY

AGE Present at birth or soon after. Can increase in size and number with age.
GENDER M = F.
PREVALENCE Present in 10% to 28% of the normal population.
RACE Blacks > whites.
ETIOLOGY Unclear.

PATHOPHYSIOLOGY

The defect leading to CALM formation has not been identified. CALM hyperpigmentation is caused by increased melanogenesis and subsequent higher melanin content in the keratinocytes.

PHYSICAL EXAMINATION

Skin Findings

TYPE Macule to patch.
SIZE 2 mm to 15 to 20 cm (Fig. 7-14).
COLOR Light brown: "coffee with milk."
SHAPE Round to oval.
DISTRIBUTION May occur anywhere on the body except mucous membranes.

LABORATORY EXAMINATIONS

DERMATOPATHOLOGY Increase in basal layer pigmentation with giant pigment granules in both the melanocytes and keratinocytes. Giant macromelanosomes (up to 5 μm in diameter) are usually present.
WOOD'S LAMP May accentuate and reveal CALM unapparent to visible light.

DIFFERENTIAL DIAGNOSIS

A CALM can be confused with an early nevus spilus, linear nevoid hyperpigmentation, Becker's nevus, postinflammatory hyperpigmentation, or a phytophotodermatitis.

COURSE AND PROGNOSIS

One to three CALM are common in normal individuals. They appear at or near birth, grow proportionally with the child, and are asymptomatic for life.

More than three CALM in one individual is rare (0.5% of the population) and can be a sign of a neurocutaneous disease such as neurofibromatosis, tuberous sclerosis, Albright's syndrome (polyostotic fibrous dysplasia), ataxia telangiectasia, Silver's syndrome, basal cell nevus syndrome, Turner's syndrome, or Cowden's disease.

MANAGEMENT

CALM are asymptomatic, benign, and do not require treatment. Cosmetically, CALM can be masked by cover-up makeup, or lightened/cleared with laser.

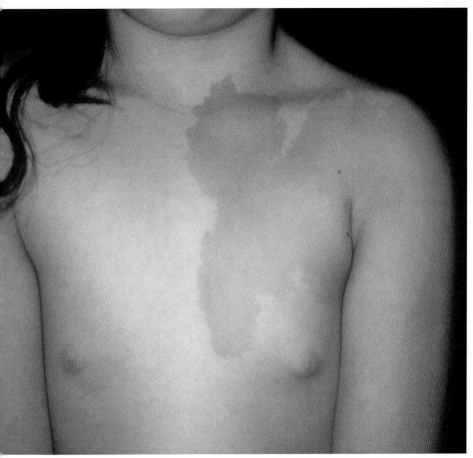

FIGURE 7-14 Café au lait macule (CALM) Large brown macule with irregular "coast of Maine" jagged borders in a girl with McCune–Albright syndrome.

TABLE 7-2 Café Au Lait Macules and Associated Syndromes

Disorder	Synonyms	Etiology	Cutaneous Findings	Associated Features
Neurofibromatosis type 1 (NF-1)	von Recklinghausen's disease	*NF1* gene mutation; AD	CALM, axillary/intertriginous freckling, cutaneous neurofibromas, peripheral nerve sheath tumors, large congenital nevi, xanthogranulomas	Lisch nodules, optic gliomas, macrocephaly, CNS tumors, seizures, kyphoscoliosis, sphenoid wing dysplasia, thinning of ribs, bowing deformity of the tibia and ulna, pseudoarthroses
Watson syndrome		*NF1* gene mutation; AD-likely; Variant of NF-1	CALM, intertriginous freckling	Intellectual deficit, short stature, pulmonary valve stenosis
Neurofibromatosis type 2 (NF-2)	Central neurofibromatosis	*NF2* gene mutation; AD	CALM may occur, few or absent neurofibromas	Acoustic neuromas (schwannomas), intracranial and intraspinal tumors, lens opacities
Neurofibromatosis type 5 (NF-5)	Segmental neurofibromatosis	Postzygotic *NF1* gene mutation	CALM, intertriginous freckling, neurofibromas in a segmental distribution	Deeper involvement within the involved body segment (bony or soft tissue growths)
Neurofibromatosis type 6 (NF-6)	Familial café au lait macules		CALM, intertriginous freckling	Rarely skeletal or learning abnormalities, Lisch nodules
McCune–Albright syndrome	Polyostotic fibrous dysplasia, Albright's syndrome	Mosaic *GNAS₁* gene mutation	CALM with more jagged "coast of Maine" borders (Fig. 7-14); CALMs usually end at midline	Polyostotic fibrous dysplasia, endocrine dysfunction, sexual precocity
Jaffe–Campanacci syndrome		*NF1* gene mutation; likely NF-1 variant	CALM with more jagged "coast of Maine" borders, nevi, perioral freckle-like macules	Non-ossifying fibromas, mental retardation, hypogonadism, precocious puberty; ocular, skeletal, and cardiac abnormalities

Disorder		Gene mutation	Cutaneous findings	Systemic features
Piebaldism		KIT gene mutation; AD	CALM, congenital depigmented patches	Rarely mental retardation, aganglionic megacolon, Hirschsprung disease
Tuberous sclerosis	Epiloa, Bourneville disease	TSC1 and TSC2 gene mutations; AD	CALM, hypomelanotic macules, adenoma sebaceum, periungual fibromas, shagreen patches	Seizures, mental retardation, rhabdomyomas, calcified brain nodules
Ataxia telangiectasia	Louis-Bar syndrome	ATM gene mutation; AR	CALM, telangiectasia of conjunctiva, neck: hyper- and hypopigmentation	Ataxia, myoclonus, choreoathetosis, impaired cell-mediated and humoral immunity
Silver–Russell syndrome	Russell–Silver syndrome		CALM, diffuse brown patches, achromic macules may be present	IUGR, macrocephaly, triangular facies, ambiguous genitalia, clinodactyly, hyperhidrosis, dwarfism
Bloom syndrome		BLM gene mutation; AR	CALM, photosensitivity, telangiectatic rash	Stunted growth, dolichocephaly, high-pitched voice, testicular atrophy, immune deficiencies
Multiple endocrine neoplasia type IIb (MEN-IIb)	MEN type III	RET gene mutation; AD	CALM; multiple mucosal neuromas on lips, oral cavity, and eyelids; abnormal pigmentation	Marfanoid habitus, thickened corneal nerves, GI ganglioneuromatosis, pheochromocytoma, medullary thyroid carcinoma
Turner's syndrome	Gonadal dysgenesis, XO syndrome	45, X karyotype	CALM, epicanthal folds, hypertelorism, webbed neck, redundant neck skin, lymphedema, alopecia areata	Short stature, deafness, gonadal dysgenesis (with sexual retardation), bicuspid aortic valve, PDA, coarctation of aorta, renal abnormalities
Cowden's syndrome	Multiple hamartoma syndrome	PTEN gene mutation; AD	CALM, multiple trichilemmomas, oral papillomatosis, acral keratoses	Breast cysts/malignancy, thyroid malignancies, GI polyps, ovarian cysts, uterus adenocarcinomas, lentigines

DERMAL MELANOCYTIC DISORDERS

CONGENITAL DERMAL MELANOCYTOSIS (MONGOLIAN SPOT)

Lesions of congenital dermal melanocytosis are benign, blue–black large macular lesions characteristically located over the lumbosacral area most commonly seen in Asian, black, and Hispanic populations. They typically self-resolve during childhood.

EPIDEMIOLOGY

AGE Present at birth and fades during first 1 to 2 years of life.
GENDER M = F.
RACE Seen in 90% to 100% of Asian infants, 65% to 95% of black infants, 85% of South American Indian infants, 63% of Indian infants, 46% of Hispanic infants, and <13% of white infants.
ETIOLOGY Dermal location of melanocytes results in blue–gray appearance to the skin (Tyndall's phenomenon).

PATHOPHYSIOLOGY

Melanocytes undergo embryonic migration from the neural crest to the epidermis. It is thought that these lesions represent migrational arrest with resultant ectopic melanocytes in the dermis, which appear blue–black from the Tyndall's phenomenon (longer wavelength colors including red, orange, and yellow are absorbed, but shorter wavelengths colors such as blue and violet are reflected, giving these lesions the blue color).

HISTORY

Lesions of dermal melanocytosis develop in utero and are most noticeable at birth. They are asymptomatic, benign, and darker in color until age 1 year, enlarge in size until age 2 years, and then spontaneously disappear by age 10 to 12 years. Fewer than 5% of these lesions persist for life. No melanomas have been reported to occur arising from congenital dermal melanocytosis.

PHYSICAL EXAMINATION

Skin Findings
TYPE Poorly circumscribed macule to patch.
COLOR Deep brown, slate gray to blue–black.
SIZE Ranges from 1 cm to extensive areas (85% of cases occupy <5% of the body and only 5% involve >15% of the body surface area).
NUMBER Typically single lesion, rarely multiple.
DISTRIBUTION Anywhere especially buttock, back, shoulders.
SITES OF PREDILECTION Lumbosacral region (Fig. 7-15) > back > rest of body.

DIFFERENTIAL DIAGNOSIS

Lesions of dermal melanocytosis are sometimes mistaken for ecchymoses, but the areas are nontender. Congenital dermal melanocytosis must also be differentiated from a nevus of Ota, a nevus of Ito, and blue nevus.

LABORATORY EXAMINATIONS

DERMATOPATHOLOGY Elongated spindle-shaped melanocytes are present in the mid- to deep dermis.
ELECTRON MICROSCOPY Dermal melanocytes have a preponderance of mature melanosomes.

MANAGEMENT

Treatment is unnecessary because these lesions tend to fade by age 10 to 12 in the majority of individuals. Lesions of congenital dermal melanocytosis persist in fewer than 5% of the population. Cosmetically, lesions can be covered with makeup or lightened by laser treatment. Extensive dermal melanocytosis should raise the possibility of phakomatosis pigmentovascularis types II and IV.

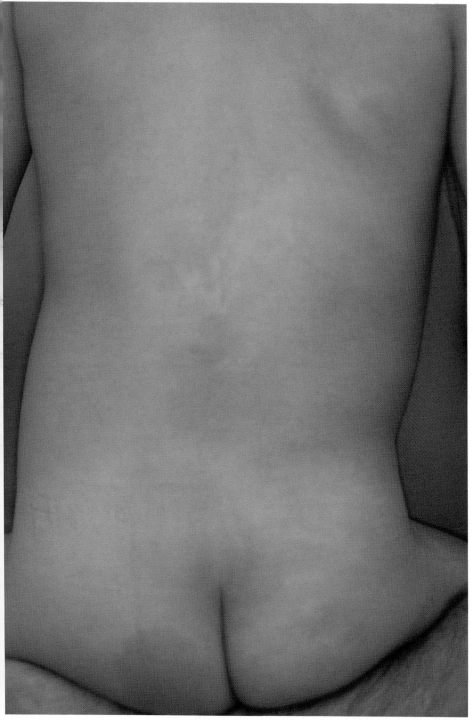

FIGURE 7-15 Congenital dermal melanocytosis Asymptomatic macular blue–gray pigmentation on the back of a child.

NEVUS OF OTA, NEVUS OF ITO

The nevus of Ota is a unilateral bluish-gray macular discoloration in the periorbital region (trigeminal nerve, first and second branches). The nevus of Ito is a similar blue–gray discoloration located on the neck and shoulder.

SYNONYMS Nevus fuscocaeruleus ophthalmomaxillaris (Ota), nevus fuscocaeruleus acromiodeltoideus (Ito), oculodermal melanocytosis, congenital melanosis bulbi, melanosis bulborum, aberrant dermal melanocytosis, progressive melanosis oculi, persistent aberrant dermal melanocytosis, oculomucodermal melanocytosis.

EPIDEMIOLOGY

AGE Bimodal age distribution: 50% are present at birth or in the first year of life, 36% appear between the ages of 11 and 20 years.
GENDER F > M, 5:1.
RACE More prevalent in Asians (75% of cases); less commonly seen in East Indians and blacks; and rarely seen in whites.
PREVALENCE Primary complaint in 0.4% to 0.8% of outpatient visits in Japan.
ETIOLOGY Dermal location of melanocytes results in blue–gray appearance of the skin (Tyndall's phenomenon).

PATHOPHYSIOLOGY

During embryonic development, melanocytes migrate from the neural crest to the epidermis. It is thought that the nevus of Ota and nevus of Ito represent melanocytes that have experienced migrational arrest in the dermis. Some have speculated that there is a hormonal influence as well, accounting for the lesions that appear at puberty and the female predominance. Trauma has also been reported as a triggering mechanism.

The nevi of Ota and Ito appear blue–black from the deep dermal location of the melanocytes and the optical Tyndall's phenomenon (longer wavelength colors such as red, orange, and yellow are not reflected, but shorter wavelengths colors such as blue and violet are reflected, resulting in a visibly blue–black in color).

HISTORY

Nevi of Ota/Ito are sometimes present at birth, or can appear during childhood/puberty. They may increase in intensity and extent during the first year of life. They persist for life. Most nevi of Ota/Ito are benign. There are rare reports of sensorineural deafness and melanoma associated with these lesions.

PHYSICAL EXAMINATION

Skin Findings

TYPE Poorly demarcated macules to patches with speckled or mottled appearance.
COLOR Patchy blue–gray, blue–black.
SIZE 1 to 10 cm.
DISTRIBUTION *Ota:* Typically unilateral, periorbital region, can involve ipsilateral sclera (Fig. 7-16). Fifty percent of cases involve the ophthalmic and maxillary branches of the fifth cranial nerve. Rarely, pigmentation can also involve conjunctiva, cornea, retina, lips, palate, pharynx, or nasal mucosa. *Ito:* Typically unilateral neck/shoulder region in the distribution of the posterior supraclavicular and lateral cutaneous nerves. In <5% of cases, these nevi can be bilateral. Nevi of Ota and Ito may also coexist in the same patient.

General Findings

Most nevi of Ota and Ito are seen as an isolated cutaneous findings; 9% of congenital nevi of Ota are associated with open-angle glaucoma. Other rare associations include cellular blue nevi, nevus flammeus (phakomatosis pigmentovascularis), and melanoma.

Differential Diagnosis

Nevi of Ito and Ota are sometimes mistaken for ecchymoses, but the areas are nontender. Nevi of Ito and Ota must also be differentiated from congenital dermal melanocytosis, blue nevi, melasma, and vascular malformations.

LABORATORY EXAMINATIONS

DERMATOPATHOLOGY Skin biopsy demonstrates increased number of dendritic melanocytes in the mid-to-deep dermis.

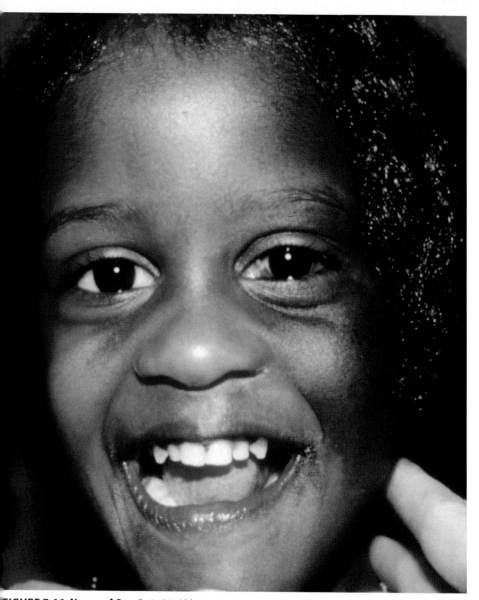

FIGURE 7-16 Nevus of Ota Periorbital blue–gray pigmentation with scleral involvement.

MANAGEMENT

Nevi of Ota and Ito do not require treatment. Cosmetically, they can be masked by cover-up makeup. They can also be lightened by laser. Because of their risk of malignancy, these nevi should be followed annually and new subcutaneous nodules should be biopsied for histologic examination. If ocular pigmentation is present, routine ophthalmologic examination (checking for glaucoma and/or ocular melanoma) is recommended.

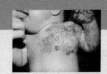
DISORDERS OF BLOOD AND LYMPH VESSELS

CONGENITAL VASCULAR LESIONS

INSIGHT It is important to differentiate between the three most common vascular anomalies in new-borns: capillary stains that self-resolve, port-wine stains that benefit from laser treatment, and hemangiomas, which spontaneously involute.

CAPILLARY STAIN (SALMON PATCH)

The salmon patch is the most common benign vascular lesion seen in infants, typically on the forehead, glabella, or nape of neck. Salmon patches are most prominent during infancy, then self-resolve during childhood.

SYNONYMS Nevus simplex, telangiectatic nevus, "stork bite," nuchal nevus, Unna's nevus, evanescent macule, angel kiss, or aigrette.

EPIDEMIOLOGY

AGE Present at birth, fades with time.
GENDER M = F.
INCIDENCE Occurs in 30% to 40% of newborns.
ETIOLOGY Thought to be a persistence of fetal circulation, gradually becomes less prominent.

HISTORY

Present at birth, these benign lesions fade with time. In lighter skin types, the patch may be more persistent or evident during episodes of crying or physical exertion. Fifty percent of salmon patches in the nuchal region persist for life. They are asymptomatic and benign.

PHYSICAL EXAMINATION

Skin Findings

TYPE Macular with telangiectasias.
COLOR Dull pink to red.
DISTRIBUTION Head and neck.
SITES OF PREDILECTION Nape of neck (22%), glabella (20%) (Fig. 8-1A), and eyelids (5%).

DIFFERENTIAL DIAGNOSIS

Salmon patch is the most common vascular birthmark. Its classic locations and self-resolving tendencies should differentiate it from other vascular birthmarks such as capillary malformations and hemangiomas.

LABORATORY EXAMINATIONS

HISTOPATHOLOGY Skin biopsy reveals dilated dermal capillaries.

COURSE AND PROGNOSIS

Facial salmon patches fade with time (Fig. 8-1B) and only become evident in lighter skin types with crying or physical exertion. Nuchal salmon patches can persist but are asymptomatic and not usually of cosmetic concern because they are covered by the posterior hairline.

MANAGEMENT

Unlike capillary malformations, facial salmon patches fade almost completely and usually do not require treatment. Persistent lesions can occur in the nuchal area, but these are typically covered with hair and not a cosmetic concern. Rare bothersome persistent lesions can be treated with laser ablation.

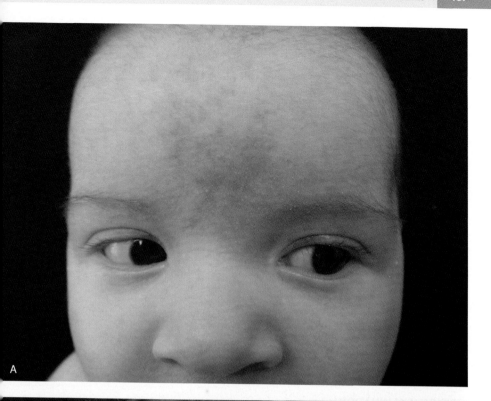

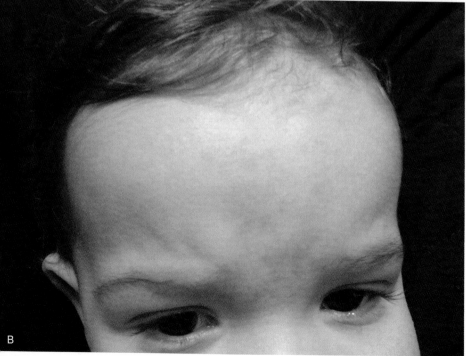

FIGURE 8-1 **Salmon patch** **A:** Salmon patch on the glabella of a newborn. **B:** Same child at age 1 year with barely any residual vascular lesion.

CAPILLARY MALFORMATIONS (PORT-WINE STAIN) AND ASSOCIATED SYNDROMES

The most common capillary malformation is a port-wine stain (PWS): a lesion comprising dilated capillaries, which are macular at onset, but become plaque-like with time as the capillaries dilate. The majority are present at birth, and unlike salmon patches, they persist for life. PWS are benign, but rarely may be associated with underlying syndromes such as Sturge–Weber (Table 8-1).

SYNONYMS Nevus flammeus, telangiectasia.

EPIDEMIOLOGY

AGE Present at birth, persists throughout life.
GENDER M = F.
RACE Whites > Asians > blacks.
ETIOLOGY Mutation in vascular morphogenesis.

PATHOPHYSIOLOGY

Given the occasional association of a PWS with Sturge–Weber or Klippel–Trenaunay syndromes (Table 8-1), it is postulated that the PWS is caused by a mutation in the anterior neural crest or mesoderm during embryogenesis. Activating mutations in the gene GNAQ have been linked with both PWSs and the Sturge–Weber syndrome.

PHYSICAL EXAMINATION

Skin Lesions

TYPE Infancy: macular. Adulthood: nodular, plaque-like.

COLOR Infancy: pink. Adulthood: red, purple.
SHAPE Segmental. Large lesions follow a dermatomal distribution and rarely cross the midline (Fig. 8-2A).
DISTRIBUTION Localized or diffuse. Most commonly involve the face in a trigeminal nerve distribution (V1, V2, or V3).

DIFFERENTIAL DIAGNOSIS

The diagnosis of a PWS is made clinically. The differential diagnosis of a PWS includes a hemangioma, salmon patch, venous malformation, lymphatic malformation, or arteriovenous malformation. Doppler ultrasound, CT, MRI, or other imaging studies may be needed if the diagnosis is unclear.

LABORATORY EXAMINATIONS

HISTOPATHOLOGY Dilated capillaries and increased ectasias in the deep reticular dermis.
IMMUNOHISTOCHEMISTRY GLUT-1-negative, differentiating PWS from hemangiomas.

TABLE 8-1 Port-Wine Stains and Associated Syndromes

Syndrome	Synonyms	Cutaneous Findings	Associated Features
Sturge–Weber syndrome	Encephalofacial angiomatosis	V1/V2 PWS, can have oral telangiectatic hypertrophy	Vascular malformation of ipsilateral meninges and cerebrum, intracranial calcifications, seizures, hemiplegia, glaucoma, mental retardation. Associated with mutations in GNAQ.
Klippel–Trenaunay syndrome	Nevus vasculosus hypertrophicus hemangiomas, varicosities	PWS over a limb (leg much more commonly than arm) as well as venous dilation or varicosities	Associated limb hypertrophy. Sporadic inheritance.
Parkes Weber syndrome		Findings of Klippel–Trenaunay, as well as additional arteriovenous malformation or arteriovenous fistula	Associated limb hypertrophy. Associated with mutations in RASA1.

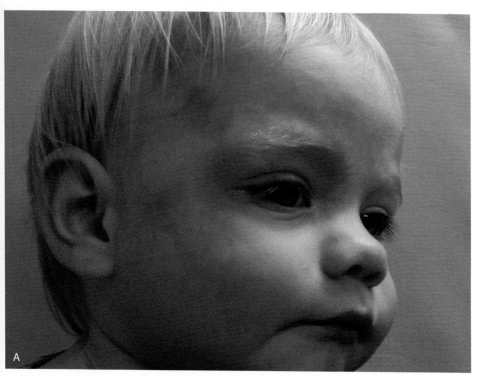

FIGURE 8-2 Capillary malformation A: Macular capillary malformation on the face of an infant.
(continued)

COURSE AND PROGNOSIS

PWS do not regress spontaneously. The area of involvement tends to increase in proportion to the size of the child. In adulthood, PWS can turn darker red–purple in color and thicken, which leads to more severe cosmetic disfigurement. In some cases, the thickening is associated with hyperplastic skin changes and asymmetric overgrowth of the area underlying the PWS (face > trunk and limbs).

MANAGEMENT

Isolated PWS are benign but can be disfiguring and distressing to the patient. Multiple treatments with a pulsed dye laser are very effective and should be considered in childhood before the lesion progresses to a more severe nodular, disfiguring form. Alternatively, a PWS can be covered up with makeup.

The majority of PWS have no associated abnormalities. Infrequently, a midline PWS of the lumbosacral, back, or nape area may be a hallmark for spinal dysraphism especially if seen in conjunction with other skin signs (pit, dimple, sinus, fibroma, lipoma, or hypertrichosis). Dysraphism can be detected with ultrasound or MRI.

Rarely, PWS can be associated with Sturge–Weber syndrome (Fig. 8-2B) or Klippel–Trenaunay syndrome (Table 8-1). It is estimated that 10% to 15% of infants with a V1 PWS will develop the ocular glaucoma and neurologic seizures of Sturge–Weber syndrome. The risk of Sturge–Weber is increased with multiple dermatomal involvement (e.g., V1, V2, and V3) or with bilateral PWSs. If suspected, internal imaging with radiography (calcifications), CT (cortical and leptomeningeal brain lesions), MRI (myelination), SPECT (blood flow), or PET (glucose metabolism) may be helpful. Klippel–Trenaunay syndrome is the association of limb hypertrophy with an overlying PWS and venous malformation or varicosity. Again, Doppler ultrasound or MRI can better detect the extent of tissue involvement in these patients.

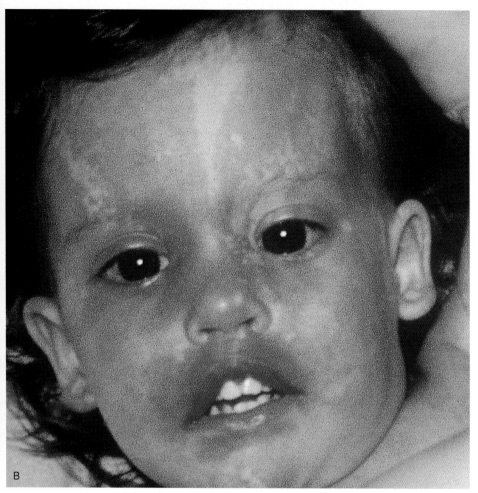

FIGURE 8-2 *(Continued)* **Capillary malformation B:** Facial capillary malformation in a child with Sturge–Weber syndrome.

HEMANGIOMAS AND ASSOCIATED SYNDROMES

Hemangiomas are benign, vascular proliferations that rapidly enlarge during the first year of life and slowly spontaneously involute by age 5 to 10 years. Superficial hemangiomas have a bright red, nodular surface and deeper lesions may be blue–purple in color. Rarely, they may be associated with systemic malformations (Table 8-2).

SYNONYMS Infantile hemangioma, hemangioma of infancy, strawberry nevus, angioma cavernosum, capillary hemangioma.

EPIDEMIOLOGY

AGE Rarely present at birth, but arise in the first weeks to months of life.
GENDER F > M, 5:1
PREVALENCE Seen more in premature infants (<30 weeks gestational age or birthweight < 1,500 g), infants of mothers' status postchorionic villus sampling, infants of older mothers, and infants of multiple gestation.
RACE More common in Caucasians.
INCIDENCE Most common tumor of infancy. Seen in 2.6% of all newborns. Occur in 10% to 12% of Caucasian infants, with nearly all present by age 1 year.
ETIOLOGY Abnormally increased vascular proliferation. Reports of familial cases with autosomal dominant inheritance.

PATHOPHYSIOLOGY

Hemangiomas are localized proliferations of blood vessels. Extensive study is underway to understand the signaling mechanisms that cause this benign tumor to grow, plateau, and then spontaneously involute. Several proposed mechanisms for hemangioma formation include the following:

1. A mutation in endothelial cells,
2. A mutation in other cells influencing endothelial proliferation,
3. Placental origin of proliferative cells, and/or
4. Dysregulation of immature endothelial progenitor cells.

It seems that a combination of these mechanisms, multiple genes, and local effects all influence the development, growth, and involution of hemangiomas. Endothelial cells from infantile hemangiomas stain positive for $GLUT1$, a specific glucose transporter, though its exact role in the pathogenesis of infantile hemangiomas remains to be determined.

HISTORY

Lesions present soon after birth during the first few weeks of life (Fig. 8-3A). The lesions proliferate 6 to 18 months (Fig. 8-3B), and then spontaneously involute, typically by age 9 years (Fig. 8-3C). Thirty percent of lesions involute by age 3, 50% by age 5, 70% by age 7, and 90% by age 9. At the end of involution, most lesions are cosmetically undetectable, but a few can leave atrophic, fibrofatty, or telangiectatic markings. Rarely, a hemangioma proliferates in utero, is present at birth, and undergoes rapid spontaneous resolution ("rapidly involuting congenital hemangioma" or "RICH") in the first year of life. Even more rare is a noninvoluting congenital hemangioma ("NICH"), which will not go away spontaneously. Both of these latter hemangioma variants are the exception rather than the rule.

Solitary hemangiomas are asymptomatic, benign, and rarely bleed. Possible complications include the following:

1. Ulceration (seen in 10% of hemangiomas, Fig. 8-3B), most common on lip, neck, or anogenital locations.
2. Location near critical structures (periorbital, nasal tip, lip, pinna, breast, and anogenital area) causing obstruction.
3. Association with internal abnormalities (CNS, laryngeal obstruction, and spinal dysraphism).

TABLE 8-2 Hemangiomas and Associated Syndromes

Disorder	Synonyms	Cutaneous Findings	Associated Features
Rapidly involuting hemangioma	RICH	Hemangioma proliferates in utero, involutes first year of life	
Noninvoluting congenital hemangioma	NICH	Hemangioma proliferates in utero, never involutes	
Diffuse neonatal hemangiomatosis		Multiple hemangiomas	Hemangiomas of GI tract, liver, CNS, lungs. Risk of high-output cardiac failure, GI bleeding, hydrocephalus, visceral hemorrhage, ocular abnormalities, and hypothyroidism.
Benign neonatal hemangiomatosis		Multiple hemangiomas	No visceral involvement
PHACES syndrome		Large cervicofacial hemangioma	Posterior fossa abnormalities, Hemangiomas, Arterial abnormalities, Cardiac defects, Eye anomalies, Sternal defects
LUMBAR syndrome		Lower body hemangioma	Lower body hemangioma, Urogenital anomalies/ulceration, Myelopathy, Bony deformities, Anorectal malformations/arterial anomalies, Renal anomalies
PELVIS syndrome		Sacral region hemangioma	Perineal hemangioma, External genitalia malformations, Lipomyelomeningocele, Vesicorenal abnormalities, Imperforate anus, Skin tag

PHYSICAL EXAMINATION

Skin Findings

TYPE Nodule, plaque, may be ulcerated.
COLOR Superficial: pink, red. Deep: blue–purple. Involuting: white/gray.
FREQUENCY 50% to 60% superficial, 25% to 35% combined, 15% deep.
SIZE Average 2 to 5 cm but can grow up to 20 cm in size.
PATTERN Focal or segmental.
PALPATION Superficial lesions are soft/compressible; deeper lesions are more firm.
SITES OF PREDILECTION Face, trunk, legs, oral, and genital mucous membranes.

DIFFERENTIAL DIAGNOSIS

Hemangiomas are sometimes confused with other vascular abnormalities such as capillary malformations, infantile myofibromatosis, or pyogenic granulomas. Deeper lesions can mimic dermal or subcutaneous masses such as fibrosarcoma, rhabdomyosarcoma, neuroblastoma, dermatofibrosarcoma protuberans, nasal glioma, lipoblastoma, venous, lymphatic, or AV malformations. The characteristic proliferative and involuting phase can clinically differentiate hemangiomas from other vascular lesions. Radiographic studies or histologic examination may be necessary in most difficult cases.

LABORATORY EXAMINATIONS

HISTOPATHOLOGY Proliferating: endothelial cell hyperplasia, lobule formation, mast cells, and prominent basement membrane. Involuting: fibrofatty tissue, decreased mast cells.
IMMUNOHISTOCHEMISTRY GLUT1-positive staining differentiates infantile hemangiomas from all other vascular malformations.
DOPPLER EVALUATION Can determine slow flow hemangiomas versus fast flow AV malformations.
CT SCAN Uniformly enhancing soft tissue mass with dilated feeding and draining vessels.
MRI Soft tissue mass which is iso- or hypointense to muscle with flow voids.

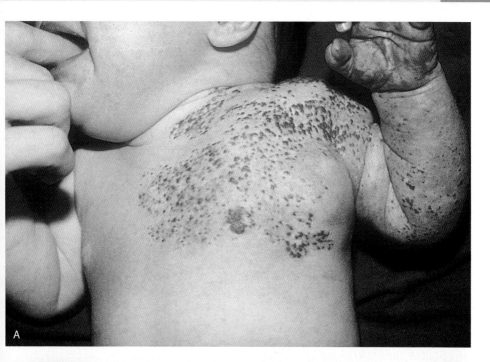

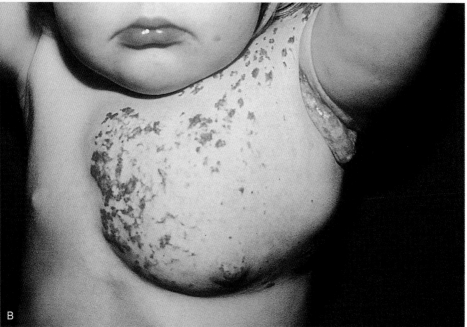

FIGURE 8-3 Hemangioma, infancy A: A 10-week-old infant with a vascular lesion noted at birth.
Hemangioma, age 1 B: Same child 1 year later with a fully proliferated hemangioma. *(continued)*

COURSE AND PROGNOSIS

Hemangiomas spontaneously involute by age 5 to 9 years. The residual skin changes are barely detectable but can include skin atrophy, fibrofatty tissue, telangiectasia, or depigmentation (Fig. 8-3C). Typical spontaneous involution leaves the best cosmetic results, and thus nonintervention in uncomplicated lesions is recommended.

Focal hemangiomas are typically small, arise from one locus and spontaneously involute without any complications. Larger segmental hemangiomas may be associated with systemic anomalies such as spinal dysraphism, GI or GU anomalies, or PHACES syndrome (Table 8-2).

A midline hemangioma of the lumbosacral, back, or nape area may be a hallmark for spinal dysraphism especially if seen in conjunction with other skin signs (pit, dimple, sinus, fibroma, lipoma, or hypertrichosis) or other malformations (imperforate anus, GI fistulae, skeletal, and renal abnormalities). An MRI can detect these underlying defects. Hemangiomas in this region have been associated with the LUMBAR and PELVIS syndromes as well (Table 8-2).

Ten to twenty-five percent of patients will have multiple hemangiomas, and numerous cutaneous hemangiomas can be a marker for internal involvement. A child with numerous cutaneous hemangiomas should be evaluated for the possibility of hemangiomas of the visceral organs, GI tract, liver, CNS, lungs, mucous membranes, or eyes. Complications include high-output cardiac failure, GI bleeding, hydrocephalus, visceral hemorrhage, and ocular abnormalities. Radiologic evaluation (ultrasound, CT, or MRI) may be helpful in determining the extent of internal involvement. Infants with large or multiple hemangiomas should also be screened for hypothyroidism due to overproduction of type III iodothyronine deiodinase.

MANAGEMENT

Treatment for the majority of simple hemangiomas is unnecessary because they are asymptomatic and self-resolve with a good cosmetic result.

Less than 2% of hemangiomas require intervention (for ulceration/bleeding, blocking facial structures or GI/GU tracts). Ulcerations can be managed with local wound care: saline soaks, topical antibiotics (mupirocin or metronidazole), and occlusive dressings. Pain associated with the ulcers can be alleviated with oral acetaminophen. Superinfected lesions may require a course of oral antibiotics (such as a first-generation cephalosporin).

Intralesional steroids can be used to treat small hemangiomas, but periocular injections can be complicated by ophthalmic artery occlusion and can lead to blindness. Topical steroids are safer, but their efficacy is unclear. Topical 5% imiquimod cream reportedly helps proliferating hemangiomas, but the cream can cause erosions as a complication.

Over the last decade, the use of systemic and topical beta blockers for the treatment of infantile hemangiomas has become increasingly prevalent for large, ulcerating, or high-risk hemangiomas. Systemic propranolol has been demonstrated to be effective and well-tolerated for the management of infantile hemangiomas. Dosing of 3 mg/kg/d of propranolol for 24 weeks has demonstrated efficacy in complete resolution of hemangiomas in the majority of patients; some may require a second or prolonged course. Doses of 1 to 3 mg/kg/d in divided doses have shown efficacy in smaller series. Adverse reactions associated with propranolol use include bradycardia, hypoglycemia, and bronchospasm. The use of topical beta blockers including timolol has also been explored for the management of infantile hemangiomas with promising results. Systemic steroids, such as prednisolone or prednisone, are used for life-threatening obstructive hemangiomas; 2 to 3 mg/kg/d is recommended until cessation of hemangioma growth or shrinking is achieved, followed by steroid taper. Adverse reactions to systemic steroid include cushingoid facies, irritability, GI symptoms, and decreased growth rate.

Systemic IFN-α (angiogenesis inhibitor) can be used for refractory, severe life-threatening hemangiomas at a dose of 1 to 3 million U/m^2/d injected subcutaneously. Adverse effects include spastic diplegia, fever, irritability, diarrhea, neutropenia, elevated LFTs, and skin necrosis. Systemic vincristine is a chemotherapy approach for resistant life-threatening hemangiomas, but its effectiveness is unclear. Adverse effects include peripheral neuropathy, jaw pain, anemia, and leukopenia.

Pulsed dye laser is effective in lightening the surface of proliferative red lesions; however, there was no change in clearance compared to children not treated with laser by age 1, and the PDL-treated children were more likely to develop atrophy, hypopigmentation, ulceration, and scarring. Argon and Nd:YAG lasers are

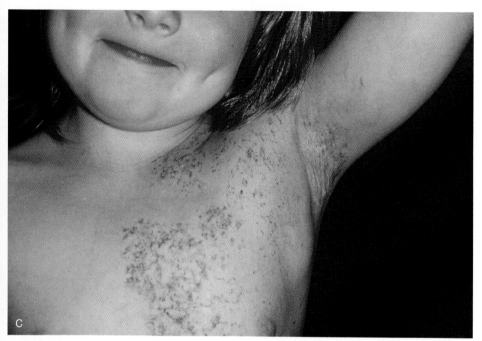

FIGURE 8-3 *(Continued)* **Hemangioma, age 3 C:** Same child 3 years later with an involuting hemangioma.

capable of treating deeper hemangiomas, but the risk of scarring is even higher with these lasers.

Surgical management (with or without embolization) is difficult, and should be reserved for proliferating hemangiomas in life-threatening locations. The timing of surgical intervention might be most helpful after complete involution (for any residual fibrofatty component), which may leave a preferable cosmetic outcome to surgical scarring.

BENIGN VASCULAR PROLIFERATIONS

SPIDER ANGIOMA

A spider angioma is a localized area of dilated capillaries, radiating from a central arteriole, occurring in healthy children.

SYNONYMS Nevus araneus, spider nevus, arterial spider, spider telangiectasia, vascular spider.

EPIDEMIOLOGY

AGE Young childhood and early adulthood.
GENDER F > M.
INCIDENCE May occur in up to 15% of normal individuals.
ETIOLOGY Usually idiopathic dilated blood vessel. May be associated with hyperestrogen states such as pregnancy or estrogen therapy (e.g., oral contraceptives) or hepatocellular disease (such as subacute and chronic viral hepatitis and alcoholic cirrhosis).

PHYSICAL EXAMINATION

Skin Findings

TYPE Central papule at the site of the feeding arteriole with radiating telangiectatic vessels (legs).
SIZE 2 mm to 1.5 cm in diameter. Usually solitary (Fig. 8-4).
COLOR Red.
SHAPE Round to oval.
PALPATION On diascopy, radiating telangiectasia blanches and central arteriole may pulsate.

SITES OF PREDILECTION Face, neck, upper trunk, arms, hands, fingers, and mucous membranes of lip or nose.

DIFFERENTIAL DIAGNOSIS

Spider angiomas can be confused with other vascular lesions such as cherry angiomas or telangiectasias.

COURSE AND PROGNOSIS

Few spider angiomas may regress spontaneously. However, the majority of lesions will persist. They are benign and asymptomatic, but often occur on the face and are cosmetically distressing to patients. Rarely, they may be associated with systemic diseases such as hereditary hemorrhagic telangiectasia (HHT), ataxia telangiectasia, progressive systemic sclerosis, and CREST syndrome.

MANAGEMENT

Spider angiomas are benign and thus do not require treatment. Lesions that are of cosmetic concern may be eradicated with electrodesiccation, electrocoagulation, or laser therapy. Patients should be forewarned that the lesions often recur.

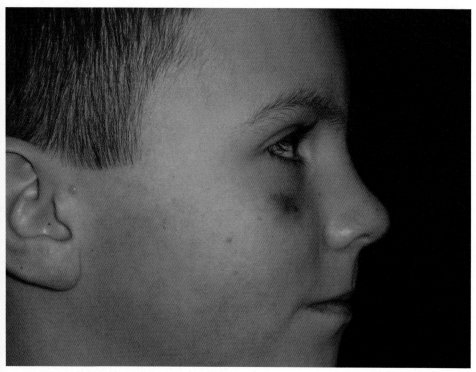

FIGURE 8-4 Spider angioma Vascular papule with radiating arterioles on the cheek of a child.

CHERRY ANGIOMA

Cherry angiomas are benign, bright red, dome-shaped vascular lesions that usually occur on the trunk.

SYNONYMS Campbell de Morgan spots, senile angioma, cherry hemangioma.

EPIDEMIOLOGY

AGE Any age, more commonly seen in adults.
GENDER M = F.
INCIDENCE Common, seen in most adults by age 60 years.
ETIOLOGY Increased number in elderly and during pregnancy.

PHYSICAL EXAMINATION

Skin Findings

TYPE Small macule to dome-shaped papule (Fig. 8-5).
COLOR Bright red to violaceous.
SIZE 1 to 8 mm in size.
NUMBER Elderly adults may have 50 to 100.
PALPATION Soft, compressible. Often blanches completely with pressure.
SITES OF PREDILECTION Trunk, proximal extremities.

DIFFERENTIAL DIAGNOSIS

The diagnosis of cherry angiomas is made clinically. They may sometimes be confused with petechiae. Larger lesions may look like a pyogenic granuloma, hemangioma, or angiokeratoma.

LABORATORY EXAMINATIONS

DERMATOPATHOLOGY Numerous dilated, congested capillaries; edematous stroma with homogenization of collagen. Epidermis thinned.

COURSE AND PROGNOSIS

Cherry angiomas begin to appear in adolescence, becoming more numerous with advancing age. They are asymptomatic, but may bleed when traumatized. Rare cases of eruptive cherry angiomas can be associated with systemic disease.

MANAGEMENT

Cherry angiomas in children are benign and hence no treatment is necessary. Lesions that are of cosmetic concern can be treated with electrodesiccation, laser therapy, or surgical removal.

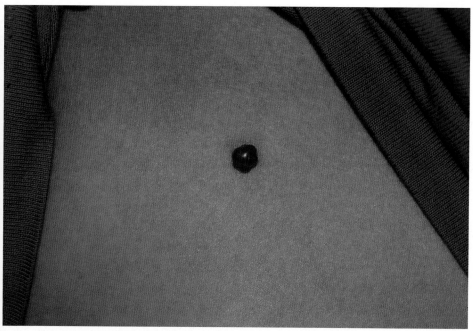

FIGURE 8-5 Cherry angioma Benign 4-mm vascular papule on the torso of a child.

ANGIOKERATOMA

An angiokeratoma is a benign skin lesion comprised of dilated dermal capillaries with overlying epidermal hyperkeratosis. There are five variants:

1. Solitary or multiple angiokeratomas: result from injury or irritation to the wall of a venule in the papillary dermis.
2. Angiokeratomas or the scrotum or vulva (Fordyce): may be associated with thrombophlebitis, varicoceles, inguinal hernias, varicosities, hemorrhoids, OCPs, or increased venous pressure from pregnancy.
3. Angiokeratoma corporis diffusum: clustered angiokeratoma on the trunk usually secondary to hereditary lysosomal storage diseases such as Fabry's disease (α-galactosidase deficiency), α_1 fucosidase deficiency.
4. Angiokeratoma of Mibelli: may be AD inheritance with lesions on the fingers and toes. This variant may be associated with chilblains or acrocyanosis.
5. Angiokeratoma circumscriptum: a capillary–lymphangioma malformation that occurs on the trunk or extremities of children.

EPIDEMIOLOGY

AGE Angiokeratoma circumscriptum can be seen at birth, in infancy, and in childhood. The other forms appear later in life.

GENDER F > M: Angiokeratoma circumscriptum, angiokeratoma of Mibelli.

PREVALENCE Angiokeratoma of Fordyce is common. The other forms are uncommon.

ETIOLOGY Unclear. Solitary angiokeratomas are sometimes associated with trauma.

GENETICS Angiokeratoma of Mibelli may have AD inheritance with variable penetrance. Angiokeratoma corporis diffusum of Fabry's disease demonstrates X-linked recessive inheritance. Angiokeratoma corporis diffusum may also be linked with autosomal recessive diseases such as GM1 gangliosidosis, galactosialidosis, β-mannosidosis, and aspartylglycosaminuria.

PHYSICAL EXAMINATION

Skin Findings

TYPE Verrucous papules coalescing into plaques (Fig. 8-6).

COLOR Dark red to black.

SIZE 1 mm to several centimeters.

SHAPE Round to stellate, can be in streaks or bands.

PALPATION Soft.

Sites of Predilection

1. Solitary or multiple angiokeratomas: lower extremities.
2. Angiokeratomas or the scrotum or vulva (Fordyce): scrotum in males, labia in females.
3. Angiokeratoma corporis diffusum: clustered angiokeratomas on the trunk (bathing suit distribution).
4. Angiokeratoma of Mibelli: dorsa of hands, feet, fingers, toes, elbows, and knees.
5. Angiokeratoma circumscriptum: trunk, arms, and legs.

DIFFERENTIAL DIAGNOSIS

Angiokeratomas are diagnosed and categorized by clinical presentation. Numerous angiokeratomas should alert one to check for more systemic disease.

LABORATORY EXAMINATIONS

HISTOPATHOLOGY Dilated papillary dermal blood vessels with overlying acanthosis and hyperkeratosis of the epidermis. Angiokeratoma circumscriptum: capillary–lymphatic malformation. Fabry's disease: glycolipid vacuoles (PAS- and Sudan black-positive staining) in endothelial cells and pericytes.

COURSE AND PROGNOSIS

Angiokeratomas are typically asymptomatic but persist for life and grow proportionately with the child. Occasionally, they may bleed or warrant removal for cosmetic reasons.

Angiokeratoma corporis diffusum has more widespread lesions and may be associated with hereditary lysosomal storage diseases such as Fabry's disease (α-galactosidase deficiency) or other enzymatic deficiencies.

MANAGEMENT

Angiokeratomas are benign and thus do not need treatment. They may, however, bleed or warrant removal for cosmetic reasons. They can be treated with surgical excision, electrodesiccation, or laser therapy.

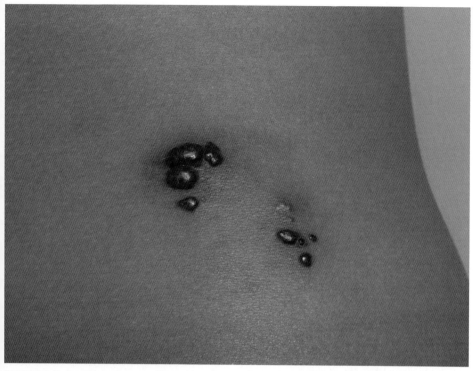

FIGURE 8-6 Angiokeratoma, solitary Vascular papules coalescing into a plaque on the torso of a child.

PYOGENIC GRANULOMA

A pyogenic granuloma is a rapidly developing, bright red papule or nodule usually occurring at a site of trauma.

 INSIGHT Although the clinical diagnosis of pyogenic granuloma can often be readily made, it is always reasonable to send the lesions for histologic confirmation, because of the worrisome differential diagnosis.

SYNONYMS Granuloma telangiectaticum, granuloma pyogenicum, lobular capillary hemangioma, tumor of pregnancy, eruptive hemangioma.

EPIDEMIOLOGY

AGE Usually children or young adults; most common in the second decade of life.
GENDER M = F.
ETIOLOGY Reactive vascular proliferation. One-third seen with posttraumatic injury. Can be seen with systemic retinoids, indinavir, EGFR inhibitors, PWS, and pregnancy.

HISTORY

Pyogenic granulomas are rapidly proliferating vascular nodules that typically arise at a site of minor trauma. They are benign but have a tendency to get traumatized easily and bleed copiously.

PHYSICAL EXAMINATION

Skin Lesions

TYPE Solitary vascular papule or nodule with smooth or warty surface (Fig. 8-7).
COLOR Bright red, dusky red, violaceous, and brown–black.
SIZE 5 mm to 2 cm. Usually <1 cm.

SHAPE Usually lesion is pedunculated, base slightly constricted, or sessile.
SITES OF PREDILECTION Area of trauma: fingers, face, lips, face, tongue. Gingiva in pregnant women.

DIFFERENTIAL DIAGNOSIS

The diagnosis of a pyogenic granuloma is typically made on history and clinical examination. The differential diagnosis includes a hemangioma, amelanotic melanoma, metastatic carcinoma, glomus tumor, irritated nevus, or wart.

DERMATOPATHOLOGY

HISTOPATHOLOGY Well-circumscribed, usually exophytic, proliferation of small capillaries in a fibromyxoid matrix surrounded by hyperplastic epithelial collarette.

COURSE AND PROGNOSIS

Pyogenic granulomas are benign, but have a tendency to get traumatized easily and bleed copiously. They are often precipitated by minor trauma and have a tendency to recur after (traumatic) removal or sprout new satellite lesions.

MANAGEMENT

Surgical shave excision with electrosurgery of the base under local anesthesia is recommended. Surgical specimens should be sent for histopathologic examination to confirm the diagnosis. Patients should be forewarned that the lesions can recur.

Some pyogenic granulomas have been treated with pulsed dye lasers successfully, providing another treatment option.

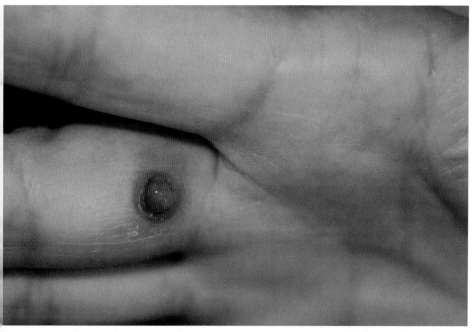

FIGURE 8-7 Pyogenic granuloma Sudden appearance of a vascular nodule on the palm of a child.

VASCULAR CHANGES ASSOCIATED WITH SYSTEMIC DISEASE

LIVEDO RETICULARIS

Livedo reticularis (LR) is common physiologic finding of a mottled bluish (livid) discoloration of the skin that occurs in a net-like pattern.

SYNONYMS AND CLOSELY RELATED CONDITIONS Livedo racemosa, livedo annularis.

CLASSIFICATION

1. LR with no systemic disease:
   a. *Physiologic LR (cutis marmorata):* normal LR response to cold in neonates, young children, some adults with chilblains, or acrocyanosis.
   b. *Benign idiopathic LR.* Permanent bluish mottling from persistent vasospasm of arterioles for which no underlying disease is found.
2. LR secondary to systemic disease:
   a. Vasospasm: occurs with Raynaud's and connective tissue disease.
   b. Intravascular obstruction: cryoglobulins, cold agglutinins, paraproteins, polycythemia vera, thrombocytosis, antiphospholipid syndrome, protein C deficiency, protein S or antithrombin III deficiencies, emboli, heparin or warfarin necrosis. Stasis may also result from paralysis, cardiac failure, Sneddon's syndrome, extensive LR, hypertension, cerebrovascular accidents, and transient ischemic attacks.
   c. Vasculitis: polyarteritis nodosa, cryoglobulinemic vasculitis, rheumatoid vasculitis, lupus erythematosus, dermatomyositis, lymphoma, syphilis, tuberculosis, pancreatitis, calciphylaxis.
   d. Others: drugs [such as amantadine (Fig. 8-8), norepinephrine, quinine, and quinidine], infections, or with neoplasms.

EPIDEMIOLOGY

AGE Adolescence to adulthood.
GENDER M = F.

PATHOPHYSIOLOGY

Livedo pattern is caused by vasospasm of the arterioles in response to cold, leading to hypoxia and dilation of the capillaries and venules. Decreased perfusion of the skin and/or decreased blood drainage leads to pooling of deoxygenated blood in the venous plexus, creating the mottled cyanotic reticular pattern that persists after rewarming.

HISTORY

LR appears or worsens with cold exposure, sometimes with associated numbness and tingling.

PHYSICAL EXAMINATION

Skin Findings

TYPE Net-like, blotchy, or mottled macular cyanosis (Fig. 8-8). Ulceration may occur.
COLOR Reddish-blue.
PALPATION Skin feels cool.

Distribution

1. Physiologic/benign idiopathic LR: symmetrical, arms/legs; less commonly, body; lower legs.
2. Secondary LR: patchy, asymmetrical on extremities.

DIFFERENTIAL DIAGNOSIS

The differential diagnosis for LR includes other reticulated skin disorders such as erythema ab igne, erythema infectiosum, or poikiloderma. Fixed lesions persistent from birth and minimally variable with temperature should raise suspicion for cutis marmorata telangiectatica congenita (CMTC) (see next section).

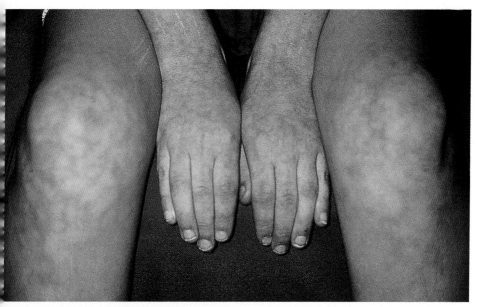

FIGURE 8-8 Livedo reticularis Net-like mottled vascular pattern secondary to amantadine in a young patient.

LABORATORY EXAMINATIONS

DERMATOPATHOLOGY Can vary, as causes for LR vary: arteriolar intimal proliferation with dilated numerous capillaries; thickening of walls of venules; lymphocytic perivascular infiltration.

COURSE AND PROGNOSIS

Physiologic or benign idiopathic LR recurs with cold exposure but rarely becomes permanent. Secondary LR is a precursor to more serious systemic sequelae.

MANAGEMENT

Physiologic or benign idiopathic LR:

1. Keep extremities from cold temperature exposure.
2. Low-dose aspirin (3–5 mg/kg/d po divided qid).
3. Pentoxifylline (Trental) for severe refractory cases.

In cases of secondary LR, treatment should be directed at the underlying disorder.

CUTIS MARMORATA TELANGIECTATICA CONGENITA

CMTC is a reticulated mottling of the skin that is more extensive and persistent than cutis marmorata. CMTC can lead to skin ulceration and atrophic scarring.

SYNONYM Congenital generalized phlebectasia.

EPIDEMIOLOGY

AGE Onset at birth.
GENDER M = F.
PREVALENCE Rare.
ETIOLOGY Unknown.
GENETICS Autosomal dominant with low penetrance.

PATHOPHYSIOLOGY

Ectasia of capillaries and veins may represent a mesodermal defect, which would explain CMTC's association with other mesodermal congenital abnormalities.

PHYSICAL EXAMINATION

Skin Findings

TYPE Macular reticulated mottling. Ulceration may be present over the reticulated vascular pattern and may heal with depressed scars (Fig. 8-9).
COLOR Red to blue.
SIZE Dilated venous channels 3 to 4 mm in diameter.
DISTRIBUTION Typically generalized. Localized forms have been seen confined to the trunk or one extremity.

General Findings

Generalized CMTC: can be associated with neurologic, vascular, ocular, skeletal abnormalities.
Localized CMTC: can be associated with decreased limb girth.

DIFFERENTIAL DIAGNOSIS

CMTC needs to be differentiated from cutis marmorata, which has a more short-lived, transient course and does not scar. Both are diagnosed by clinical history and physical examination.

LABORATORY EXAMINATIONS

HISTOPATHOLOGY Skin biopsy may show dilated capillaries and venules in all layers of the dermis and subcutaneous tissue. Histology may also be subtle and nondiagnostic.

COURSE AND PROGNOSIS

Typically mottled pattern is present at birth and improves but persists with age. Most cases are localized to one extremity possibly with hypoplasia of the affected limb, but no systemic abnormalities. Fifty percent of CTMC cases have other congenital abnormalities, particularly diffuse CMTC (vascular, skeletal, ocular, neurologic, or soft tissue defects). Rarely, CMTC can be seen in infants with neonatal lupus.

MANAGEMENT

The skin lesions do not require therapy and the mottled vascular pigmentation usually improves. Reticulated scarring, however, is permanent. With localized CMTC, limb hypoplasia can develop. For generalized CMTC, ocular, skeletal, and neurologic issues should be screened for and addressed accordingly.

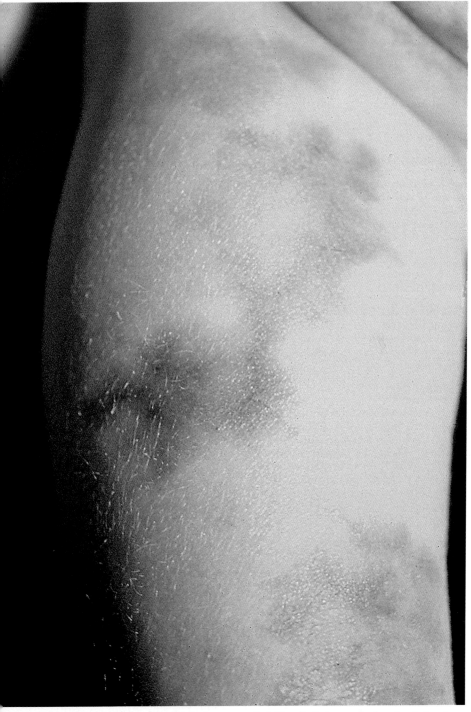

FIGURE 8-9 Cutis marmorata telangiectatica congenital Vascular lesion on the leg of an infant that resolves leaving depressed scars.

HEREDITARY HEMORRHAGIC TELANGIECTASIA

HHT is an autosomal dominant condition that affects blood vessels, especially in the mucous membranes of the mouth and the GI tract. The disease often manifests itself by recurrent epistaxis appearing in childhood. The telangiectasias of the skin and mucous membranes appears later in life and the clinical spectrum can range from cosmetic, asymptomatic lesions to severe pulmonary, GI, GU, and CNS hemorrhages.

SYNONYMS Osler–Weber–Rendu disease, Osler's disease.

EPIDEMIOLOGY

AGE Epistaxis may appear in childhood (average age 8 to 10 years) but cutaneous telangiectasias typically develop after puberty.
PREVALENCE Rare.
GENETICS Autosomal dominant. Mutations in *ENG* (endoglin gene) and *ACVRL1* have been identified.

PATHOPHYSIOLOGY

HHT blood vessels lack adequate perivascular support (pericytes, smooth muscle, and elastic fibers). Thus, the telangiectatic capillaries rupture easily and cause repeated nasal and GI hemorrhages.

HISTORY

The typical skin lesions (punctate red macules and papules) begin to appear after puberty but peak in the third or fourth decade. Bouts of recurrent epistaxis often begin in childhood; GI bleeding in HHT patients usually presents in adulthood. Up to 30% of HHT patients develop hepatic AVMs, up to 30% develop pulmonary AVMs, and 10% to 20% develop cerebral AMVs.

PHYSICAL EXAMINATION

Skin Findings

TYPE Macules or papules.
SIZE 1 to 3 mm in diameter.
COLOR Red.
SHAPE Punctate (most frequent; Fig. 8-10A), stellate, or linear.
ARRANGEMENT OF MULTIPLE LESIONS Symmetrical and scattered, nonpatterned.
DISTRIBUTION Upper half of the body; begin on the mucous membranes of the nose, later develop on the lips, (Fig. 8-10B); mouth (tongue), conjunctivae (Fig. 8-10C), trunk,

upper extremities, palms, soles, hands, fingers, and toes.
NAILS Nail beds of fingers and toes.
MUCOUS MEMBRANES Telangiectases appear on nasal septum, on the tip and dorsum of the tongue, nasopharynx, and throughout the GI tract.

General Findings

Up to 30% have hepatic AVMs, up to 30% have pulmonary AVMs, and 10% to 20% have cerebral AMVs.

LABORATORY EXAMINATIONS

HEMATOLOGY Anemia from chronic blood loss.
DERMATOPATHOLOGY Skin biopsy reveals dilated capillaries and venules located in the dermis, lined by flattened endothelial cells.
IMAGING X-ray, CT, or MRI to rule out pulmonary AV fistulae.

DIFFERENTIAL DIAGNOSIS

Clinical diagnosis made if triad is present of (1) typical telangiectases on skin (fingers and palms) and mucous membranes (lips and tongue), (2) repeated GI hemorrhages, and (3) family history.

MANAGEMENT

In mild cases of HHT, treatment of the telangiectases is not necessary; however, iron supplementation for anemia is recommended. Troublesome or cosmetically unwanted telangiectases can be destroyed with laser therapy or cauterization.

In severe cases of HHT, there may be extensive systemic involvement. Pulmonary AVMs can lead to hypoxemia, hemorrhages, and cerebral events. Hepatic AVMs may cause liver fibrosis and cirrhosis, which leads to coagulation defects increasing the severity of hemorrhage. Surgical resection or embolization of involved pulmonary and GI segments may be necessary.

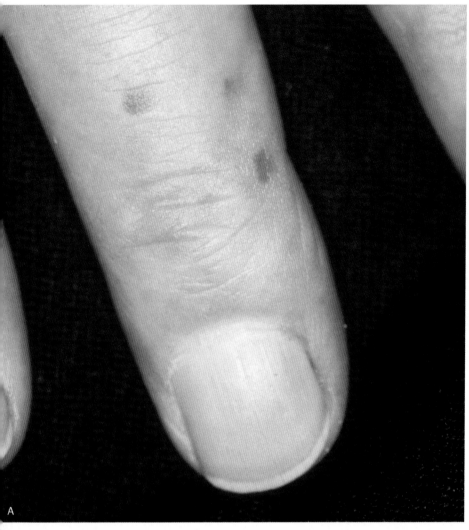

A

FIGURE 8-10 Hereditary hemorrhagic telangiectasia A: Punctate hemorrhagic macules on the finger. *(continued)*

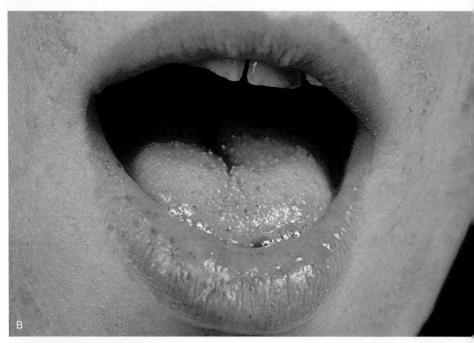

FIGURE 8-10 *(Continued)* **B:** Punctate hemorrhagic macules on the lips.

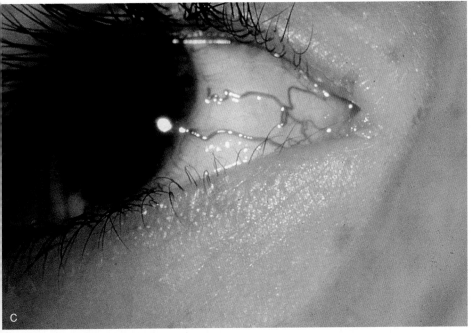

FIGURE 8-10 *(Continued)* **C:** Telangiectasias on the bulbar conjunctiva.

DISORDERS OF LYMPHATIC VESSELS

MICROCYSTIC LYMPHATIC MALFORMATION

A microcystic lymphatic malformation is a benign tumor of the lymphatic system characterized by groups of deep-seated vesicles that have been likened to "frog spawn." Often there is a hemangiomatous component.

SYNONYMS Hemangiolymphoma, lymphangioma circumscriptum.

EPIDEMIOLOGY

AGE Present at birth or infancy.
GENDER M = F.
PREVALENCE Uncommon.
ETIOLOGY Unclear.

HISTORY

Appear at birth or soon after; can remain stable or slowly grow with time.

PHYSICAL EXAMINATION

Skin Findings

TYPE Deep-seated, crops of vesicles coalescing into plaques (Fig. 8-11).
COLOR Clear or red–purple.
SIZE 2- to 4-mm vesicles.
SHAPE Grouped vesicles.
SITES OF PREDILECTION Proximal extremities, shoulder, neck, axillae, mouth (cheek, tongue, floor).

LABORATORY EXAMINATIONS

DERMATOPATHOLOGY Skin biopsy reveals dilated lymph vessels with associated blood vessel dilation in the upper dermis.

DIFFERENTIAL DIAGNOSIS

The diagnosis of microcystic lymphatic malformation can be made clinically, radiologically, or by biopsy. The differential diagnosis includes angiokeratoma, hemangioma, recurrent herpetic lesion, contact dermatitis, and molluscum contagiosum.

COURSE AND PROGNOSIS

Many microcystic lymphatic malformations are asymptomatic and so slow-growing that no systemic effects are seen. More extensive lesions can increase in size and if bleeding (from a hemangiomatous component) occurs, they can require intervention.

MANAGEMENT

Asymptomatic, stable microcystic lymphatic malformations do not need treatment. Lesions are often much more extensive than is clinically visible and have a tendency to recur, thus attempts at removal can sometimes worsen the outcome. Symptomatic lesions due to leaking lymph, inflammatory flares, or infections can be removed by surgical excision, fulguration, coagulation, or CO_2 laser ablation. It may be more difficult to remove larger/deeper lesions, because they can be extensive and recurrent. Multiple surgical excisions may be necessary.

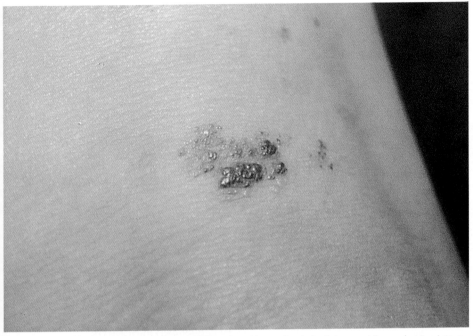

FIGURE 8-11 **Microcystic lymphatic malformation** Hemorrhagic and clear vesicles coalescing into a well-circumscribed plaque on the back of a young child.

MACROCYSTIC LYMPHATIC MALFORMATION

Macrocystic lymphatic malformations are interconnected, large, loculated lymphatic proliferations that are often detectable in utero. They are benign, but can become symptomatic with hemorrhage and sudden swelling. They can also be associated with abnormal karyotypes, malformation syndromes, or teratogen exposure.

SYNONYMS Hygroma colli, cystic hygroma, cavernous lymphangioma.

EPIDEMIOLOGY

AGE May be present at birth or infancy.
GENDER M = F.
PREVALENCE Rare.

HISTORY

Lesions appear later in life as subcutaneous swellings that involve large body surface areas. They can be quite deep and debilitating (Fig. 8-12).

PHYSICAL EXAMINATION

Skin Findings

TYPE Translucent nodular or cystic swellings.
COLOR Flesh colored to pink–red.
SIZE 1 to several centimeters in size.
SITES OF PREDILECTION Neck, axillae, lateral chest, groin, or popliteal fossa.

General Findings

Can be associated with karyotype abnormalities (Down syndrome, Turner syndrome, and Noonan syndrome).

LABORATORY EXAMINATIONS

DERMATOPATHOLOGY Histologic examination shows a uniloculated or multiloculated nodule of numerous dilated lymph channels lined with flat or cuboidal endothelial cells.
RADIOLOGIC Ultrasound, CT, or MRI reveals large, cystic spaces in the dermis, subcutis, or muscles.
SPECIAL TESTS Lesions enhance with transillumination.

DIFFERENTIAL DIAGNOSIS

The diagnosis of a macrocystic lymphatic malformation is made by history and clinical findings and can be confirmed by imaging studies and/or tissue diagnosis. The differential diagnosis includes a cavernous hemangioma and soft tissue proliferation.

COURSE AND PROGNOSIS

Macrocystic lymphatic malformations can involve large parts of the face, trunk, or extremities and can be very debilitating.

MANAGEMENT

Percutaneous sclerotherapy is the treatment of choice for macrocystic lymphatic malformations and multiple treatments may be necessary to induce inflammation and encourage scarred shrinkage of the cysts. Surgical removal is the second approach and may require split-thickness grafts and/or tissue expanders to fill in the wound. Severe, extensive macrocystic lesions may be untreatable.

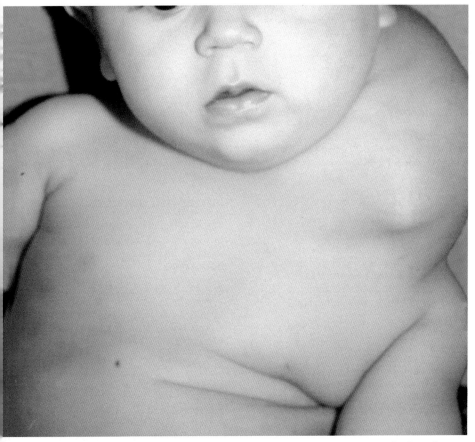

FIGURE 8-12 Macrocystic lymphatic malformation Large, cystic swelling on the neck of an infant.

LYMPHEDEMA

Lymphedema is diffuse soft tissue swelling caused by poor lymphatic drainage. It may be a primary disease (congenital) or secondary (e.g., postsurgical) to pathologic obstruction of the lymph vessels. Primary disease manifests at birth or during childhood and secondary (acquired) disease typically presents later.

EPIDEMIOLOGY

AGE Primary lymphedema: 13% congenital, most manifest age 9 to 25 years. Secondary lymphedema: any age.
GENDER F > M.

Etiology

Primary:

1. Milroy's disease: mutation in genes that encode vascular endothelial growth factor receptor. Autosomal dominant inheritance.
2. Meige lymphedema: mutation in genes that encode for forkhead family transcription factor C2. Autosomal dominant inheritance.

Secondary: Postsurgery, postinfection, filariasis.

PATHOPHYSIOLOGY

The lymphatic drainage to an extremity is impaired either primarily (e.g., congenital lymphedema) or secondarily (e.g., postsurgical) and leads to swelling of the affected extremity.

HISTORY

Lymphedema of the involved area results in swelling that fluctuates in severity and gradually worsens with age. Milroy's disease is an autosomal dominant disorder with an inherited tendency for lymphedema of the legs. The etiology is unclear.

PHYSICAL EXAMINATION

Skin Findings

TYPE Diffuse swelling (Fig. 8-13).

PALPATION Firm with pitting under pressure.
SITES OF PREDILECTION Lower extremities, upper extremities.
OTHER FINDINGS Stemmer sign—inability to tent the skin at the base of involved digits due to lymphedema.

DIFFERENTIAL DIAGNOSIS

The diagnosis of lymphedema is made by history and clinical examination. The differential diagnosis includes cellulitis and deep tissue infection.

COURSE AND PROGNOSIS

Lymphedema slowly progresses with age, and repeated swelling of the affected area leads to worsening of the disease.

MANAGEMENT

Maintenance therapy consists of the following:

1. Rest and limb elevation.
2. Compression with elastic support stockings, wraps, or pneumatic compression devices.
3. Reducing sodium intake.
4. Diuretics can also be helpful.
5. Subcutaneous lymphangiectomy can be attempted, but scarring is extensive and unsightly.

Supportive care measures such as physical therapy with lymphedema massage may offer symptomatic relief.

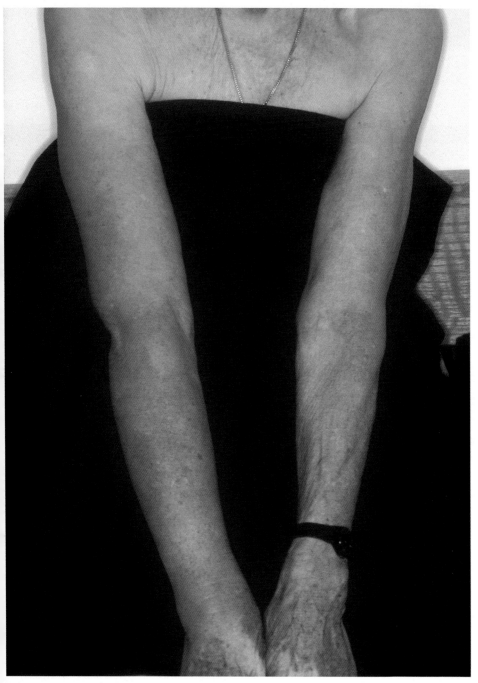

FIGURE 8-13 Lymphedema Postsurgical swelling of the right arm compared to the left arm.

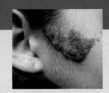

BENIGN EPIDERMAL PROLIFERATIONS

EPIDERMAL NEVUS

Epidermal nevi are benign, well-circumscribed proliferations of the epidermis and papillary dermis appearing in the distribution of Blaschko's lines.

INSIGHT When examining a lesion that appears linear, consider the swirled or undulating pattern of Blaschko's lines; if present, this will immediately focus the differential diagnosis.

SYNONYMS Nevus verrucosus, nevus unius lateris, ichthyosis hystrix, and linear nevus sebaceous.

EPIDEMIOLOGY

AGE 80% present in the first year of life. Most of them appear from birth to 18 years. May become more prominent during puberty, increasing in thickness and darkening in color.
GENDER M = F.
PREVALENCE 1 in 1,000 infants.
ETIOLOGY Most cases sporadic, some cases familial. Mutations in gene for fibroblast growth factor receptor 3 (FGFR3) identified. Some exhibit a chromosomal break at 1q23. Mutations in PIK3CA and HRAS have also been identified in keratinocytic epidermal nevi.

PATHOPHYSIOLOGY

Epidermal nevi arise from the pluripotent embryonic basal cell layer. There are likely many different candidate gene mutations that result in epidermal nevi, including those mentioned above.

HISTORY

Epidermal nevi are present at or soon after birth. Solitary small lesions are common. Larger lesions can affect an entire limb or side

of the body with associated adnexal tissue proliferations or hypertrophy. Growth or darkening of the lesion during puberty can occur.

PHYSICAL EXAMINATION

Skin Findings

TYPE At birth: macular/velvety. Later: warty/papillomatous plaques (Fig. 9-1).
NUMBER Solitary or multiple.
COLOR At birth: white. Later: flesh-colored, light, or dark brown. Rarely hypopigmented.
SIZE Few millimeters to several centimeters.
DISTRIBUTION Typically unilateral. Rarely can be bilateral.
ARRANGEMENT Linear following the lines of Blaschko.
SITES OF PREDILECTION Trunk or limb > head or neck. Flexural areas are more verrucous.

DIFFERENTIAL DIAGNOSIS

The diagnosis of an epidermal nevus is made based upon history and physical examination. The differential diagnosis includes linear and whorled hypermelanosis, nevus sebaceus, seborrheic keratosis, wart, psoriasis, acanthosis nigricans, lichen striatus, incontinentia pigmenti, hypomelanosis of Ito, or an inflammatory linear verrucous epidermal nevus (ILVEN).

LABORATORY EXAMINATIONS

DERMATOPATHOLOGY Skin biopsy shows epidermal hyperplasia, hyperkeratosis, acanthosis, papillomatosis, and parakeratosis. There may be increased melanin in the basal layer in places. There may be ballooning of the cells (epidermolytic hyperkeratosis) in places.

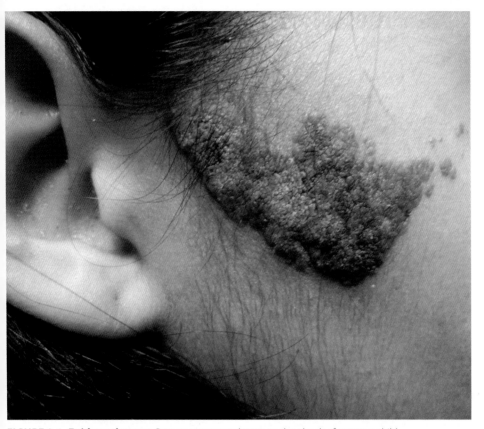

FIGURE 9-1 Epidermal nevus Brown verrucous plaque on the cheek of a young child.

COURSE AND PROGNOSIS

Epidermal nevi are typically asymptomatic and grow proportionately with the child. May start macular and become more verrucous over time. Malignant degeneration of epidermal nevi is rare, and can occur after puberty. Case reports of basal cell carcinomas, squamous cell carcinomas, keratoacanthomas, and trichoblastomas have been reported to develop within epidermal nevi. Adults with the variant of epidermolytic epidermal nevi can have a keratin mutation in their germ line (KRT1 or KRT10) genes resulting in offspring with epidermolytic hyperkeratosis.

MANAGEMENT

Treatment of the skin lesions is not necessary. Symptomatic or cosmetically unwanted lesions can be treated with shave excision, dermabrasion, laser ablation, electrodesiccation, and cryotherapy. Recurrence is common especially if only the epidermis is removed, but deeper attempts to remove epidermis and papillary dermis risk greater scarring. Test sites are recommended. Surgical removal is curative but may be extensively scarring and risks possible keloid formation.

INFLAMMATORY LINEAR VERRUCOUS EPIDERMAL NEVUS

ILVEN is a psoriasiform, pruritic, erythematous epidermal nevus appearing in a Blaschko linear distribution.

SYNONYM Dermatitis epidermal nevus.

EPIDEMIOLOGY

AGE 75% present by age 5 years, 95% present by age 7 years.
GENDER F > M.
PREVALENCE Uncommon.
ETIOLOGY Unclear. May be a clonal dysregulation of keratinocytes. Rare familial cases.

PATHOPHYSIOLOGY

Possible psoriasiform pathophysiology. Possible dysregulation of keratinocyte growth.

HISTORY

Initial presentation of ILVEN is of a barely palpable lesion or a confluence of smooth-topped papules. This progresses to a more psoriasiform erythematous and scaly lesion. It persists for years with episodes of inflammation. Other skin findings include an increased number of cutaneous lesions including café au lait spots, congenital hypopigmented macules, and congenital nevocellular nevi. Rarely, there may also be associated ipsilateral limb reductions, arthritis, neurological problems, skeletal defects, seizure disorders, mental retardation, or ocular abnormalities. When ILVEN occurs with ipsilateral limb defects, the acronym PENCIL (psoriasiform epidermal nevus, congenital ipsilateral limb defects) may be used.

PHYSICAL EXAMINATION

Skin Findings

TYPE Scaling papules coalescing into plaques.
COLOR Erythematous.
SIZE 2 to several cm in length.
SHAPE Linear along the lines of Blaschko.

DISTRIBUTION Lower extremities > upper extremities > trunk (Fig. 9-2).

DIFFERENTIAL DIAGNOSIS

The diagnosis of ILVEN is made on morphologic appearance of lesions, intense pruritus, and resistance to therapy. ILVEN can be confused with warts, psoriasis, lichen simplex chronicus, lichen striatus, lichen planus, incontinentia pigmenti, linear and whorled hypermelanosis, or hypomelanosis of Ito.

LABORATORY EXAMINATIONS

DERMATOPATHOLOGY Skin biopsy reveals hyperkeratosis, focal parakeratosis, acanthosis with elongation of the rete ridges, spongiosis, and a perivascular lymphocytic and histiocytic infiltrate.

COURSE AND PROGNOSIS

Most ILVEN lesions resolve by adulthood, but may last for years with episodes of intense pruritus that is refractory to treatment.

MANAGEMENT

Pruritus and inflammatory episodes may benefit from topical steroids but patients need to be cautioned about steroid overuse given the persistence of the lesion for many years. The verrucous ILVEN appearance can be improved with emollients (such as hydrated petrolatum, Vaseline, mineral oil, moisturizers), keratolytics (hydroxy acids, tretinoin, 5-fluorouracil creams), or topical calcipotriol. With noncompliance or discontinuation of therapy, lesions revert to their hyperkeratotic form. Curative attempts can be made with pulsed dye laser, dermabrasion, laser ablation, and surgical removal, but test patches are recommended to evaluate the scarring from these procedures.

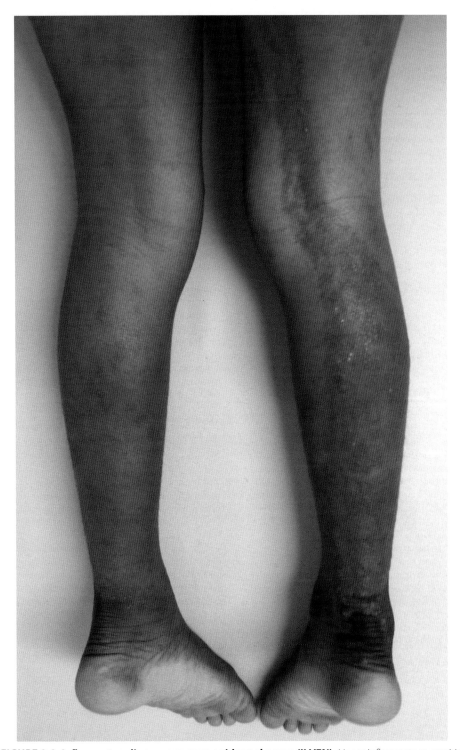

FIGURE 9-2 Inflammatory linear verrucous epidermal nevus (ILVEN) Linear inflammatory, pruritic plaque on the right posterior leg of young child.

EPIDERMAL NEVUS SYNDROMES

Epidermal nevus syndrome encompasses a number of clinical entities, which have in common the presence of an epidermal nevus (or nevus sebaceus) with skin, skeletal, cardiovascular, and/or CNS abnormalities.

SYNONYMS Schimmelpenning–Feuerstein–Mims syndrome, nevus sebaceus syndrome, Solomon syndrome, Jadassohn syndrome, Phakomatosis pigmentokeratotica.

EPIDEMIOLOGY

AGE Birth to 40 years of age.
GENDER M = F.
INCIDENCE Up to 33% of patients with epidermal nevi.
GENETICS Believed to occur sporadically. Likely lethal disorder rescued by mosaicism.

PATHOPHYSIOLOGY

Proposed mechanisms for the wide range of phenotypes seen include abnormal induction producing ectodermal and mesodermal malformations or abnormal neuroectoderm development.

HISTORY

A spectrum of epidermal nevi may be represented in this syndrome: verrucous epidermal nevus, nevus sebaceus, wooly hair nevus, Becker nevus, nevus spilus, and nevus comedonicus. Other mucocutaneous lesions include hypo- or hyperpigmentation, café au lait macules, hemangiomas, aplasia cutis congenita, hair and dental abnormalities, and dermatomegaly (increase in skin thickness, warmth, and hairiness).

Associated systemic abnormalities may be seen in the CNS (hemimegalencephaly, seizures, hemiparesis, mental retardation), skeleton (limb dysplasia or overgrowth, bone deformities, cysts, atrophies, and hypertrophies), ocular, cardiac, and/or GU system.

PHYSICAL EXAMINATION

Skin Findings

TYPE Hypertrophic warty papules coalescing into plaques.

COLOR Orange, brown, or dark brown.
SIZE AND SHAPE 2- to 4-mm papules coalescing to larger plaques.
DISTRIBUTION May be single linear lesion or more extensive Blaschkoid lesion, unilateral (Fig. 9-3) or bilateral.
SITES OF PREDILECTION Trunk, extremities, head, neck.

LABORATORY EXAMINATIONS

DERMATOPATHOLOGY Skin biopsy shows findings consistent with an epidermal nevus.

DIFFERENTIAL DIAGNOSIS

Diagnosis should be suspected on presentation with extensive epidermal nevi or epidermal nevi associated with systemic abnormalities. Differential diagnosis includes Proteus syndrome, CHILD syndrome, Goltz syndrome, incontinentia pigmenti, and other disorders with Blaschkoid skin findings.

COURSE AND PROGNOSIS

Rarely, malignant transformation of epidermal nevi may occur (basal cell carcinomas, squamous cell carcinomas, keratoacanthomas, and trichoblastomas). Transformation most common with nevus sebaceus syndrome. This syndrome may also be associated with various visceral malignancies: Wilms' tumor, astrocytoma, adenocarcinoma, ameloblastoma, ganglioneuroblastoma, esophageal and stomach carcinoma, and squamous cell carcinoma. In addition, hypophosphatemic rickets may be seen in epidermal nevus syndrome, thought to be due to overproduction of fibroblast growth factor 23 (FGF23).

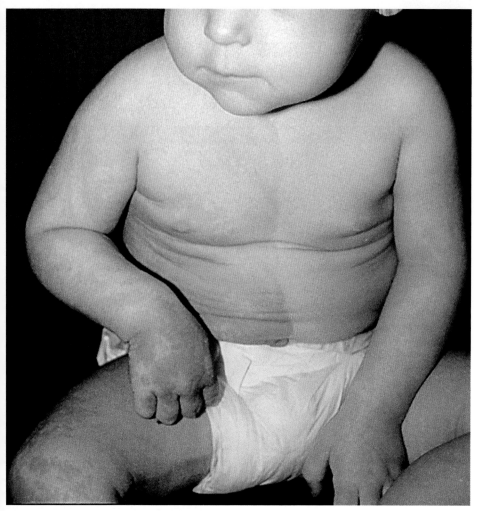

FIGURE 9-3 Epidermal nevus syndrome Large, unilateral whorled hyperpigmented plaques in a young infant.

MANAGEMENT

The treatment of skin lesions in the epidermal nevus syndrome is difficult given their extensive distribution. Symptomatic or cosmetically unwanted lesions can be treated with shave excision, dermabrasion, laser ablation, electrodesiccation, and cryotherapy. Recurrence is common especially if only the epidermis is removed, but deeper attempts to remove epidermis and papillary dermis risk greater scarring. Test sites are recommended. Surgical removal is curative but is extensively scarring and risks possible keloid formation.

Pertinent medical history includes developmental history, specifically attainment of developmental milestones, history of seizures, and abnormalities of bones, eyes, and urinary tract. Screening for hypophosphatemic rickets should be considered. Mucocutaneous, neurologic, ophthalmologic, and orthopedic examinations must be performed. Regular follow-up should be instated. Periodic electroencephalograms and skeletal radiologic analysis may be important to the long-term care of the patient.

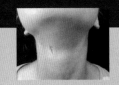

BENIGN APPENDAGEAL PROLIFERATIONS

NEVUS SEBACEUS

A nevus sebaceus is a solitary, well-circumscribed, yellow-orange hairless plaque located on the face or scalp that is a hamartoma of follicular, sebaceous, and apocrine origin.

SYNONYMS Nevus sebaceus of Jadassohn, organoid nevus.

EPIDEMIOLOGY

AGE Usually present near birth. May appear in childhood or adulthood. Increase in prominence at onset of puberty.
GENDER M = F.
PREVALENCE Uncommon.
GENETICS Usually sporadic, rare familial forms reported. Mutations in the HRAS and KRAS genes have been identified in sebaceus nevi.

HISTORY

A nevus sebaceus is typically present near birth and has two stages: a prepubertal/infantile stage (Fig. 10-1) and pubertal/adolescent phase (Fig. 10-2).

PHYSICAL EXAMINATION

Skin Findings

TYPE Hairless plaque surface may be velvety, verrucous, or papillomatous.
COLOR Yellow, yellow-brown, orange, pink.
SIZE Few millimeters to several centimeters.
SHAPE Round, oval, or linear.
DISTRIBUTION Head and neck.
ARRANGEMENT Solitary lesion; rarely, multiple lesions have been reported.

General Findings

Typically there are no systemic symptoms. In the scalp, the lesion remains hairless. Rarely, extensive lesions can be associated with ocular, CNS, or skeletal abnormalities. This constellation of extensive sebaceus nevi and associated abnormalities is termed nevus sebaceus syndrome (also known as Schimmelpenning syndrome). The association of nevus sebaceus, CNS malformations, aplasia cutis congenita, ocular limbal dermoid, and pigmented nevus has also been rarely reported and termed SCALP syndrome.

DIFFERENTIAL DIAGNOSIS

The differential diagnosis includes other appendageal tumors; smaller lesions can resemble warts. Juvenile xanthogranuloma is another benign proliferation with a yellowish-hue also presenting in infancy.

LABORATORY EXAMINATION

DERMATOPATHOLOGY Infancy: numerous immature sebaceous glands with irregular morphology and cords or buds of undifferentiated hair follicles. Adult: papillomatous hyperplasia of the epidermis with hyperkeratosis and hypergranulosis. There are also typically ectopic apocrine glands located deep in the dermis.

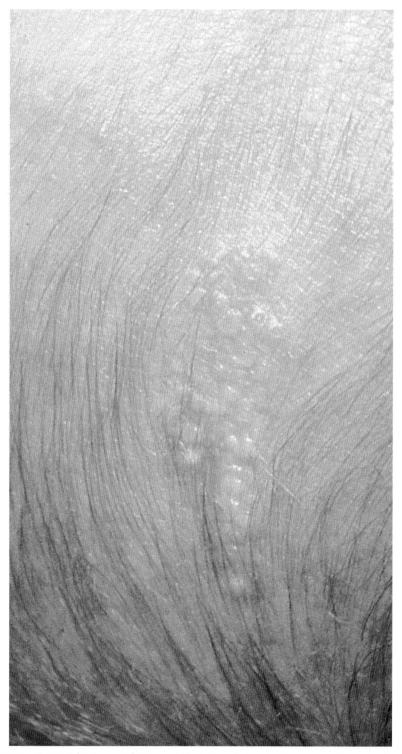

FIGURE 10-1 Nevus sebaceous, infant A pebbly, hairless flesh-colored plaque on the scalp of an infant.

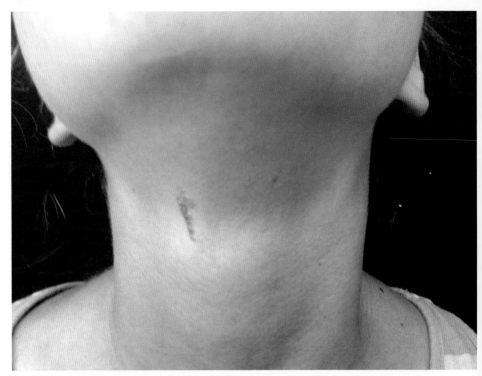

FIGURE 10-2 Nevus sebaceus, prepubertal child An elevated orange, hairless plaque with pebbly surface in a prepubertal child.

COURSE AND PROGNOSIS

Nevus sebaceus tends to grow slowly and become thicker and more papillomatous with age. Approximately 10% may have benign or, rarely, malignant neoplastic changes that manifest as nodules or ulcers within the lesion: trichoblastoma, trichilemmoma, syringo-cystadenoma papilliferum (Fig. 10-3) are the most common neoplasms. Other possible growths include sebaceous adenoma, apocrine adenoma, poroma, basal cell carcinoma, and squamous cell carcinoma.

MANAGEMENT

Nevus sebaceus lesions before puberty can be observed regularly for any signs or symp-toms of neoplastic change. While there is an increased risk of neoplasms such as syringo-cystadenoma or trichoblastoma arising within nevus sebaceus, these neoplasms are benign. Only 1% of nevus sebaceus lesions will develop a carcinoma in its lifetime.

More worrisome for the patient is often the progressively verrucous appearance of the lesion or the difficulty of monitoring the lesions in the scalp. Thus deep surgical excision may be warranted. More superficial shave excisions, dermabrasion, or laser ablation are usually not successful, with risk of recurrence for incompletely excised lesions.

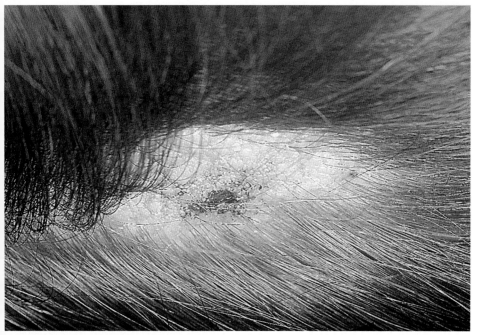

FIGURE 10-3 Nevus sebaceus, adult Central ulceration and crusting in an adult nevus sebaceus. Skin biopsy revealed neoplastic changes of a syringocystadenoma papilliferum.

NEVUS COMEDONICUS

A nevus comedonicus is a rare, localized proliferation of the pilosebaceous unit resulting in a well-circumscribed area of comedones.

SYNONYM Comedo nevus.

EPIDEMIOLOGY

AGE Present at birth in 50%; others appear before age 10 years.
GENDER M = F.
PREVALENCE Rare.
ETIOLOGY Some familial cases reported. FGFR2 gene mutations identified.

PATHOPHYSIOLOGY

A mesodermal developmental defect of the pilosebaceous unit, the nevus comedonicus is incapable of forming mature terminal hairs. As a result, the sebaceous glands within a nevus comedonicus accumulate cornified debris in numerous dilated follicular ostia.

PHYSICAL EXAMINATION

Skin Findings

TYPE Papules, open (blackheads) and closed (whiteheads) comedones (Fig. 10-4). Rarely papules, cysts.
ARRANGEMENT Linear or band-like configuration.
SIZE Individual comedones are on the order of 1 to 2 mm. The extent of the entire nevus comedonicus may range from a few millimeters to several centimeters.
DISTRIBUTION Unilateral solitary lesion on any part of the body. Rarely may have extensive lesions which can present in association with CNS, ocular, or musculoskeletal abnormalities (so-called nevus comedonicus syndrome).
SITES OF PREDILECTION Face, neck > trunk > extremities.

DIFFERENTIAL DIAGNOSIS

Nevus comedonicus can be confused clinically with comedonal acne, dilated pore, hidradenitis suppurativa, but the congenital onset and localized nature are diagnostic.

LABORATORY EXAMINATIONS

DERMATOPATHOLOGY Skin biopsy shows dilated invaginations filled with cornified debris. Associated acute or chronic inflammation may be variably present. Hair shafts are absent.

COURSE AND PROGNOSIS

Nevi comedonicus are usually asymptomatic but can occasionally become inflamed and painful, typically with the hormones of puberty. Pustules, abscesses, and scarring may occur. The lesions persist throughout life but are benign. Rarely, they may be associated with systemic abnormalities (ipsilateral cataract and skeletal defects).

MANAGEMENT

A nevus comedonicus is benign and requires no treatment. Cosmetically, manual comedo extraction can improve the appearance of the lesion. Topical salicylic acid, hydroxy acids, or retinoid preparations help prevent follicular blockage, but the results are not permanent.

Active inflammatory episodes can be managed with topical antibiotics (clindamycin, erythromycin), benzoyl peroxide, or sulfur. In severe cases, oral antibiotics may be helpful.

More permanent results can be achieved with surgical excisions, dermabrasion, or laser ablation, but scarring can result.

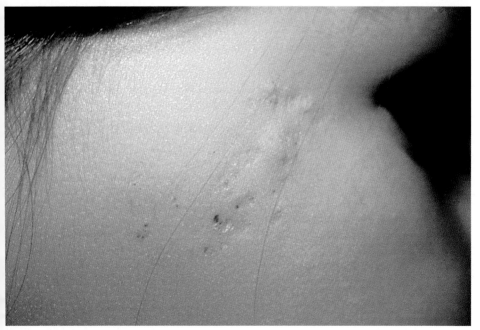

FIGURE 10-4 Nevus comedonicus Localized area of open comedones on the cheek of a child present since birth.

TRICHOEPITHELIOMA

Trichoepitheliomas are benign proliferations of follicular germinative (basaloid) cells that appear in childhood as numerous flesh-colored papules on the face and, less often, on the scalp, neck, or trunk.

SYNONYMS Brooke's disease (multiple familial trichoepitheliomas), epithelioma adenoides cysticum, multiple benign cystic epithelioma.

EPIDEMIOLOGY

AGE Early childhood or puberty.
GENDER M = F.
PREVALENCE Uncommon.
GENETICS Autosomal dominant inheritance. Brooke's disease mapped to multiple gene loci, including 9p21 and CYLD gene at 16q12–13.

HISTORY

Multiple trichoepitheliomas appear during early childhood or at puberty and are asymptomatic but permanent. Multiple trichoepitheliomas are a component of Brooke–Spiegler syndrome and Rombo syndrome when arising alongside other cutaneous neoplasms.

PHYSICAL EXAMINATION

Skin Findings

TYPE Firm papules and nodules.
COLOR Flesh-colored, pink.
SIZE Individual lesions typically 2 to 5 mm on face. Lesions may enlarge to 2 to 3 cm on other sites.
SHAPE Round.
NUMBER Few at onset to multiple after puberty (Fig. 10-5).
DISTRIBUTION Face, ears, and trunk.

SITES OF PREDILECTION Nasolabial folds, nose, forehead, upper lip, and eyelids.

DIFFERENTIAL DIAGNOSIS

The diagnosis of trichoepitheliomas is based on clinical findings and confirmed by skin biopsy. Trichoepitheliomas are most commonly confused with basal cell carcinomas or other appendageal tumors.

LABORATORY EXAMINATIONS

DERMATOPATHOLOGY Solitary classical trichoepitheliomas histologically show numerous horn cysts and abortive attempts to form hair papillae and hair shafts. The follicular germinative cells are grouped in clusters or cribriform cords of basaloid cells.

COURSE AND PROGNOSIS

Trichoepitheliomas are benign lesions that persist for life. Clinically, more lesions may appear on the face, but patients are otherwise asymptomatic.

MANAGEMENT

Trichoepitheliomas are benign and treatment is not necessary. Given the prominent facial location in many patients, trichoepitheliomas cosmetically may be treated with laser, electrosurgical destruction, or less commonly with multiple small surgical excisions.

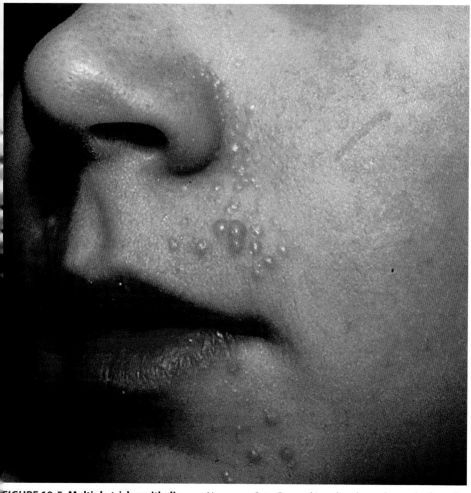

FIGURE 10-5 Multiple trichoepitheliomas Numerous 2- to 5-mm skin-colored papules on the face of a child.

SYRINGOMA

Syringomas are benign tumors of the apocrine or eccrine duct that appear as multiple tiny papules on the upper and lower eyelids.

EPIDEMIOLOGY

AGE Typically appear at puberty or adolescence.
GENDER F > M.
INCIDENCE Uncommon, estimated up to 1% of the population.
OTHER FACTORS Higher incidence (up to 37%) in patients with Down's syndrome.

HISTORY

Syringomas are asymptomatic benign skin lesions that appear and proliferate at puberty. They may be influenced by hormones and commonly present in multiples or eruptively.

PHYSICAL EXAMINATION

Skin Findings

TYPE Tiny firm papules.
COLOR Flesh-colored to yellow.
SIZE 1 to 5 mm.
NUMBER Few to numerous.
DISTRIBUTION Eyelids, neck, chest, abdomen, back, upper arms, thighs, genitalia, palms, and soles.
SITES OF PREDILECTION Lower eyelids (Fig. 10-6).

DIFFERENTIAL DIAGNOSIS

The diagnosis of syringomas is usually made clinically. The differential diagnosis includes other appendageal tumors, milia, or acne.

LABORATORY EXAMINATIONS

DERMATOPATHOLOGY Skin biopsy reveals many small tubular ducts (with central lumina lined by an eosinophilic cuticle) in the dermis. Some cross sections appear as ducts with comma-like tails commonly referred to as "tadpoles."

COURSE AND PROGNOSIS

Syringomas appear and proliferate during puberty and then typically persist asymptomatically for life. Rare cases of spontaneous regression are reported.

MANAGEMENT

Syringomas are benign and treatment is not necessary. Therapeutic methods of removal for cosmetic purposes include electrosurgical destruction, surgical removal, cryotherapy, and laser ablation.

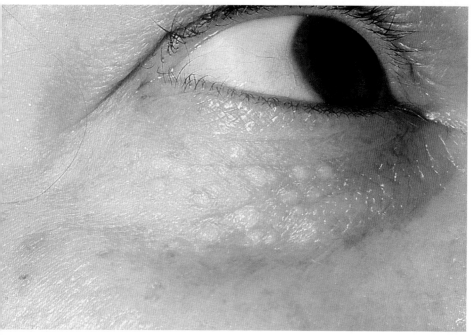

FIGURE 10-6 Syringomas Small 3- to 5-mm yellowish papules on the lower eyelid of a young adult.

PILOMATRIXOMA

A pilomatrixoma is a benign tumor of the hair follicle that clinically presents as a solitary calcified nodule on the face, neck, or arms of children or young adults.

SYNONYMS Calcifying epithelioma of Malherbe, pilomatricoma, trichomatrioma.

EPIDEMIOLOGY

AGE Childhood and adolescence.
GENDER F > M.
PREVALENCE Uncommon.
GENETICS Mutation in the CTNNB1 gene encoding β-catenin. Usually not inherited although rare familial forms have been reported.

HISTORY

Pilomatrixomas are not present at birth, appear suddenly, and persist throughout life. They are caused by a mutation in the CTNNB1 gene leading to a defective β-catenin, which disrupts the normal signaling pathway for cellular differentiation.

PHYSICAL EXAMINATION

Skin Findings

TYPE Solitary firm papule or nodule (Fig. 10-7).
COLOR Flesh-colored or reddish-blue hue.
SIZE 0.5 to 3 cm.
NUMBER Usually solitary, rare cases of multiple in number.
PALPATION Firm and lobular. May have dense, rock-like hard quality if extremely calcified. When skin is stretched lesion has a "tent" appearance with multiple angles.
DISTRIBUTION Face, neck, arms, or genital area.
SITES OF PREDILECTION More than 50% on head or neck.

General Findings

Rare familial forms associated with myotonic dystrophy (Steinert's disease).

DIFFERENTIAL DIAGNOSIS

The differential diagnosis includes other dermal tumors and cysts. The firmness to palpation and distinct color of a pilomatrixoma can help differentiate it from other entities.

LABORATORY EXAMINATIONS

DERMATOPATHOLOGY Skin biopsy reveals sheets of compact basal cells alternating with "ghost" or "shadow" eosinophilic, anucleate, cornified matrical cells. Calcification and ossification may also be present.

COURSE AND PROGNOSIS

Pilomatrixomas are typically asymptomatic. Occasionally, lesions may become inflamed or swollen. They may self-resolve and calcified material may perforate through the skin.

MANAGEMENT

Pilomatrixomas can slowly extrude with calcified material perforating through the skin. Alternatively, surgical excision can be done for both cosmetic and therapeutic purposes. Patients should be warned that recurrences are possible.

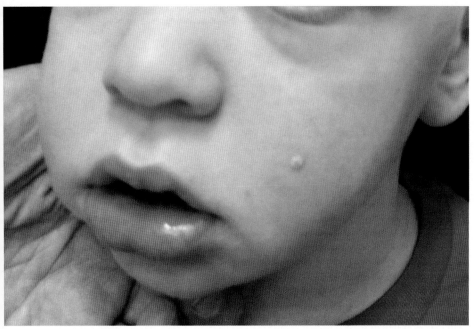

FIGURE 10-7 Pilomatrixoma Firm flesh-colored papule on the left cheek of a young boy.

STEATOCYSTOMA MULTIPLEX

Steatocystoma multiplex is a benign disorder characterized by multiple cutaneous cystic nodules with sebaceous glands that drain oily material when punctured. They are usually multiple and located mainly on the chest of affected individuals.

 INSIGHT A diagnostic pearl for steatocystomas is to gently nick a lesion with a #11 blade; a yellowish, oily substance will be expressed, confirming the diagnosis.

SYNONYM Sebocystomatosis.

EPIDEMIOLOGY

AGE Adolescence.
GENDER M = F.
PREVALENCE Uncommon.
GENETICS AD inheritance; mutation of keratin 17 gene.
OTHER FEATURES May occur concomitantly with eruptive vellus hair cysts and pachyonychia congenita.

PATHOPHYSIOLOGY

Steatocystoma multiplex are hamartomas; histologic variants of dermoid or vellus hair cysts.

HISTORY

Steatocystoma multiplex arise at puberty or thereafter and persist. They may become larger at puberty but are usually asymptomatic and have no central punctum. When punctured they drain a clear oily fluid.

PHYSICAL EXAMINATION

Skin Findings

TYPE Papules and nodules (Fig. 10-8).
COLOR Flesh-colored to yellow.
SIZE 2 to 4 mm in diameter, may enlarge into nodules >1 cm in size.

SHAPE Round.
PALPATION Fleshy to firm.
DISTRIBUTION Chest, face, scalp, arms, scrotum, and thighs.
SITES OF PREDILECTION Sternal areas, axillae, neck, scrotum, and proximal extremities.

DIFFERENTIAL DIAGNOSIS

Steatocystomas are diagnosed by history and clinical findings. Steatocystomas can be confused with sebaceous, keratin-inclusion cysts or pilar cysts. Unlike the other cysts, steatocystomas have odorless, oily fluid when expressed.

LABORATORY EXAMINATIONS

DERMATOPATHOLOGY Steatocystomas have cystic spaces lined by a corrugated thin epidermal lining. Abortive hair follicles and groups of sebaceous, eccrine, or apocrine structures are often incorporated into the cyst wall. Glycogen and amylophosphorylase may be present in the invaginations and cyst wall.

COURSE AND PROGNOSIS

Steatocystomas appear at puberty and persist for life. They are asymptomatic but can become quite numerous and troublesome cosmetically.

MANAGEMENT

Steatocystomas are benign, thus no treatment is necessary. Therapeutic methods of removal for cosmetic purposes include electrosurgical destruction, surgical removal, cryotherapy, and laser ablation.

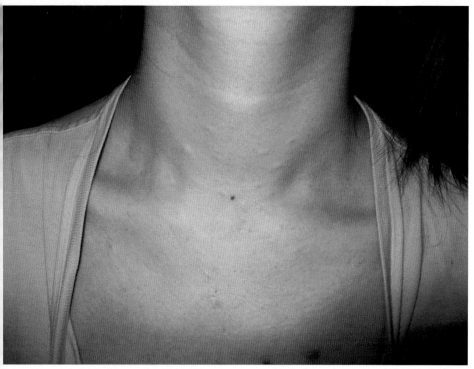

FIGURE 10-8 Steatocystoma multiplex Multiple asymptomatic flesh-colored cysts on the chest and neck of a young woman.

TRICHILEMMAL CYST

A trichilemmal cyst is the second most common type of cutaneous cyst occurring most often on the scalp. It is often an inherited trait and can be single or multiple in number.

SYNONYMS Pilar cyst, isthmus-catagen cyst, wen.

EPIDEMIOLOGY

AGE Any age.
GENDER F > M.
PREVALENCE 4 to 5 times less common than epidermal inclusion cysts (EICs).
GENETICS May be inherited as an autosomal dominant trait.

PATHOPHYSIOLOGY

Trichilemmal cysts are formed around hairs with trapping of the keratin intradermally leading to cyst formation and enlargement.

HISTORY

Trichilemmal cysts appear in the scalp and are usually asymptomatic. They lack the central punctum seen in EICs. Overlying scalp hair usually normal; may be thinned if cyst is large. They grow and then plateau in size and persist for life. Ruptured cysts may become inflamed and painful.

PHYSICAL EXAMINATION

Skin Findings

TYPE Smooth, firm, dome-shaped nodules to tumors (Fig. 10-9).
COLOR Flesh-colored.
SIZE 0.5 to 5 cm.
NUMBER Frequently multiple.
DISTRIBUTION 90% occur in the scalp.

DIFFERENTIAL DIAGNOSIS

Other cysts can mimic trichilemmal cysts, but the scalp location is usually diagnostic.

LABORATORY EXAMINATIONS

DERMATOPATHOLOGY Cyst with a stratified squamous epithelial lining and a palisaded outer layer resembling the outer root sheath of a hair follicle. The inner layer is corrugated with no granular layer and the cyst contents consist of dense keratin often with calcified cholesterol. Surrounding skin may show foreign body giant cell response and inflammation, particularly in cases of cyst rupture.

COURSE AND PROGNOSIS

Trichilemmal cysts begin on the scalp during adolescence and persist for life. They can become inflamed or painful. They may also become quite large in size.

MANAGEMENT

Trichilemmal cysts are benign, thus asymptomatic lesions can be left untreated. Symptomatic lesions can be incised and the cyst contents can be expressed; however, they often recur. Surgical excision with removal of the cyst capsule is needed for permanent cure. These surgical removals may be bloody given the well-vascularized scalp location of these lesions.

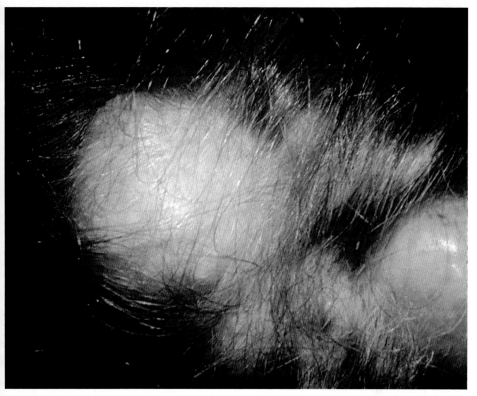

FIGURE 10-9 Trichilemmal cyst Smooth cystic growths on scalp.

EPIDERMAL INCLUSION CYST

EIC, the most common cutaneous cyst, is caused by epidermal implantation of the epidermis within the dermis. This causes a cyst filled with keratin debris to form. Cyst contents are cream-colored with a pasty consistency, and smell-like rancid cheese.

SYNONYMS Epidermoid cyst, sebaceous cyst, infundibular cyst, epidermal cyst.

EPIDEMIOLOGY

AGE Any age.
GENDER M > F.
PREVALENCE Common.

PATHOPHYSIOLOGY

Epidermal cysts are formed when skin desquamation is blocked and keratin accumulates in a subepidermal cystic enclosure instead of normally shedding to the skin surface.

HISTORY

Cysts appear, occasionally drain from a central punctum but often recur. They are benign but can intermittently become inflamed, rupture, or get infected.

PHYSICAL EXAMINATION

Skin Findings

TYPE Nodule, usually with central punctum (Fig. 10-10).
COLOR Flesh-colored to white.
SIZE Few millimeters to several centimeters.
ARRANGEMENT Usually solitary, may be multiple.
DISTRIBUTION Face, neck, upper trunk, and scrotum.

General Findings

Increased in patients with acne, Gardner syndrome.

DIFFERENTIAL DIAGNOSIS

Epidermal cysts can be confused with other cysts, however the rancid white-yellow cyst contents are diagnostic.

LABORATORY EXAMINATIONS

DERMATOPATHOLOGY Skin excisions reveal a cyst lined by stratified squamous epithelium and the cyst space filled with keratin. Surrounding tissue may have acute or chronic granulomatous inflammation, especially in cases of cyst rupture.

COURSE AND PROGNOSIS

EICs are benign; however, they may grow to disfiguring sizes or become recurrently inflamed. If the cyst ruptures, the irritating cyst contents initiate an inflammatory reaction, and the lesion becomes painful. Very rarely, a basal cell or squamous cell carcinoma can arise within an EIC.

MANAGEMENT

Asymptomatic lesions can be left untreated. Inflamed lesions can be injected with intralesional corticosteroid injection to decrease the pain and swelling. Secondarily infected lesions may require systemic antibiotics. Recurrent symptomatic lesions can be incised and cyst contents can be expressed; however, they often recur. Surgical excision of the entire area with removal of the cyst capsule is required for permanent cure.

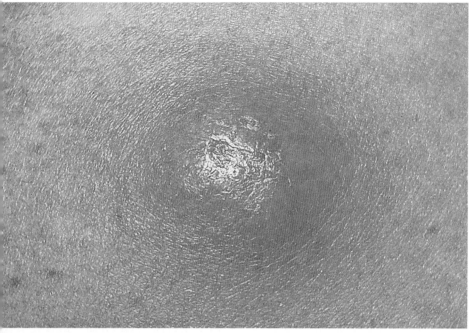

FIGURE 10-10 Epidermal inclusion cyst A 1-cm erythematous painful ruptured cyst with a central punctum on the arm.

DERMOID CYST

Dermoid cysts are ectopic rests of ectodermal tissue that occur along fusion planes during embryonic development. They are present at birth but may not become visible until they enlarge or become inflamed.

EPIDEMIOLOGY

AGE Present at birth, may become more prominent during childhood.
GENDER M = F.
PREVALENCE Rare.

PATHOPHYSIOLOGY

Dermoid cysts are formed when the ectoderm is accidentally sequestered along the embryonic fusion plane during development. They are benign but can intermittently become inflamed, rupture, or get infected.

PHYSICAL EXAMINATION

Skin Findings

TYPE Doughy-to-firm nodule (Fig. 10-11).
COLOR Flesh-colored.
SIZE 1 to 4 cm.
DISTRIBUTION Common periorbitally, especially lateral eyebrow. Also can be seen on nose, scalp, neck, sternum, sacrum, and scrotum.

General Findings

Cysts on the midline nose or scalp have higher likelihood of sinus tract or intracranial extension.

DIFFERENTIAL DIAGNOSIS

Dermoid cysts can be confused with other cysts, however the location along an embryonic fusion plane (particularly the common lateral eyebrow location) can be helpful.

LABORATORY EXAMINATIONS

DERMATOPATHOLOGY Dermoid cysts are lined by keratinized squamous epithelium with mature adnexal structures including hair follicular and sebaceous contents. Hair shafts may be found within the dermoid cyst contents.

COURSE AND PROGNOSIS

Dermoid cysts are benign, however, those located on the midline nose or scalp have a higher risk of intracranial extension. A sinus ostium (marked by protruding hairs or discharge) increases the likelihood of intracranial involvement. Dermoid cysts that communicate with the CNS put the patient at risk for infections, chemical meningitis, or hydrocephalus should the cyst rupture. Finally, dermoid cysts over the spine may be associated with occult spinal dysraphism.

MANAGEMENT

Dermoid cysts are managed by surgical excision. Presurgical imaging should be performed to exclude a connection to the CNS.

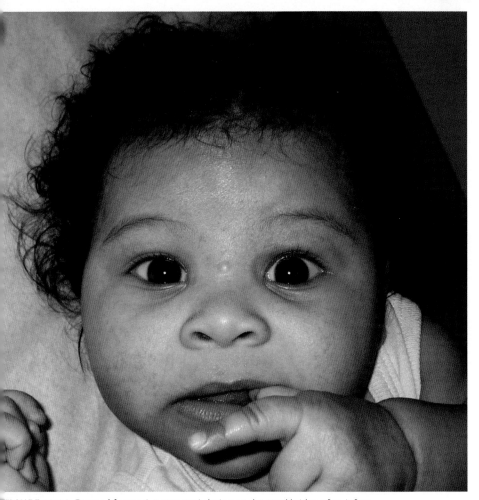

FIGURE 10-11 Dermoid cyst A 4-mm cystic lesion on the nasal bridge of an infant.

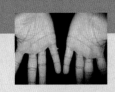

BENIGN DERMAL PROLIFERATIONS

CONNECTIVE TISSUE NEVUS

Connective tissue nevi are benign, slightly elevated, well-circumscribed plaques that are often seen as an isolated skin finding, but can also be associated with systemic disease (Table 11-1).

SYNONYMS Nevus elasticus, juvenile elastoma, collagenoma, collagen hamartomas.

EPIDEMIOLOGY

AGE Present at birth or childhood.
GENDER M = F.
PREVALENCE Uncommon.
GENETICS May have an autosomal dominant inherited form; see Table 11-1.

PATHOPHYSIOLOGY

Connective tissue nevi are localized malformations of dermal collagen and/or elastic fibers.

HISTORY

Connective tissue nevi appear in childhood or adolescence and are asymptomatic but can be disfiguring.

PHYSICAL EXAMINATION

Skin Findings

TYPE Slightly raised plaque (Fig. 11-1). May have a pebbly surface.
COLOR Flesh-colored to yellow.
SIZE Few millimeters to several centimeters.
NUMBER Solitary or multiple.
DISTRIBUTION Symmetrically over abdomen, back, buttocks, arms, thighs. Occasionally linear configuration.

General Findings

Can be associated with systemic disease (Table 11-1).

DIFFERENTIAL DIAGNOSIS

Connective tissue nevi can be diagnosed clinically and confirmed by skin biopsy. They can

be confused with other dermal or subcutaneous processes such as fibromatoses, fibrous hamartoma of infancy, infantile myofibromatosis, dermatofibromas, lipomas, scars, keloids, pseudoxanthoma elasticum, or mucopolysaccharidoses.

LABORATORY EXAMINATIONS

DERMATOPATHOLOGY Skin biopsy reveals disorganized collagen and/or elastin fibers in the dermis. Typically, there is an increase in collagen and a decrease or normal amount of elastin. Biopsies of the lesion can be easily mistaken for normal skin. Special staining for collagen or elastic fibers may aid in the diagnosis.

COURSE AND PROGNOSIS

Connective tissue nevi are benign. They persist for life and can increase in number during pregnancy. They are typically asymptomatic but can be cosmetically troublesome. The presence of connective tissue nevi should alert the clinician to check carefully for other signs of tuberous sclerosis or other associated syndromes (Table 11-1).

MANAGEMENT

Treatment for connective tissue nevi is not necessary. Early recognition and evaluation for possible associated syndromes (Table 11-1), such as tuberous sclerosis, is recommended. Cosmetically, the lesions tend to be too large yet subtle to warrant treatment. Cosmetic improvement can be attempted by surgical excision, dermabrasion, electrosurgery, curettage, and laser ablation.

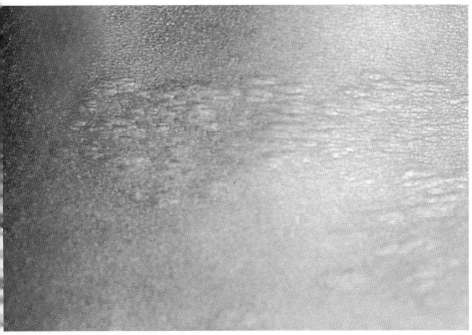

FIGURE 11-1 **Connective tissue nevus** Flesh-colored, slightly raised plaque on the torso of an infant.

TABLE 11-1 Connective Tissue Nevi and Associated Syndromes

Syndrome	Inheritance	Cutaneous Findings	Associated Features
Familial cutaneous collagenomas	Autosomal dominant (possible *LEMD3* gene mutation)	Multiple collagenomas	May have associated cardiomyopathy
Tuberous sclerosis collagenomas	Autosomal dominant (*TSC1* or *TSC2* gene mutation)	Shagreen patch, adenoma sebaceum, ash leaf macules, café au lait spots, periungual fibromas	Epilepsy, mental retardation, rhabdomyomas, calcified brain nodules
Buschke–Ollendorff syndrome	Autosomal dominant (*LEMD3* gene mutation)	Dermatofibrosis lenticularis disseminata	Osteopoikilosis seen on x-ray, dysplasia of bone (leg bones, pelvis, hands, feet)
Proteus syndrome	Mosaic mutation (*AKT* gene mutation)	Cerebriform connective tissue nevus, often on the feet (plantar collagenoma)	Areas of sporadic, progressive overgrowth, vascular malformations, linear epidermal nevi, dysregulated adipose tissue

BECKER'S NEVUS

Becker's nevus is a common acquired benign hamartoma that occurs as a unilateral brown pigmented plaque, typically on the shoulder of adolescent boys. Over time, the lesion becomes hairy and may become slightly raised.

SYNONYMS Becker's melanosis, Becker's pigmentary hamartoma, nevoid melanosis, pigmented hairy epidermal nevus.

EPIDEMIOLOGY

AGE Pigmentation onset 50% before 10 years, 25% between 10 and 15 years, and 25% after 15 years. Hypertrichosis may follow.
GENDER M > F, estimated 6:1.
INCIDENCE 0.5% in adolescent males. Incidence much less in females.
ETIOLOGY Hamartoma of mesoderm and ectoderm tissues.
GENETICS May be familial in some cases, with lesions expressing heightened sensitivity to androgens.

HISTORY

Becker's nevi are thought to have an increased number of androgen receptors accounting for their onset at/around puberty and the clinical appearance of smooth muscle thickening with hypertrichosis, hypertrophic sebaceous glands, and acne.

PHYSICAL EXAMINATION

Skin Findings

TYPE Isolated macule or plaque, smooth or verrucous surface, often with increased hair growth (Fig. 11-2).
COLOR Flesh-colored to tan to brown, blotchy.
SIZE One to several centimeters (average size approximately 125 cm²).
SHAPE Large, irregular shape.
NUMBER Typically solitary, may be multiple.
DISTRIBUTION Unilateral on shoulder or back; less commonly on extremities.
SIDE-LIGHTING Oblique lighting of the lesion will help to detect subtle elevation.

General Findings

Associated findings are uncommon. In rare instances, underlying hypoplasia of the tissue may be present (i.e., shortened extremity, breast hypoplasia), termed Becker's nevus syndrome.

DIFFERENTIAL DIAGNOSIS

The diagnosis of a Becker's nevus is often made by history and clinical examination. The increased hair growth (seen in 56% and predominantly in males) is distinctive for Becker's nevi. Becker's nevi can be confused with café au lait macules, congenital nevi, plexiform neurofibromas, or congenital smooth muscle hamartomas.

LABORATORY EXAMINATIONS

DERMATOPATHOLOGY Epidermal papillomatosis, acanthosis, hyperkeratosis, and occasional horn cysts. Hypertrichosis may be noted. No nevomelanocytes are present. Melanocyte numbers are not increased. Basal cell keratinocytes are packed with melanin. Occasionally, a concomitant smooth muscle hamartoma may be seen.

COURSE AND PROGNOSIS

Pigmentation occurs in adolescence usually followed by increased coarse hair growth in over half of affected males. Females with Becker's nevi have less of a tendency to have hair growth in the lesion. After 2 years, the lesion tends to stabilize and may fade slightly but persists for life. Becker's nevi may be associated with a smooth muscle hamartoma. They are typically asymptomatic, but may be pruritic. Becker's nevi are benign and malignant transformation has not been reported. Very rarely, Becker's nevi can have associated underlying anomalies: hypoplasia of the ipsilateral breast, arm, lumbar spina bifida, thoracic scoliosis, pectus carinatum, scrotal abnormalities, or enlargement of the ipsilateral foot.

MANAGEMENT

Becker's nevi are benign and thus no treatment is necessary. Lesions tend to be quite large and treatment becomes impractical. Cosmetically, lesions can be lightened or the hair can be removed with laser therapy, but recurrence rates are high, and frequent treatments may be necessary. Patients with Becker's nevi should also be examined for the rarely associated soft tissue or bony abnormalities.

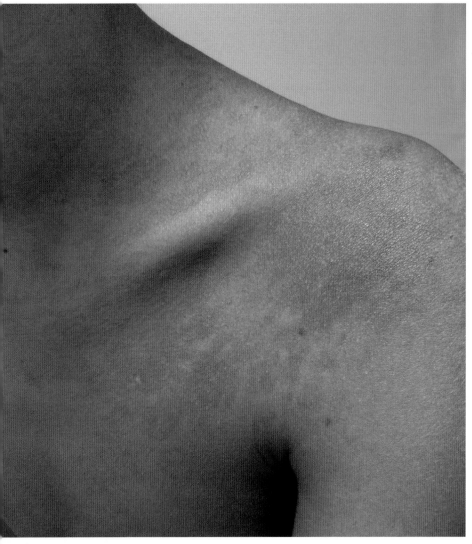

FIGURE 11-2 Becker's nevus Large, brown plaque that has become more noticeable with puberty.

RECURRENT INFANTILE DIGITAL FIBROMA

Recurrent infantile digital fibromas are single or multiple fibrous nodules occurring on the fingers and toes, during infancy, or early childhood.

SYNONYMS Infantile digital fibromatosis, Reye's tumor, inclusion body fibromatosis.

EPIDEMIOLOGY

AGE At birth or during the first years of life.
GENDER M = F.
ETIOLOGY Unknown.

PATHOPHYSIOLOGY

Immunohistochemical and ultrastructural studies have shown that the fibroblasts contain myofilaments and demonstrate mitotic activity. Eosinophilic inclusions are suggestive of a possible viral etiology.

PHYSICAL EXAMINATION

Skin Findings

TYPE Nodules (Fig. 11-3).
SIZE Few millimeters to 3.5 cm.
COLOR Flesh-colored to pink.
NUMBER Most often solitary but can be multiple.
PALPATION Firm.
DISTRIBUTION Dorsolateral aspects of fingers or toes. Thumbs and great toes usually spared. Rarely on hands or feet without digital involvement.

DIFFERENTIAL DIAGNOSIS

History, physical examination, and skin biopsy can differentiate recurrent digital fibromas from verrucae, periungual fibromas, supernumerary digits, fibroepithelial polyps, or other dermal proliferations.

LABORATORY EXAMINATIONS

DERMATOPATHOLOGY Skin biopsy reveals many spindle cells and collagen bundles arranged in interlacing fascicles in the dermis. The cells contain characteristic perinuclear eosinophilic inclusions measuring 3 to 10 μm in diameter (collection of actin microfilaments by ultrastructural studies) that are visible on routine hematoxylin/eosin stains and highlighted by trichrome staining.

COURSE AND PROGNOSIS

The lesions of recurrent infantile digital fibromas appear in infancy and spontaneous involution may occur after several years.

MANAGEMENT

For smaller asymptomatic lesions, no treatment is necessary and spontaneous regression is possible. Larger lesions can lead to functional impairment or deformity. For cosmetic and functional purposes, removal of these lesions by surgical excision can be performed. In up to 75% of cases, recurrences are observed in late childhood, at which time wide surgical excision may be required.

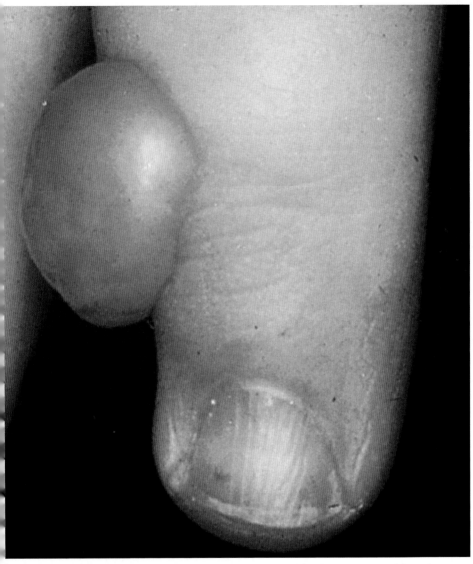

FIGURE 11-3 Recurrent infantile digital fibroma Two-year-old with a recurrent nodule in the index finger. (Reproduced with permission from IM Freedberg et al., *Dermatology in General Medicine.* 5th ed. McGraw-Hill; 1999.)

RUDIMENTARY SUPERNUMERARY DIGITS

Rudimentary supernumerary digits are soft tissue reduplicates that typically occur on the lateral sides of normal digits.

SYNONYM Rudimentary polydactyly.

EPIDEMIOLOGY

AGE At birth.
GENDER M = F.
RACE Black >> white, up to 10:1.
PREVALENCE 1 per 1,000 in whites, 10 per 1,000 in blacks.
GENETICS AD inheritance.

PATHOPHYSIOLOGY

Most cases of rudimentary supernumerary digits occur as an isolated AD inherited malformation. Rarely, they may be manifestations of a larger intrauterine growth that may have been amputated.

PHYSICAL EXAMINATION

Skin Findings

TYPE Papules, nodules.
SIZE Few millimeters to 2 cm.
COLOR Flesh-colored.
PALPATION Fleshy to firm texture.
OTHER May contain cartilage or vestigial nail.
DISTRIBUTION Bilateral. Most common: ulnar side of the fifth digit (Fig. 11-4).

DIFFERENTIAL DIAGNOSIS

Family history and the bilateral, symmetric appearance of rudimentary supernumerary digits can differentiate them from recurrent digital fibromas, verrucae, periungual fibromas, fibroepithelial polyps, or other dermal proliferations.

LABORATORY EXAMINATIONS

DERMATOPATHOLOGY Skin biopsy reveals disorganized fascicles of nerve fibers. May contain cartilage or vestigial nail.

COURSE AND PROGNOSIS

Rudimentary supernumerary digits are present at birth and persist for life. Most are asymptomatic, but some can be painful. They are benign and not associated with any systemic abnormalities.

MANAGEMENT

For smaller asymptomatic lesions, no treatment is necessary. For larger and/or painful lesions, surgical removal is recommended. Attempts at removal should encompass the base of the lesions since residual papules at the site may lead to painful neuromas later in life.

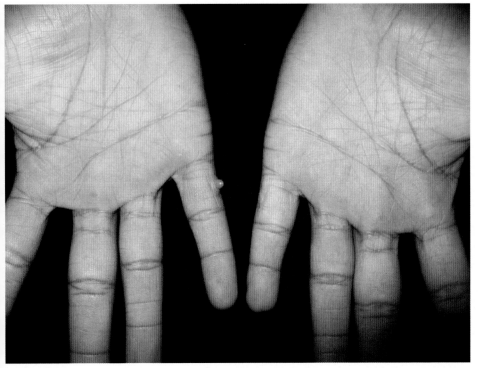

FIGURE 11-4 Supernumerary digit Small flesh-colored papules bilaterally on the hands present since birth.

HYPERTROPHIC SCARS AND KELOIDS

Hypertrophic scars and keloids are formed when there is an exaggerated fibrous tissue response to cutaneous injury. A hypertrophic scar remains confined to the site of original injury; a keloid, however, extends beyond this site with claw-like extensions.

 INSIGHT Hypertrophic scars and keloids can be very refractory to treatment and may arise seemingly spontaneously in predisposed individuals.

EPIDEMIOLOGY

AGE Puberty to 30 years of age.
GENDER M = F.
RACE Much more common in darker skin types.
ETIOLOGY Unknown. Usually follow injury to skin (i.e., surgical scar, laceration, abrasion, cryosurgery, electrocoagulation, as well as vaccination, acne, ear piercing, etc.). May also arise spontaneously without history of injury.

HISTORY

Scars or keloids appear and are usually asymptomatic. May be pruritic or painful at onset. Symptoms fade with time.

PHYSICAL EXAMINATION

Skin Findings

TYPE Papules, nodules (Fig. 11-5).
COLOR Flesh-colored to pink.
SHAPE May be linear. Hypertrophic scars: dome-shaped, confined. Keloids extend claw-like beyond the site.
PALPATION Firm to hard; surface smooth.
SITES OF PREDILECTION Ear lobes, shoulders, upper back, chest.

DIFFERENTIAL DIAGNOSIS

The diagnosis of a hypertrophic scar or keloid is made clinically. A biopsy is usually not warranted unless there is clinical doubt, because it may induce new hypertrophic scarring or keloid formation. The differential diagnosis includes a dermatofibroma, dermatofibrosarcoma protuberans, desmoid tumor, sarcoidosis, foreign body granuloma, or lobomycosis.

LABORATORY EXAMINATIONS

DERMATOPATHOLOGY A hypertrophic scar appears as whorls of young fibrous tissue and fibroblasts in haphazard arrangement. A keloid has an added feature of thick, eosinophilic, acellular bands of collagen.

COURSE AND PROGNOSIS

Hypertrophic scars tend to regress in time becoming flatter and softer. Keloids, however, may continue to slowly expand in size for years.

MANAGEMENT

A person with a history of hypertrophic scars and/or keloids should avoid skin trauma and elective procedures (e.g., ear piercing) to reduce the risk of scar formation. Once formed, the treatment for hypertrophic scars and keloids includes topical steroids with or without occlusion (such as flurandrenolide-impregnated tape) or intralesional steroids [such as triamcinolone (3–40 mg/mL, intralesional 0.1–1 mL q6 weeks)]. Steroid treatment often reduces pruritus or sensitivity of lesions, decreases lesion volume, and leads to lesion flattening. Combined treatment of intralesional triamcinolone and cryotherapy may be slightly more effective. Lesions that are excised surgically often recur larger than the original lesion. Thus, careful plastic surgery and occlusive wound care is recommended if excision is to be attempted. Radiation therapy has also been used for treatment of recalcitrant keloids.

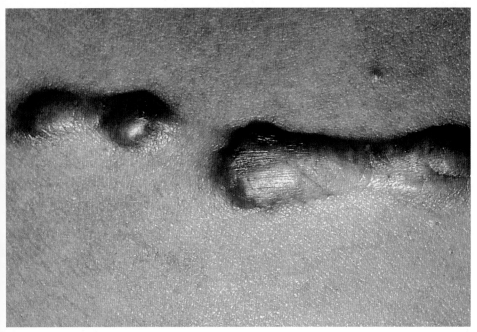

FIGURE 11-5 Keloid Spontaneous keloid on the chest of a child.

DERMATOFIBROMA

Dermatofibromas are very common, benign, dimpling skin lesions, usually occurring on the extremities, important only because of their cosmetic appearance or their being mistaken for other lesions.

SYNONYMS Solitary histiocytoma, sclerosing hemangioma, histiocytoma cutis, fibroma simplex, benign fibrous histiocytoma, nodular subepidermal fibrosis, dermal dendrocytoma.

EPIDEMIOLOGY

AGE Occasionally seen in children, more common in adolescence and adulthood.
GENDER F > M.
ETIOLOGY Unknown, may be chronic histiocytic–fibrous reaction to insect bite, skin injury, ingrown hair, or other minor trauma.

PHYSICAL EXAMINATION

Skin Findings
TYPE Papule or nodule (Fig. 11-6).
SIZE 3 to 10 mm in diameter.
COLOR Flesh-colored, pink, brown, tan, dark brown.
PALPATION Firm.
NUMBER Usually solitary, may be multiple.
DIMPLE SIGN Lateral compression with thumb and index finger produces a depression or dimple known as the "Fitzpatrick sign."
DISTRIBUTION Legs > arms > trunk. Uncommonly occur on head, palms, soles.

DIFFERENTIAL DIAGNOSIS

Dermatofibromas are diagnosed clinically and the dimple sign is a useful clinical diagnostic tool. Dermatofibromas may be confused with nevi, scars, cysts, lipomas, or histiocytomas.

LABORATORY EXAMINATIONS

DERMATOPATHOLOGY Skin biopsy shows a proliferation of spindle-shaped fibroblasts/collagen fibers and/or histiocytes. Thick, hyalinized collagen bundles seen at the periphery and the overlying epidermis are usually hyperplastic with flat confluent rete ridges and hyperpigmentation of the basal layer.
IMMUNOHISTOCHEMISTRY Positive for vimentin, factor XIIIa, muscle-specific actin, and histiocytic markers such as KP-1 and HAM-56. Negative for CD-34.

COURSE AND PROGNOSIS

Lesions appear gradually over several months and persist for years to decades; few lesions regress spontaneously.

MANAGEMENT

Dermatofibromas are benign and typically best left untreated. Surgical removal is not usually indicated because the resulting scar is often worse cosmetically. Indications for excision include repeated trauma, unacceptable cosmetic appearance, or uncertainty of clinical diagnosis. Cryotherapy may be used to flatten raised lesions.

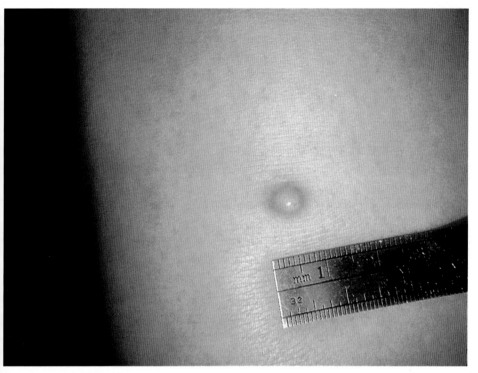

FIGURE 11-6 Dermatofibroma Raised dome-shaped 5-mm papule on the leg of a child.

SKIN TAG

A skin tag is a benign, pedunculated lesion with the color of the skin or darker, occurring at intertriginous sites.

 INSIGHT Although totally benign, skin tags can be associated with acanthosis nigricans and, in this context, can suggest an underlying malignancy or insulin-resistant state.

SYNONYMS Acrochordon, cutaneous papilloma, soft fibroma, fibroepithelial polyp.

EPIDEMIOLOGY

AGE Adolescence and adulthood.
GENDER F = M.
INCIDENCE 50% of all adults have at least one skin tag.
ETIOLOGY Unknown. Often familial. More common in overweight individuals and in setting of insulin resistance.

HISTORY

Usually asymptomatic, but skin tags may become inflamed or irritated. Occasionally, they may become tender or bleed following trauma or torsion.

PHYSICAL EXAMINATION

Skin Findings

TYPE Pedunculated papules.
SIZE Few millimeters to 2 cm.
COLOR Flesh-colored or darker.
SHAPE Usually round to oval.

NUMBER One (Fig. 11-7) to several.
PALPATION Soft, pliable.
DISTRIBUTION Intertriginous areas.
SITES OF PREDILECTION Neck, axillae, inframammary, groin, eyelids.

DIFFERENTIAL DIAGNOSIS

The diagnosis of skin tags is typically made clinically. The differential diagnosis includes a pedunculated dermal or compound melanocytic nevus, neurofibroma, seborrheic keratosis, or wart.

LABORATORY EXAMINATIONS

DERMATOPATHOLOGY Skin biopsy shows a pedunculated lesion of dense collagenous stroma with thin-walled dilated blood vessels in the center.

COURSE AND PROGNOSIS

Skin tags tend to become larger and more numerous over time. They are benign and asymptomatic, but on occasion can torse with ensuing infarction and autoamputation.

MANAGEMENT

Skin tags are benign thus no treatment is necessary. Symptomatic skin tags can be removed by snipping them off with scissors, tangential shave removal, electrodesiccation, or cryosurgery.

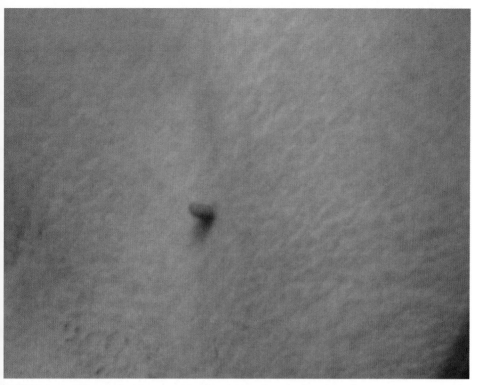

FIGURE 11-7 Skin tag One 3-mm pedunculated skin color growth in the axilla.

LEIOMYOMA

Leiomyomas are benign dermal tumors arising from the smooth muscle cells of the arrectores pilorum and are clinically characterized by solitary or multiple red–brown dermal nodules subject to episodes of paroxysmal pain.

There are three types of leiomyomas:

1. Piloleiomyoma: solitary from the arrector pili muscles or multiple with AD inheritance.
2. Genital leiomyomas: from the dartoic, vulvar, or mamillary muscles of the scrotum, labia, or nipple.
3. Angioleiomyomas: arising from vascular smooth muscle.

SYNONYMS Leiomyoma cutis, superficial benign smooth muscle tumor.

EPIDEMIOLOGY

AGE Can be seen in childhood. More common in adolescence or adulthood.
GENDER M = F.
PREVALENCE Uncommon.
ETIOLOGY Usually acquired, except multiple piloleiomyomas.
GENETICS Multiple piloleiomyomas are inherited in an autosomal dominant trait.
SKIN SYMPTOMS Chronic lesions can be sensitive to touch or cold; spontaneously painful.

PHYSICAL EXAMINATION

Skin Findings

TYPE Papules, nodules (Fig. 11-8).
SIZE 1 mm to 2 cm.
COLOR Flesh-colored to reddish-brown.
PALPATION Firm, fixed to skin but freely movable over the underlying structures. May be tender to palpation.
SHAPE Round.
ARRANGEMENT Grouped when multiple; tend to coalesce into plaques with arciform or linear configuration.
DISTRIBUTION Extremities, trunk greater than the face, neck, vulva, penis, scrotum, nipple, and areola.
GENETICS Mutation of the fumarate hydratase gene on chromosome 1q42.3–43 in hereditary cases.

General Findings

Leiomyomas typically have no associated systemic findings. Rarely, women with multiple inherited piloleiomyomas may have associated painful smooth muscle tumors of the uterus (familial leiomyomatosis cutis et uteri). Hereditary leiomyomatosis may rarely also be

associated with a familial predilection for renal cell cancer due to mutations in the fumarate hydratase gene (Reed syndrome).

DIFFERENTIAL DIAGNOSIS

History, physical examination, and skin biopsy can help differentiate leiomyomas from angiolipomas, dermatofibromas, schwannomas, neurofibromas, glomus tumors, osteoma cutis, eccrine spiradenomas, neuromas, and neurilemmomas. Rarely, there can be leiomyosarcomas, which are typically larger than their benign counterparts.

LABORATORY EXAMINATIONS

DERMATOPATHOLOGY Pilar leiomyomas reveal a proliferation of haphazardly arranged smooth muscle fibers in the dermis, separated from the epidermis with a Grenz zone. Angioleiomyomas reveal a well-demarcated dermal nodule composed of concentrically arranged smooth muscle fibers around numerous slit-like vascular spaces.

COURSE AND PROGNOSIS

Leiomyomas are benign and are typically asymptomatic. Some lesions are painful. They have a high incidence of recurrence (50%) following removal but are not at risk of malignant transformation.

MANAGEMENT

Leiomyomas are benign and thus no treatment is necessary. For symptomatic lesions, possible treatments include surgical excision but the recurrence rate is high (50%). Other management options include topical nitroglycerine, systemic nifedipine, acetaminophen, or lidocaine for symptomatic relief or CO_2 ablation for removal with varied reported success.

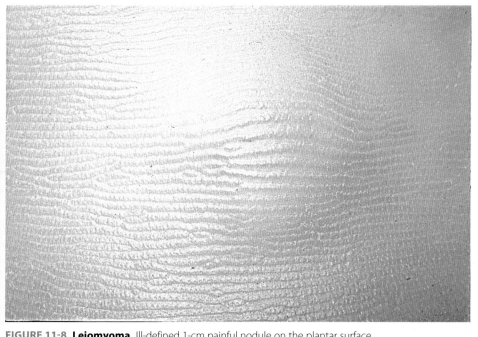

FIGURE 11-8 **Leiomyoma** Ill-defined 1-cm painful nodule on the plantar surface.

LIPOMA

A lipoma is a common benign tumor characterized by an asymptomatic, well-demarcated, soft nodule of mature fat cells. They are typically solitary lesions and benign, but can be multiple and associated with more diffuse disease (Table 11-2).

EPIDEMIOLOGY

AGE Any age, most onset postpuberty.
GENDER M > F.
INCIDENCE Very common.
ETIOLOGY Familial multiple lipomatosis: AD inheritance. Increased in individuals with obesity, diabetes, or hypercholesterolemia. Some are posttraumatic. Postulated HMGIC gene mutation with translocations on 12q13–15 associated with familial lipomatosis.

HISTORY

Lipomas are typically isolated asymptomatic nodules that are stable or slowly growing in size for years. Rates of growth seem to increase with weight gain and enlarging lesions may compress nerves and become painful. Multiple lipomas may be seen with associated disease (Table 11-2).

PHYSICAL EXAMINATION

Skin Findings

TYPE Single or multiple nodules.
SIZE Few millimeters to 10 cm.
COLOR Flesh-colored.
SHAPE Round, disc-shaped, or lobulated.
PALPATION Soft, mobile.
DISTRIBUTION Anywhere.

SITES OF PREDILECTION Neck, shoulders, trunk (Fig. 11-9), and buttocks.

DIFFERENTIAL DIAGNOSIS

The diagnosis of a lipoma is made by history and clinical examination. It can be confused with a cyst, or other subcutaneous masses.

LABORATORY EXAMINATIONS

DERMATOPATHOLOGY Encapsulated tumors composed of mature fat cells (large polygonal or spherical cells with lipid vacuole and peripherally displaced nucleus) intersected by thin strands of fibrous tissue.

COURSE AND PROGNOSIS

Most lipomas remain stable and asymptomatic. They may enlarge, impinge on nerve, and become tender. Malignant transformation (liposarcoma) is extremely rare and typically occurs in large lesions (>10 cm).

MANAGEMENT

Lipomas are usually benign and asymptomatic and thus no treatment is required. For symptomatic or enlarging lesions, surgical excision or liposuction can be performed.

TABLE 11-2 Lipomas and Associated Syndromes

Syndrome	Synonyms	Cutaneous Findings	Associated Features
Familial multiple lipomatosis		Multiple asymptomatic diffuse lipomas	Inherited in an autosomal dominant fashion, potential
Adiposis dolorosa	Dercum's disease	Tender lipomas on arms and legs	Usually in postmenopausal women; paresthesias, weakness, arthralgias, obesity, mental disturbances, amenorrhea, alcoholism
Benign symmetric lipomatosis	Madelung's disease	Symmetric neck and upper trunk lipomas	Usually in alcoholic men, mutation in tRNA lysine gene
CLOVE syndrome	Congenital lipomatous overgrowth, vascular malformation, epidermal nevi	Congenital lipomas, nevi	Gigantism, hemihypertrophy, mesenchymal neoplasms, mosaic PIK3CA gene mutation

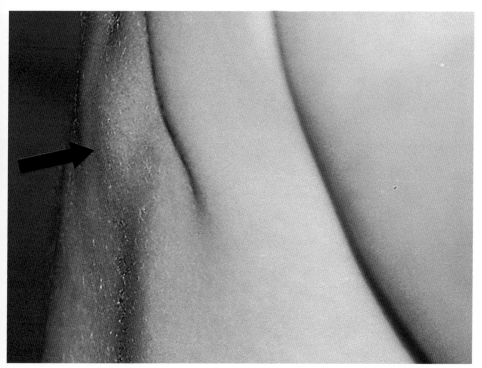

FIGURE 11-9 Lipoma Soft, asymptomatic nodule on the midback of an infant. Imaging studies were normal.

GIANT CELL TUMOR OF THE TENDON SHEATH

A giant cell tumor of the tendon sheath is a usually benign lesion that presents with a firm enlarging nodule on the finger.

SYNONYMS Localized nodular tenosynovitis, giant cell synovioma, pigmented villonodular synovitis.

EPIDEMIOLOGY

AGE Any age, most onset between 30 and 50 years.
GENDER F > M.
INCIDENCE Common.

HISTORY

Giant cell tumors are typically isolated asymptomatic nodules that are stable or slowly growing in size for years. Enlarging lesions may compress nerves and become painful or impair mobility.

PHYSICAL EXAMINATION

Skin Findings

TYPE Single nodule (Fig. 11-10).
SIZE Few millimeters to 1.5 cm.
COLOR Flesh-colored.
SHAPE Round.
PALPATION Firm, immobile.
DISTRIBUTION Finger > hand > toes.

DIFFERENTIAL DIAGNOSIS

The diagnosis of a giant cell tumor is made by history and clinical examination. It can be confused with a rheumatoid nodule, cyst, or subcutaneous granuloma annulare.

LABORATORY EXAMINATIONS

DERMATOPATHOLOGY Well-circumscribed lobular growth attached to the tendon sheath with cellular areas of polygonal cells blending with hypocellular areas of spindle cells, with characteristic multinucleate giant cells scattered throughout.

COURSE AND PROGNOSIS

Giant cell tumors of the tendon sheath are benign, and may be reactive or neoplastic in nature.

MANAGEMENT

Giant cell tumors are benign and asymptomatic and thus no treatment is required. For symptomatic or enlarging lesions, surgical excision can be performed, but there is a recurrence rate up to 30%.

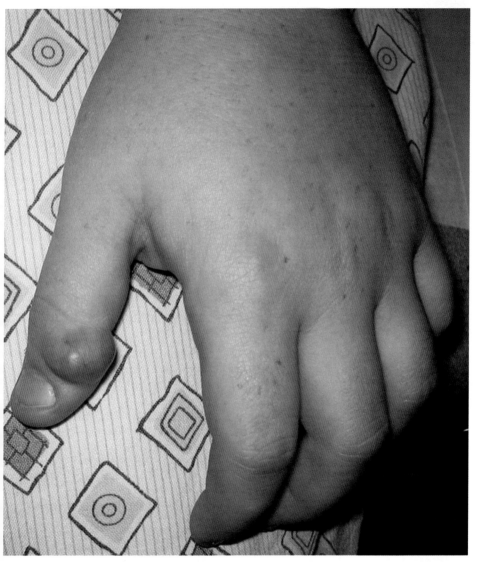

FIGURE 11-10 Giant cell tumor of the tendon sheath Enlarging firm nodule on the thumb of a child.

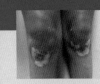

DISORDERS OF PIGMENTATION

Skin color is genetically determined and is caused by the total amount of melanin pigment in the skin. Normal constitutive melanin pigmentation determines skin type, which is classified by the Fitzpatrick skin phototypes as follows:

Skin Phototypes	Ability to Tan	Susceptibility to Burns
SPT I	Never tans, white skin	Sunburns easily
SPT II	Tans with difficulty	Sunburns easily
SPT III	Can tan with time	Occasionally burns
SPT IV	Tans easily	Rarely burns
SPT V	Tans easily, brown skin	Rarely burns
SPT VI	Tans easily, black skin	Rarely burns

Disorders of hypopigmentation are caused by decreased melanin content in the skin owing to decreased or absent melanin production or melanocytes (specialized cells of the epidermis that produce and store melanin). Disorders of hyperpigmentation are caused by increased melanin content in the skin owing to an increase in melanin production or melanocytes.

DISORDERS OF HYPOPIGMENTATION

Decreased or absent melanin in the skin can lead to hypomelanosis and can occur by two main mechanisms.
1. Melanocytopenic hypomelanosis: absent or decreased number of melanocytes (e.g., vitiligo).
2. Melanopenic hypomelanosis: absent or decreased melanin production, but normal number of melanocytes [e.g., oculocutaneous albinism (OCA)].

PITYRIASIS ALBA

Pityriasis alba is a common asymptomatic, sometimes scaly, hypopigmentation of the face, neck, and body.

INSIGHT Pityriasis alba entails both mild dermatitis and pigment alteration; generally, the former responds quickly while the latter continues to be an issue for many months or years.

EPIDEMIOLOGY

AGE Young children, often between the ages of 3 and 16 years.
GENDER M = F.
RACE All races, more noticeable in darker skin types.
PREVALENCE Common.
ETIOLOGY Likely a form of atopic dermatitis.

PATHOPHYSIOLOGY

Pityriasis alba is thought to be an eczematous dermatosis, with hypomelanosis resulting from postinflammatory changes and ultraviolet screening effects of the hyperkeratotic (increased thickness) and parakeratotic (inappropriately maturing) epidermis.

HISTORY

Hypopigmented areas are usually stable then gradually disappear with age. Some lesions may persist into adulthood. The areas are typically asymptomatic, but can sometimes burn or itch.

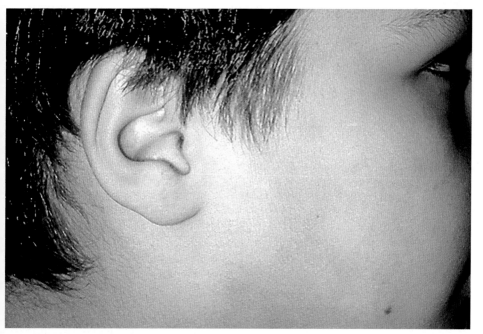

FIGURE 12-1 Pityriasis alba Faint hypopigmented slightly scaly macules located on the cheeks and preauricular area of a child.

PHYSICAL EXAMINATION

Skin Findings

TYPE Macules, may have slight scale.
NUMBER One to twenty lesions may be present.
COLOR Pink, then off-white to tan-white. Can repigment over time.
SIZE AND SHAPE 5 to 30 mm or larger.
DISTRIBUTION Face (malar region), neck, trunk, extremities.
SITES OF PREDILECTION Face, especially the cheeks (Fig. 12-1), midforehead, and around the eyes and mouth.

General Findings

May be associated with atopy (eczema, allergies, hay fever, asthma).

DIFFERENTIAL DIAGNOSIS

Pityriasis alba can be confused with other hypopigmented skin disorders such as vitiligo, tinea versicolor, tinea corporis, pityriasis lichenoides, and postinflammatory hypopigmentation.

LABORATORY EXAMINATIONS

DERMATOPATHOLOGY Histology reveals hyperkeratosis, parakeratosis, moderately dilated vessels of the superficial dermis, slight perivascular infiltrate, and edema of the papillary dermis.

On electron microscopy or immunohistochemistry, the number of melanocytes is normal or slightly reduced and those melanocytes present contain fewer and smaller melanosomes.
WOOD'S LAMP Accentuates hypopigmentation. Lesions are NOT depigmented.

COURSE AND PROGNOSIS

Pityriasis alba is a benign condition and often is self-limited, clearing at puberty. It is usually asymptomatic, but can be itchy or have a burning sensation.

MANAGEMENT

Treatment is unnecessary. The condition improves with age. For cosmetic reasons, emollient creams (hydrated petrolatum, Vaseline, mineral oil, moisturizers) may be useful to diminish the dry scales and ambient UV exposure can help repigment the area. In severely symptomatic cases of pityriasis alba, a mild topical steroid can be used sparingly in appropriate strengths for short durations (bid for 2 weeks). Topical calcineurin inhibitors and topical vitamin D analogs have also been reported to offer some relief for individuals with pityriasis alba and can be used for longer durations.

POSTINFLAMMATORY HYPOPIGMENTATION

A common cause of benign hypopigmentation characterized by decreased melanin formation following cutaneous inflammation.

SYNONYM Postinflammatory hypomelanosis.

EPIDEMIOLOGY

AGE Any age.
GENDER M = F.
ETIOLOGY Usually follows involution of any inflammatory skin disorders (e.g., eczematous or psoriatic lesions, pityriasis rosea, burns, bullous disorders, infections, etc.).

PATHOPHYSIOLOGY

Inflammatory conditions of the epidermis may result in transient alterations in melanosome biosynthesis, melanin production, and transport. Keratinocyte injury may render them temporarily unable to accept melanin from melanocytic dendrites. Severe inflammation or cutaneous injury (e.g., freezing) may even lead to a complete loss of melanocytes or melanocyte function.

HISTORY

SKIN SYMPTOMS None.

PHYSICAL EXAMINATION

Skin Findings

TYPE Macules, patches.
COLOR Off-white.
SHAPE Linear, oval, round, punctate depending on primary process (Fig. 12-2).
DISTRIBUTION Localized or diffuse depending on primary process.
WOOD'S LAMP Accentuates hypopigmentation. Lesions are NOT depigmented.

DIFFERENTIAL DIAGNOSIS

A clinical history of an antecedent inflammatory dermatosis is helpful to differentiate postinflammatory hypopigmentation from tinea versicolor, tuberous sclerosis, vitiligo, albinism, or infectious disease (e.g., leprosy). A careful clinical examination can also aid in distinguishing hypopigmented areas from entirely depigmented lesions.

LABORATORY EXAMINATIONS

DERMATOPATHOLOGY Skin biopsy may show decreased melanin in keratinocytes; inflammatory infiltrate may or may not be present depending on the etiologic primary process.
WOOD'S LAMP Accentuates hypopigmentation. Lesions are NOT depigmented.

COURSE AND PROGNOSIS

Hypopigmentation gradually self-resolves over a period of months provided that the affected areas are kept disease-free. Common inflammatory conditions that lead to postinflammatory hypopigmentation include psoriasis, seborrheic dermatitis, atopic dermatitis, lichen sclerosus, lichen striatus, lupus, and pityriasis lichenoides chronica.

MANAGEMENT

Postinflammatory hypopigmentation is a benign reactive condition, thus no treatment is necessary. Prevention would focus on eliminating the primary inflammatory process, allowing the melanocytes to recover and the hypopigmentation to slowly self-resolve. Patients should be counseled that hypopigmentation may take weeks to months of inflammation-free periods to improve. Judicious ambient UV exposure may be helpful in repigmenting affected areas.

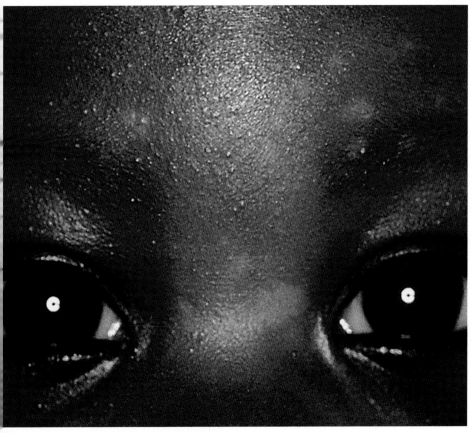

FIGURE 12-2 Postinflammatory hypopigmentation Residual hypopigmented macules after a rash on the face of a child.

VITILIGO

Vitiligo is an acquired pigmentary disorder characterized clinically by the development of completely depigmented macules, microscopically by the absence of melanocytes, and medically by the increased risk of autoimmune mediated disease (e.g., thyroid disorders).

 INSIGHT Visible depigmentation carries deep cultural and religious stigma for many and, while not life-threatening, vitiligo should be approached with this understanding.

EPIDEMIOLOGY

AGE Any age, 50% begin between ages 10 and 30 years.
GENDER M = F.
RACE All races. More noticeable in darker skin types.
INCIDENCE Common. Affects up to 2% of the population.
GENETICS Up to 30% of patients have a first-degree relative with vitiligo. Families with thyroid disease, Type 1 diabetes, and other autoimmune processes are at increased risk of developing vitiligo. Several genetic loci have been implicated: AIS1 (FOXD3), PTPN22, VIT1 (FBXO11), CTLA4, MITF, MHC (HLA-DRB1, HLA-DRB4, HLA-DQB1), ESR1, AIS2, AIS3, MLB2, CAT, VDR, MYG1, GCH1, NALP1 (SLEV1), ACE, AIRE, COMT.
ETIOLOGY Likely autoimmune mediated.

PATHOPHYSIOLOGY

In lesions of vitiligo, there is a decrease or absence of functional melanocytes in the skin. Numerous pathophysiologic mechanisms for vitiligo have been proposed: an autoimmune destruction of melanocytes, a defect in the structure and function of melanocytes, defective-free radical defenses, decreased melanocyte survival, autocytotoxic metabolites, faulty membrane lipid proteins in the melanocyte, defective melanocyte growth factors, neurochemical destruction of melanocytes, and viral etiologies.

HISTORY

Both genetics and environment play a role in vitiligo. Many patients attribute the onset of

their vitiligo to trauma, as with cuts, suture sites, etc. (Koebner or isomorphic phenomenon). Emotional stress (e.g., grief over lost partner) is also mentioned by patients as a cause. The depigmented areas gradually appear and 30% or more of individuals with vitiligo can undergo spontaneous repigmentation.

PHYSICAL EXAMINATION

Skin Findings

TYPE OF LESION Macule, patch.
SIZE Variable presentation from 1- to 5-mm confetti macules, to large several centimeter confluent patches.
COLOR White depigmentation.
SHAPE Oval, geographic patterns; linear.
DISTRIBUTION Face (periorificial), dorsa of hands, nipple, axillae, umbilicus, sacrum, inguinal, anogenital areas, extremities (elbows, knees, digits, wrists, ankles, shins), bony prominences (Fig. 12-3).

Associated Cutaneous Findings

HAIR White hair and premature gray hair, alopecia areata.
NEVI Halo nevi may be associated with vitiligo.
EYE Iritis in 10%, but may not be symptomatic; retinal changes consistent with healed chorioretinitis in up to 30% of patients.
PERIFOLLICULAR REPIGMENTATION Repigmentation occurs around hair follicles (Fig. 12-4) with macules that enlarge and eventually fuse to a confluent skin color. When areas of partial repigmentation are observed, the skin may have a "trichrome" appearance (normally pigmented, depigmented, and repigmenting areas).

General Examination

Hyper- or hypothyroidism is present in up to 30% of patients with vitiligo. Uncommon associations include diabetes mellitus, pernicious anemia, Addison's disease, gonadal failure, polyendocrinopathy, halo nevi, alopecia areata, and lichen sclerosis.

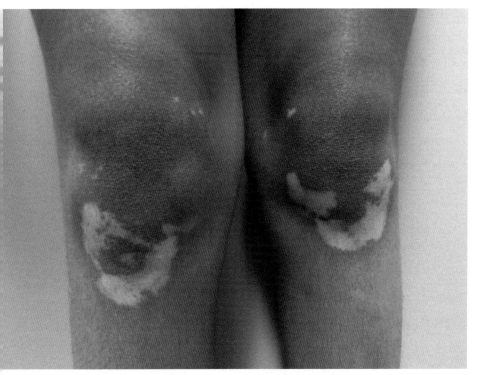

FIGURE 12-3 Vitiligo Areas of depigmentation on the knees of a child.

DIFFERENTIAL DIAGNOSIS

The differential diagnosis of completely depigmented skin lesions include lupus erythematosus, pityriasis alba, tinea versicolor, piebaldism, chemical leukoderma, scleroderma, leprosy, nevus depigmentosus, tuberous sclerosis, leukoderma with metastatic melanoma, and postinflammatory hypopigmentation.

LABORATORY EXAMINATIONS

DERMATOPATHOLOGY On skin biopsy, melanocytes are completely absent in fully developed vitiligo macules, but at the margin of the lesions, there may be melanocytes present with a mild surrounding lymphocytic response.

LABORATORY EXAMINATION OF BLOOD Blood tests for T4, TSH, glucose, CBC, and cortisol (in high-risk patients) may be indicated to rule out concurrent autoimmune diseases. Workup for additional autoimmune conditions as indicated based on the past medical and family histories.

WOOD'S LAMP Depigmented areas will light up brightly with the Wood's lamp examination.

COURSE AND PROGNOSIS

The course of vitiligo is unpredictable; lesions may remain stable for years or progress rapidly. Approximately 30% of patients have some degree of sun-induced or spontaneous repigmentation. Children tend to have a better prognosis and have fewer associated endocrinopathies as compared to adults.

MANAGEMENT

Ambient sunlight with sunscreen can help repigmentation, especially in cosmetically noticeable areas such as the face or hands. In older children that are sunlight responsive and compliant, phototherapy (narrowband UVB > PUVA) is useful. Limited use of topical steroids to the affected areas has been successful, but should be discontinued if there is no clinical improvement after 2 months. Topical tacrolimus 0.1% ointment has reported success without the adverse effects of light or steroid therapy and can be tried alone or in conjunction with other treatment modalities. In older refractory adults, suction blisters and autologous small skin punch grafts from normal skin areas can be grafted to depigmented areas, but scarring and dyspigmentation may result. Camouflage cosmetics may also be helpful for cosmetically noticeable areas.

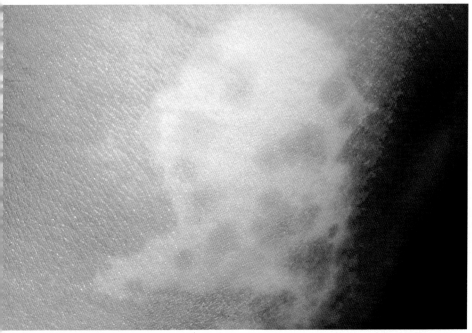

FIGURE 12-4 Vitiligo Depigmented area with characteristic "islands of repigmentation" indicative of follicular regeneration of pigment.

OCULOCUTANEOUS ALBINISM

OCA is a rare group of inherited disorders that present as a congenital absence of pigment in the skin, eyes, and hair. The pigment deficiency is caused by decreased or absent melanin, despite normal numbers of melanocytes in the skin.

OCA is primarily AR-inherited and can be categorized into four forms:

1. OCA type 1: absent (OCA1A) or decreased (OCA1B) tyrosinase activity.
2. OCA type 2: mutations in the P gene (resulting in defective molecular transporters).
3. OCA type 3: mutations in tyrosinase-related protein 1 (TYRP1) gene.
4. OCA type 4: mutations in membrane-associated transported protein (MATP) gene.

Ocular albinism (OA) patients primarily have XLR-inherited retinal depigmentation caused by a mutation in the ocular albinism type 1 (OA1) gene.

EPIDEMIOLOGY

AGE Present at birth.
INCIDENCE 1:20,000 in whites. 1:1,500 in some African tribes.
GENETICS OCA: AR (rare cases of AD). OA: XLR (rare cases of AR).

PATHOPHYSIOLOGY

OCA1 and OCA3 are endoplasmic reticulum (ER) retention diseases where the mutated proteins (tyrosinase or TYRP1, respectively) cannot leave the ER to become part of the melanosomes. OCA2 leads to a dysfunctional P protein which leads to abnormal processing or transport of tyrosinase. OCA4 leads to a defective transporter protein. OA has a mutated membrane glycoprotein that is thought to influence melanosomal growth and maturation.

PHYSICAL EXAMINATION

Skin Findings

TYPE Macular depigmentation of entire body (Fig. 12-5).
COLOR White or light tan (tyrosinase-negative).
HAIR White or light brown (tyrosinase-positive), red.
EYES Iris translucency, reduced visual acuity, photophobia, strabismus, nystagmus, lack of binocular vision.

LABORATORY EXAMINATIONS

Dermatopathology

LIGHT MICROSCOPY Melanocytes are present in normal numbers in the skin and hair bulb in all types of albinism. The dopa reaction is markedly reduced or absent in melanocytes of the skin and hair depending on the type of albinism.
IMMUNOHISTOCHEMISTRY AND ELECTRON MICROSCOPY Melanosomes are present in melanocytes in all types of albinism but, depending on the type of albinism, there is a reduction of the melanin content within melanosomes, with many completely lacking melanin.
TYROSINE HAIR BULB TEST Hair bulbs are incubated in tyrosine solutions for 12 to 24 hours and develop new pigment formation from normal and tyrosinase-positive OCA patients, but no new pigment formation is present in tyrosinase-negative OCA types.

DIFFERENTIAL DIAGNOSIS

The differential diagnosis would be whole-body vitiligo, but iris translucency and the presence of other eye findings in the fundus are reliable signs of albinism.

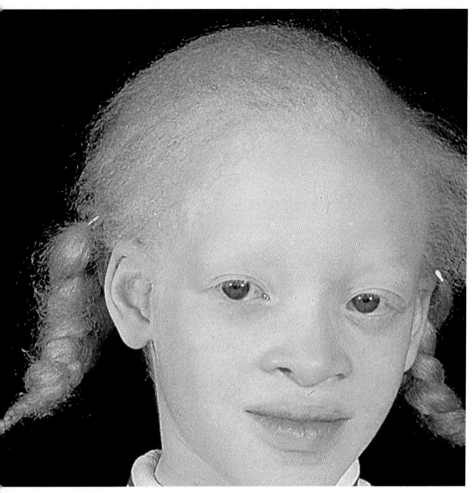

FIGURE 12-5 Albinism An African American child with albinism. Note the light-colored hair, skin and eyes in a child whose familial constitutional skin color is much darker.

COURSE AND PROGNOSIS

Depending upon the OCA type and degree of tyrosinase activity, patients may vary in severity from complete loss of pigment to subtle pigmentary dilution (Table 12-1). Patients with OCA learn early in life to avoid the sun because of repeated sunburns, especially as toddlers. They have a normal life span but can have problems with vision, to the point of blindness, and skin cancers later in life: squamous cell carcinomas (with metastases), basal cell carcinomas, and melanomas (typically amelanotic).

MANAGEMENT

Recognition of OCA early in life is important to begin early patient education about rigor-ous protective skin care. Daily application of topical, potent, broad-spectrum sunblocks, including lip protection (SPF higher than 30) is necessary. Special UV protective clothing and wide brim hats help to reduce sun exposure.

Avoidance of direct sun exposure between the hours of 10 AM and 2 PM, especially in high-intensity seasons or climates is recommended. OCA patients should have regular periodic skin examinations to detect skin cancers as early as possible. Patients should also have UV protective eyewear and regular ophthalmologic care.

TABLE 12-1 Classification of Albinism

Type	Subtypes	Gene Locus	Includes	Clinical Findings
OCA1	OCA1A	TYR - 11q14–q21	Tyrosinase-negative OCA	White hair and skin, eyes (pink at birth → blue). Skin cancers common.
	OCA1B	TYR - 11q14–q21	Minimal pigment OCA Platinum OCA Yellow OCA Temperature-sensitive OCA, tyrosinase loses activity at 35°C. Autosomal recessive OA (some)	White to near-normal skin and hair pigmentation Platinum (pheomelanin) hair Yellow (pheomelanin) hair, light red or brown hair May have near-normal pigment but not in axillas
OCA2		P - 15q11–q12	Tyrosinase-positive Brown OCA	Yellow hair, "creamy" white (Africa) Light brown/tan skin (Africa)
OCA3		TYRP1 - 9p23	Autosomal recessive OCA (some) Rufous OCA	Red and red-brown skin and brown eyes (African/African American population)
OCA4		MATP/SLC45A2 - 5p13		Generalized hypopigmentation (Japanese/East Asian population)
OA1		OA1/GPR143 - Xp22.3	X-linked OA, Nettleship–Falls ocular albinism	Normal pigmentation of skin, hair Hypopigmented eyes
OA2		OA2/CACNA1F - Xp11.23	X-linked OA, Forsius–Eriksson ocular albinism	Nystagmus, astigmatism, changes in color vision, retinal pigment changes

OCA, oculocutaneous albinism; OA, ocular albinism; TRPI, tyrosine-related protein I.

NEVUS DEPIGMENTOSUS

Nevus depigmentosus is a congenital hypomelanotic lesion characterized by a single depigmented spot, a segmental absence of pigment, or a Blaschkoid streak of hypopigmentation with a chronic persistent course.

SYNONYMS Nevus achromicus, nevoid linear hypopigmentation.

EPIDEMIOLOGY

AGE Present at birth.
GENDER M = F.
PREVALENCE 1 in 75 people.

PATHOPHYSIOLOGY

Proposed mechanism for nevus depigmentosus is chromosomal mosaicism.

HISTORY

Individuals are born with the depigmented area of skin and the area is asymptomatic but persists for life.

PHYSICAL EXAMINATION

Skin Findings

TYPE Macules or patches.
COLOR Depigmented white or light tan (Fig. 12-6).
SIZE Few millimeters to several centimeters.
SHAPE Isolate, segmental, or linear following Blaschko's lines.
DISTRIBUTION Trunk, buttocks, lower abdomen, proximal extremities > face, neck.

DIFFERENTIAL DIAGNOSIS

An isolated nevus depigmentosus must be differentiated from vitiligo, nevus anemicus, and lesions of tuberous sclerosis. Very extensive lesions, multilinear Blaschkoid hypomelanosis should raise the possible diagnosis of hypomelanosis of Ito in which the pigmentation is associated with abnormalities of the hair, CNS, eyes, or musculoskeletal system.

LABORATORY EXAMINATIONS

DERMATOPATHOLOGY Lesions may show normal or decreased melanocyte numbers.
ELECTRON MICROSCOPY Melanin density within melanocytes is decreased or normal, with a normal number of melanocytes.
WOOD'S LAMP Accentuation of depigmented areas.

COURSE AND PROGNOSIS

Lesions persist for life, but remain asymptomatic.

MANAGEMENT

A nevus depigmentosus is asymptomatic and for small lesions, treatment is not necessary. Extensive lesions, or those on the face, can be cosmetically upsetting to the patient. Since nevus depigmentosus lesions do not tan as well as the surrounding skin, they become more noticeable with UV exposure. Thus rigorous sun protection (SPF 30 of higher) helps keep lesions less cosmetically detectable.

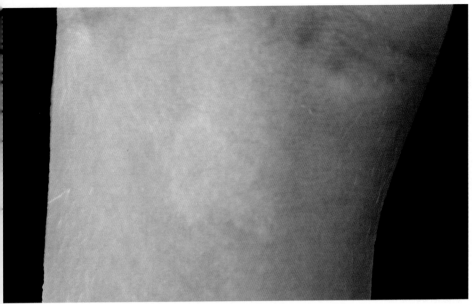

FIGURE 12-6 Nevus depigmentosus Depigmented area on the posterior leg of a child.

NEVUS ANEMICUS

Nevus anemicus is a rare congenital area of pale skin that represents localized, decreased perfusion.

SYNONYM Pharmacologic nevus.

EPIDEMIOLOGY

AGE Newborn.
GENDER F > M.
PREVALENCE Rare.

PATHOPHYSIOLOGY

It has been suggested that nevus anemicus arises from a focal increased blood vessel sensitivity to vascular catecholamines and thus are permanently vasoconstricted.

HISTORY

Lesions are present at birth and persist asymptomatically for life.

PHYSICAL EXAMINATION

Skin Findings

TYPE Macule or patch (Fig. 12-7).
SIZE Few millimeters to several centimeters, typically up to 5 to 10 cm in size.
COLOR Hypopigmented, avascular appearing.
DISTRIBUTION Chest > face and extremities.

DIFFERENTIAL DIAGNOSIS

The differential diagnosis includes nevus depigmentosus, tuberous sclerosis, vitiligo, hypomelanosis of Ito, and incontinentia pigmenti. Three factors may be helpful for differentiating a nevus anemicus from a pigmentary problem: (1) a nevus anemicus does not accentuate by Wood's lamp; (2) pressure on the lesion by a glass slide makes the lesion unapparent from surrounding normal skin; and (3) stroking or heat application fails to induce erythema in the lesion (Fig. 12-7).

LABORATORY EXAMINATIONS

DERMATOPATHOLOGY A skin biopsy reveals normal numbers of blood vessels and melanocytes. The biopsy would most likely be interpreted as normal skin.
WOOD'S LAMP Does not enhance the lesion.

COURSE AND PROGNOSIS

Nevus anemicus persists for life and is usually asymptomatic. They are usually only noticeable when there is surrounding vasodilation because of heat or stress. In individuals with multiple café au lait macules and a nevus anemicus—particularly on the neck or upper chest—evaluation for an association with neurofibromatosis type 1 may be considered.

MANAGEMENT

No treatment is effective or necessary.

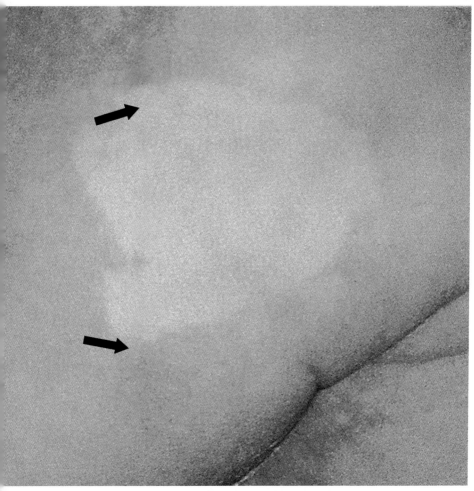

FIGURE 12-7 Nevus anemicus Hypopigmented macule present since birth. Stroking of the lesion produces a normal erythematous response at the periphery (*arrows*) but not within the lesion, indicative of its avascularity.

DISORDERS OF HYPERPIGMENTATION

Increased melanin in the skin can lead to hypermelanosis and can occur by two main mechanisms:

1. Increased melanocytes in the epidermis producing melanocytic hypermelanosis.
2. Normal melanocyte numbers in the epidermis, but increased amounts of *melanin-producing melanotic hypermelanosis* [e.g., postinflammatory hyperpigmentation (PIH)].

POSTINFLAMMATORY HYPERPIGMENTATION

PIH is a common entity characterized by increased melanin formation and deposition following cutaneous inflammation.

SYNONYM Postinflammatory hypermelanosis.

EPIDEMIOLOGY

AGE Any age.
GENDER M = F.
RACE More severe and longer lasting in darker skin types.
ETIOLOGY An acquired increase of melanin pigment can follow any inflammatory process (physical trauma, acne, friction, irritant dermatitis, eczematous dermatitis, lichen simplex chronicus, psoriasis, pityriasis rosea, fixed drug eruptions, lichen planus, pyoderma, photodermatitis, dermatitis herpetiformis, lupus erythematosus).

PATHOPHYSIOLOGY

Inflammatory conditions of the skin may result in increased melanin within the epidermis or dermis. The epidermal forms of PIH are caused by an increase in melanin synthesis and/or transfer to the keratinocytes. The dermal forms of PIH are caused by dermal melanophages phagocytosing melanosomes after skin injury.

PHYSICAL EXAMINATION

Skin Findings

TYPE Macules, patches (Fig. 12-8).
SIZE Few millimeters to several centimeters.
COLOR Epidermal PIH: tan to dark brown. Dermal PIH: gray-blue to gray-brown.
SHAPE Linear, oval, round, punctate depending on primary process.

DISTRIBUTION Localized or diffused depending on primary process.

DIFFERENTIAL DIAGNOSIS

A clinical history of a previous inflammatory process is helpful to distinguish PIH from melanocytic proliferations (ephelides, lentigines, nevi), endocrine abnormalities (Addison's disease, estrogen therapy, ACTH and MSH producing tumors, hyperthyroidism), metabolic disorders (hemochromatosis, porphyria cutanea tarda, ochronosis), melasma, melanoma, scleroderma, pregnancy, drug-induced hyperpigmentation, ashy dermatosis, and macular amyloidosis.

LABORATORY EXAMINATIONS

DERMATOPATHOLOGY Epidermal PIH: increased melanin in the epidermal keratinocytes. Dermal PIH: increased melanin within the dermal melanophages.
WOOD'S LAMP Accentuation of epidermal pigmentation.

COURSE AND PROGNOSIS

Epidermal hyperpigmentation gradually fades over a period of months provided the underlying dermatosis is kept under good control. Dermal hyperpigmentation is more difficult to clear, and may persist for life. Darker skin types have a more refractory course.

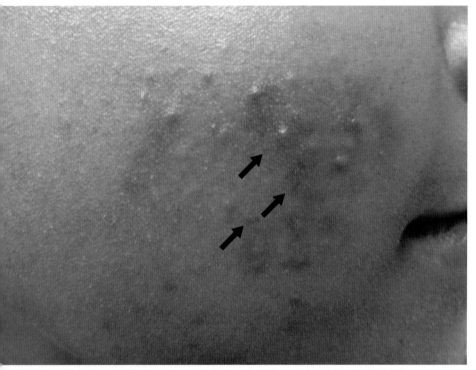

FIGURE 12-8 Postinflammatory hyperpigmentation Hyperpigmented areas (*arrows*) resulting from inflammatory lesions in an adolescent with acne.

MANAGEMENT

Treatment is not necessary and with good control of the underlying dermatosis, the hyperpigmentation (epidermal PIH > dermal PIH) will fade over time. To hasten the resolution of PIH, several topical approaches have limited success: sun protection (SPF 30 of higher), azelaic acid, hydroxy acid peels, hydroquinone (2–4%), or a steroid/hydroquinone/retinoid combination. Patients should be warned that with all therapies, worsening of the hyperpigmentation is possible. They should also be informed about sun protection when using these products as well as about their slow therapeutic action (3–4 months are required before a therapeutic effect is achieved).

Laser treatments are more successful for epidermal PIH than dermal PIH. Lasers have their limitations, especially in darker skin types where constitutive pigment can be lost.

LINEAR AND WHORLED NEVOID HYPERMELANOSIS

Linear and whorled nevoid hypermelanosis is a benign, congenital, streaky hyperpigmentation along Blaschko's lines resulting from mosaicism.

SYNONYMS Linear nevoid hyperpigmentation, zebra-like hyperpigmentation in whorls and streaks, reticulate, and zosteriform hyperpigmentation.

EPIDEMIOLOGY

AGE At or soon after birth.
GENDER M = F.
RACE No racial predilection.
PREVALENCE Rare.
ETIOLOGY Chromosomal mosaicism may be present.

PATHOPHYSIOLOGY

Nevoid hyperpigmentation along Blaschko's lines is thought to be due to somatic mosaicism during embryogenesis likely because of a heterogeneous group of genetic abnormalities rather than just one specific entity. The whorled lines of pigment likely represent the clonal migration and proliferation of embryonic melanocyte precursors.

HISTORY

Whorled "marble cake-like" streaks of hyperpigmentation appear soon after birth with no antecedent rash, persist asymptomatically for life, and may become less prominent with time. There are rare reports of associated cardiac, neurologic, or musculoskeletal defects.

PHYSICAL EXAMINATION

Skin Findings

TYPE Macular whorled hyperpigmentation (Fig. 12-9).

COLOR Hyperpigmentation. Occasionally hypopigmentation.
SIZE Several centimeters to entire body.
DISTRIBUTION Localized area, entire limb, quadrant, or the whole body. Mucous membranes, palms, soles spared.

DIFFERENTIAL DIAGNOSIS

History and physical examination with no antecedent rash and no associated anomalies differentiates linear and whorled nevoid hypermelanosis from incontinentia pigmenti (third stage), hypomelanosis of Ito, epidermal nevi, or other reticulated pigmentary syndromes.

LABORATORY EXAMINATIONS

DERMATOPATHOLOGY Skin biopsy shows basilar hyperpigmentation with a slight increase in basal melanocytes without incontinence of pigment.

COURSE AND PROGNOSIS

Skin findings are congenital, asymptomatic, and persist for life without complications. A few cases fade in pigmentation with time.

MANAGEMENT

Linear and whorled hyperpigmentation is benign and asymptomatic, but can be cosmetically distressing to the patient. Topical treatments are not effective. Camouflage cosmetics may be helpful. Laser treatments as a possible treatment modality are being investigated.

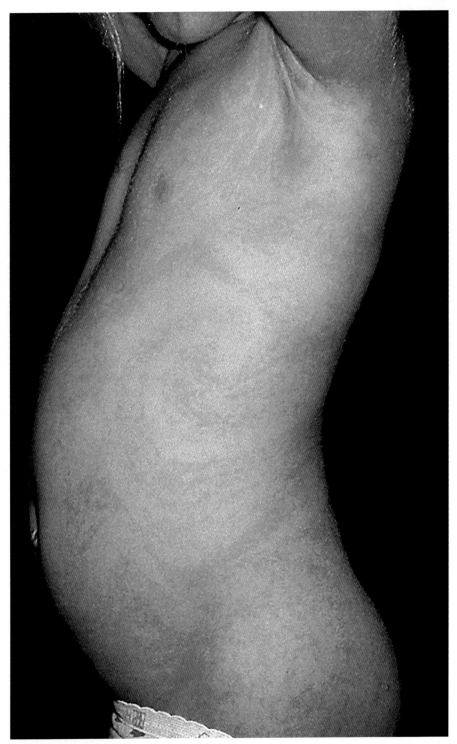

FIGURE 12-9 Linear and whorled hypermelanosis Congenital whorled pigmentation present since birth in an otherwise well child.

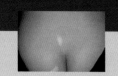

NEUROCUTANEOUS DISORDERS

The neurocutaneous disorders are a group of inherited conditions associated with skin, peripheral and central nervous system (CNS), and other systemic abnormalities. Embryologi-cally, the skin and nervous system are derived from the same neural crest origin, and thus it is not surprising that many neurologic disorders have associated skin abnormalities.

NEUROFIBROMATOSIS

Neurofibromatosis (NF) is an autosomal dominant disorder characterized cutaneously by café au lait macules (CALMs), axillary freckling, cutaneous neurofibromas, and tumors of the nervous system. NF has seven recognized subtypes:

1. NF-1: von Recklinghausen disease, mutation in NF1 gene, abnormal neurofibromin.
2. NF-2: Acoustic neuroma, mutation in NF2 gene abnormal merlin/neurofibromin 2.
3. NF-3: Mixed NF with central and peripheral neurofibromas.
4. NF-4: Variant NF.
5. NF-5: Segmental NF.
6. NF-6: CALMs only.
7. NF-7: Late-onset NF.

SYNONYM von Recklinghausen disease (NF Type 1).

EPIDEMIOLOGY

AGE Birth: plexiform neurofibromas may be present (25%). Aging from 2 to 3 years: CALM (>90%), axillary or inguinal freckling (80%). Puberty: other cutaneous neurofibromas (up to 90%).
GENDER M > F.
RACE All races.
INCIDENCE **NF-1,** 1:3,000 people; **NF-2,** 1:40,000 people.
HEREDITY AD, with variable expressivity.

PATHOPHYSIOLOGY

NF-1 is an autosomal dominantly inherited disorder caused by a mutation in chromosome 17q11.2. The gene product, neurofibromin, negatively regulates the *Ras*-family of signal-ing molecules through GTP-activating protein (GAP) function. NF-2 is also an autosomal dominantly inherited disorder caused by a mutation in chromosome 22q12.2. The gene product, merlin (also known as neurofibromin 2), is thought to be involved in actin cytoskeletal signaling.

HISTORY

CALMs are not usually present at birth but appear during the first 3 years; neurofibromas appear during late adolescence and may be tender to palpation. Clinical manifestations can vary depending on which organ is affected: hypertensive headache (pheochromocytomas), pathologic fractures (bone cysts), mental retardation, brain tumors (astrocytoma), short stature, or precocious puberty (early menses, clitoral hypertrophy) may develop.

PHYSICAL EXAMINATION

Skin Findings

CALMS 2-mm to >20-cm brown "coffee-with-milk" colored macules (90%). Often with an ovoid appearance (Fig. 13-1).

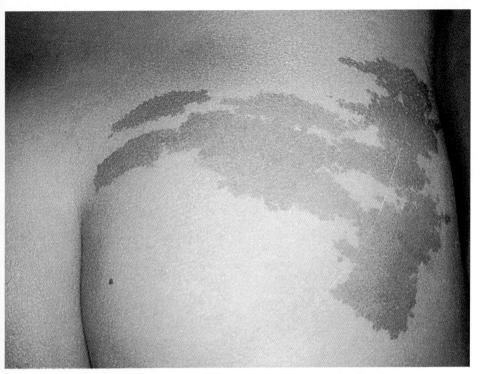

FIGURE 13-1 Neurofibromatosis, café au lait macule Well-demarcated uniform brown macule on the buttock of a patient with neurofibromatosis.

CROWE'S SIGN Freckle-like macules in the axillary or inguinal folds (80%) (Fig. 13-2).

NEUROFIBROMAS Soft tan-to-pink nodules with "button hole sign"—invagination with the tip of finger (60–90%) (Fig. 13-3). Occasionally may be subcutaneous, below the surface of the skin.

PLEXIFORM NEUROFIBROMAS Soft tan loose lesions, described as a "bag of worms" (25%).

NEVUS ANEMICUS Patch of relatively hypopigmented-appearing skin resulting from vasoconstriction of overly sensitive cutaneous blood vessels. Seen in the neck and upper chest of individuals with NF (up to 50%).

GLOMUS TUMORS Multiple blue-red painful vascular papules on the fingers and toes, often associated with the nail bed.

JUVENILE XANTHOGRANULOMAS Yellow-orange verrucous papules with a stuck-on appearance (15%).

DISTRIBUTION OF LESIONS Randomly distributed but may be localized to one region (segmental NF).

General Findings

EYE Lisch nodules—pigmented iris hamartomas (>90%), hypertelorism (25%), glaucoma.

MUSCULOSKELETAL Macrocephaly (20–50%), sphenoid wing dysplasia (<5%), scoliosis (10%), spina bifida, pseudoarthrosis (2%), thinning of long bone cortex, local bony overgrowth, absent patellae.

TUMORS Optic glioma (15%), malignant peripheral nerve sheath tumors (arise from plexiform neurofibromas) (15%), pheochromocytoma (1%), juvenile myelomonocytic leukemia (especially in patients with juvenile xanthogranulomas), rhabdomyosarcoma, duodenal carcinoid, somatostatinoma, parathyroid adenoma.

CNS Learning disorder (50%), seizures (5%), mental retardation (5%), hydrocephalus (2%).

CARDIOVASCULAR Hypertension (30%), pulmonary stenosis (1%), renal artery stenosis (2%).

LABORATORY EXAMINATIONS

Dermatopathology

CALM Increased melanin within the epidermis, increased melanocytes, giant melanosomes.

NEUROFIBROMAS Dermal small nerve fibers with surrounding fibroblasts, Schwann cells, and perineural cells.

PLEXIFORM NEUROFIBROMAS Large hypertrophied nerves with spindle-shaped fibroblasts and Schwann cells in a myxoid matrix.

WOOD'S LAMP CALMs are more easily visualized with Wood's lamp examination.

DIFFERENTIAL DIAGNOSIS

CALMs can also be present in McCune–Albright syndrome (polyostotic fibrous dysplasia). The CALMs in McCune–Albright syndrome frequently have a jagged "coast of Maine" border as compared to the CALMs in NF-1, which have smooth "coast of California" borders. Other criteria listed above are required to establish a diagnosis of NF.

COURSE AND PROGNOSIS

There is a variable involvement of the organs affected over time, with NF-1 patients being most severely involved. Skin problems can range from just a few pigmented macules to marked disfigurement with thousands of nodules, segmental hypertrophy, and plexiform neurofibromas. The mortality rate is higher than in the normal population, principally because of the development of systemic tumors and complications during adult life.

MANAGEMENT

It is important to establish the diagnosis to follow patients with a multidisciplinary approach.

NF-1 The diagnosis of NF-1 can be made if **two** of the following NIH criteria are met:

1. Six or more CALMs (<5 years old: CALM >5 mm each; >5 years old: CALM >1.5 cm each).

2. Multiple freckles in the axillary and/or inguinal regions (Crowe's sign).
3. Two or more neurofibromas of any type, or one plexiform neurofibroma.
4. Bony lesion (sphenoid wing dysplasia, thinning of long bone cortex, with or without pseudoarthrosis).
5. Optic nerve glioma(s).
6. Two or more Lisch nodules (iris hamartomas) on slit lamp examination.
7. First-degree relative (parent, sibling, or child) with NF-1 by the above criteria.

Ninety-seven percent of NF-1 patients meet these criteria by age 8 years, 100% by 20 years. In NF-1, support groups help with social adjustment in severely affected persons. An orthopedic physician should manage the two major bone problems: kyphoscoliosis and tibial bowing. A plastic surgeon can do reconstructive surgery on the facial asymmetry. The language disorders and learning disabilities should be evaluated by psychological assessment. Close follow-up annually should be mandatory to detect sarcomas and leukemias and to screen for new dermatologic lesions, neurologic symptoms, or onset of hypertension. Regular ophthalmologic evaluation is also encouraged.

NF-2 The diagnosis of NF-2 can be made by:

1. CT scan or MRI demonstrating bilateral acoustic neuromas or
2. A first-degree relative (parent, sibling, child) with NF-2 and either:
   a. Unilateral nerve VIII mass or
   b. Two of the following: neurofibroma, meningioma, glioma, schwannoma, juvenile posterior subcapsular lenticular opacity.

Cutaneous schwannomas are seen in the majority of patients with NF-2 (67%).

NF-5 In NF-5, the disease has a segmental distribution because of postzygotic mutations and mosaicism. The cutaneous lesions characteristically respect the midline. Involvement of the gonads in these individuals can result in offspring with full-blown NF-1, thus genetic counseling is recommended.

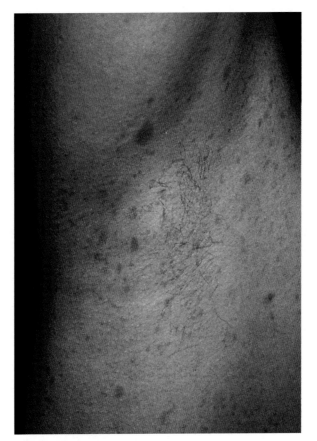

FIGURE 13-2 Neurofibromatosis, Crowe's sign Axillary freckling in an adolescent with neurofibromatosis.

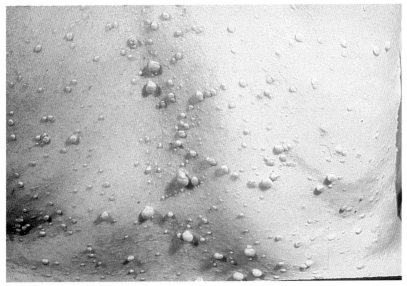

FIGURE 13-3 Neurofibromatosis, neurofibromas Skin-colored soft papules and nodules on the back are neurofibromata appearing in late adolescence in a patient with neurofibromatosis.

TUBEROUS SCLEROSIS

Tuberous sclerosis is an autosomal dominant disease characterized by the triad of seizures, mental retardation, and skin findings (congenital hypopigmented spots, facial angiofibromata).

SYNONYMS Epiloia (**epi**lepsy, **lo**w **i**ntelligence, **a**ngiofibroma), Bourneville disease.

EPIDEMIOLOGY

AGE Infancy.
GENDER M = F.
RACE All races.
INCIDENCE 1:10,000.
GENETICS AD, more than 75% of cases are new mutations.

PATHOPHYSIOLOGY

Gene defects in chromosome 9p34 (termed TSC1, 33–50% of patients) and chromosome 16p13 (termed TSC2, 50–64% of patients) have been identified. Chromosome 9q34 affects the gene product hamartin, a protein that interacts with tuberin in some fashion. Chromosome 16p13 affects the gene product tuberin—a protein that negatively regulates *Rab5* and *Rheb* proteins through GAP domains and impacts *Ras* and *MAP kinase* signaling. Both chromosome mutations lead to genetic alterations of ectodermal and mesodermal cells with hyperplasia and a disturbance in embryonic cellular differentiation.

HISTORY

White macules appear at birth or in infancy (90% occur by 1 year of age, 100% appear by the age of 2 years) followed by a shagreen patch, a form of a connective tissue nevus (seen in 40% of patients between 2 and 5 years of age) and facial angiofibromas at puberty. The skin changes often precede the systemic symptoms. Seizures (95%) and infantile spasms (70%) follow skin signs, and earlier-onset seizures lead to more marked mental retardation.

PHYSICAL EXAMINATION

Skin Findings (96%)

1. Hypomelanotic macules (ash leaf spot, confetti macules, and thumbprint macules), 90% by 1 year (Fig. 13-4 A and B). Classic ash leaf macules have one tapered end and one ovoid or rounded end.

2. Facial red papules/nodules (adenoma sebaceum, angiofibromas), <20% at 1 year, 80% by adulthood (Fig. 13-5).
3. Truncal yellow–brown plaques (Shagreen "leather" patch, connective tissue nevus) in 40%—favors buttock area (Fig. 13-6).
4. Peri/subungual papules (fibromas, "Koenen tumors") in 30% to 60% (Fig. 13-7).
5. Forehead fibrous plaque (hamartomas) in 20% (Fig. 13-8).
6. CALMs in 30%. See section above on "Neurofibromatosis" for description of CALMs.

General Findings

EYE Retinal hamartomas (40%), achromic retinal patches (40%), retinal astrocytoma.
MUSCULOSKELETAL Cystic bone rarefaction.
DENTAL Pitted enamel (90%), gingival fibromas.
PULMONARY Lymphangioleiomyomatosis (30% females).
RENAL Bilateral angiomyolipomas (90%), cysts, carcinoma.
ENDOCRINE Precocious puberty, hypothyroidism.
CNS Seizures (95%), subependymal nodules (80%), cortical tubers (90%), infantile spasms (70%), mental retardation, intracranial calcification, giant cell astrocytoma.
CARDIAC Myocardial rhabdomyoma (80%), Wolff–Parkinson–White syndrome.

LABORATORY EXAMINATIONS

DERMATOPATHOLOGY White macules: decreased number of melanocytes, decreased melanosome size, decreased melanin in melanocytes, and keratinocytes. Angiofibromata: dermal fibrosis, capillary dilation, absence of elastic tissue. CALM: Increased melanin within the epidermis, increased melanocytes, giant melanosomes.
WOOD'S LAMP Accentuates depigmented and hyperpigmented lesions.
SKULL X-RAY Multiple calcific densities are seen in 50% to 75% of individuals.
MRI OR CT SCAN In smaller children, when skull radiographs are not diagnostic, small calcifications (often paraventricular) and ventricular dilation are helpful in diagnosis.

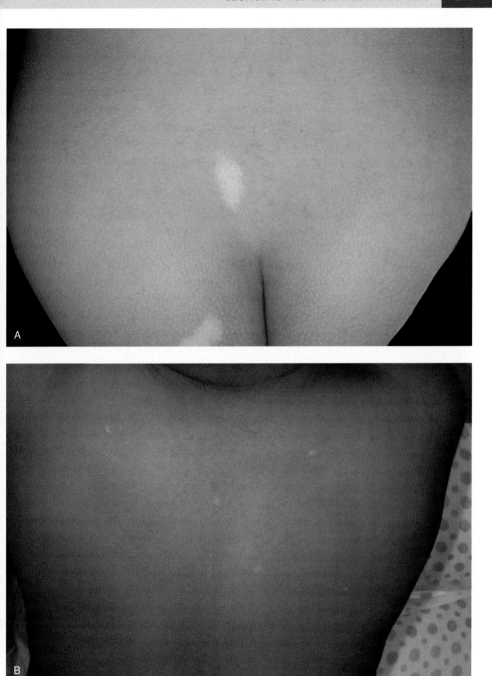

FIGURE 13-4 Tuberous sclerosis, ash leaf macule A: Oval-shaped hypopigmented macules on the lower back of a child with tuberous sclerosis. **B:** Scattered hypopigmented macules on the back of a child.

DIFFERENTIAL DIAGNOSIS

The diagnosis may be difficult or impossible in an infant or child when white macules are the only cutaneous finding. Initially, TS may be confused with nevus depigmentosus, vitiligo, or piebaldism. The angiofibromata (adenoma sebaceum) of the face are almost pathognomonic but do not appear until late infancy or older.

Even when typical white ash leaf or thumbprint macules are present, it is necessary to confirm the diagnosis. A pediatric neurologist can then evaluate the patient with a study of the family members, and by obtaining various types of imaging. It should be noted that mental retardation and seizures may be absent.

COURSE AND PROGNOSIS

Diagnostic criteria for tuberous sclerosis complex have either **two major features** as listed below or **one major feature** plus **two minor features**:

1. **Major features** include facial angiofibromas or forehead plaque; ungual or periungual fibromas; three or more hypomelanotic macules; shagreen patch (connective tissue nevus); retinal nodular hamartomas; cortical tubers; subependymal nodules; subependymal giant cell astrocytoma; renal angiomyolipoma; cardiac rhabdomyoma; and pulmonary lymphangioleiomyomatosis.
2. **Minor features** include confetti skin lesions; dental pits; gingival fibromas; retinal achromic patches; cerebral white matter radial migration lines; renal cysts; rectal polyps; bone cysts; or nonrenal hamartomas.

MANAGEMENT

Treatment is targeted at affected organs. In severe cases of TS, 30% of patients die before the fifth year of life and 50% to 75% before reaching adult age. Most die from CNS tumors or status epilepticus.

Every newly diagnosis TS patient should have either a CT scan or MRI to look for confirmatory subependymal nodules or cortical tubers in the brain. Seizures can be controlled with anticonvulsant therapy. Renal ultrasounds should be obtained to monitor for polycystic kidney disease or rarely malignant renal cell carcinoma. ECGs can be abnormal before arrhythmias appear clinically. In women, a lung CT scan will detect lymphangioleiomyomatosis. Additionally, ophthalmologic examination, neurodevelopmental testing, genetic counseling, and support groups are recommended.

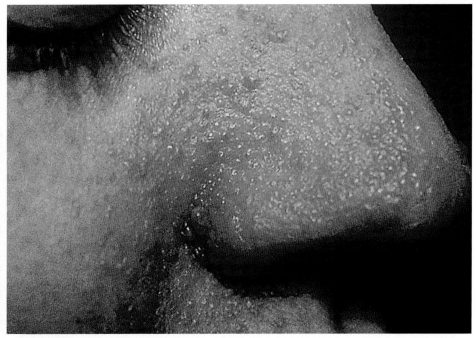

FIGURE 13-5 Tuberous sclerosis, adenoma sebaceum Small erythematous papules on the nose and cheeks of an adolescent representing angiofibromata.

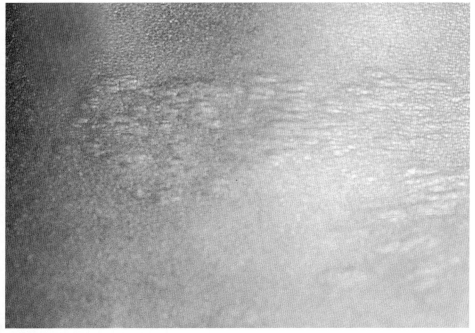

FIGURE 13-6 Tuberous sclerosis, Shagreen patch Raised skin-colored plaque on the torso of a child representing a connective tissue nevus.

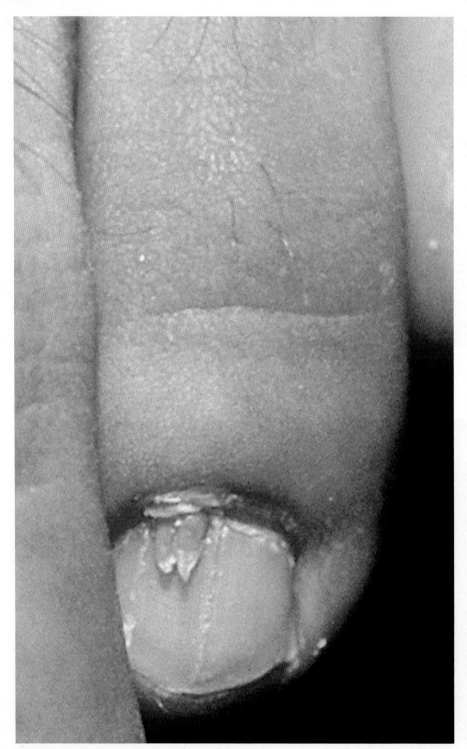

FIGURE 13-7 Tuberous sclerosis, periungual fibromas Flesh-colored periungual papule appearing in adolescence in an individual with tuberous sclerosis.

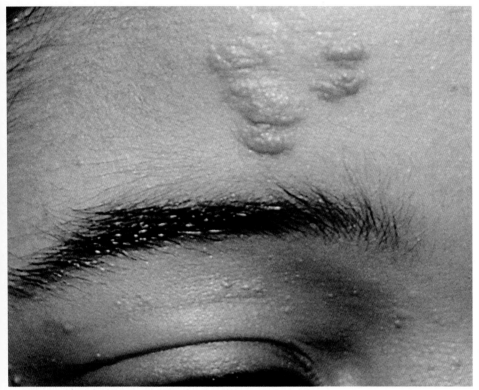

FIGURE 13-8 Tuberous sclerosis, forehead fibrous plaque   Raised skin-colored plaque on the forehead of a child representing a connective tissue nevus.

INCONTINENTIA PIGMENTI

Incontinentia pigmenti (IP) is an X-linked dominant (male lethal) disease affecting the skin, CNS, eyes, and skeletal system. The skin of affected females has "marble cake" lines of Blaschkoid pigmentation with four distinct stages: inflammatory/vesicular, verrucous, hyperpigmented, and hypopigmented/atrophic. Eighty percent of IP patients have eye, CNS, or skeletal manifestations.

SYNONYMS Bloch–Sulzberger syndrome, Bloch–Siemens syndrome.

EPIDEMIOLOGY

AGE Vesiculobullous stage: first days to weeks of life.
GENDER Females, 97%. Disease is prenatally lethal to males.
PREVALENCE Rare.
GENETICS XLD, some sporadic.

PATHOPHYSIOLOGY

The linear skin lesions in IP reflect mosaicism from lyonization (X inactivation).
Two gene loci for IP have been identified:

1. IP1 with Xp11/autosome translocations causing pigmentary abnormalities without a preceding inflammatory phase.
2. IP2 with XLD mutations in the NEMO gene (Xq28). These mutations are suspected to produce a failure of immune tolerance in ectodermal tissues resulting in an autoimmune-like reaction in heterozygote girls and a fatal graft-versus-host-like disease in homozygous boys.

PHYSICAL EXAMINATION

Skin Findings

INFLAMMATORY STAGE (newborn to few months) Linear vesicles/bullae on trunk or extremities at birth or shortly thereafter (Fig. 13-9).
VERRUCOUS STAGE (few months to 1 year) Linear verrucous lesions, resolves after several months (Fig. 13-10).
HYPERPIGMENTED STAGE (1 year to adolescence) Reticulate hyperpigmented streaks (seen in 100% of patients, Fig. 13-11).
HYPOPIGMENTED STAGE (adulthood) Hypopigmented atrophic linear streaks, devoid of hair, and sweat pores.

General Findings

EYE Microphthalmia, retinal vascular abnormalities, pseudoglioma, cataracts, optic atrophy.
MUSCULOSKELETAL Skull abnormalities, scoliosis.
CNS Mental retardation (16%), seizures (3%), spastic abnormalities (13%).
OTHER Pulmonary hypertension, asymmetric breast development, supernumerary nipples, conical/missing teeth (64%), nail dystrophy (7%), nail tumors, and peripheral eosinophilia during inflammatory phase (74%).

DIFFERENTIAL DIAGNOSIS

The differential can vary from stage to stage.
INFLAMMATORY STAGE Can be confused with herpes, epidermolysis bullosa, linear IgA, childhood bullous pemphigus.
VERRUCOUS STAGE Can be confused with an epidermal nevus.
HYPERPIGMENTED STAGE Can be confused with linear and whorled nevoid hypermelanosis, lichen planus, lichen nitidus.
HYPOPIGMENTED STAGE Can be confused with hypomelanosis of Ito.

LABORATORY EXAMINATIONS

Dermatopathology

INFLAMMATORY STAGE Intraepidermal vesicles with eosinophils, focal dyskeratosis.
VERRUCOUS STAGE Acanthosis, irregular papillomatosis, hyperkeratosis, basal cell vacuolization.
HYPERPIGMENTED STAGE Extensive deposits of melanin in melanophages in the upper dermis.
HYPOPIGMENTED STAGE Decreased melanin as well as appendages in affected skin.
HEMATOLOGY Peripheral eosinophilia in inflammatory stage.
RADIOGRAPHY Lytic effects on distal phalanges.

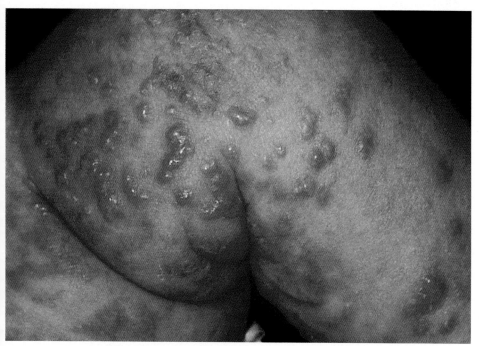

FIGURE 13-9 Incontinentia pigmenti, inflammatory stage Inflammatory papules and vesicles on the leg of a newborn.

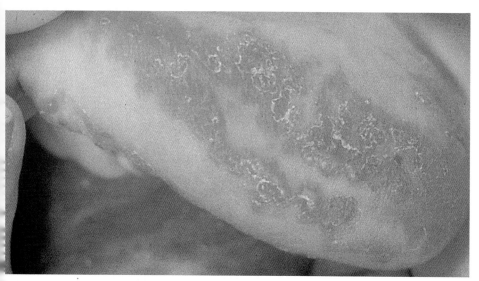

FIGURE 13-10 Incontinentia pigmenti, verrucous stage Verrucous linear streaks on the trunk of an infant.

COURSE AND PROGNOSIS

Up to 80% of patients have systemic disease. There is a poor prognosis and developmental delay in patients who develop seizures during the first week of life. Absence of seizures and normal developmental milestones appears to predict a good prognosis. The pigmentary changes may persist for many years and gradually fade, completely disappearing in adolescence or early adulthood.

MANAGEMENT

No treatment is effective or required for the cutaneous lesions of IP, other than symptomatic relief. Neurologic, dental, ophthalmic evaluations, and genetic counseling/support groups for carrier females are advisable because up to 80% of affected children have associated congenital defects.

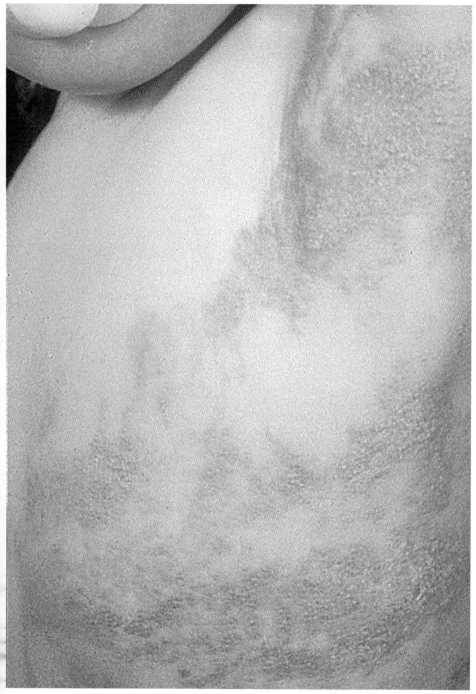

FIGURE 13-11 Incontinentia pigmenti, hyperpigmented stage Hyperpigmentation along the lines of Blaschko in a child with incontinentia pigmenti.

HYPOMELANOSIS OF ITO

A heterogenous group of disorders that have in common: hypopigmented streaks in a Blaschkoid distribution associated with CNS, ocular or musculoskeletal abnormalities.

SYNONYMS IP achromians, pigmentary mosaicism, linear nevoid hypopigmentation.

EPIDEMIOLOGY

AGE Birth, early infancy or childhood.
GENDER M = F.
PREVALENCE 1:8,000.
RACE Equal, but more noticeable in darker skin types.
GENETICS Usually sporadic, AD cases reported.

PATHOPHYSIOLOGY

Chromosomal mosaicism has been detected in 30% of patients. The mosaic karyotype can be in autosomes or X chromosomes, and can be a wide variety of chromosomal defects including aneuploidies. The pigmentary streaks may be caused by two cellular clones with different pigment potential or reflect a number of pigmentary gene mutations.

HISTORY

Skin hypopigmentation is in a whorled, Blaschkoid pattern; present at birth or early childhood. It is asymptomatic but persists for life. Associated systemic disease may include seizures, mental retardation, skeletal abnormalities, and strabismus.

PHYSICAL EXAMINATION

Skin Findings

TYPE Macular.
COLOR Tan to off-white.
SHAPE Linear, streaked, whorled. "Marble cake" following lines of Blaschko (Fig. 13-12).

DISTRIBUTION Ventral trunk, flexor surfaces of limbs. Scalp, palms, soles spared.

General Findings

Internal manifestations occur in 75% to 94% of patients.
CNS Seizures, mental retardation, macrocephaly.
EYE Strabismus, heterochromia iridis, microphthalmia, nystagmus.
MUSCULOSKELETAL Scoliosis, asymmetry of limbs, dwarfism, small stature, polydactyly, syndactyly, spina bifida occulta.
HAIR Alopecia, hirsutism, facial hypertrichosis.
DENTAL Anodontia, dental dysplasia.
OTHER Hepatomegaly, diaphragmatic hernia.

DIFFERENTIAL DIAGNOSIS

Diagnosis is made on history and physical examination. The differential diagnosis includes IP, Goltz syndrome, nevus depigmentosus, depigmented lichen striatus, or vitiligo.

LABORATORY EXAMINATIONS

DERMATOPATHOLOGY Skin may appear normal or have decreased areas of melanin. There is no pigment incontinence in contrast to IP.

MANAGEMENT

No treatment for the skin lesions is needed. The skin lesions may slowly repigment in late childhood. Therapeutics are directed toward controlling neurologic symptoms and correcting skeletal malformations.

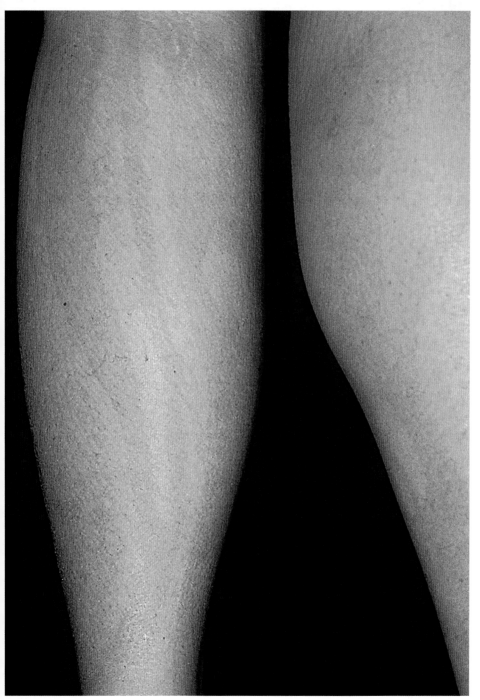

FIGURE 13-12 Hypomelanosis of Ito Whorled hypopigmented streaks along the lines of Blaschko, a negative image of the hyperpigmented stage of IP.

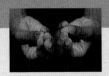

MISCELLANEOUS INFLAMMATORY DISORDERS

PAPULOSQUAMOUS ERUPTIONS

PITYRIASIS ROSEA

Pityriasis rosea (PR) is a common, benign, self-limited whole body rash with a seasonal prevalence that is clinically characterized by a solitary "herald patch" lesion followed by a whole body exanthem.

 INSIGHT Particularly in patients with darker skin types, pityriasis rosea may be more papular and present in an "inverse pattern" (favoring the body folds such as axillae and inguinal creases).

SYNONYMS Pityriasis rosea Gibert, roseola annulata (historical).

EPIDEMIOLOGY

AGE 10 to 35 years. Rare in <2 years.
INCIDENCE Up to 2% of all dermatology visits.
GENDER F > M, 2:1.
PREVALENCE Common, especially in fall and spring.
ETIOLOGY Human herpes viruses HHV6 and HHV7 have been postulated, but not proven.

HISTORY

A solitary "herald" patch (Fig. 14-1) typically precedes the exanthematous phase by 1 to 2 weeks. The exanthem develops over a period of a week and self-resolves in 6 to 14 weeks without intervention. A generalized prodrome similar to viral infection—upper respiratory symptoms, fevers, myalgias—may be present in more than 60% of individuals.

PHYSICAL EXAMINATION

Skin Lesions

HERALD PLAQUE Ovoid patch or plaque with collarette of scale (80%). May rarely have ≥2 herald patches or individual presents for evaluation after patch has faded.

EXANTHEM Papules and plaques with fine scale.
COLOR Pink or red.
SIZE Herald patch: 1 to 10 cm. Exanthem: 5 mm to 3 cm.
SHAPE Round to oval.
ARRANGEMENT Lesions follow the lines of cleavage in a "Christmas tree" distribution.
DISTRIBUTION Trunk > proximal arms, legs. Head, face (Fig. 14-2), palms and soles typically spared. Herald patch most often on the trunk but rarely can occur on limbs.
SITES OF PREDILECTION Axillae, back, inguinal areas.

General Findings

Headache, malaise, pharyngitis, or lymphadenitis (5%).

DIFFERENTIAL DIAGNOSIS

The diagnosis of PR is made on history of herald patch and clinical findings. PR can be confused with tinea corporis, secondary syphilis, guttate psoriasis, tinea versicolor, parapsoriasis, pityriasis lichenoides (PL), nummular eczema, seborrheic dermatitis, or a drug eruption (gold, ACE inhibitors, metronidazole, isotretinoin, arsenic, β-blockers, barbiturates, sulfasalazine, bismuth, clonidine, imatinib and other tyrosine kinase inhibitors, mercurials, D-penicillamine, tripelennamine, ketotifen).

LABORATORY EXAMINATIONS

DERMATOPATHOLOGY Small mounds of parakeratosis, spongiosis, lymphohistiocytic infiltrate.

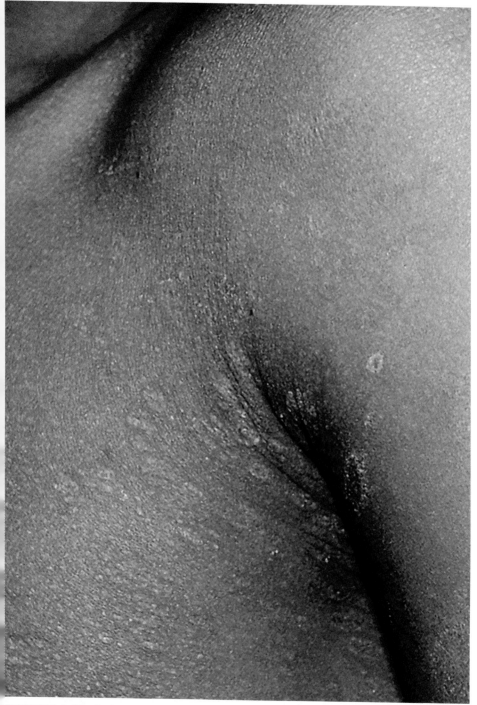

FIGURE 14-1 Pityriasis rosea Scattered erythematous plaques with a collarette of scale concentrated in the axillary area.

COURSE AND PROGNOSIS

PR is typically asymptomatic and self-resolves in 6 to 14 weeks. Atypical cases may have severe pruritus, have a more vesicular, purpuric, or pustular presentation, or may last as long as 5 months. Once cleared, it is uncommon for PR to recur.

MANAGEMENT

Because PR is benign and self-limited, no treatment is needed. In atypical PR or at-risk individuals, serologic testing for syphilis (RPR) should be performed as secondary syphilis can have a similar presentation. Pruritus can be improved with topical steroids, judicious ambient sunlight exposure, and/or oral antihistamines. Systematic reviews regarding the use of oral erythromycin or oral acyclovir for PR have not yielded any definitive benefit from either agent. In more severe, prolonged cases, UVB light therapy or a short course of oral steroids may be indicated for symptomatic relief and eruption clearance.

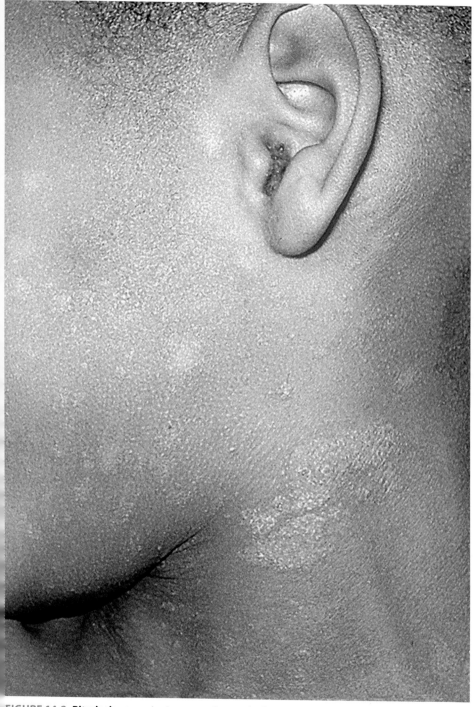

FIGURE 14-2 Pityriasis rosea Lesions spreading to the face which is uncommon but can be seen in childhood PR.

PITYRIASIS LICHENOIDES

PL is a papular, clonal T-cell disorder, characterized by recurrent crops of spontaneously regressing papules. Clinically, the spectrum ranges from an acute form, pityriasis lichenoides et varioliformis acuta (PLEVA), to a more chronic form, pityriasis lichenoides chronica (PLC).

 INSIGHT Pityriasis lichenoides chronica may manifest as predominantly hypopigmented patches, which are akin to postinflammatory hypopigmentation from primary lesions.

SYNONYMS Acute guttate parapsoriasis, parapsoriasis varioliformis, Mucha–Habermann disease, guttate parapsoriasis of Juliusberg.

EPIDEMIOLOGY

Age

1. PLEVA: Any age.
2. PLC: Adolescents and adults.

GENDER M > F.
ETIOLOGY Clonal T-cell disorder.

PATHOPHYSIOLOGY

The etiology of PLEVA and PLC is unclear. Theories include an infectious course, a postinfectious hypersensitivity reaction, an autoimmune mechanism, or an adverse reaction to drugs. PLEVA shows a predominance of CD8+ T cells. PLC shows a predominance of CD4+ T cells.

HISTORY

Self-resolving skin lesions tend to appear in crops over a period of weeks or months. Cutaneous lesions are usually asymptomatic, but may be pruritic or sensitive to touch.

PHYSICAL EXAMINATION

Skin Lesions

TYPE PLEVA: Papules (Fig. 14-3), vesicles, pustules, scale. PLC: Papules, crusts, scars.
COLOR PLEVA: Pink, red. May have a hemorrhagic appearance. PLC: Red, brown. White scars.
DISTRIBUTION Generalized distribution (Fig. 14-4), including palms, soles, and mucous membranes.

General Findings

Rare fever, malaise, and headache.

DIFFERENTIAL DIAGNOSIS

PLEVA can be confused with lymphomatoid papulosis, vasculitis, drug reaction, bites, scabies, varicella, folliculitis, impetigo, or prurigo nodularis. PLC can be confused with parapsoriasis, lichen planus (LP), guttate psoriasis, PR, or secondary syphilis.

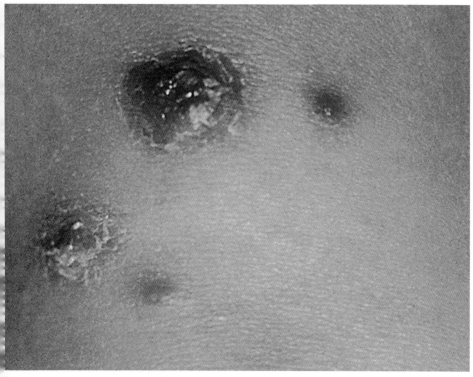

FIGURE 14-3 Pityriasis lichenoides et varioliformis acuta Inflammatory edematous papules on the forearm of a child.

LABORATORY EXAMINATIONS

DERMATOPATHOLOGY Skin biopsy shows epidermal spongiosis, keratinocyte necrosis, vesiculation, ulceration, and exocytosis. There is also dermal edema, a wedge-shaped inflammatory cell infiltrate extending to deep reticular dermis; hemorrhage; vessels congested with blood, and swollen endothelial cells.

COURSE AND PROGNOSIS

PL skin lesions continue to appear in crops, but both disorders tend to have a relapsing benign course. PLEVA may last a few weeks to months, and PLC may last years. Individuals with PL should have continued follow-up because rare cases have been reported to progress to cutaneous T-cell lymphoma (CTCL).

MANAGEMENT

PL episodes are self-limited and most patients do not require any therapeutic intervention. For symptomatic relief or for individuals with extensive disease, judicious ambient sunlight exposure, topical steroids, topical coal tar, oral antihistamines, oral tetracycline, or oral erythromycin have had reported success.

In more severe, prolonged cases, UVB light therapy or a short course of oral steroids/methotrexate may be indicated. Follow-up of these children (acutely: every few months, then chronically: an annual skin examination) is needed to monitor for possible development of CTCL.

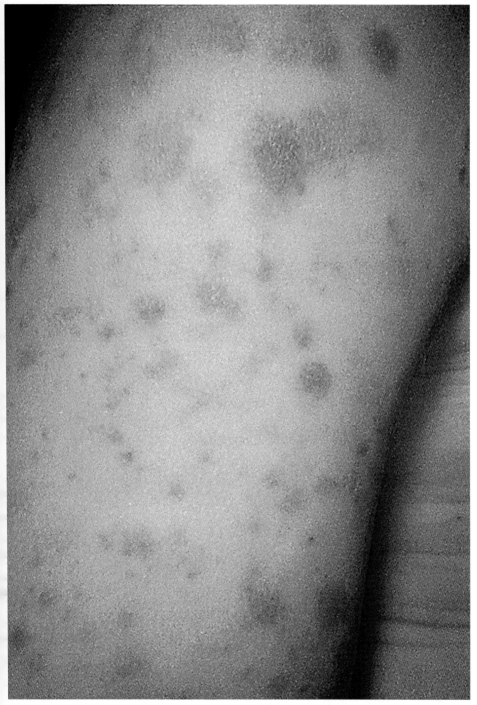

FIGURE 14-4 Pityriasis lichenoides Scattered inflammatory papules on the right arm of a child. The lesions are in different stages of evolution characteristic of PLEVA.

LICHENOID ERUPTIONS

LICHEN SCLEROSUS

Lichen sclerosus (LS) is a benign mucocutaneous disorder, characterized by sclerotic white plaques with epidermal atrophy.

SYNONYMS Guttate morphea, guttate sclero-derma, white-spot disease, lichen sclerosus et atrophicus, balanitis xerotica obliterans (BXO; lichen sclerosus of the penis).

EPIDEMIOLOGY

AGE 1 to 13 years. 70% before age 7 years. Also 50- to 60-year-old women.
GENDER F > M, 10:1.
ETIOLOGY Genetic predisposition. HLA-DQ7 association. Possible increased incidence in individuals with autoimmune diseases.

HISTORY

LS is an inflammatory dermal disease that causes white scar-like atrophy. In nongenital skin, it may be pruritic or cosmetically upsetting. Symptoms of advanced genital disease may include genital pruritus, dysuria, or dyspareunia.

Asymptomatic genital lesions may be present for years prior to detection. Often the skin findings are mistaken for sexual abuse in young children and are thus brought to medical attention. Older patients are diagnosed when atrophic changes are noted by a gynecologist or internist during pelvic examination. Spontaneous involution occurs in children more than adults.

PHYSICAL EXAMINATION

Skin Lesions

TYPE Papules, plaques. Ulcers or fissuring may develop.
COLOR Papules: pink. Plaques: ivory "mother-of-pearl."
NONGENITAL DISTRIBUTION Trunk, periumbilical, neck, axillae, thighs; flexor surface of wrists.
GENITAL DISTRIBUTION Females: "figure-of-eight" or "hourglass" perivulvar/perianal/perineum (Fig. 14-5) with most frequent involvement of the labia. Males: prepuce and glans (Fig. 14-6).
ORAL MUCOSA Buccal, palate, tongue: bluish-white plaques, erosions, macerated lesions.

DIFFERENTIAL DIAGNOSIS

LS can be confused with morphea, lichen simplex chronicus, discoid lupus erythematosus, leukoplakia, LP, condyloma acuminatum, intertrigo candidiasis, pinworm infestation, or bacterial vulvovaginitis. Most importantly, genital LS in children can be confused with sexual abuse which is often what brings the lesions to medical attention.

LABORATORY EXAMINATIONS

DERMATOPATHOLOGY Early lesions: hyperkeratosis, follicular plugging, edema with a lymphocytic band-like infiltrate subepidermally. Later lesions: epidermal atrophy, band of homogenized dermal collagen below epidermis.

COURSE AND PROGNOSIS

The prognosis is good for patients with childhood onset. Most clear in 1 to 10 years and 60% to 70% improve substantially by puberty. A small number persist into adulthood. Persistent lesions can be sensitive especially while walking; pruritus and pain can occur especially if erosions are present. Other complications include dysuria, dyspareunia, and stricture of the introitus. In males, chronic BXO can lead to phimosis and recurrent balanitis. Rarely, chronic scarred lesions can show malignant degeneration into squamous cell carcinoma.

MANAGEMENT

1. Topical steroids are effective in the treatment of genital LS. A short course of medium or strong steroid ointment once or twice daily for 12 to 24 weeks has the best reported clinical outcomes. Intralesional steroids have also been used.
2. Emollients and antipruritic agents can also be tried for symptomatic relief.
3. Topical calcineurin inhibitors (tacrolimus 0.1% ointment or pimecrolimus cream) have reported success.
4. Topical vitamin D (calcipotriene cream) and vitamin A have anecdotal success.
5. Use of 2% testosterone propionate in petrolatum or 1% progesterone (100 mg/30 g of petrolatum) can be tried, but often yields little success.
6. Surgical interventions may be warranted for GU complications such as stricture of the introitus in females and phimosis in males.
7. Involution in adults is uncommon and LS needs to be chronically monitored for progression toward malignant degeneration (estimated 4.4% of adult cases). In adults, new nodules or ulcers that persist for weeks warrant a skin biopsy to rule out leukoplakia or carcinoma.

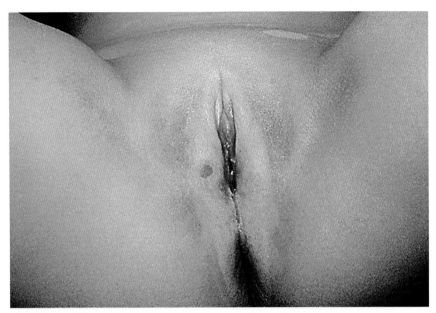

FIGURE 14-5 Lichen sclerosus Hypopigmented "hourglass" or "figure-of-eight" configuration around the vulva and the perianal area of a young girl. Lichen sclerosis is often mistaken for child abuse.

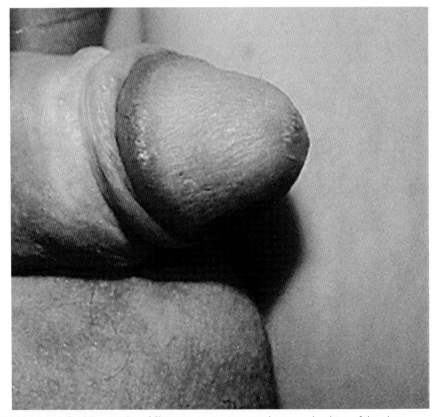

FIGURE 14-6 Balanitis xerotica obliterans Hypopigmented area on the dorsa of the glans.

LICHEN PLANUS

LP is an inflammatory disorder of the skin and mucous membranes with characteristic flat-topped (Latin *planus*, "flat"), violaceous, shiny, pruritic papules, and milky-white papules and plaques in the mouth.

SYNONYM Lichen ruber planus.

EPIDEMIOLOGY

AGE Rare in children. More common in 30 to 60 years old.
GENDER F = M.
PREVALENCE 1% of the population.
ETIOLOGY Unknown. Triggers: viral infections, autoimmune diseases, medications, vaccinations, and dental materials.
GENETICS Sporadic. Rare familial cases.

PATHOPHYSIOLOGY

LP is thought to be caused by T-cell–mediated autoimmune damage to basal keratinocytes, which have been altered by viruses, medications, or other allergens. Several exogenous antigens thought to trigger LP include viruses (hepatitis C, transfusion-transmitted virus, HHV-6, HHV-7, HSV, VZV), vaccinations (hepatitis B), bacteria (*Helicobacter pylori*), dental materials (amalgam, mercury, copper, gold), and drugs (captopril, enalapril, labetalol, methyldopa, propranolol, chloroquine, hydroxychloroquine, quinacrine, chlorothiazide, hydrochlorothiazide, gold salts, penicillamine, quinidine). Autoimmune diseases may also be associated with LP (increased frequency of HLA-B27, HLA-B51, HLA-Bw57, HLA-DR1, and HLA-DR9 alleles).

HISTORY

LP is a pruritic eruption involving the wrists, forearms, genitalia, distal lower extremities, and presacral areas. Clinical variants range from annular, bullous, hypertrophic, linear, to ulcerative lesions, which may spontaneously remit, or persist for life.

PHYSICAL EXAMINATION

Skin Lesions

TYPE Papules (Fig. 14-7) or plaques.
SIZE 1 to 10 mm.
SHAPE Polygonal.
COLOR Violaceous, with white lines (Wickham's striae).
ARRANGEMENT Grouped, linear, annular, or disseminated.
DISTRIBUTION Wrists, forearms, genitalia, distal lower extremities, and presacral areas.
MUCOUS MEMBRANES White papules/lines on the buccal mucosa, tongue, lips (60%).
SCALP Atrophic scalp skin with scarring alopecia (lichen planopilaris).
NAILS Destruction of the nail fold and nail matrix (10%) (Fig. 14-8), including the potential for twenty-nail dystrophy involving all fingernails and toenails.
KOEBNER PHENOMENON Lesions may present in areas of cutaneous trauma such as linear arrays consistent with scratching.

DIFFERENTIAL DIAGNOSIS

LP can be a reaction pattern to various exogenous antigens. Thus, identifying potential triggers such as viruses, medications, vaccinations, immunizations, and dental materials is important, before labeling the condition idiopathic LP. Other diseases that resemble LP include lupus erythematosus, lichen nitidus, lichen striatus, LS, PR, and psoriasis.

LABORATORY EXAMINATIONS

DERMATOPATHOLOGY Hyperkeratosis, hypergranulosis, irregular acanthosis, liquefactive degeneration of the basal cell layer, and a band-like mononuclear infiltrate that hugs the epidermis.

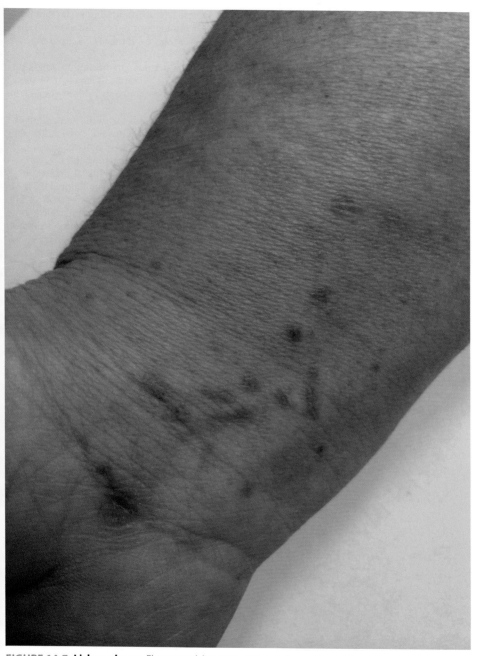

FIGURE 14-7 Lichen planus Flat-topped, linear pruritic papules on the wrist.

COURSE AND PROGNOSIS

Spontaneous resolution of LP in weeks is possible; two-thirds of patients self-resolve after 1 year. LP lesions may also persist for years, especially on the shins and in the mouth where the mean duration is longer (5 years). Careful follow-up for oral LP and hypertrophic LP are recommended since the potential exists for malignant transformation (1–2%).

MANAGEMENT

Therapies for LP include the following:

1. Topical corticosteroids with or without occlusion or intralesional steroids. Patients should be forewarned that occlusion increases the steroid strength and cautioned about steroid side effects.

2. Topical calcineurin inhibitors (tacrolimus 0.1% ointment or pimecrolimus cream) have reported success for some cases of refractive oral LP.

3. Systemic steroids (prednisone 1–2 mg/kg/d divided qid–bid for 5–14 days) can be used in severe cases, and only in short courses, for disease flares.

4. Systemic retinoids (acitretin 30 mg/kg/d or etretinate 50 mg/d in adult-sized patients for 8 weeks) can be used in difficult cases.

5. Phototherapy with narrowband UVB or PUVA (psoralen plus artificial UVA exposure) may be used in older children or in generalized, severe, resistant cases.

6. Systemic griseofulvin, metronidazole, sulfasalazine, cyclosporine, mycophenolate mofetil, and thalidomide have had anecdotal reported successes.

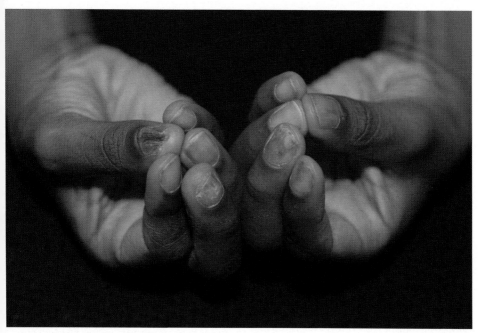

FIGURE 14-8 Lichen planus, nails Destruction of the nail fold and nail matrix in a child with LP.

LICHEN NITIDUS

Lichen nitidus is a benign dermatosis commonly seen in childhood, characterized by asymptomatic, small, flesh-colored pinpoint papules located on the flexor surface of the arms and wrists, lower abdomen, genital, and submammary region.

EPIDEMIOLOGY

AGE Preschool and school-age children; often age 1 to 6 years old.
GENDER Equal predilection.
PREVALENCE Uncommon.
ETIOLOGY Possibly a form of LP.

PATHOPHYSIOLOGY

Because of ultrastructural and immunophenotypic studies, lichen nitidus is thought to share a similar pathogenesis to LP: a T-cell–mediated autoimmune damage to basal keratinocytes.

HISTORY

The skin lesions appear suddenly and are typically asymptomatic (rare cases have pruritus). Lesions may regress spontaneously after weeks to months but other cases persist for years.

PHYSICAL EXAMINATION

Skin Findings

TYPE Numerous monomorphic papules. Shiny with fine scale.
COLOR Flesh-colored, pink, or brown.
SIZE Pinpoint to pinhead in size (Fig. 14-9).
SHAPE Round or polygonal.
SITES OF PREDILECTION Flexor surface of the arms, anterior wrist surface, lower abdomen, shaft and glans of the penis, and breasts.
DISTRIBUTION In groups and in linear lesions in lines of trauma (Koebner reaction). Rare generalized form.
NAILS Pitting, ridging, splitting (10%). More common in individuals with palmar involvement.

DIFFERENTIAL DIAGNOSIS

Lichen nitidus can be confused with LP, lichen striatus, LS, papular eczema, psoriasis, flat warts, keratosis pilaris, lichen spinulosus, or an id reaction.

LABORATORY EXAMINATIONS

DERMATOPATHOLOGY Sharply circumscribed nests of lymphocytes and histiocytes in the uppermost dermis (often confined to two to three dermal papillae) with overlying thin, scaling epidermis. Dermis and epidermis are often detached at central portion of lesion. Rete ridges extend down around the infiltrate in a "claw-and-ball"-like manner.

COURSE AND PROGNOSIS

Typical lichen nitidus lesions self-resolve in 1 to 2 years. In other instances, lesions may persist for several years despite treatment. There are rare reports of lichen nitidus seen in association with Crohn's disease, but the majority of cases have no associated systemic abnormalities. After papules clear, the skin heals without atrophy or pigmentary changes.

MANAGEMENT

Given the benign, self-limited clinical course of lichen nitidus, no treatment is necessary. In rare cases with pruritus, topical corticosteroids with or without occlusion may be helpful. Patients should be forewarned that occlusion increases the steroid strength and cautioned about steroid side effects. Topical calcineurin inhibitors have also had reported success.

In severe, refractory, generalized forms of lichen nitidus, narrowband UVB, PUVA, oral etretinate, and oral itraconazole have anecdotal reported success.

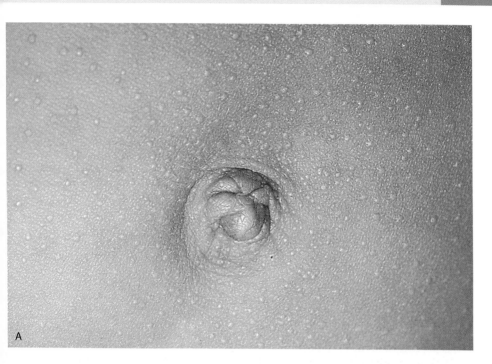

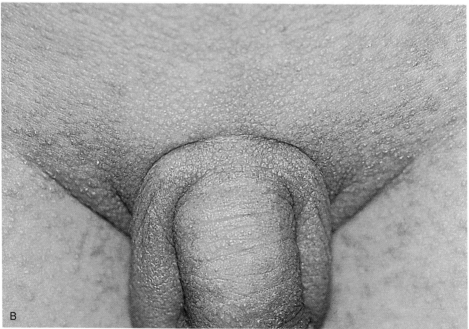

FIGURE 14-9 Lichen nitidus A: Scattered small pinpoint on the abdomen of a child. **B:** Same child with extensive groin involvement.

LICHEN STRIATUS

A benign, self-limited dermatitis characterized by a unilateral papular eruption on the extremity of a child in a Blaschkoid distribution.

SYNONYMS Linear lichenoid dermatosis, Blaschko linear acquired inflammatory skin eruption (BLAISE).

EPIDEMIOLOGY

AGE Onset 4 months to 15 years of age. Median age: 2 to 3 years.
GENDER F > M.
INCIDENCE Uncommon.
SEASONAL PREVALENCE Spring and summer.
ETIOLOGY Somatic mosaicism. ? Viral trigger. Possible association with atopy.

HISTORY

Lichen striatus appears suddenly, reaches its maximum extent within several days to weeks and then regresses spontaneously within 6 to 12 months. Lesions are asymptomatic. Nail involvement can be limited to a single digit and lead to onycholysis, splitting, fraying, and nail loss.

PHYSICAL EXAMINATION

Skin Findings

TYPE Papules, slight fine scale.
SIZE Papules: 1 to 4 mm.
COLOR Hypopigmented, pink or red.
SHAPE Small, flat-topped lesions.
ARRANGEMENT Linear following Blaschko lines (Fig. 14-10).
DISTRIBUTION Extremities, face, neck, trunk, and buttocks.
SITES OF PREDILECTION Often unilateral on an extremity.

DIFFERENTIAL DIAGNOSIS

Characteristic Blaschko linear arrangement of lesions located on an extremity or other common sites is indicative of lichen striatus. Lichen striatus needs to be differentiated from other linear disorders such as nevus unius lateris, psoriasis, lichen nitidus, an epidermal nevus, or linear LP.

LABORATORY EXAMINATIONS

DERMATOPATHOLOGY A dense perivascular or band-like lymphohistiocytic infiltrate appears in the dermis. The epidermis reveals a small lymphocytic invasion with focal areas of acanthosis, parakeratosis, and spongiosis.

COURSE AND PROGNOSIS

Lichen striatus is typically an asymptomatic, self-limiting disorder of short duration (6–12 months).

MANAGEMENT

Given the benign, self-limited clinical course of lichen striatus, no treatment is necessary. In rare cases with pruritus, topical corticosteroids with or without occlusion may be helpful. Patients should be forewarned that occlusion increases the steroid strength and cautioned about steroid side effects.

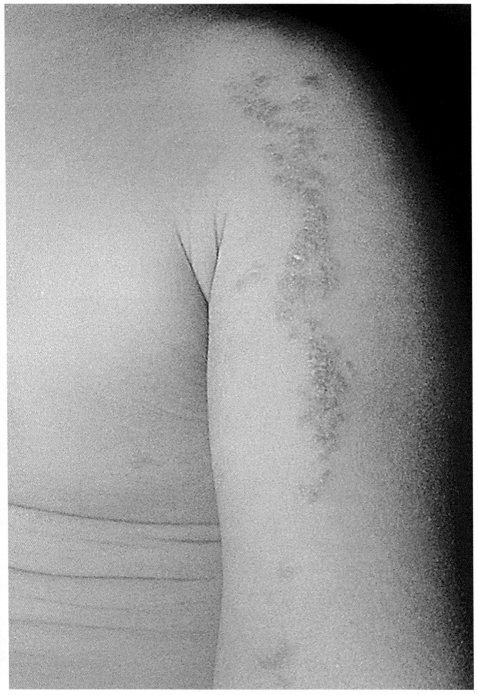

FIGURE 14-10 **Lichen striatus** Erythematous papules coalescing into a linear plaque on the arm of a child.

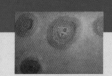

HYPERSENSITIVITY REACTIONS

DRUG HYPERSENSITIVITY ERUPTIONS

A drug hypersensitivity reaction is an adverse, allergic response to an ingested or parenterally administered drug characterized by a cutaneous eruption.

There are several different immune mechanisms thought to play a role:

1. **Type I: IgE-dependent drug reactions** characterized by urticaria, angioedema, and anaphylaxis.

2. **Type II: Cytotoxic drug-induced reactions** characterized by petechiae from drug-induced thrombocytopenia.

3. **Type III: Immune complex-mediated drug reactions** characterized by vasculitis, serum sickness, urticaria.

4. **Type IV: Delayed-type, cell-mediated drug reactions** characterized by exanthematous, fixed drug eruptions (FDEs), Stevens–Johnson syndrome (SJS), and toxic epidermal necrolysis (TEN).

EXANTHEMATOUS DRUG REACTION

An exanthematous drug reaction is an adverse, allergic response to an ingested or parenterally administered drug characterized by a morbilliform cutaneous eruption that mimics a viral exanthem.

INSIGHT In the appropriate clinical setting, an exanthematous drug reaction, a viral exanthem, and acute graft-versus-host disease (GVHD) are all clinically and histologically indistinguishable.

SYNONYMS Morbilliform drug eruption, maculopapular drug eruption, drug rash.

EPIDEMIOLOGY

AGE Children < adolescents < adults.
GENDER F > M.
INCIDENCE 1% of population on a systemic medication.
ETIOLOGY Numerous drugs have been associated with the development of exanthematous drug eruptions—see Table 15-1 for a partial list. Antibiotics are the most frequent class of medications associated with exanthematous drug eruptions.

PATHOPHYSIOLOGY

Exanthematous drug hypersensitivity reactions are likely type IV, cell-mediated immune responses. Viral infections may increase the incidence (e.g., aminopenicillins cause a morbilliform rash in nearly 100% of patients concurrently infected with EBV).

HISTORY

The exanthematous rash typically appears 7 to 14 days (peak incidence ninth day) after drug administration; however, skin lesions can appear anytime between day 1 and 21 after drug exposure. The rash starts on the trunk and typically spreads to the face and extremities. It can be quite pruritic and distressing. Fever and malaise are variably present.

PHYSICAL EXAMINATION

Skin Findings

TYPE OF LESION Macules, papules, plaques (Fig. 15-1A).
SIZE Individual lesions 1 mm to 1 cm with diffuse body surface area involvement possible.
COLOR Pink/red to dusky purple/brown, especially in darker skin types.
DISTRIBUTION OF LESIONS Trunk, spreads centrifugally to face (Fig. 15-1B) and extremities. Confluent in intertriginous areas (axilla, groin, inframammary area). Palms and soles may be involved.

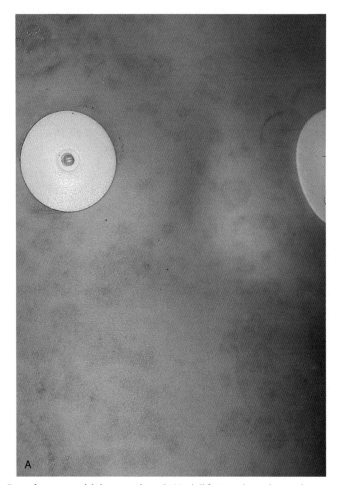

FIGURE 15-1 Drug hypersensitivity reaction A: Morbilliform rash on the trunk occurring 1 week after the administration of a systemic antibiotic. *(continued)*

TABLE 15-1 Drugs Associated with Exanthematous Drug Eruptions

Drugs with High Probability of Reaction	Penicillins, amoxicillin, ampicillin Cephalosporins Carbamazepine Allopurinol Gold salts Trimethoprim-sulfamethoxazole
Drugs with Medium Probability of Reaction	Sulfonamides (bacteriostatic, antidiabetic, diuretic) Nitrofurantoin Hydantoin derivatives Isoniazid Chloramphenicol Erythromycin Streptomycin
Drugs with Low Probability of Reaction	Barbiturates Benzodiazepines Phenothiazines Opioids (morphine, codeine)

MUCOUS MEMBRANES ± Exanthem on buccal mucosa.

General Findings

± Fever, malaise

DIFFERENTIAL DIAGNOSIS

An exanthematous drug reaction can be confused with a viral exanthema, allergic contact dermatitis, pityriasis rosea, psoriasis, toxic shock syndrome, scarlet fever, acute GVHD, eczema, or secondary syphilis.

LABORATORY EXAMINATION

DERMATOPATHOLOGY Perivascular inflammation with scattered eosinophils.

COURSE AND PROGNOSIS

Exanthematous drug reactions can occur 1 to 21 days after drug exposure. With discontinuation of the drug, the rash begins to fade (often after a 2- to 3-day lag time following drug discontinuation). The fiery red rash gradually fades to a dull purple and then desquamates. A rechallenge with the drug often elicits a faster, more severe response. Ten percent of patients sensitive to penicillins given cephalosporins will exhibit cross-drug sensitivity and develop an eruption. Similarly, patients sensitized to one sulfa-based drug (bacteriostatic, antidiabetic, diuretic) may cross-react with another category of that drug.

MANAGEMENT

Correct identification and discontinuation of the offending drug is needed. Symptomatic relief for pruritic skin lesions can be obtained with systemic antihistamines (diphenhydramine, hydroxyzine HCl, cetirizine HCl), oatmeal baths, emollients (hydrated petrolatum, Vaseline, camphor-menthol creams, moisturizers), and topical steroids. Severe cases may benefit from a limited course of systemic steroids (prednisone or methylprednisolone). Steroid use may not speed ultimate resolution of the eruption but can offer symptomatic relief from pruritus.

PREVENTION

The patient should be made aware of the possible drug allergen and cross-reactants. His or her medical chart should be updated accordingly. For morbilliform eruptions, the drug can be readministered, though the eruption may recur upon reexposure. It is possible to "treat through" an exanthematous drug hypersensitivity rash in cases where the offending drug is critical or life-sustaining and there are no appropriate non–cross-reacting alternative medications.

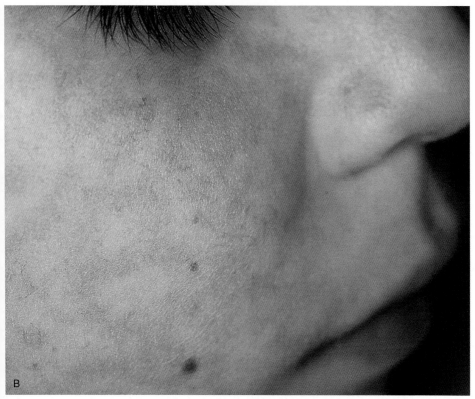

B

FIGURE 15-1 *(Continued)* **Drug hypersensitivity reaction B:** Morbilliform rash eventually spread to the face and extremities of the same child.

URTICARIA: WHEALS AND ANGIOEDEMA

Urticaria is a transient allergic response characterized by edematous plaques (wheals) and/or deep dermal swelling (angioedema). In some cases, urticaria is accompanied by respiratory symptoms, vascular collapse, and/or shock (anaphylaxis).

 INSIGHT The hallmark of urticaria is its transience. An individual lesion should not persist for more than 24 hours.

SYNONYMS Wheals, hives, nettle rash.

EPIDEMIOLOGY

AGE Any age.
GENDER F > M, 2:1.
INCIDENCE 5% of the population.
ETIOLOGY >50% of urticaria is idiopathic. Urticaria can result from immune (autoimmune, IgE-mediated, immune complex, or complement/kinin-dependent) or nonimmune (direct mast cell degranulators, vasoactive stimuli, ASA, NSAIDs, dietary pseudoallergens, ACE inhibitors) mechanisms.

PATHOPHYSIOLOGY

The mast cell is the primary cell type responsible for urticaria. IgE, opiates, C5a anaphylatoxin, quinolones, vancomycin, and some neuropeptides can cross-link or bind receptors on the surface of mast cells leading to degranulation of its contents. Mast cells release histamine and other proinflammatory mediators which bind to receptors on the postcapillary venules in the skin. This leads to vasodilation and plasma leakage clinically seen as wheals and/or angioedema.

HISTORY

In urticaria, wheals are transient skin lesions that come and go in <24 hours. Skin symptoms can include pruritus, flushing, or burning. In angioedema, deeper swelling of the dermis, subcutaneous, or submucosal tissue occurs and may persist for 3 to 4 days. Systemic symptoms can include respiratory symptoms, arthralgias, fatigue, abdominal pain, fever, and diarrhea.

PHYSICAL EXAMINATION

Skin Findings

TYPE Wheal: edematous papule, plaque (Fig. 15-2).

SIZE 1 mm to 10 cm.
SHAPE Round, oval, annular, or polycyclic.
COLOR Pink to red, with surrounding or central pallor.
DISTRIBUTION Typically generalized (Fig. 15-3).

Angioedema Skin Findings

TYPE Diffuse swelling.
COLOR Pink-red.
SITES OF PREDILECTION Face (eyelids, lips, tongue).

General Findings

Malaise, fever, arthralgias, respiratory symptoms, hypotension, and shock.

DIFFERENTIAL DIAGNOSIS

The transient edematous plaques are diagnostic for urticaria, although often parents can mistake blisters or insect bites for urticaria. Urticaria also needs to be differentiated from dermatographism (present in 5% of the normal population), eczema, contact dermatitis, mastocytosis, erythema multiforme (EM), and allergic vasculitis.

LABORATORY EXAMINATIONS

DERMATOPATHOLOGY Dermal or subcutaneous edema, vascular dilation, and mild perivascular infiltrate.
BLOOD TESTS In evaluating patients with urticaria or angioedema, a complete blood count with differential, chemistry panel, liver function tests, and complement levels should be obtained to evaluate for systemic causes. Complement levels, particularly C4, will be depressed in individuals with C1-inhibitor deficiencies. Serum tryptase—a marker of mast cell activation—may be elevated in episodes of angioedema associated with anaphylaxis.

COURSE AND PROGNOSIS

Urticaria self-resolves in 1 year in 50% of cases. Up to 20% of cases can have a chronic relapsing course.

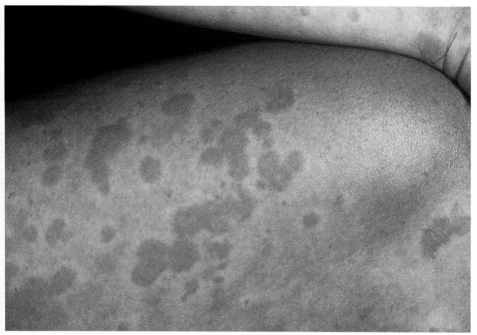

FIGURE 15-2 Urticaria Erythematous papules and plaques with surrounding blanched halos characteristic of urticarial lesions on the knee of a child.

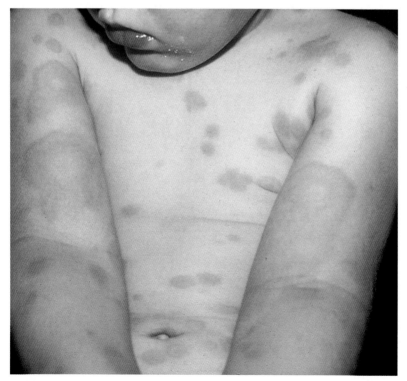

FIGURE 15-3 Urticaria Transient well-circumscribed, erythematous and annular plaques characteristic of urticaria.

MANAGEMENT

Identification and elimination of any causative agent is most helpful. Several drugs have been associated with urticaria, as listed in Table 15-2. Foods that can cause urticaria include milk, eggs, wheat, shellfish, and nuts. Other forms include physical urticaria (dermatographism, cold; Fig. 15-4); solar, cholinergic, pressure, vibratory, and hereditary angioedema (autosomal dominantly inherited disorder caused by a low level of, or dysfunctional, plasma protein C1 inhibitor). In up to 50% of cases, the etiology is undetermined. Urticaria can be precipitated by stress.

TREATMENT Treatment is primarily symptomatic with one or more antihistamines (chlorpheniramine, hydroxyzine, diphenhydramine, doxepin, acrivastine, cetirizine, loratadine, mizolastine, desloratadine, fexofenadine, levocetirizine, cimetidine, or ranitidine). Topical regimens include oatmeal baths, calamine or 1% menthol cream, and/or topical steroids.

More refractory cases may require systemic steroids (prednisone or methylprednisolone), but only short courses are recommended and rebound is possible. Chronic urticaria may require long-term management.

Epinephrine, intravenous fluid resuscitation, and airway protection are the treatments of choice for anaphylaxis, and it can be reassuring for patients with urticaria to carry an epinephrine pen for self-administration during severe episodes if necessary.

TABLE 15-2 Drugs Associated with Urticaria

Antibiotics	Penicillins
	Sulfonamides
Cardiac medications	Amiodarone
	Procainamide
Immunotherapeutics	Serum-derived products
Chemotherapies	L-asparagine
	Bleomycin
	Cisplatin
	Daunorubicin
	5-fluorouracil
	Thiotepa
ACE inhibitors	Captopril, Enalapril, Lisinopril
Calcium channel blockers	Nifedipine, Diltiazem, Verapamil
Direct histamine releasers	Morphine
	Radiocontrast dye
	Muscle relaxants
	Salicylates
	Sympathomimetics
	Various antimicrobials

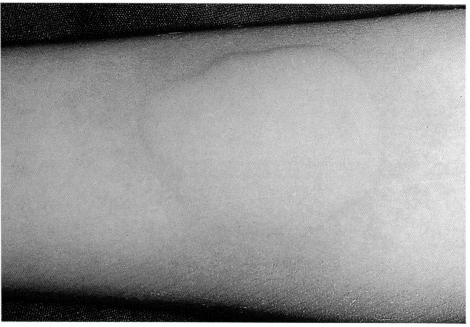

FIGURE 15-4 Urticaria, cold-induced Cold urticaria can be reproduced by placing an ice cube on the forearm for 2 to 5 minutes with a resultant urticarial wheal.

ERYTHEMA MULTIFORME, STEVENS–JOHNSON SYNDROME, AND TOXIC EPIDERMAL NECROLYSIS

Acute blistering reactions can be classified as follows:

1. EM is a reactive syndrome most often precipitated by infectious agents such as herpes simplex virus (HSV).

2. SJS and TEN are reactive syndromes along the same clinical spectrum most often triggered by systemic drugs.

ERYTHEMA MULTIFORME SYNDROME

EM is a reactive syndrome characterized by "target" lesions of the skin and mucous membranes most commonly precipitated by an infection (usually HSV).

SYNONYM EM von Hebra.

CLASSIFICATION

EM MINOR Mild, sudden onset of papules, some of which evolve into target lesions. No prodrome or mucosal involvement. Recurrences common.
EM MAJOR EM associated with mucosal lesions and systemic symptoms. Historically erroneously synonymous with SJS, which is probably a separate disease with distinct pathophysiology.

EPIDEMIOLOGY

AGE 50% of patients are older than 20 years of age. Rare under 2 years of age.
GENDER M > F.
INCIDENCE Uncommon, less than 1% of individuals affected.
ETIOLOGY Most common precipitant is HSV (>50%); reported association with other infections, drugs, or systemic disease.
GENETICS May see increased incidence in HLA-DQw3, HLA-DRw53, HLA-Aw33 populations, particularly with HSV-triggered EM.

PATHOPHYSIOLOGY

Likely an aberrant immune response to select precipitants in certain predisposed individuals. Possible precipitants include infections (HSV >>> *Mycoplasma pneumoniae*, *Histoplasma capsulatum*, parapoxvirus, vaccinia, VZV, adenovirus, EBV, CMV, hepatitis viruses, Coxsackie virus, parvovirus B19, HIV, *Chlamydophila psittaci*, salmonella, *Mycobacterium tuberculosis*, dermatophytes), rarely drugs (NSAIDs, sulfonamides, antiepileptics, antibiotics), or systemic disease (IBD, SLE, Behçet's).

HISTORY

Skin lesions appear abruptly 3 to 14 days after precipitant (HSV-induced herpes labialis in >50%) and new lesions can continue to appear for up to 10 days. Fever, malaise, and mucous membrane involvement may also be present in EM Major.

PHYSICAL EXAMINATION

Skin Lesions

TYPE Macules, papules, scale, vesicles, bullae.
COLOR Red ring, dusky purple center (Fig. 15-5).
SIZE 5 mm to 3 cm.
SHAPE Target or iris lesions are typical. Classic target lesions contain a dusky or violaceous center, an edematous inflammatory zone, and an erythematous periphery, though atypical target or "targetoid" lesions may be seen.
DISTRIBUTION Upper body, extremities. Grouped on elbows, knees.
SITES OF PREDILECTION Upper extremities and face > palms, neck, trunk > legs. Lesions often start acrally and spread centripetally.
MUCOUS MEMBRANES Oral, ocular, and genital blistering and ulceration may be present.

DIFFERENTIAL DIAGNOSIS

EM can be confused with viral exanthems, bullous diseases, urticaria, secondary syphilis, psoriasis, FDE, subacute cutaneous lupus erythematosus, vasculitis, polymorphous light eruption, or pityriasis rosea. The "target lesions" are classic for EM, but may be confused with erythema annulare centrifugum (EAC), tinea corporis, or other annular eruptions.

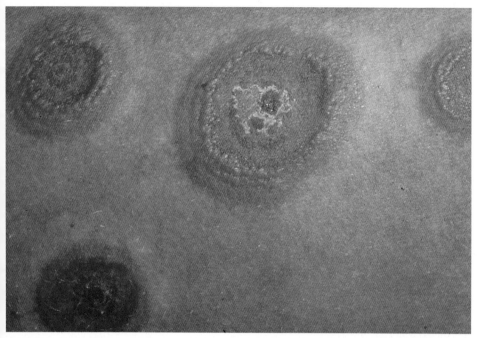

FIGURE 15-5 Erythema multiforme Polycyclic target lesions with alternating rings of erythema and dusky desquamation on the arm.

LABORATORY EXAMINATIONS

DERMATOPATHOLOGY Interface dermatitis, spongiosis, exocytosis, vacuolar degeneration of the basal keratinocytes, dermal edema, perivascular mononuclear infiltrate.

INFECTIOUS DISEASE EVALUATION If lesions suggestive of primary HSV are present, direct fluorescence antibody, viral culture, or PCR may be used to confirm the etiology of the primary lesion. Serology for *M. pneumoniae* is generally positive in associated eruptions.

COURSE AND PROGNOSIS

EM appears abruptly 3 to 14 days after insult (HSV, infection, drug, etc.); skin lesions fully evolve in 72 hours and persist for 1 to 2 weeks. Lesions can be pruritic or painful, systemic symptoms and mucosal involvement may be present. EM typically resolves after 2 weeks with no sequelae, but recurrences are common.

MANAGEMENT

For EM management, if a precipitant can be identified, it should be treated or removed. In recurrent EM cases secondary to HSV, daily prophylactic acyclovir, valacyclovir, or famciclovir may be necessary.

In most cases of EM, the rash will self-resolve in 5 to 15 days without treatment. Symptomatic relief for pruritic skin lesions can be obtained with systemic antihistamines (diphenhydramine, hydroxyzine HCl, cetirizine HCl), oatmeal baths, emollients (hydrated petrolatum, Vaseline, moisturizers), and topical steroids.

In severe EM, systemic steroids (prednisone, methylprednisolone) can be added. Open skin lesions can be treated with topical antibiotics and topical petrolatum-impregnated gauze if needed for prevention of secondary bacterial infection. Oral lesions can benefit from anesthetic rinses. Ocular lesions need topical treatment in conjunction with an ophthalmologist.

In severe refractory or recurrent EM cases, azathioprine, thalidomide, dapsone, cyclosporine, mycophenolate mofetil, or PUVA have had reported successes.

STEVENS–JOHNSON SYNDROME AND TOXIC EPIDERMAL NECROLYSIS

SJS and TEN are rare, severe cutaneous drug reactions characterized by tenderness of the skin/mucosa, followed by extensive exfoliation that is potentially life-threatening.

SYNONYM Lyell's syndrome.

CLASSIFICATION

SJS and TEN are considered as two clinical ends along a spectrum of adverse drug reaction severity with:
SJS <10% body surface area skin sloughing.
SJS/TEN OVERLAP 10% to 30% body surface area skin sloughing.
TEN >30% body surface area skin sloughing.

EPIDEMIOLOGY

AGE Older children. More common in adults older than 40 years.
GENDER SJS: M = F. TEN: F > M.
INCIDENCE SJS: 6 per million, TEN: 1 per million. Markedly increased incidence in individuals with HIV.
GENETICS Genetic susceptibility in HLA-B12 (particularly with NSAIDs), HLA-B*5801 (particularly with allopurinol), HLA-B*1502 (particularly with anticonvulsants).
ETIOLOGY SJS: Drugs (≥50%); TEN: Drugs (>95%); NSAIDs, antibiotics, and anticonvulsants are most common triggers. Antiretroviral agents may trigger SJS/TEN in individuals with HIV.

PATHOPHYSIOLOGY

SJS/TEN develops because of a host's impaired capacity to metabolize reactive drug metabolites. The metabolites then trigger an interaction between the cell-death receptor Fas and its ligand (FasL) causing extensive keratinocyte death (apoptosis), loss of cohesion, necrosis resulting in full-thickness epidermal necrosis. Drugs implicated include NSAIDs (phenylbutazone, piroxicam), antibiotics (amithiozone, aminopenicillins) sulfa drugs (sulfadoxine, sulfadiazine, sulfasalazine, trimethoprimsulfamethoxazole), allopurinol, antiretrovirals, and antiepileptics (barbiturates, carbamazepine, phenytoin, and lamotrigine).

HISTORY

One to three weeks after drug exposure, SJS/TEN begins with fever, pain with swallowing, and stinging eyes. Dysuria may be present. Up to 3 days later, the skin lesions appear on the trunk spreading to the upper extremities and face. The skin turns dusky purple-red before dermal–epidermal detachment with sheets of skin falling off leaving raw, red denuded areas. Systemic symptoms include fever, malaise, myalgia, arthralgias, dysuria, nausea and vomiting, diarrhea, and conjunctival burning.

PHYSICAL EXAMINATION

Skin Findings

TYPE Macules, papules, plaques, blisters, desquamation (Fig. 15-6).
COLOR Red/purple to gray.
PALPATION Nikolsky sign: lateral mechanical pressure causes epidermal detachment manifesting as blister extension.
DISTRIBUTION Often truncal initially, spreading to upper extremities and face. Palms/soles can be involved.
MUCOUS MEMBRANES (≥90%, especially in SJS) Erosions on buccal (Fig. 15-7A), ocular (Fig. 15-7B), genital mucosae.

General Findings

Fever, Lymphadenopathy (LAD)
OCULAR (85%) Conjunctival hyperemia, keratitis, pseudomembrane formation, erosions.
RESPIRATORY (25%) Epithelial damage, erosions.
GASTROINTESTINAL Diarrhea, esophagitis.
RENAL Tubular necrosis, renal failure.
OTHER Hepatitis, cytopenia.

DIFFERENTIAL DIAGNOSIS

SJS/TEN can be confused with EM, staphylococcal scalded skin syndrome (SSSS), severe acute GVHD, DRESS, Kawasaki disease (KD), thermal burns, phototoxic eruptions, generalized FDE, LE, or generalized erythroderma (from severe psoriasis, atopic dermatitis, mycosis fungoides, etc.).

LABORATORY EXAMINATIONS

DERMATOPATHOLOGY Early: necrosis of the basal cell layer with subepidermal bullae formation. Late: full-thickness epidermal necrosis, sparse perivascular infiltrate. Analysis of frozen cryostat sections on "jelly roll" skin samples demonstrating full-thickness necrosis can expedite SJS/TEN diagnosis for more rapid clinical intervention.

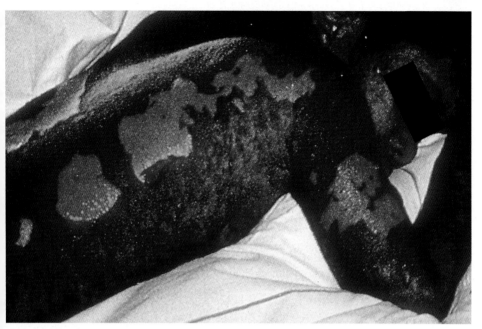

FIGURE 15-6 Toxic epidermal necrolysis Whole-body desquamation characteristic of toxic epidermal necrolysis.

COURSE AND PROGNOSIS

Course is similar to that of severe widespread thermal burns. Outcome is worse in patients who are older, or have more extensive skin involvement. Mortality rate is 5% for SJS and 35% for TEN as is typically caused by sepsis (*Staphylococcus aureus*, *Pseudomonas aeruginosa*) or fluid and electrolyte imbalances.

MANAGEMENT

SJS/TEN management consists of rapid diagnosis and elimination of the causative agent. Patients should be monitored closely and those with extensive skin involvement are best cared for in a burn or intensive care unit with IV fluid and electrolyte replenishment, temperature control, and vigilant wound care. Careful daily wound care (wash with isotonic sterile sodium chloride, mupirocin on orifices, Vaseline-impregnated gauze or silicone dressings, antibiotic eye drops to cornea) with

minimal manipulation can lead to regrowth of epidermis in 1 to 3 weeks. Pressure points and perioral areas heal more slowly.

The use of systemic steroids for SJS/TEN management is controversial as large randomized controlled trials demonstrating efficacy are lacking. High-dose IV immunoglobulins may be of some benefit if administered early. Cyclosporine, cyclophosphamide, plasmapheresis, *N*-acetyl-cysteine have had anecdotal successes.

PREVENTION

Those who do recover from TEN need to be aware of their drug sensitivity and possible cross-reactants. Reexposure to the offending agent or structurally similar drugs can lead to a faster, more severe TEN episode, thus drugs should not be readministered. The patient's medical chart should clearly document the severe drug reaction and the patient should wear a medical alert bracelet.

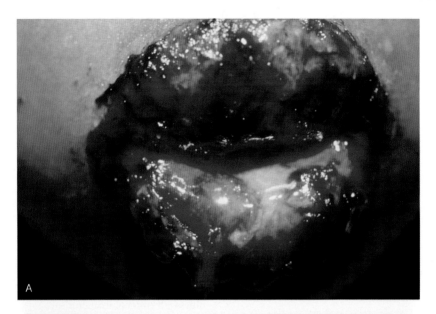

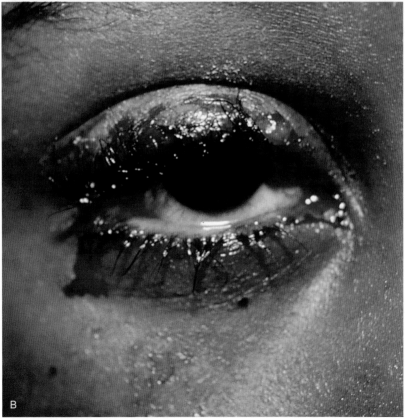

FIGURE 15-7 Stevens–Johnson syndrome A: Debilitating mucosal involvement with hemorrhagic ulcerations and crusting requiring hospital admission for IV fluids and supportive care. **B:** Ocular involvement with erosions and ulcerations in the same child.

FIXED DRUG ERUPTION

An FDE is a recurrent cutaneous reaction to an ingested drug characterized by the formation of a fixed plaque, bulla, or erosion at the same site, hours after the offending drug is ingested.

EPIDEMIOLOGY

AGE Any age.
GENDER M = F.
INCIDENCE Uncommon.
ETIOLOGY The drugs most commonly implicated are phenolphthalein, antimicrobial agents (tetracycline, minocycline, sulfonamides, trimethoprim-sulfamethoxazole, metronidazole), nystatin, anti-inflammatory agents (salicylates, NSAIDs, naproxen, acetaminophen, dipyrone, dimenhydrinate, phenylbutazone, phenacetin), psychoactive agents (barbiturates, carbamazepine), quinine and quinidine. The foods most commonly implicated are peas, beans, and lentils.

HISTORY

An FDE will first present as an erythematous plaque that occurs 1 to 2 weeks after exposure to the offending agent. With subsequent exposures, the violaceous plaque recurs within minutes to 24 hours and recurs at the same site. The patient typically reports seeing the lesion at seemingly random intervals. Careful history will usually elicit the sporadic use of an over-the-counter or PRN medication that is causing the recurrent rash (i.e., ibuprofen, aspirin, eye drops, laxatives, etc.).

PHYSICAL EXAMINATION

Skin Findings

TYPE Macule, plaque, bullae, erosion.
SHAPE Round to oval (Fig. 15-8).
COLOR Red, purple, brown.
SIZE 0.5 to 20 cm in diameter.
NUMBER Solitary lesion. With repeated attacks, multiple lesions may occur. Occasionally generalized FDEs with disseminated multiple lesions may occur.
SITES OF PREDILECTION Lips, hands, face, feet, genitalia.

DIFFERENTIAL DIAGNOSIS

FDE can be confused with recurrent herpetic lesions, arthropod bite, other drug reactions such as EM, a contact dermatitis, or other eczematous processes.

LABORATORY EXAMINATIONS

DERMATOPATHOLOGY Perivascular and interstitial dermal lymphohistiocytic infiltrate, at times with eosinophils and/or subepidermal vesicles and bullae with overlying epidermal necrosis. Between outbreaks, the site shows marked pigmentary incontinence with melanin in macrophages in the upper dermis.

COURSE AND PROGNOSIS

The cutaneous lesions of FDE resolve within a few weeks of withdrawing the offending agent. The lesions often heal with hyperpigmentation given the pigmentary incontinence that occurs during the inflammatory phase of the lesions. A notable exception is pseudoephedrine, which classically causes a non-pigmented FDE. The rash recurs within hours following ingestion of a single dose of the drug.

MANAGEMENT

The management for an FDE is to identify and withhold the offending drug. The hyperpigmented postinflammatory changes will slowly resolve with time.

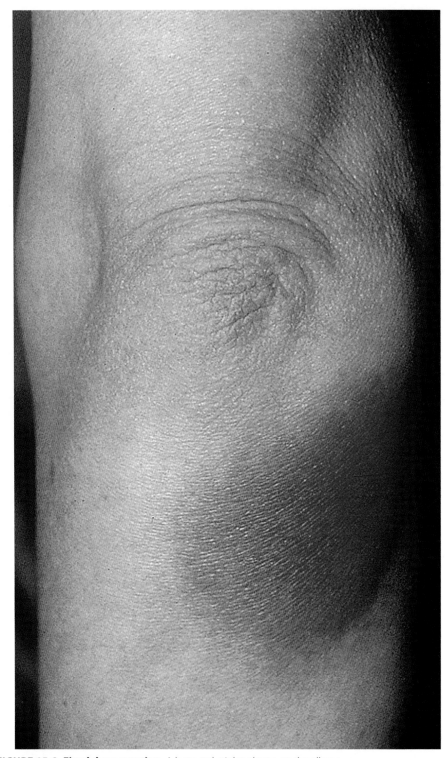

FIGURE 15-8 Fixed drug eruption A large red–violet plaque on the elbow.

SERUM SICKNESS

Serum sickness is an allergic reaction characterized by urticaria, malaise, fever, LAD, splenomegaly, and arthralgias. It originally was seen most in treatment with horse or rabbit antiserum; it is now seen with drugs or vaccinations.

EPIDEMIOLOGY

AGE Any age.
GENDER M = F.
INCIDENCE Uncommon.
ETIOLOGY Type-III (immune-complex mediated) hypersensitivity reaction.

PATHOPHYSIOLOGY

Serum sickness is mediated by circulating antigen–antibody complexes (type III Arthus reaction), in which IgG is the predominant immunoglobulin.

HISTORY

Urticarial rash and low-grade fever, usually 7 to 21 days following administration of offending agent, or earlier in individuals previously sensitized to the agent. Agents derived from nonhuman animals (such as horse or rabbit antithymocyte globulin or mouse-based monoclonal antibodies) are common triggering drugs.

PHYSICAL EXAMINATION

Skin Findings

TYPE Wheals, edema (Fig. 15-9).
COLOR Pink, red, or violaceous.
SHAPE Round, oval, and polycyclic.
ARRANGEMENT Scattered, discrete lesions or dense, confluent areas.
DISTRIBUTION Trunk, extremities, face. Mucous membranes may be involved. A predilection for the lateral aspects of the hands and feet may be observed.

General Findings

LYMPHADENOPATHY (often in epitrochlear region).
MUSCULOSKELETAL (50%) Arthralgia, polyarthritis.
NEUROLOGIC Peripheral neuritis, radiculitis, optic neuritis, cerebral edema.
RENAL Glomerulonephritis.

DIFFERENTIAL DIAGNOSIS

Serum sickness can be confused with urticaria, angioedema, urticarial vasculitis, a viral exanthem, TEN, or subacute bacterial endocarditis.

LABORATORY EXAMINATIONS

DERMATOPATHOLOGY Engorged blood vessels with edema and perivascular inflammation.
HEMATOLOGY ± Eosinophilia, elevated ESR, hypocomplementemia.

COURSE AND PROGNOSIS

Serum sickness has a self-limited course, progression may continue for several days, and then disappear within 2 to 3 weeks. Most cases resolve with no permanent sequelae. In rare instances, coronary artery vasculitis or neuropathy may persist.

MANAGEMENT

The triggering agent should be promptly discontinued. Symptomatic treatment of serum sickness includes analgesics and one or more antihistamines (chlorpheniramine, hydroxyzine, diphenhydramine, doxepin, acrivastine, cetirizine, loratadine, mizolastine, desloratadine, fexofenadine, levocetirizine, cimetidine, or ranitidine). Antihistamines should be continued for 1 to 2 weeks beyond clinical clearance to avoid recurrences or relapses and may need to be tapered slowly over several months.

Although their efficacy has not been proven, systemic steroids (prednisone, prednisolone) are used if common measures fail to comfort patient. More refractory cases may require systemic steroids (prednisone or methylprednisolone), but only short courses are recommended and rebound is possible. For anaphylactic or life-threatening situations (individuals with facial edema or respiratory symptoms), subcutaneous epinephrine is effective. The triggering agent and reaction should be carefully documented in the patient's medical record and reexposure should be avoided.

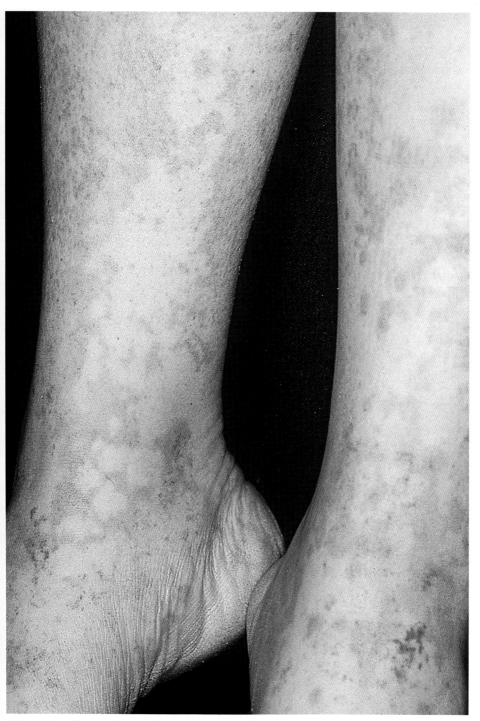

FIGURE 15-9 Serum sickness Urticarial, coalescing plaques on the lower legs of an adolescent with serum sickness.

ERYTHEMA ANNULARE CENTRIFUGUM

EAC is a cutaneous eruption characterized by migratory erythematous annular lesions with raised borders and central clearing. The etiology of EAC is unknown but it has been speculated that it occurs as a hypersensitivity reaction to an underlying infectious, inflammatory, or neoplastic process.

SYNONYMS Erythema perstans, erythema figuratum perstans, gyrate erythema, palpable migrating erythema.

EPIDEMIOLOGY

AGE Any age.
GENDER M = F.
GENETICS Rare case reports of autosomal dominant inheritance.
ETIOLOGY Likely hypersensitivity reaction to drugs (diuretics, NSAIDs, antimalarials, gold), foods, infections (dermatophytes, *Candida albicans, Penicillium*, poxvirus, EBV, molluscum contagiosum, parasites, *P. pubis*), blood dyscrasias, immunologic disorders (neonatal lupus, Sjögren's syndrome, autoimmune endocrinopathies, hypereosinophilic syndrome), liver disease, hyperthyroidism, or neoplasms (lymphomas, leukemias).

HISTORY

Rash appears and spreads centrifugally over a period of 1 to 2 weeks. It is typically asymptomatic or mildly pruritic and can recur for months to years depending upon its etiologic process.

PHYSICAL EXAMINATION

Skin Findings

TYPE Papules or plaques with fine circumferential scale.
SIZE 1 to 10 cm.
COLOR Pink, red, purple.
NUMBER Solitary or multiple.
SHAPE Oval, circinate, semiannular, targetlike, or polycyclic (Fig. 15-10).
DISTRIBUTION Trunk, buttocks, thighs, and lower legs. Rarely palms, soles, mucous membranes.

DIFFERENTIAL DIAGNOSIS

The differential diagnosis of EAC is other annular rashes including pityriasis rosea, EM, erythema marginatum, erythema chronicum migrans, dermatophyte infections, urticaria, urticarial vasculitis, granuloma annulare, sarcoidosis, psoriasis, and annular LE.

LABORATORY EXAMINATIONS

DERMATOPATHOLOGY Skin biopsy shows parakeratosis and focal infiltration of lymphocytes around dermal blood vessels and adnexal structures in a "coat–sleeve" pattern. There is minimal papillary edema and mild spongiosis.

COURSE AND PROGNOSIS

The duration of EAC is extremely variable; new lesions may continue to form for months or even years, appearing in successive forms.

MANAGEMENT

The treatment of EAC depends on the etiology and eradication of the causative agent is curative. Even in the absence of an identifiable cause, empiric treatment with antibiotics or antifungals may be helpful. Pruritic symptoms of EAC can be treated with antihistamines (chlorpheniramine, hydroxyzine, diphenhydramine, doxepin, acrivastine, cetirizine, loratadine). Topical regimens include antipruritics (calamine or 1% menthol cream) and/or topical steroids. Improvement with topical tacrolimus and topical calcipotriol has been reported.

Systemic steroids (prednisone, prednisolone) may suppress EAC but the disorder frequently recurs after cessation. Anecdotally, systemic metronidazole and subcutaneous interferon-α have had some success.

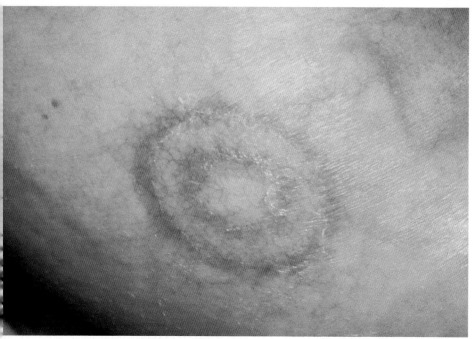

FIGURE 15-10 Erythema annulare centrifugum Polycyclic lesions on the thigh of a child.

GRAFT-VERSUS-HOST DISEASE

GVHD is an immune disorder caused by the response of histoincompatible, immunocompetent donor cells against the tissues of an immunoincompetent host.

CLASSIFICATION

Acute Cutaneous GVHD

1. Stage 1: Maculopapular eruption involving <25% of body surface area.
2. Stage 2: Maculopapular eruption involving 25% to 50% of body surface.
3. Stage 3: Erythroderma with greater than 50% body surface area involvement.
4. Stage 4: Erythroderma with bulla formation.

Acute cutaneous GVHD is often accompanied by gastrointestinal tract and liver involvement, marked by diarrhea and hyperbilirubinemia, respectively.

Chronic Cutaneous GVHD

1. Lichenoid or lichen planus-like type
2. Sclerodermoid or sclerotic type
3. Poikilodermatous type

EPIDEMIOLOGY

AGE Any age, increased risk with older donor or recipient.
GENDER Increased risk with F donor/M recipient.
INCIDENCE Acute: 25% to 50%. Chronic: 50% of allogeneic peripheral blood stem cell transplantation (PBSCT) or bone marrow transplantation (BMT) recipients.
ETIOLOGY Immune-mediated reaction in the graft-recipient from immunocompetent donor cells.

PATHOPHYSIOLOGY

GVHD is an immunologic reaction induced by a graft of allogeneic lymphoid cells into a recipient with antigens not present in the donor. It is one of the major complications of allogeneic BMT or PBSCT with clinical manifestations in the skin, liver (cholestatic hepatitis), and/or GI tract (diarrhea). Severity of GVHD is related to histocompatibility mismatch between donor and recipient and preparatory regimen used.

HISTORY

ACUTE GVHD Rash and pruritus typically occur 14 to 21 days (usually <3 months) after BMT or PBSCT.
CHRONIC GVHD Rash typically appears later than 40 days (average: 4 months) post-BMT or PBSCT, either evolving from acute GVHD or arising de novo.

Both acute and chronic GVHD may also be triggered by donor lymphocyte infusions following the initial transplantation.

PHYSICAL EXAMINATION

Skin Findings (Acute GVHD)

TYPE Maculopapular, papules, bullae.
COLOR Red.
DISTRIBUTION Acral: palms, soles, pinna (Fig. 15-11), cheeks, neck, upper back, or generalized (Fig. 15-12). Perifollicular accentuation may occur.

General Findings (Acute GVHD)

High fever, hepatitis, jaundice, diarrhea, serositis, pulmonary insufficiency.

Skin Findings (Chronic GVHD)

TYPE Papules, plaques (Fig. 15-13), ulcers.
COLOR Purple, hypopigmented.
PALPATION Sclerotic.
DISTRIBUTION Dorsal hands, forearms. Sclerosis on trunk, buttocks, hips, thighs.

General Findings (Chronic GVID)

Hair loss; anhidrosis, oral LP-like lesions; erosive stomatitis, oral and ocular sicca-like syndrome; esophagitis, serositis, fasciitis, bronchiolitis obliterans, chronic liver disease; wasting.

DIFFERENTIAL DIAGNOSIS

Acute GVHD can be confused with an exanthematous drug reaction, viral exanthem, or TEN. Chronic GVHD can be confused with lichen planus, lichenoid drug reaction, PLC, scleroderma, or poikiloderma.

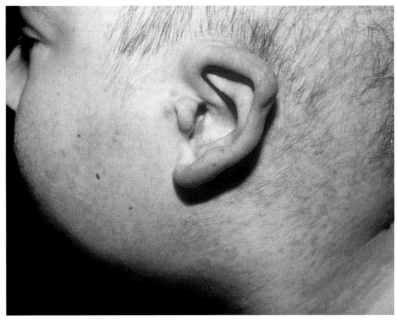

FIGURE 15-11 Graft-versus-host disease, acute Red-to-violaceous hue on the pinna of a child with acute GVHD.

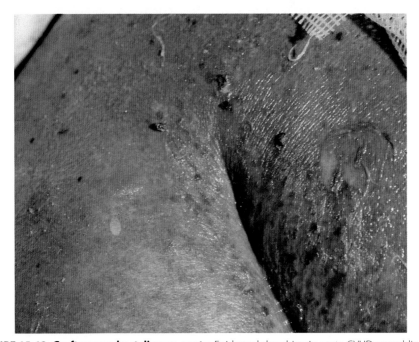

FIGURE 15-12 Graft-versus-host disease, acute Epidermal sloughing in acute GVHD resembling TEN-like changes. (Reproduced with permission from Fitzpatrick TB et al. *Color Atlas and Synopsis of Clinical Dermatology*. 2nd ed. New York, NY: McGraw-Hill; 1992.)

LABORATORY EXAMINATIONS

Dermatopathology

ACUTE GVHD Basal cell vacuolization and necrosis of individual keratinocytes with a mild perivenular mononuclear cell infiltrate. Apposition of lymphocytes to necrotic keratinocytes can be seen and vacuoles coalesce forming subepidermal clefts and/or complete dermoepidermal separation.

CHRONIC GVHD Hyperkeratosis, mild hypergranulosis, mild acanthosis, moderate basal vacuolization, band-like lymphocytic infiltrate next to the epidermis, melanin incontinence, loss of hair follicles, entrapment of sweat glands, and dense dermal sclerosis.

COURSE AND PROGNOSIS

ACUTE GVHD Profoundly decreases survival after PBSCT or BMT. Mild-to-moderate acute GVHD responds well to treatment. Severe GVHD patients are susceptible to infections (bacterial, fungal, or viral) and those with TEN-like skin changes have a very poor prognosis. Acute GVHD has mortality rate up to 45% in BMT and PBSCT patients.

CHRONIC GVHD Sclerodermoid changes, tight skin, and joint contractures may result in impaired mobility and ulcerations. There is also associated hair loss, xerostomia, and xerophthalmia which can result in corneal ulcers and blindness. GI disease leads to malabsorption. Mild chronic cutaneous GVHD may resolve spontaneously. Severe changes are usually permanent and debilitating. Chronic GVHD has an overall survival rate of approximately 40% at 10 years owing to infections and immunosuppression.

MANAGEMENT

ACUTE GVHD The current strategy is to treat the BMT or PBSCT recipient with an immunosuppressive regimen including methotrexate, cyclosporine, mycophenolate, or other agents for 180 days posttransplant, followed by an immunosuppressive taper to prevent acute GVHD. If GVHD develops while on this regimen, systemic steroids are added. Other treatment possibilities include thalidomide, hydroxychloroquine, clofazimine, or azathioprine. Topical steroids can provide adjunctive symptomatic relief for cutaneous involvement.

CHRONIC GVHD Treatment for chronic GVHD is difficult and consists of systemic steroids alone or in combination with cyclosporine or tacrolimus. Topical agents may be of limited value in sclerotic disease. Other treatment possibilities include PUVA, photopheresis, etretinate, acitretin, infliximab, daclizumab and investigational systemic agents are currently being studied.

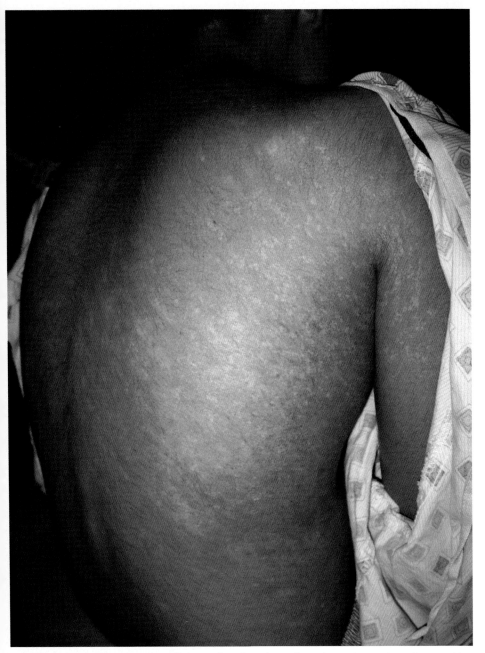

FIGURE 15-13 Graft-versus-host-disease, chronic Lichenoid papules coalescing into plaques with significant hypopigmentation 4 months after an allogeneic BMT.

ERYTHEMA NODOSUM

Erythema nodosum (EN) is a cell-mediated, hypersensitivity reaction characterized by tender red nodules usually on the pretibial area.

INSIGHT

EN is sometimes mistaken for multifocal cellulitis.

SYNONYMS Erythema contusiformis, EN migrans.

EPIDEMIOLOGY

AGE Any age. Most commonly seen in patients aging from 15 to 30 years.
GENDER F > M, 3:1.
INCIDENCE Uncommon.
SEASON Spring and fall prevalence.
ETIOLOGY Up to 40% or more cases are idiopathic. Associated triggers include infections (streptococcus, mycoplasma, tuberculosis, coccidioidomycosis, histoplasmosis, leprosy, leishmaniasis, cat scratch disease, mycobacterium marinum, yersinia, lymphogranuloma venereum, hepatitis B, brucellosis, meningococcus, gonococcus, pertussis, syphilis, *Chlamydia*, blastomycosis, HIV), drugs (estrogens, birth control pills, sulfonamides, penicillin, bromides, iodides, phenytoin), pregnancy, underlying systemic diseases (sarcoidosis, Crohn's, ulcerative colitis, Behçet's, Sweet's, regional ileitis), or internal malignancy.

PATHOPHYSIOLOGY

EN represents a delayed-type hypersensitivity reaction to a variety of different stimuli.

HISTORY

Skin lesions appear over a few days as warm tender red nodules, most often on the pretibial area. The skin lesions slowly heal over 3 to 6 weeks but can recur, especially with recurrent infection. Associated arthralgias (50%), fever, and malaise may be present.

PHYSICAL EXAMINATION

Skin Findings

TYPE Nodules (Fig. 15-14).
COLOR Bright to deep red followed by purple to brown.
SIZE 1 to 5 cm.
SHAPE Round, oval.

DISTRIBUTION Pretibial area > thighs/forearms > trunk, neck, face.

General Findings

FEVER
MUSCULOSKELETAL Arthritis, myalgias.

DIFFERENTIAL DIAGNOSIS

The differential diagnosis includes ecchymoses, cellulitis, erysipelas, deep fungal infections, insect bites, thrombophlebitis, erythema induratum, and other panniculitides.

LABORATORY EXAMINATIONS

DERMATOPATHOLOGY Septal panniculitic inflammation involving the dermis and subcutaneous fat with perivascular inflammatory spillover into some adjacent fat lobules.

COURSE AND PROGNOSIS

Most cases of EN resolve spontaneously in 3 to 6 weeks, especially with rest and leg elevation. Ultimately, the course depends upon the underlying etiology and elimination of the precipitant when possible (i.e., discontinue triggering drug, treat underlying infection or systemic disease, etc.). Recurrences are also dependent on etiology and recurrent EN in children is primarily seen with recurrent streptococcal infection.

MANAGEMENT

Identification and elimination of the etiologic agent is most helpful. Recommended workup for an etiologic agent includes a careful drug history, throat culture to rule out streptococcus, chest x-ray to rule out sarcoidosis, tuberculin test to rule out primary tuberculosis, or other tests as deemed necessary by history.

Symptomatic treatment of the skin lesions includes bed rest, leg elevation, and compressive bandages, salicylates, and other NSAIDs (indomethacin, naproxen). Intralesional or systemic steroids can be used only if the etiologic agent is known (and infectious agents have been excluded). Other possible treatments include potassium iodide, colchicine, hydroxychloroquine, cyclosporine, and thalidomide. NSAIDs should be avoided in patients with IBD since these can flare the bowel symptoms.

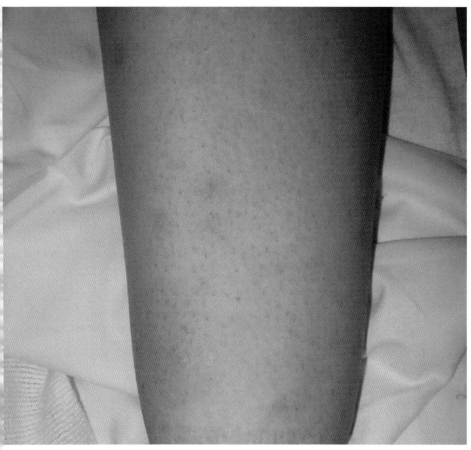

FIGURE 15-14 Erythema nodosum Tender red nodules on the pretibial area of an adolescent.

COLD PANNICULITIS

Cold panniculitis is characterized by erythematous plaques or nodules that appear on exposure to the cold.

SYNONYM Popsicle panniculitis.

EPIDEMIOLOGY

AGE Infants, small children.
GENDER M = F.
ETIOLOGY Cold (weather, ice, popsicles) causes the fat to solidify with resultant plaque or nodule formation. Also seen on the lateral thighs of female equestrians.

PATHOPHYSIOLOGY

Cold panniculitis occurs when the body fat solidifies and then liquifies on rewarming, with resulting inflammatory changes. The higher prevalence in infants and children is thought to be related to the fact that the subcutaneous fat in young children solidifies more easily than it does in adults.

HISTORY

Erythematous plaques or nodules develop on the exposed area hours after exposure to the cold. The areas may be painful or asymptomatic.

PHYSICAL EXAMINATION

Skin Findings

TYPE Plaques, nodules.
COLOR Pink to red.

SHAPE Round to oval.
DISTRIBUTION Bilateral cheeks (Fig. 15-15), chin, lateral thighs.

DIFFERENTIAL DIAGNOSIS

The differential diagnosis for cold panniculitis includes other forms of panniculitis, cellulitis, erysipelas, insect bites, or ecchymoses.

LABORATORY EXAMINATIONS

DERMATOPATHOLOGY Nonspecific inflammation of septa and lobules of the deep dermis and subcutaneous fat.

COURSE AND PROGNOSIS

Cold panniculitis lesions can appear 5 minutes to 3 days after cold exposure, and regress over weeks to months with postinflammatory pigmentation changes that can persist for up to 1 year.

MANAGEMENT

Cold panniculitis self-resolves with cold avoidance and treatment is unnecessary.

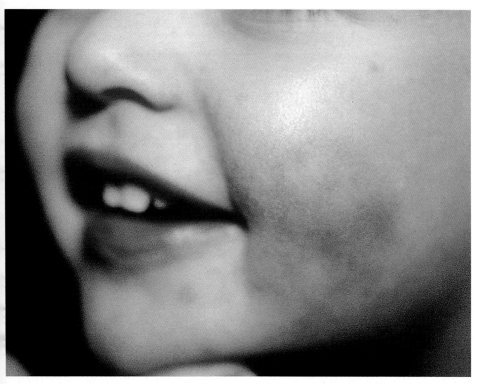

FIGURE 15-15 Cold panniculitis Erythematous nodules on the cheeks of a child a few days after cold exposure.

NEUTROPHILIC DERMATOSES

SWEET'S SYNDROME

Sweet's syndrome (SS) is a rare, recurrent skin disease characterized by painful papules, plaques, and nodules on the limbs, face, and trunk, accompanied by fever and leukocytosis.

INSIGHT

In the initial stage, SS may present as vesiculating papules; varicella must be excluded at this stage.

SYNONYM Acute febrile neutrophilic dermatosis.

EPIDEMIOLOGY

AGE Infants, children, adults aging from 30 to 60 years.
GENDER F > M, 4:1.
INCIDENCE Rare.
ETIOLOGY 50% idiopathic. Possible hypersensitivity reaction to infection. In adults, SS can be seen as an immunologic response to IBD, drugs, autoimmune disorders, pregnancy, or malignancy (particularly AML).

PATHOPHYSIOLOGY

SS is thought to represent a hypersensitivity reaction to an infection (*Streptococcal, Yersinia,* atypical mycobacteria, CMV, hepatitis, HIV, BCG vaccination), malignancy (acute myeloid leukemia, transient myeloid proliferation, GU carcinoma, breast carcinoma, colon carcinoma), autoimmune disease (Behçet's, autoimmune thyroiditis, sarcoidosis, dermatomyositis, SLE, rheumatoid arthritis, relapsing polychondritis, Sjögren's), pregnancy, IBD (ulcerative colitis), or drugs (G-CSF, furosemide, hydralazine, minocycline, and trimethoprim-sulfamethoxazole).

HISTORY

In cases of SS, upper respiratory tract infection or flu-like symptoms with high fevers often precede the skin lesions by 1 to 3 weeks. Then, there is a sudden appearance of tender and painful papules and plaques on the face, neck, and limbs (usually spares torso), associated with a leukocytosis and polyarthritis. SS can rarely occur in the setting of profound leukopenia or neutropenia in response to a drug or infectious trigger.

PHYSICAL EXAMINATION

Skin Findings

TYPE Papules, nodules, bullae (Fig. 15-16). Papule may take on a pseudovesiculated appearance due to the associated edema.
COLOR Red, bluish-red.
SIZE 1 to 2 cm.
PALPATION Lesions are tender.
SHAPE Annular or arcuate.
ARRANGEMENT Single lesion or multiple lesions, asymmetrically distributed.
DISTRIBUTION Face, neck, and extremities. Spares torso.

General Findings

FEVER (80%).
MUSCULOSKELETAL (30%) Arthralgias, arthritis, myalgias.
OCULAR (50%) Conjunctivitis, episcleritis, limbal nodules, iridocyclitis.
OTHER Neutrophilic alveolitis, multifocal sterile osteomyelitis (SAPHO syndrome), glomerulonephritis, hepatitis, myositis, meningitis, encephalitis, pancreatitis, gastritis.

DIFFERENTIAL DIAGNOSIS

The differential diagnosis of SS includes EM, EN, prevesicular herpes simplex infection, preulcerative pyoderma gangrenosum (PG), bowel-bypass syndrome, urticaria, serum sickness, other vasculitides, SLE, and panniculitis.

LABORATORY EXAMINATIONS

DERMATOPATHOLOGY Edema and a dense, perivascular infiltration with polymorphonuclear leukocytes in the upper and middermis without vasculitis.
HEMATOLOGY Leukocytosis (>10,000/mm^3), increased ESR, and C-reactive protein. Absence of these features does not eliminate possibility of SS.

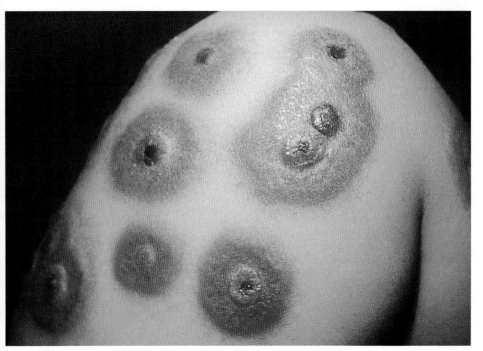

FIGURE 15-16 Sweet's syndrome Erythematous plaques and nodules with central bullous changes on a child's knee.

COURSE AND PROGNOSIS

Untreated, SS lesions enlarge over a period of days or weeks, and eventually resolve without scarring after 1 to 12 months. The skin lesions exhibit an excellent response to systemic steroids, usually resolving in days. Recurrences are seen in 50% of patients, often in previously involved sites, especially in patients with associated hematologic disorders.

MANAGEMENT

If an infection is identified, proper antimicrobial therapy is necessary.

Both the skin lesions and systemic symptoms of SS respond dramatically to steroids (prednisone or prednisolone). Solitary lesions can be treated with topical steroids, and/or topical calcineurin inhibitors. Other effective SS treatments include potassium iodide, clofazimine, colchicine, indomethacin, naproxen, sulindac, cyclosporine, thalidomide, a-interferon, and dapsone.

PYODERMA GANGRENOSUM

PG is a rapidly evolving, chronic, and severely debilitating skin disease characterized by painful ulcers with undermined borders and a purulent necrotic base. It occurs most commonly in association with systemic disease, especially inflammatory bowel disease or myeloproliferative disorders.

SYNONYM Phagedenisme geometrique.

CLASSIFICATION

1. Ulcerative: Classic PG associated with IBD or inflammatory arthritis.
2. Bullous: Atypical or bullous PG associated with AML, myelodysplasia, and other myelo-proliferative disorders (CML).
3. Pustular: Sterile pustular eruption ± PG associated with IBD.
4. Superficial granulomatous: Localized ulcerative and vegetative lesion following trauma (surgery).

EPIDEMIOLOGY

AGE Infants, children, adults ranging from 20 to 50 years.
GENDER F > M.
INCIDENCE Rare.
ETIOLOGY Idiopathic (25–50%), immunologic abnormality suspected.

HISTORY

Acute onset with painful hemorrhagic pustule or nodule arising either de novo or following minimal trauma (pathergy), typically on the lower legs.

PATHOPHYSIOLOGY

An underlying immunologic abnormality in patients is suspected since PG is often associated with illnesses such as large and small bowel disease, arthritis, paraproteinemia, multiple myeloma, leukemia, active chronic hepatitis, and Behçet's syndrome.

PHYSICAL EXAMINATION

Skin Findings

TYPE Papule, pustule, nodule, or ulcer with undermined borders (Fig. 15-17).
SIZE 1 to 10 cm.
COLOR Red or purple, with classic "gun-metal gray" border appearance.
SHAPE Irregular or serpiginous.
ARRANGEMENT Usually solitary. May form in clusters that coalesce.
DISTRIBUTION Lower extremities > genitals/buttocks > abdomen > face.

MUCOUS MEMBRANES Rarely, aphthae; ulcers of oral mucosa and conjunctivae.

General Findings

FEVER
GASTROINTESTINAL (30%) Ulcerative colitis or Crohn's syndrome.
MUSCULOSKELETAL (20%) Arthritis.
HEMATOLOGIC (25%) AML, CML, hairy cell leukemia, myelodysplasia, monoclonal gammopathy.

DIFFERENTIAL DIAGNOSIS

The differential diagnosis of PG includes furuncle, carbuncle, cellulitis, panniculitis, gangrene, ecthyma gangrenosum, atypical mycobacterial infection, clostridial infection, deep mycoses, amebiasis, bromoderma, pemphigus vegetans, stasis ulcers, and Wegener's granulomatosis.

LABORATORY EXAMINATION

DERMATOPATHOLOGY Nonspecific, nondiagnostic. Neutrophilic inflammation, engorgement, and thrombosis of the small and medium vessels. Necrosis, hemorrhage may be present. The presence of infectious organisms must be excluded on histopathology and tissue culture.

COURSE AND PROGNOSIS

Untreated, PG may last months to years. Lesions undergo necrosis and ulceration can expose underlying tendons or muscles. Ulceration may extend rapidly within a few days, or slowly and new ulcers may appear as older lesions resolve. Reepithelialization begins at the margins of the lesion and the lesions heal with atrophic scars.

MANAGEMENT

PG is best managed by identification and treatment of any associated underlying disease. For cutaneous lesions, management consists of decreasing inflammation, reducing pain, and promoting healing.

Topical regimens for mild disease include gentle cleansing (0.25% acetic acid soaks, whirlpool baths), wet dressings with potassium permanganate, silver sulfadiazine cream, cromolyn sodium solution, nicotine patch,

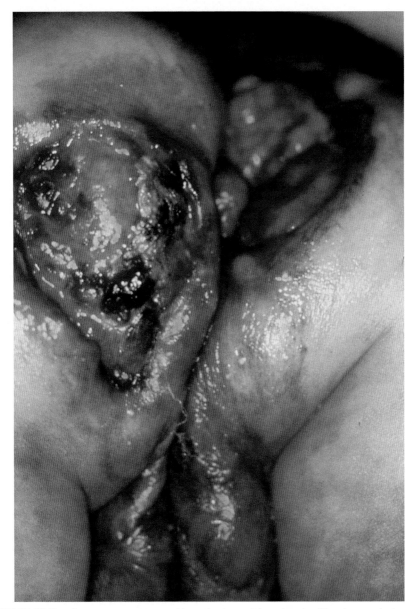

FIGURE 15-17 Pyoderma gangrenosum Necrotic ulcers with undermined borders on the buttocks of an infant.

topical or intralesional steroids, or topical tacrolimus.

For moderate disease or severe disease, oral steroids (prednisone, prednisolone) are the most effective. Systemic cyclosporine or tacrolimus can be used for PG refractory to steroids. Other treatment modalities include oral antibiotics, colchicine, infliximab, dapsone, clofazimine, potassium iodide, thalidomide, methotrexate, azathioprine, mycophenolate mofetil, cyclophosphamide, chlorambucil, intravenous immunoglobulin (IVIg), and plasmapheresis.

Surgical debridement and excision of the ulcers should be avoided because PG is subject to pathergy in 20% of cases.

SARCOIDOSIS

Sarcoidosis is a chronic granulomatous inflammatory process of unknown etiology that affects the skin, eye, lungs, and reticuloendothelial system.

SYNONYMS Lofgren's syndrome—erythema nodosum, hilar adenopathy, fever, arthritis; Heerfordt's syndrome—parotid gland enlargement, uveitis, fever, cranial nerve palsy; Darier–Roussy disease—subcutaneous sarcoidosis.

Special Types

1. *Lupus pernio:* Soft, violaceous plaques on the nose, cheek, and earlobes, associated with pulmonary sarcoidosis (75%).
2. *Scar sarcoidosis:* Purple nodules occurring in an old scar.

EPIDEMIOLOGY

AGE Uncommon in children. Adults: Aging between 25–35 years and 45–65 years.
GENDER 2:1 Female:Male.
INCIDENCE African American women: 107 per 100,000. Sweden 64 per 100,000. United Kingdom 20 per 100,000.
RACE African Americans > Caucasians.
GEOGRAPHY United States: Southeast states, Northern Europe.
SEASONAL Increased in winter and spring.
GENETICS Familial cases reported. HLA-1, HLA-B8, HLA-DR3 associations. Polymorphism for gene encoding angiotensin-converting enzyme (ACE).
ETIOLOGY Multifactorial with host response/delayed hypersensitivity and abnormal immunoregulation all playing a role.

PATHOPHYSIOLOGY

An autoimmune or infectious trigger leads to granuloma formation in susceptible hosts with hyperactivity of their cell-mediated immune system.

HISTORY

Young children with sarcoidosis develop asymptomatic eczematous or infiltrated papules, plaques, and pustules. They tend to have polyarthritis, uveitis, and not as many pulmonary symptoms. Older children and adolescent symptoms resemble the adult form of sarcoidosis with fever, cough, weight loss, abdominal pain, adenopathy, lung disease, hypergammaglobulinemia, and hypercalcemia.

PHYSICAL EXAMINATION

Skin Lesions

TYPE Maculopapules, plaques. Ulceration may occur in chronic lesions.
SIZE 0.5 to 1 cm.
COLOR Red-brown to purple.
PALPATION Blanching with glass slide (diascopy) reveals "apple-jelly" yellowish-brown color.
SHAPE Annular, polycyclic, serpiginous.
DISTRIBUTION Face (Fig. 15-18), lips, neck, upper trunk extremities.

General Findings

FEVER LAD (90%) Bilateral hilar adenopathy on chest x-ray.
MUSCULOSKELETAL Arthralgias.
GASTROINTESTINAL Abdominal pain.
PULMONARY (90%) Alveolitis, granulomatous infiltration, bronchiolectasis.
OCULAR Uveitis and iritis.
OTHER Parotid gland enlargement, facial nerve paralysis, and CNS involvement are rare.

DIFFERENTIAL DIAGNOSIS

The differential diagnosis of sarcoid includes infections with granulomatous inflammation (leprosy, tuberculosis), lupus erythematosus, foreign body reactions, granulomatous mycosis fungoides, granulomatous rosacea, granuloma annulare, necrobiosis lipoidica, rheumatoid nodule, and interstitial granulomatous dermatitis.

LABORATORY EXAMINATIONS

DERMATOPATHOLOGY Superficial and deep non-caseating epithelioid granulomas without surrounding lymphocytic inflammation ("naked" tubercles). Multinucleated giant cells with nuclei in a peripheral arc with eosinophilic "asteroid bodies" or basophilic "Schaumann bodies."
BLOOD CHEMISTRY Increase in serum ACE (60%), hypergammaglobulinemia, hypercalcemia.

COURSE AND PROGNOSIS

Sarcoidosis in children tends to regress completely over several years. Mortality is less than 5%.

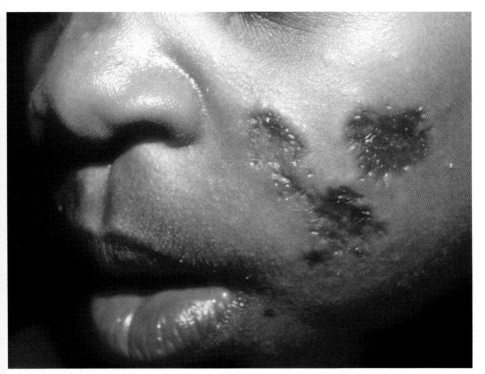

FIGURE 15-18 Sarcoidosis Violaceous scarred plaques on the cheek of a child.

MANAGEMENT

MILD DISEASE Topical corticosteroids under plastic dressings, intralesional steroids, or systemic corticosteroids (prednisone, methylprednisolone) help skin lesions.

MODERATE-TO-SEVERE DISEASE Systemic corticosteroids (prednisone, methylprednisolone) help skin, ocular disease, active pulmonary disease, cardiac arrhythmia, CNS involvement, facial palsy, and hypercalcemia. Other drugs include hydroxychloroquine, oxyphenbutazone, chloroquine, potassium-*p*-aminobenzoate, azathioprine, chlorambucil, methotrexate, thalidomide, isotretinoin, minocycline, allopurinol, infliximab, adalimumab, and etanercept.

CUTANEOUS VASCULITIS

Cutaneous vasculitis represents a specific pattern of inflammation which can affect small, medium, or large vessels of the arterial or venous system. Small vessel disease occurs in capillaries, arterioles, and postcapillary venules as seen in Henoch–Schönlein purpura (HSP) and urticarial vasculitis. Medium-sized vessel disease affects arteries and veins within the dermis or subcutis as seen in polyarteritis nodosa (PAN). Large vessel disease occurs in named arteries and the aorta as seen in KD.

HENOCH–SCHÖNLEIN PURPURA

HSP is a cutaneous small vessel vasculitis of children characterized by a diffuse vasculitis of the skin, joints, GI tract, CNS, and kidneys following an upper respiratory infection.

SYNONYMS Anaphylactoid purpura, purpura rheumatica, cutaneous small vessel vasculitis secondary to circulating IgA complexes.

EPIDEMIOLOGY

AGE Up to 90% of cases in pediatric age group; peak age 3 to 10 years.
GENDER M = F. Intussusception in M > F.
INCIDENCE 180 cases per million.
SEASONAL PREVALENCE Fall and winter.
ETIOLOGY IgA-mediated hypersensitivity reaction to an upper respiratory tract infection (sometimes β-hemolytic streptococci).

PATHOPHYSIOLOGY

HSP vasculitis is caused by deposition of immune complexes of IgA class in the capillaries, pre- and postcapillary venules of the upper dermis, GI tract, glomeruli, and synovial membrane, lungs, and CNS. The immune complex deposition results in complement activation and vascular damage.

HISTORY

HSP presents as acute-onset purpura, joint pain, and abdominal symptoms, 1 to 2 weeks after an upper respiratory tract infection. Purpura is often the presenting sign of the disease. Renal involvement may or may not occur.

PHYSICAL EXAMINATION

Skin Findings

TYPE Macules (petechiae), patches (ecchymoses), tender papules (palpable purpura) (Fig. 15-19).
SIZE 2 to 10 mm.
COLOR Red, purple, brown.
SHAPE Annular, oval, arciform.
ARRANGEMENT Discrete or confluent.
DISTRIBUTION Lower extremities, buttocks.

General Findings

FEVER (40%).
GASTROINTESTINAL Abdominal pain (85%), vomiting, GI bleeding, intussusception (2%).

MUSCULOSKELETAL Swelling of the ankles and knees.
RENAL Gross or microscopic hematuria, proteinuria.

DIFFERENTIAL DIAGNOSIS

The differential diagnosis for HSP includes acute rheumatic fever, disseminated intravascular coagulation (DIC), meningococcal septicemia, Rocky Mountain spotted fever, pigmented purpuric dermatoses, and other small vessel vascular reactions to drugs, neoplasms, inflammatory disorders, autoimmune disorders, and infections.

LABORATORY EXAMINATIONS

DERMATOPATHOLOGY Leukocytoclastic vasculitis with fibrinoid degeneration of small dermal vessel walls, perivascular and intramural infiltrate of neutrophils and/or lymphocytes, nuclear dust, and RBC extravasation with deposits of hemosiderin.
IMMUNOFLUORESCENCE Deposition of IgA, C3, and fibrin.
URINALYSIS Hematuria, proteinuria, red cell casts.
HEMATOLOGY Leukocytosis, anemia, thrombocytosis, elevated sedimentation rate.
OTHER Antistreptolysin O (ASLO) may be positive, throat culture may be positive, stools may be guaiac positive, complement may be reduced or normal.

COURSE AND PROGNOSIS

HSP is self-limited and typically resolves over the course of weeks to months. Recurrent attacks may occur (5–10%). Younger children tend to have a milder disease course of shorter duration with less GI and renal involvement and reduced recurrence rate. Up to 5% of patients with HSP-associated nephritis will progress to ESRD, more commonly seen in adult patients. Mortality is estimated to be less than 1% to 3%, usually because of renal or GI complications.

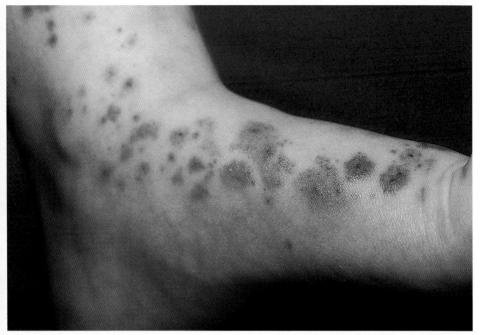

FIGURE 15-19 Henoch–Schönlein purpura Hemorrhagic macules, papules, and urticarial lesions on the foot of a child.

MANAGEMENT

The skin and systemic symptoms of HSP are usually self-limited, thus treatment consists of bed rest and supportive care. Antibiotics may be given if an upper respiratory infection is suspected. Systemic steroids may be useful for complicated noninfectious cases of HSP with GI, renal, CNS, or pulmonary manifestations though data regarding their efficacy are mixed.

Renal vasculitis is the only potential chronic problem in a patient with HSP. Corticosteroids, cyclophosphamide, or azathioprine may be used to treat severe renal involvement. IVIg, plasmapheresis, and aminocaproic acid have anecdotal effectiveness.

URTICARIAL VASCULITIS

Urticarial vasculitis is a multisystem disease characterized by cutaneous lesions resembling urticaria and biopsy findings of a leukocytoclastic vasculitis, accompanied by varying degrees of arthritis, arthralgia, angioedema, uveitis, myositis, abdominal or chest pain.

 INSIGHT While purpura is the classical *sine qua non* of vasculitis, in urticarial vasculitis, especially early lesions, there may be deep dusky areas that are not truly purpuric clinically.

SYNONYMS Hypocomplementemic vasculitis, usually lupus-like syndrome, chronic urticaria as a manifestation of venulitis.

EPIDEMIOLOGY

AGE 30 to 50 years. Rare in children.
GENDER F > M.
INCIDENCE 10% of patients with urticaria.
ETIOLOGY Immune complex disorder or non-specific reaction pattern to different etiologic agents.

PATHOPHYSIOLOGY

Thought to be an immune complex disease, similar to cutaneous vasculitis with deposition of antigen–antibody complexes in cutaneous blood vessel walls leading to complement activation and neutrophil chemotaxis. Collagenase and elastase released from neutrophils cause vessel wall and cell destruction. It can be associated with autoimmune connective tissue diseases (Sjögren's syndrome, SLE), infections (HBV, HCV, EBV), medications (potassium iodide, fluoxetine), hematologic disorders (IgM or IgM monoclonal gammopathies), and malignancies (multiple myeloma, colon, and renal cell carcinoma).

HISTORY

Recurrent papules, plaques, or wheals that last more than 24 hours with itching, burning, or stinging ± arthritis, or other constitutional symptoms.

PHYSICAL EXAMINATION

Skin Findings

TYPE OF LESION Macules, plaques, or wheals.
COLOR Early: pink, red; late: purple, yellow-green, brown.
DISTRIBUTION Trunk, proximal extremities (Fig. 15-20).
PALPATION Blanch when pressed, but purpura remains.

General Examination

FEVER (15%) LAD: (5%).
MUSCULOSKELETAL Arthralgias ± arthritis (70%).
GASTROINTESTINAL Nausea, abdominal pain (30%).
PULMONARY Cough, dyspnea, hemoptysis.
CNS Pseudotumor cerebri (10%).
RENAL Diffuse glomerulonephritis (20%).
OCULAR Conjunctivitis, episcleritis, iritis, uveitis (10%).

DIFFERENTIAL DIAGNOSIS

Urticarial vasculitis may be confused with urticaria, serum sickness, EM, angioedema, SLE, and other vasculitides.

LABORATORY EXAMINATIONS

DERMATOPATHOLOGY Early: leukocytoclastic vasculitis with perivascular infiltrate consisting primarily of neutrophils; leukocytoclasis; fibrinoid deposition in and around vessel walls; endothelial cell swelling; and extravasation of RBCs. Pigmentary incontinence may be observed.
OTHER Hypocomplementemia (70%) with low C1q, C3, and C4; circulating immune complexes; elevated sedimentation rate; microhematuria/proteinuria (10%), positive ANA.

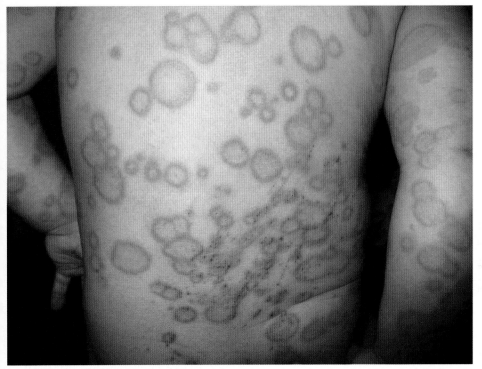

FIGURE 15-20 Urticarial vasculitis Urticarial plaques that last >24 hours and do not blanch with diascopy (gentle pressure with a glass slide).

COURSE AND PROGNOSIS

Urticarial vasculitis has a chronic (months to years) but benign course. Episodes recur over periods ranging from months to years. Systemic disease occurs in 50% of the hypocomplementemic patients, which is termed hypocomplementemic urticarial vasculitis syndrome (HUVS).

MANAGEMENT

First-line treatment includes H$_1$-blockers (diphenhydramine, hydroxyzine, cetirizine, loratadine, fexofenadine), H$_2$-blockers (cimetidine, ranitidine hydrochloride), and NSAIDs (ibuprofen, indomethacin, naproxen). Second-line treatment would be systemic steroids (prednisone, prednisolone) which may be useful for more severe disease. Systemic colchicine, dapsone, hydroxychloroquine, mycophenolate mofetil, and pentoxifylline have reported successes. Rituximab may be helpful for hypocomplementemic urticarial vasculitis. Anakinra and canakinumab are newer biologic agents which block interleukin-1 activity and appear efficacious in select patients with urticarial vasculitis.

POLYARTERITIS NODOSA

PAN is a multisystem, necrotizing vasculitis of predominantly medium-sized arteries with cutaneous and systemic variants. Infantile cases are typically more severe and life-threatening than the adult cases. Skin-limited cutaneous PAN may be seen in older children as well.

SYNONYMS Periarteritis nodosa, panarteritis nodosa.

EPIDEMIOLOGY

AGE *Infantile PAN:* In children younger than 2 years. *Adult PAN:* Occurring from 40 to 60 years of age.
GENDER Infantile PAN: M < F. Adult PAN: M > F.
INCIDENCE 16 cases per million.
GENETICS Mutations in the CECR1 gene encoding the growth factor adenosine deaminase 2 (ADA2) have been associated with hereditary PAN.
ETIOLOGY Hypersensitivity reaction from infection or inflammatory disease that leads to IgM, C3 deposition in affected vessel walls.

PATHOPHYSIOLOGY

Necrotizing inflammation of medium-sized muscular arteries associated with infections (HBV, streptococcus, parvovirus B19, HIV), inflammatory conditions (inflammatory bowel disease, SLE, familial Mediterranean fever), and malignancies (hairy cell leukemia).

HISTORY

INFANTILE PAN Febrile illness, cardiac arteritis leading to fatal coronary disease. Renal and CNS arteries are also diseased with severe sequelae. May be a severe form of KD.
PEDIATRIC CUTANEOUS PAN Subcutaneous painful nodules, livedo reticularis, preceding upper respiratory or febrile illness.
ADULT PAN Painful nodules, fever, arthritis, abdominal pain, hypertension, peripheral neuropathy, and myocardial infarction.

PHYSICAL EXAMINATION

Skin Findings (15%)

TYPE Macules, nodules, ulcers.
PATTERN Livedo reticularis pattern (Fig. 15-21).
SIZE 0.5 to 2 cm.
COLOR Red, purple.
DISTRIBUTION Lower legs > thighs > arms > trunk > head and neck > buttocks.

General Examination

FEVER WEIGHT LOSS
MUSCULOSKELETAL Arthralgias, myalgias.
CNS Cerebrovascular accidents.
NEUROLOGICAL Motor/sensory involvement, mononeuritis multiplex, peripheral neuropathy.
EYE Hypertensive, ocular vasculitis, retinal artery aneurysm, optic disc edema, atrophy.
RENAL Renovascular hypertension, renal failure.
OTHER Abdominal pain, congestive heart failure, orchitis in males.

DIFFERENTIAL DIAGNOSIS

The diagnosis of PAN is made by tissue biopsy findings (in skin, muscle, nerve, tissue) or detection of microaneurysms (in kidney or GI tract) by imaging such as magnetic resonance angiography. The differential diagnosis includes cryoglobulinemia-associated vasculitis, connective tissue diseases, microscopic polyangiitis, Wegener's granulomatosis, and Churg–Strauss syndrome.

LABORATORY EXAMINATIONS

DERMATOPATHOLOGY Segmental necrotizing vasculitis of medium-sized vessels with polymorphonuclear neutrophils infiltrating all layers of the vessel wall and perivascular areas. Fibrinoid necrosis of vessel wall occurs with occlusion of lumen, thrombosis, and infarction of tissues supplied by involved vessel.
IMMUNOFLUORESCENCE Deposits of C3, IgM, and fibrin within vessel walls.
ARTERIOGRAPHY Aneurysms in kidney, hepatic, and visceral vasculature.
OTHER Leukocytosis, eosinophilia, anemia, elevated ESR, elevated BUN/creatinine. Tests for antineutrophil cytoplasmic antibodies (ANCA) may be positive in a small percentage of patients with PAN.

COURSE AND PROGNOSIS

Infantile PAN has a chronic relapsing course with a poor prognosis and death related to cardiac failure. Cutaneous-limited PAN may result

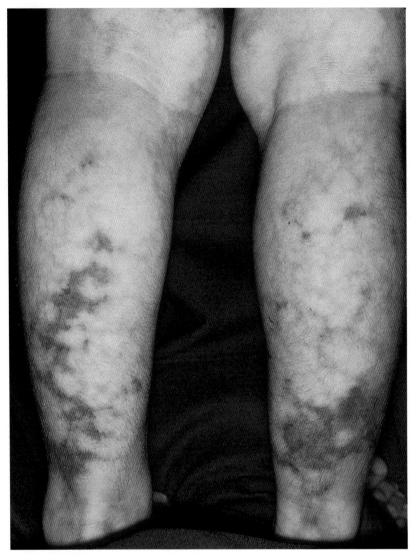

FIGURE 15-21 Infantile polyarteritis nodosa Livedo pattern of the lower legs with purpura and subcutaneous nodules on the bilateral legs of a toddler.

in high morbidity from chronic ulceration and infection unless treated. Untreated, adult PAN also has a very high morbidity and mortality characterized by fulminant deterioration or by relentless progression associated with intermittent acute exacerbations. Mortality results from renal failure, bowel perforation, cardiovascular failure, or intractable hypertension. Effective treatment reduces mortality to 50%.

MANAGEMENT

In infantile PAN, management consists of aspirin or NSAIDs (indomethacin or naproxen), and IVIg. In adult PAN, systemic corticosteroids lead to remission in half the patients. More refractory cases can be treated with cyclophosphamide, sulfapyridine, methotrexate, plasma exchange, or pentoxifylline.

IDIOPATHIC THROMBOCYTOPENIC PURPURA

Idiopathic thrombocytopenic purpura (ITP) is a common autoimmune disorder of childhood resulting in increased destruction of platelets.

SYNONYMS Immune thrombocytopenic purpura, autoimmune thrombocytopenic purpura.

CLASSIFICATION

ACUTE ITP In children, follows infection, resolves spontaneously in 2 to 3 months.
CHRONIC ITP In adults, often persists longer than 6 months without a cause.

EPIDEMIOLOGY

AGE Acute: 2 to 4 years of age. Chronic: 20 to 50 years.
GENDER Acute: M = F. Chronic: F > M, 2:1.
INCIDENCE Acute: 50 per 1,000,000 annually. Chronic: 66 per 1,000,000 annually.
SEASONALITY Slightly more common in spring and early summer.
ETIOLOGY Increased platelet destruction thought to be autoimmune and frequently follows infection (varicella, rubella, rubeola, or URI) or immunizations.

PATHOPHYSIOLOGY

Autoimmune destruction of platelets caused by antibodies against platelets.

HISTORY

Acute presentation of bleeding into the skin (from petechiae to ecchymoses) usually following a febrile illness. May be accompanied by mucosal bleeding from oral or nasal mucosal sites.

PHYSICAL EXAMINATION

Skin Findings

TYPE OF LESION Petechial macules (Fig. 15-22), ecchymoses.
SIZE 1 mm to several centimeters.
COLOR Red, purple, dark brown.
PALPATION Nonpalpable. Lesions do not blanch with pressure.
DISTRIBUTION OF LESIONS Pressure points (face and neck from crying, under elastic socks).

MUCOUS MEMBRANES Petechiae, gingival bleeding.

General Findings

CNS Intracranial hemorrhage (mortality 5% in adults, 1% in children).
OTHER Menometrorrhagia, menorrhagia, GI bleeding, retinal hemorrhages, palpable spleen.

DIFFERENTIAL DIAGNOSIS

The differential diagnosis for ITP includes telangiectasia, palpable purpura (vasculitis), purpura of scurvy, progressive pigmentary purpura (Schamberg's disease), purpura following severe Valsalva maneuver (tussive, vomiting, and retching), traumatic purpura, factitial or iatrogenic purpura, and Gardner–Diamond syndrome (autoerythrocyte sensitization syndrome).

LABORATORY EXAMINATION

DERMATOPATHOLOGY Skin biopsy may be contraindicated because of postsurgical hemorrhage in setting of thrombocytopenia.
HEMATOLOGY Thrombocytopenia (platelets below 50,000/mm^3) coagulation studies are normal (PT, PTT, fibrin split products) and exclude a consumptive process.

COURSE AND PROGNOSIS

Acute ITP of childhood is a self-limited disorder. Up to 80% of cases resolve in 4 weeks; 90% resolve in 6 months. Rarely, thrombocytopenia can last for months with a prolonged risk of hemorrhage. Only 10% of children have a more chronic course (>6 months) but these cases usually self-resolve as well. Two percent of severe childhood ITP cases have a 5-year mortality rate because of bleeding.

Older age and previous history of hemorrhage increase the risk of severe bleeding in adult, chronic ITP. Adults with severe ITP cases have the highest mortality rate because of bleeding, particularly intracranial hemorrhage.

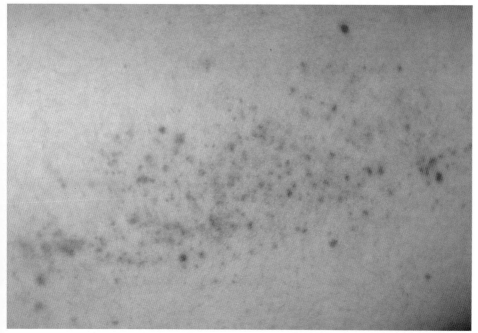

FIGURE 15-22 Idiopathic thrombocytopenic purpura Numerous petechial lesions on the leg of a child.

MANAGEMENT

Treatment is not usually needed given the high rate of spontaneous recovery in childhood acute ITP. Conservative management includes avoiding platelet inhibitors (i.e., aspirin), limiting strenuous physical activities (injury may lead to severe hemorrhage).

Persistent severe thrombocytopenia (platelets <20,000/mm^3) may warrant treatment with IVIg, systemic steroids (prednisone, methylprednisolone), platelet transfusion (for platelets <10,000/mm^3), or splenectomy for chronic cases.

DISSEMINATED INTRAVASCULAR COAGULATION

DIC is a life-threatening disorder resulting from intravascular fibrin deposition and the consumption of procoagulants and platelets. DIC is associated with a wide range of clinical circumstances (bacterial sepsis, massive trauma) characterized by both intravascular coagulation (cutaneous infarctions and/or acral gangrene) and hemorrhage.

SYNONYMS Purpura fulminans, consumption coagulopathy, defibrination syndrome, coagulation-fibrinolytic syndrome.

EPIDEMIOLOGY

AGE All ages. Purpura fulminans more common in children.
GENDER M = F.
INCIDENCE Rare; <1% of all hospitalized patients.
ETIOLOGY Conditions associated with DIC include sepsis/severe infection, massive tissue destruction (neurotrauma, organ destruction, transplant rejection), malignancy (solid tumor or myeloproliferative), transfusion reaction, rheumatologic disease (lupus), obstetric complications (amniotic fluid embolism, abruptio placentae, HELLP syndrome, retained fetal products), and vascular anomalies (Kasabach–Merritt syndrome, aneurysms).

PATHOPHYSIOLOGY

DIC is caused by the activation of the coagulation cascade leading to intravascular fibrin deposition which clogs the blood supply to the end organs. Four contributory mechanisms include increased thrombin production, anticoagulant suppression, impaired fibrinolysis, and inflammatory activation.

HISTORY

DIC typically has its onset 3 to 30 days after a resolving infection. Hemorrhagic lesions appear rapidly and systemic symptoms include fever, tachycardia, anemia, and prostration. The prognosis is grave but can be improved with therapy.

PHYSICAL EXAMINATION

Skin Findings

TYPE Ecchymoses (Fig. 15-23). May be accompanied by ulceration and frank skin necrosis.
COLOR Red, deep purple to black.
DISTRIBUTION Distal extremities; areas of pressure; lips, ears, nose, trunk.

General Findings

FEVER ± shock (14%).
BLEEDING (64%) Epistaxis, gingival/mucosal bleeding.
CNS (2%) Confusion/disorientation.
CARDIAC Hypotension, tachycardia, circulatory collapse.
PULMONARY (16%) Dyspnea/cough, ARDS.
RENAL (25%) Azotemia, renal failure.
HEPATIC (19%).

DIFFERENTIAL DIAGNOSIS

The differential diagnosis of DIC includes other diffuse hemorrhagic entities such as coumarin or heparin necrosis, thrombotic thrombocytopenic purpura-hemolytic uremic syndrome, or ITP.

LABORATORY EXAMINATIONS

DERMATOPATHOLOGY Occlusion of arterioles with fibrin thrombi and a dense polymorphonuclear infiltrate around the infarct with massive hemorrhage.
HEMATOLOGIC STUDIES *CBC:* schistocytes (fragmented RBCs) arising from RBC entrapment and damage within fibrin thrombi, seen on blood smear; thrombocytopenia. *Coagulation studies:* reduced plasma fibrinogen; elevated fibrin degradation products (D-dimer and FDPs); prolonged PT, PTT, and thrombin time.

COURSE AND PROGNOSIS

The mortality rate from DIC is high. Surviving patients require skin grafts or amputation for gangrenous tissue. Common complications include severe bleeding, thrombosis, tissue ischemia and necrosis, hemolysis, organ failure. Mortality without therapy is 90% and occurs within 48 to 72 hours. Prompt therapy can improve the prognosis and reduce mortality to as low as 18%.

MANAGEMENT

Treatment of DIC requires prompt recognition and appropriate antibiotics for management of underlying infections, clotting factor and platelet replacement, vitamin K replacement, and supportive care. Mortality ranges from 40% to 80%.

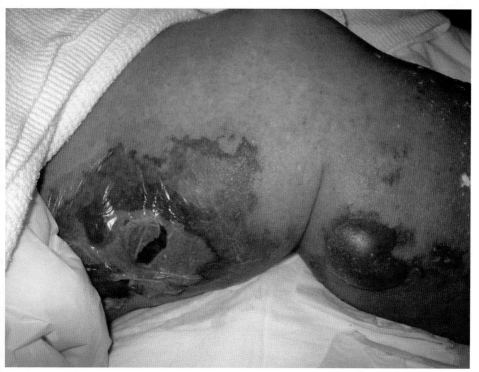

FIGURE 15-23 Disseminated intravascular coagulation, purpura fulminans Geographic and net-like areas infarction on the thigh and leg of a patient with *Pseudomonas aeruginosa* sepsis.

KAWASAKI DISEASE

KD is an acute febrile illness of infants and children, characterized by cutaneous and mucosal erythema and edema with subsequent desquamation and cervical lymphadenitis. With appropriate treatment, subsequent development of coronary artery aneurysms can be avoided.

INSIGHT The cutaneous manifestations of KD may be protean; in any child with fever for more than 5 days, this entity merits consideration.

SYNONYMS Mucocutaneous lymph node syndrome, juvenile polyarteritis nodosa.

EPIDEMIOLOGY

AGE Younger than 5 years (80%), peak incidence between ages 1 and 4 years.
GENDER M > F, 1.5:1.
RACE Japanese > other Asian ethnicity > African American > Hispanic > white children.
INCIDENCE 22 per 100,000 children under age 5 in the United States to 215 per 100,000 in Japan.
ETIOLOGY Unknown. Probably infectious with winter and spring epidemics.
GENETICS Possible genetic susceptibility, since it is much more prevalent in the Japanese population.

PATHOPHYSIOLOGY

KD is thought to be an immunologic disorder triggered by an infectious or toxic agent. This can lead to a generalized aneurysmal vasculitis.

HISTORY

Children present with fever >38.5°C for 5 days without infection plus four out of the following:

1. Bilateral conjunctival injection without exudate
2. Changes on lips and mouth (strawberry tongue, pharyngeal erythema, cheilitis)
3. Polymorphous generalized body rash
4. Hand/foot edema followed by desquamation, particularly periungually
5. Cervical LAD

Constitutional symptoms include diarrhea, arthralgias, arthritis, tympanitis, and photophobia.

PHYSICAL EXAMINATION

Skin Findings

TYPE Macules, papules, vesicles, desquamation (Fig. 15-24).
COLOR Pink, red.
DISTRIBUTION Lower abdomen, groin, perineum, buttocks, extremities, palms, soles (Fig. 15-25A).
MUCOUS MEMBRANES Hyperemic conjunctiva, red, dry fissured lips, injected pharynx, "strawberry" appearance to the tongue (Fig. 15-25B).

General Findings

FEVER LAD (80%) >1.5-cm cervical node.
MUSCULOSKELETAL Arthritis and arthralgias (knees, hips, elbows).
CARDIAC Pericardial tamponade, dysrhythmias, rubs, congestive heart failure, left ventricular dysfunction.
GI Diarrhea, vomiting, abdominal pain, jaundice, gallbladder swelling, paralytic ileus.
NEUROLOGIC Meningeal irritation, convulsions, facial palsy, paralysis of the extremities.
OTHER Cough, rhinorrhea, poor oral intake, irritability/lethargy, pyuria.

DIFFERENTIAL DIAGNOSIS

The differential diagnosis of KD includes scarlet fever, SJS, measles, juvenile rheumatoid arthritis, infectious mononucleosis, viral exanthems, leptospirosis, Rocky Mountain spotted fever, toxic shock syndrome, SSSS, EM, serum sickness, SLE, and Reiter's syndrome.

LABORATORY EXAMINATIONS

HISTOLOGY Nonspecific, perivascular infiltrates, edema, dilation of small vessels.
HEMATOLOGY Leukocytosis with left shift, anemia, thrombocytosis, elevated ESR, increased LFTs.
URINALYSIS Proteinuria, leukocytes.
ECHOCARDIOGRAPHY Pericardial effusions, coronary aneurysms.

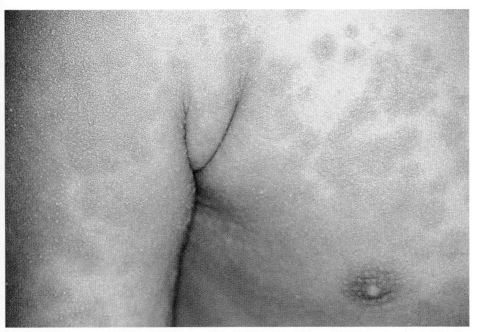

FIGURE 15-24 Kawasaki disease Blotchy erythema on the trunk of a child with Kawasaki disease. (Reproduced with permission from TB Fitzpatrick et al., *Color Atlas and Synopsis of Clinical Dermatology.* 4th ed. New York, McGraw-Hill; 2001.)

COURSE AND PROGNOSIS

The acute episode of KD self-resolves in the majority of children with no sequelae. In absence of treatment, 20% of patients will go on to develop cardiovascular complications; coronary artery aneurysms can occur 2 to 8 weeks after febrile episode. This can result in myocarditis, myocardial ischemia and infarction, pericarditis, peripheral vascular occlusion, small bowel obstruction, and stroke. Mortality rate is 1%.

MANAGEMENT

Treatment is directed at prevention of the cardiovascular complications and includes high-dose aspirin during the febrile period and high-dose IVIg. The combination of these agents has been shown in randomized controlled trials to decrease the risk of coronary artery complications. Systemic steroids may have a role in those refractory to initial management with IVIg. Due to rare instances of disease recurrence, individuals should be closely monitored by caregivers for episodes of fever or other symptoms following KD resolution.

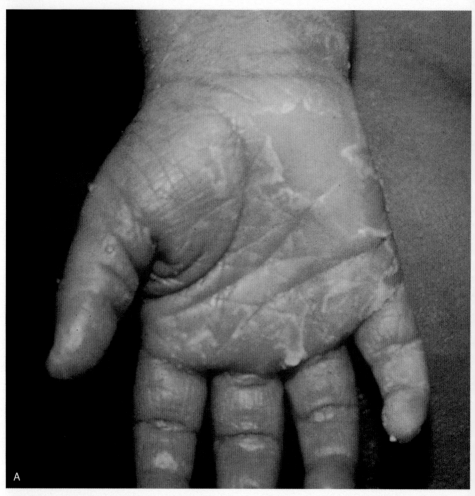

A

FIGURE 15-25 Kawasaki disease A: Palmar desquamation on the hands of a child with Kawasaki disease.

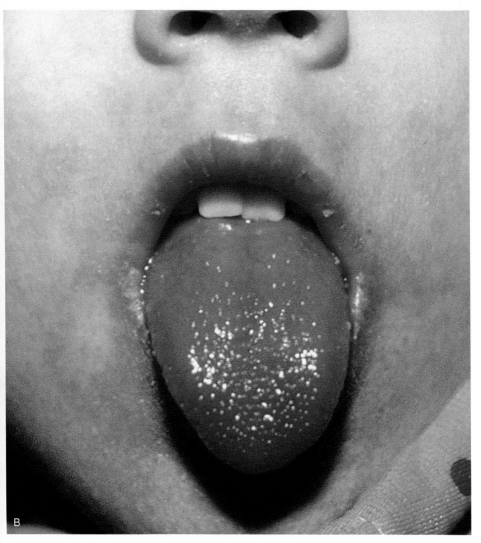

FIGURE 15-25 (*Continued*) **B:** Red "strawberry tongue" and perioral erythema in the same child.

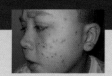

PHOTOSENSITIVITY AND PHOTOREACTIONS

PHOTOSENSITIVITY: IMPORTANT REACTIONS TO LIGHT

The term photosensitivity describes an abnormal response to light, usually referring to ultraviolet radiation (UVR). The two broad types of acute photosensitivity include the following:

1. A *sunburn* type response with the development of morphologic skin changes simulating a normal sunburn—erythema, edema, vesicles, and bullae—as seen in porphyria cutanea tarda and phytophotodermatitis.
2. A *rash* response to light exposure with development of varied morphologic expressions—macules, papules, plaques, eczematous dermatitis, urticaria—as seen in polymorphous light eruption (PMLE), solar urticaria, and eczematous drug reactions to sulfonamides.

The skin response to light exposure is strictly limited to the areas that have been exposed, and sharp borders are usually noted.

It should be noted that *sparing* of certain skin areas may provide the clue to photosensitivity—the upper eyelids (which are obscured when the eyes are open normally), the skin on the upper lip and under the chin (submental area), a triangle behind the ears, the skin under a watchband, the area covered by a bathing suit, and the skin in body creases on the back and sides of the neck or abdomen.

ACUTE SUN DAMAGE (SUNBURN)

A sunburn is an acute, delayed, and transient erythema of the skin following exposure to UVR emitted from sunlight or artificial sources. Sunburn is characterized by erythema and, if severe, by vesicles and bullae, edema, tenderness, and pain.

CLASSIFICATION

UVR sunburns can be divided into UVB (290–320 nm) erythema, which develops in 12 to 24 hours and fades within 72 to 120 hours, and UVA (320–400 nm) erythema, which peaks between 4 and 16 hours and fades within 48 to 120 hours.

EPIDEMIOLOGY

AGE All ages. Infants have an increased susceptibility.
GENDER M = F.
PHOTOTYPES Most frequently seen in skin phototypes (SPT) I, II, and III (Table 16-1).
RACE Caucasian > Asian, American Indian > Black. Individuals with light skin, blue eyes, and blond/red hair are at greatest risk of sunburn.
ETIOLOGY Overexposure to UVB (290–320 nm) leads to erythema and edema. The skin reaction can be augmented by photosensitization drugs or chemicals (psoralens, sulfonamides, tetracyclines, doxycycline, etc.). The intensity of UVR is augmented by reflective surfaces (snow, sand, water), altitude, and latitudes near the equator. UVB is most intense during the midday hours of 10 AM to 4 PM.
GENETICS SPTs are genetically determined.

PATHOPHYSIOLOGY

Sunburn-induced erythema and edema are mediated by prostaglandins, nitric oxide, histamine, and arachidonic acid. Systemic symptoms are mediated primarily by interleukins and other proinflammatory cytokines.

HISTORY

Mild reactions to sunlight begin 6 to 12 hours after the onset of exposure, peak at 24 hours, and fade within 3 to 5 days. Sunburns have a similar time course with blister formation on day 2 and desquamation on resolution. The skin usually is pruritic, painful, and warm to touch. Severe sunburn over large surfaces creates fever, chills, malaise, and even prostration.

TABLE 16-1 Fitzpatrick Classification of Skin Phototypes

Skin Phototype	Reactivity to UVR	Phenotype Examples
I	Almost always sunburns, never tans	White skin, blond hair, blue or brown eyes, freckles
II	Usually sunburns, tans with difficulty	White skin; red, blond, or brown hair, blue, hazel or brown eyes
III	Sometimes sunburns, can tan gradually	White skin, any color hair, any color eyes
IV	Occasional sunburns, tans easily	White or brown skin, dark hair, dark eyes
V	Rarely sunburns, tans well	Brown skin, dark hair, dark eyes
VI	Almost never sunburns, tans well	Dark brown or black skin, dark hair, dark eyes

PHYSICAL EXAMINATION

Skin Findings

TYPE OF LESION Macules, plaques, vesicles, and bullae (Fig. 16-1).
COLOR Bright red.
PALPATION Edematous areas are raised and tender.
DISTRIBUTION Confined to areas of exposure (rarely in covered areas, depending on the degree of exposure and the SPT of the person).

General Findings

SEVERE CASES "Toxic" appearance: Fever, weakness, tachycardia may be present.

LABORATORY EXAMINATIONS

DERMATOPATHOLOGY Necrotic keratinocytes ("sunburn cells") in the epidermis with exocytosis of lymphocytes and vacuolization of melanocytes and Langerhans cells. In the dermis, there is vascular dilation, perivascular edema, and perivascular inflammation.

DIFFERENTIAL DIAGNOSIS

Sunburns are a normal reaction of the skin to UV radiation overexposure, but airborne contact dermatitis, other photoreactions, lupus erythematosus (LE), and medication-induced photosensitivity should also be considered. Early in life, the initial presentations of photo-sensitivity disorders such as porphyria cutanea tarda or xeroderma pigmentosum may present with a sunburned appearance.

COURSE AND PROGNOSIS

Sunburns self-resolve over 2 to 4 weeks and scarring rarely results. Rarely, permanent hypomelanosis due to the destruction of melanocytes may occur.

MANAGEMENT

Photoprotection from UVA and UVB is helpful. Symptomatic treatment includes cold compresses, colloidal oatmeal baths, calamine lotion, aloe-based moisturizers, emollients (hydrated petrolatum, Vaseline), topical steroids, NSAIDs, and antihistamines. Severe cases may require systemic steroids (prednisone or methylprednisolone).

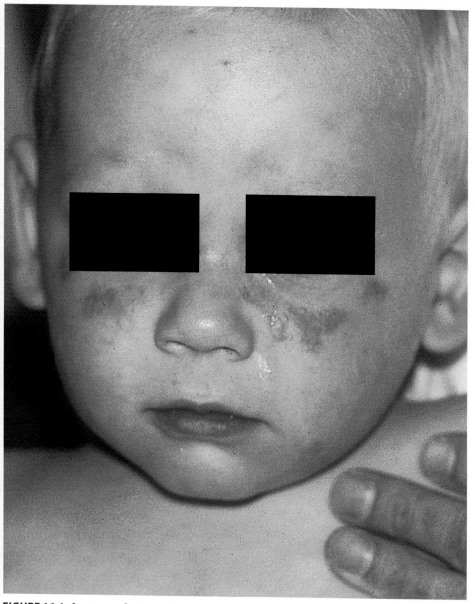

FIGURE 16-1 Acute sun damage Blistering plaques in the cheeks of a child after extended sunlight exposure.

SOLAR URTICARIA

Solar urticaria is a distinctive reaction pattern of wheals that develops within minutes after exposure to sunlight or artificial UVR and disappears within 24 hours.

EPIDEMIOLOGY

AGE Any age. More common between 30 and 50 years.
GENDER F > M, 3:1.
INCIDENCE 3/100,000.
ETIOLOGY Most likely type 1, IgE-mediated hypersensitivity reaction directed against a specific photoallergen in susceptible individuals.

PATHOPHYSIOLOGY

Solar urticaria may be induced by several different mechanisms. Some patients with solar urticaria have an inborn error of protoporphyrin metabolism. Others demonstrate passive transfer and reverse passive transfer tests supporting an allergic mechanism. For many, the mechanism is still unknown.

HISTORY

In solar urticaria, the patient experiences itching and burning that occurs within a few minutes of exposure to sunlight. Soon after, erythema and wheals appear only in the sites of exposure. The wheals disappear within several hours. Severe attacks can be associated with an anaphylactic-like reaction with nausea, headache, bronchospasm, and syncope.

PHYSICAL EXAMINATION

Skin Findings

TYPE Urticarial wheals (Fig. 16-2).
COLOR Pink, red.
DISTRIBUTION Routinely covered areas (arms, legs, and trunk) > chronically exposed areas (face and dorsa of the hands) due to skin "hardening" in areas of chronic exposure.

LABORATORY EXAMINATIONS

DERMATOPATHOLOGY Mild nonspecific changes: vascular dilatation, dermal edema, and peri-Vascular inflammation.
PHOTOTESTING Phototesting is helpful in discovering the wavelengths involved, and can aid in the management of the disorder. Solar urticaria has been classified into several types depending on the action spectrum that elicits the eruption: UVB, UVA, and visible light, or a combination of these.

DIFFERENTIAL DIAGNOSIS

Solar urticaria can be confused with PMLE, photoallergic drug reactions, or other urticarias.

COURSE AND PROGNOSIS

Solar urticaria typically undergoes spontaneous remission. Fifteen percent of patients are symptom-free after 5 years and 25% of patients are symptom-free after 10 years. Most individuals report some improvement in their symptoms over time even if complete resolution does not occur.

MANAGEMENT

Photoprotection with sun blocks and sun avoidance is helpful. Symptomatic treatment includes antihistamines (diphenhydramine, hydroxyzine, cetirizine). For severe or refractory cases, systemic steroids, antimalarials, intravenous immunoglobulin (IVIG), cyclosporine, omalizumab, extracorporeal photopheresis, or plasmapheresis may be necessary. Desensitization can be attempted with the specific wavelength light treatments with or without psoralens to slowly increase UVR tolerance ("hardening").

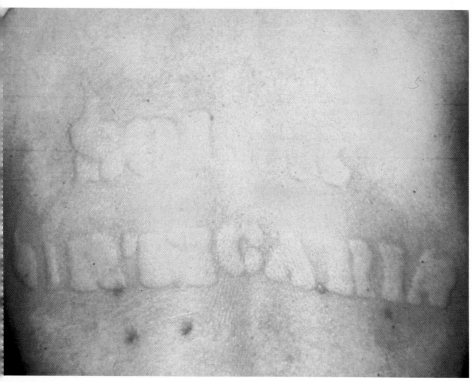

FIGURE 16-2 Solar urticaria Urticarial lesions on the back induced by solar irradiation 15 minutes prior. (Reproduced with permission from IM Freedberg et al., *Dermatology in General Medicine*. 5th ed. New York, NY: McGraw-Hill; 1999.)

POLYMORPHOUS LIGHT ERUPTION

PMLE is the most common type of photodermatosis characterized by monomorphous macules, papules, plaques, or vesicles within a few hours of sun exposure (UVB, UVA, and rarely, visible light).

 INSIGHT While PMLE can manifest differently between patients, an individual patient usually manifests with the same morphology after each exposure.

SYNONYMS Sun allergy, sun poisoning, benign summer light eruption, juvenile spring eruption.

EPIDEMIOLOGY

AGE Any age. Average age of onset: 20 to 30 years.
GENDER F > M.
INCIDENCE 22% in Scandinavia, 15% in the United States, 5% in Australia.
RACE All races.
GENETICS Up to 70% of the population has a tendency to develop PMLE, but with variable penetrance. Increased incidence of PMLE in twins and in individuals with a family history suggests an as-yet undetermined specific genetic susceptibility.

PATHOPHYSIOLOGY

The relation of the eruption to ultraviolet exposure is unknown. A delayed hypersensitivity reaction to an antigen induced by UVR is possible. UVA, UVB, and visible light have all been reported to trigger PMLE flares.

HISTORY

PMLE comes on suddenly, following minutes to days of sun exposure. The rash most often appears in vacationing persons with an acute intense exposure to sunlight. The rash appears within 18 to 24 hours after exposure and, once established, persists for 7 to 10 days, thereby limiting the vacationer's subsequent time spent outdoors. PMLE appears in spring or early summer, but will resolve by fall, suggesting a hardening response to UVR.

PHYSICAL EXAMINATION

Skin Findings

TYPE Papules, macules, vesicles, plaques (Fig. 16-3). In a given individual, one morphology tends to be dominant.

COLOR Pink to red.
SIZE 2 to 3 mm to >1 cm.
DISTRIBUTION Face (helices of ears), V of neck, outer arms, dorsal hands > covered areas (trunk).

General Findings

Fever, malaise, headache, nausea are rare. Pruritus may also be present.

LABORATORY EXAMINATIONS

DERMATOPATHOLOGY Skin biopsy shows epidermal edema, spongiosis, vesicle formation, and mild liquefaction degeneration of the basal layer, but no atrophy or thickening of the basement membrane. A dense lymphocytic infiltrate is present in the dermis, with edema and endothelial swelling.

DIFFERENTIAL DIAGNOSIS

PMLE can be difficult to distinguish from LE, solar urticaria, porphyrias, light-exacerbated atopic or seborrheic dermatoses, or erythema multiforme.

COURSE AND PROGNOSIS

The course is chronic and recurrent and may, in fact, worsen each season. Although some patients may develop "tolerance" by the end of the summer, the eruption usually recurs the following spring, and/or when they travel to tropical areas in the winter. However, spontaneous improvement or even cessation of eruptions can occur in 75% of patients after 30 years.

MANAGEMENT

To prevent PMLE, sunscreens and sun avoidance are recommended. Topical self-tanning products can help build a tan to prevent PMLE. In severe cases, phototherapy (narrowband UVB or PUVA), systemic β-carotene, antimalarials (hydroxychloroquine, chloroquine), azathioprine, or cyclosporine can be helpful.

After PMLE occurs, symptomatic relief may be obtained with topical steroids. In severe cases of PMLE, oral steroids (prednisone or methylprednisolone) may be necessary.

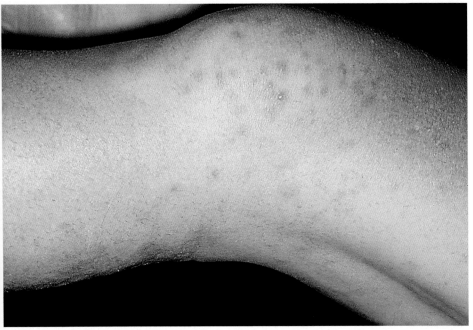

FIGURE 16-3 Polymorphous light eruption Scattered erythematous papules on the legs of a child 24 hours after sun exposure.

HYDROA VACCINIFORME

Hydroa vacciniforme (HV) is a chronic disease of childhood, of unknown etiology, characterized by recurrent vesicles on sun-exposed skin that heals with "vacciniform" scarring.

SYNONYM Bazin's HV.

EPIDEMIOLOGY

AGE 3 to 15 years.
GENDER M > F.
INCIDENCE 0.3/100,000.
RACE Caucasians, Asians > darker skin types.
GENETICS Rare familial cases reported.
ETIOLOGY Unknown.

PATHOPHYSIOLOGY

The pathogenetic mechanism for HV is unknown, and it may be a more severe scarring form of PMLE. Epstein–Barr virus has been detected in some patients. Summer UVA exposure is causal.

HISTORY

Burning, itching, stinging macules, and papules occur on sun-exposed sites 30 minutes to 2 hours after sun exposure. The papules then progress to vesicles, which umbilicate and form hemorrhagic crusts. One to two weeks later, the crusts heal with vacciniform scars. Mild fever and malaise may accompany the rash.

PHYSICAL EXAMINATION

Skin Findings

TYPE Papules, vesicles, hemorrhagic crusts, scars (Fig. 16-4).
COLOR Pink, red, hyper- and hypopigmentation.
DISTRIBUTION Face, dorsa of hands.
NAILS Photoonycholysis.

General Findings

OCULAR Keratoconjunctivitis, corneal clouding, keratitis.
SKELETAL Bone/cartilage destruction in severe HV.

DIFFERENTIAL DIAGNOSIS

The differential diagnosis for HV includes varicella, porphyrias, PMLE, and LE. Rarely, HV-like lesions have been reported as a manifestation of EBV-associated lymphoproliferative disorders in individuals with accompanying lymphadenopathy and systemic symptoms.

LABORATORY EXAMINATIONS

DERMATOPATHOLOGY Epidermal vesicles and confluent epidermal necrosis with a dense perivascular, lymphocytic infiltrate.

COURSE AND PROGNOSIS

HV has a good prognosis and typically self-resolves during adolescence. Patients are most affected by the scarring.

MANAGEMENT

There is no specific treatment for HV, and the disease self-resolves with age. Management includes sun avoidance, regular use of sunscreens, and sun-protective clothing. For severe HV, phototherapy (BB-UVB, NB-UVB, or PUVA), systemic antimalarials, β-carotene, thalidomide, azathioprine, cyclosporine, or fish oil supplementation may be helpful.

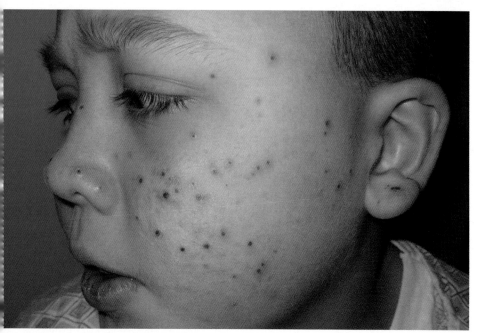

FIGURE 16-4 Hydroa vacciniforme Scarred lesions on the bilateral cheeks of a child with hydroa vacciniforme.

PHYTOPHOTODERMATITIS

Phytophotodermatitis is a streaky hyperpigmentation of the skin caused by contact with certain (furocoumarin-containing) plants and concomitant exposure to sunlight.

SYNONYMS Plant-induced photosensitivity, berloque dermatitis, Berlock dermatitis.

EPIDEMIOLOGY

AGE Any age.
GENDER M = F.
INCIDENCE Common.
ETIOLOGY Furocoumarin compounds in specific plants (parsley, celery, parsnips, lime, lemon, fig, mango, carrots, dill, meadow grass) get onto (topically) or into (by ingestion) the skin. Subsequent sunlight exposure results in photosensitive dermatitis.

HISTORY

The child usually gives a history of playing in grassy meadows or beach grass, making lemonade or limeade, followed the next day by the appearance of a streaky, erythematous (sometimes blistering) pattern leaving a residual hyperpigmentation.

PHYSICAL EXAMINATION

Skin Findings

TYPE Macules, vesicles, bullae.
SHAPE Bizarre streaks, artificial patterns that indicate an "outside job" (Fig. 16-5).
DISTRIBUTION Areas of contact: arms, legs, and face.

DIFFERENTIAL DIAGNOSIS

Phytophotodermatitis can sometimes be mistaken for child abuse with the linear hyperpigmented streaks of pigment being mistaken for resolving bruises.

COURSE AND PROGNOSIS

Most episodes of phytophotodermatitis fade spontaneously, but the pigmentation may last for weeks.

MANAGEMENT

Phytophotodermatitis is best managed by identifying and avoiding furocoumarin-containing culprits in the sun. For symptomatic relief of acute lesions, a short course of topical steroids or cooling moisturizers such as calamine or aloe may be useful. The postinflammatory hyperpigmentation will gradually fade over a period of weeks to months.

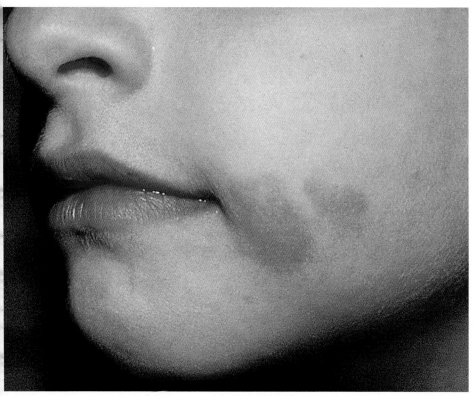

FIGURE 16-5 Phytophotodermatitis Hyperpigmentation around the mouth after exposure to limes and sunlight.

DRUG-INDUCED PHOTOSENSITIVITY

Drug-induced photosensitivity describes an adverse reaction of the skin that results from simultaneous exposure to certain drugs (via ingestion, injection, or topical application; Tables 16-2 and 16-3) and UVR or visible light. The chemicals may be therapeutic, cosmetic, industrial, or agricultural. There are two types of reaction: (1) phototoxic, which can occur in all individuals and is essentially an exaggerated sunburn response (erythema, edema, vesicles, etc.) and (2) photoallergic, which involves an immunologic response in a susceptible individual with a resultant rash.

TABLE 16-2 Drugs That Cause Phototoxicity and Photoallergy

Phototoxic Drugs	Photoallergic Drugs (Topical)	Photoallergic Drugs (Systemic)
Antiarrhythmics	Sunscreens	Antiarrhythmics
Amiodarone	Avobenzone	Quinidine
Quinidine	Benzophenones	Antimicrobials
Antimicrobials	PABA	Quinolones
Voriconazole	Fragrances	Sulfonamides
Doxycycline	Musk umbrette	Griseofulvin
Demeclocycline	Bergamot oil	Quinine
Ciprofloxacin	Oil of citron, lavender, lime	NSAIDs
Lomefloxacin	Sandalwood oil	Ketoprofen
Naladixic acid	Antimicrobials	Piroxicam
Sparfloxacin	Bithionol	
Diuretics	Chlorhexidine	
Furosemide	Fenticlor	
Thiazides	Hexachlorophene	
Antipsychotic drugs		
Chlorpromazine		
Prochlorperazine		
Psoralens		
5-methylpsoralen		
8-methylpsoralen		
4,5´,8-trimethylpsoralen		
NSAIDs		
Nabumetone		
Naproxen		
Piroxicam		
Other		
St. John's wort		
Tar		

TABLE 16-3 Xeroderma Pigmentosum Molecular Defects

XP Group	Chromosome	Gene
XPA	9q22	*XPA* nucleotide excision repair
XPB	2q21	*ERCC3* Unwinds DNA helix 3′-5′
XPC	3p25.1	*XPC* damage recognition
XPD	19q13.2	*ERCC2* Unwinds DNA helix 5′-3′
XPE	11p12	*DDB2* nucleotide excision repair
XPF	16p13.3	*ERCC4* 5′-repair endonuclease
XPG	13q32–33	*ERCC5* 3′-repair endonuclease
XP variant	6p21	*Pol-η* DNA polymerase-η

PHOTOTOXIC DRUG REACTION

Phototoxic drug reaction is an exaggerated sunburn response that can occur in all individuals exposed to UVR-induced phototoxic agents from certain medications (Table 16-2).

EPIDEMIOLOGY

AGE Any age, more common in older children and adults.
GENDER M = F.
INCIDENCE Up to 15% of photodermatology referrals.

PATHOPHYSIOLOGY

Phototoxic reactions are caused by the formation of toxic photoproducts (free radicals, superoxide anions, hydroxyl radicals, singlet oxygen) that are cytotoxic to the host's nuclear DNA or cell membranes (plasma, lysosomal, mitochondrial, microsomal). The action spectrum is typically in the UVA range. It is not known why some individuals show phototoxic reactions to a particular drug and others do not.

HISTORY

Phototoxic drug reactions are an exaggerated sunburn response (erythema, edema, burning, bullae) that develops hours after exposure to the phototoxic agent and UVR. With drug and UVR withdrawal, the reaction resolves with desquamation and hyperpigmentation.

PHYSICAL EXAMINATION

Skin Findings

TYPE Macular erythema (Fig. 16-6), edema, vesicles, bullae.
DISTRIBUTION Confined exclusively to areas exposed to light.
NAILS Photoonycholysis can occur with certain drugs (e.g., psoralens, tetracyclines, fluoroquinolones, and some NSAIDs).

LABORATORY EXAMINATIONS

DERMATOPATHOLOGY Inflammation, necrotic keratinocytes (called "sunburn cells") in the epidermis, epidermal necrobiosis, and intraepidermal and subepidermal vesiculation.

DIFFERENTIAL DIAGNOSIS

The differential diagnosis for phototoxic reactions includes sunburn, other photoreactions, airborne contact dermatitis, LE, and porphyrias.

COURSE AND PROGNOSIS

Phototoxic drug reactions disappear following cessation of drug and/or UVR. To implicate a specific drug, phototesting can be done and will exhibit a decreased minimal erythema dose (MED) to UVA. This test is especially helpful if the patient is on multiple potentially phototoxic drugs.

MANAGEMENT

Identification and elimination of the causative agent is required. Symptomatic treatment includes cold compresses, colloidal oatmeal baths, emollients (hydrated petrolatum, Vaseline, mineral oil, moisturizers), topical steroids, analgesics (aspirin, ibuprofen), and antihistamines. Severe cases may require systemic steroids (prednisone or methylprednisolone). Photoprotection from UVA and UVB is also helpful.

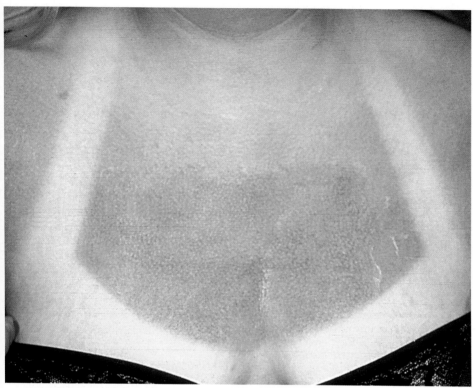

FIGURE 16-6 Phototoxic drug reaction Intense sun sensitivity induced by tetracycline in a young girl who subsequently went to a tanning booth despite precautions. (Slide used with permission from Dr. Lisa Cohen.)

PHOTOALLERGIC DRUG REACTION

Photoallergic drug reactions are a delayed hypersensitivity response after sensitization, incubation (7–10 days), and subsequent reexposure to the drug plus UVR in reactive individuals. Previous drug sensitization is necessary and photoallergy develops in only a small percentage of persons exposed to these drugs.

EPIDEMIOLOGY

AGE Any age, more common in adults.
GENDER M = F.
INCIDENCE Up to 8% of photodermatology referrals.

PATHOPHYSIOLOGY

Drug particles in the skin induce the formation of a photoproduct that conjugates with protein producing a photoallergen. The action spectrum involved is typically in the UVA range.

HISTORY

Topically applied photosensitizers are the most frequent cause of photoallergic eruptions. Sunscreen agents, antibacterial products, and fragrances account for the majority of photoallergens (Table 16-2). The causative agent may be more difficult to identify since the initial sensitization induces a delayed hypersensitivity reaction and the eruption occurs on subsequent exposures to the drug.

PHYSICAL EXAMINATION

Skin Findings

TYPE Plaques, flat-topped papules.
COLOR Pink, red, purple.
DISTRIBUTION OF LESIONS Areas exposed to light (Fig. 16-7) and adjacent nonexposed skin may also be involved.

LABORATORY EXAMINATIONS

DERMATOPATHOLOGY Skin biopsy shows epidermal spongiosis with lymphocytic infiltration.

DIFFERENTIAL DIAGNOSIS

The differential diagnosis for a photoallergic drug eruption includes sunburn, other photoreactions, airborne contact dermatitis, LE, and porphyrias.

COURSE AND PROGNOSIS

Photoallergic reactions can persist despite cessation of drugs and/or UVR. To implicate a specific chemical, photo patch testing can be done and the photoallergen will exhibit a decreased MED to UVA.

MANAGEMENT

Identification and elimination of the causative agent is required. Symptomatic treatment includes cold compresses, colloidal oatmeal baths, emollients (hydrated petrolatum, Vaseline, mineral oil, moisturizers), topical steroids, analgesics (aspirin, ibuprofen), and antihistamines. Severe cases may require systemic steroids (prednisone or methylprednisolone). Photoprotection from UVA and UVB is also helpful.

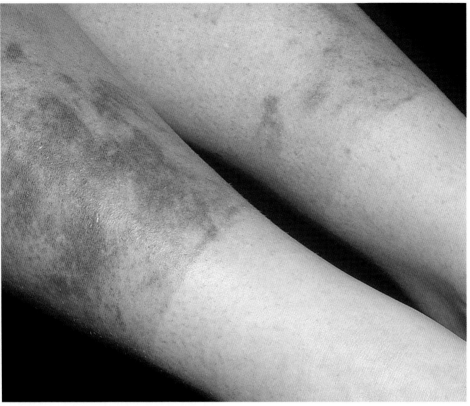

FIGURE 16-7 Photoallergic drug reaction Erythema and edema with sunlight exposure in a patient sensitized to oral sulfonamides. Note the marked cutoff between photoexposed and unexposed skin.

GENETIC DISORDERS WITH PHOTOSENSITIVITY

There are several inherited disorders with associated sensitivity or accelerated response to sun exposure. Most diseases are rare but need to be recognized at an early age so that preventative measures can be taken. These disorders can be divided into two groups:

1. Genetic disorders with prominent cutaneous malignancies:
   a. Xeroderma pigmentosum
   b. Basal cell nevus syndrome

2. Genetic disorders with prominent nonmalignant skin findings:
   a. Porphyrias (EPP being the most common pediatric form)
   b. Ataxia-telangiectasia
   c. Bloom syndrome
   d. Rothmund–Thomson syndrome

XERODERMA PIGMENTOSUM

XP is a rare autosomal recessive (AR) genodermatosis, characterized by enhanced cellular photosensitivity to UVR and early onset of cutaneous malignancies.

SYNONYM DeSanctis–Cacchione syndrome.

CLASSIFICATION

Seven complementation groups and an XP variant have been delineated (Table 16-3).

EPIDEMIOLOGY

AGE Infancy or early childhood.
GENDER M = F.
INCIDENCE 1:1,000,000 in the United States/Europe; 1:40,000 in Japan.
ETIOLOGY Defect in endonuclease—the enzyme that recognizes UV-damaged regions of DNA.
GENETICS AR; parents (obligate heterozygotes) are clinically normal.

PATHOPHYSIOLOGY

In XP, there are eight inherited forms (seven complementation groups A through G, plus a variant form; Table 16-3) each associated with a different site of impairment of genomic nucleotide excision repair. The variant form has a normal excision repair but has defective postrepair replication.

HISTORY

In approximately 50% of XP cases, there is a history of an acute sunburn reaction in infancy or early childhood with erythema that may persist for several days or weeks (in contrast to a normal sunburn, which disappears in a few days). The other patients appear to have normal sunburn reactivity. Freckle-like macules (lentigines) appear in almost all patients by age 2 (Fig. 16-8). Solar keratoses develop at an early age, and the epithelial skin cancers (basal cell or squamous cell) appear by age 8. The skin becomes dry and leathery, similar to a "farmer's skin," by the end of childhood. Most important are the series of malignancies that develop including melanoma, epithelial skin cancers, fibrosarcoma, and angiosarcoma. There is approximately a 2,000-fold increase in the frequency of basal cell carcinoma, squamous cell carcinoma, and cutaneous malignant melanoma in individuals with XP.

PHYSICAL EXAMINATION

Skin Findings

TYPES Macules, telangiectasias, nodules (BCCs, SCCs, Fig. 16-9).
COLOR Red, brown, dark brown, hypomelanotic.
DISTRIBUTION Sun-exposed areas (face, neck, forearms, and dorsa of arms, legs) > single layer of clothing areas (i.e., shirt) > double-covered areas (i.e., bathing trunk areas).
MUCOUS MEMBRANES Lips/mucous membrane telangiectasia; SCCs on the tip of the tongue.

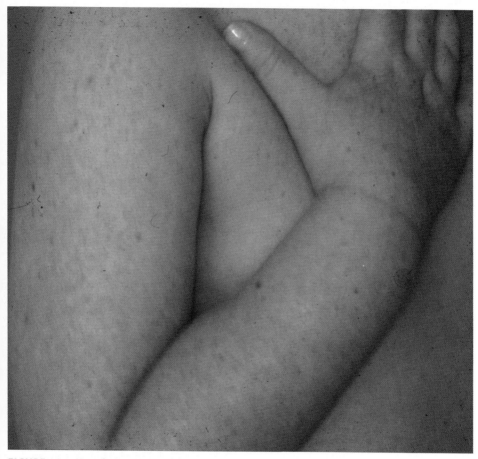

FIGURE 16-8 Xeroderma pigmentosum Diffuse lentigines on a 1-year-old with XP.

General Findings

OCULAR (40%) Photophobia, conjunctival injection, keratitis, corneal opacification, loss of eyelashes, ectropion, eyelid epithelial cancers/melanomas, blindness.
NEUROLOGIC (30%) Degeneration, mental retardation, spasticity, seizures, sensorineural deafness, diminished to absent deep tendon reflexes.
OTHER A 20-fold increase in brain sarcomas, leukemia, and lung and gastric carcinomas.

LABORATORY EXAMINATIONS

DERMATOPATHOLOGY Findings consistent with lentigines, solar damage, actinic keratoses, and basal cell and squamous cell carcinomas.
ELECTRON MICROSCOPY Abnormal melanocytes with changes in melanosomes, melanin macroglobules.

SPECIAL EXAMINATIONS

Cultured cells from XP patients exhibit a striking inhibition of growth following exposure to UVR, and cellular recovery is considerably delayed. Cell fusion studies permit a separation of the nucleotide excision repair deficient types into eight groups: XPA through XPG and a variant form.

DIFFERENTIAL DIAGNOSIS

Patients under age 10 years with severe freckling or multiple lentigines syndrome (LEOPARD syndrome) could be mistaken as having XP, but at this age, these patients do not have a history of acute photosensitivity, which is always present in XP, even in infancy.

COURSE AND PROGNOSIS

XP has a poor prognostic outcome. Metastatic melanoma or squamous cell carcinoma are the most frequent causes of death and more than 60% of patients die by age 20. Some patients with mild involvement, however, may live beyond middle age. Early diagnosis and careful protection from sun exposure may prolong life substantially.

MANAGEMENT

XP is a very serious disease requiring constant attention from the time it is first diagnosed, not only to prevent exposure to UVR but to closely monitor the patient for the detection of skin malignancies, especially melanoma. Rigorous sun protection involves wearing strong UVA/UVB sun blocks daily, protective hats, clothing, sunglasses with side shields, and avoiding the sun between the hours of 10 AM and 4 PM. Patients with XP need oral calcium and vitamin D supplements.

Destruction of actinic keratoses, basal cell and squamous cell carcinomas can be achieved with cryotherapy, electrodessication/curettage, surgical excision, topical 5-fluorouracil, topical imiquimod, or oral 13-*cis*-retinoic acid. Topical bacterial DNA repair enzyme T4 endonuclease V (T4N5) in a lipophilic vehicle has also been studied as a treatment in clinical trials.

Ophthalmologic care with methylcellulose eye drops and contact lenses are needed to protect the eyes from mechanical trauma in patients with deformed eyelids. Vision can be restored with corneal implants. Genetic counseling and prenatal diagnosis by amniocentesis (measuring UV-induced DNA damage in cultured amniotic fluid cells) and support groups are available to XP patients.

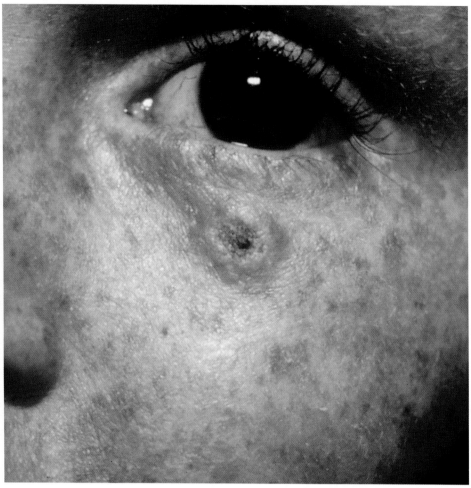

FIGURE 16-9 Xeroderma pigmentosum Large nodular basal cell carcinoma on the cheek of a child with XP.

BASAL CELL NEVUS SYNDROME

Basal cell nevus syndrome is an autosomal dominant (AD) disorder characterized by the childhood onset of multiple basal cell carcinomas and associated abnormalities of the bones, soft tissue, eyes, CNS, and endocrine organs. Diagnostic criteria for basal cell nevus syndrome are presented in Table 16-4.

SYNONYMS Nevoid basal cell carcinoma syndrome, multiple nevoid basal cell carcinoma syndrome, Gorlin syndrome, Gorlin–Goltz syndrome.

EPIDEMIOLOGY

AGE From 2 to 35 years; bony abnormalities are congenital.
GENDER M = F.
RACE Mostly Caucasian, but also occurs in blacks and Asians.
INCIDENCE Rare.
GENETICS AD, gene on chromosome 9q22.3–31.

PATHOPHYSIOLOGY

Basal cell nevus syndrome is caused by a mutation in the tumor suppressor gene *PTCH*. The *PTCH* gene encodes for a protein that binds and inhibits a transmembrane protein, SMO. Inhibition of SMO signaling is critical for tumor suppression. Thus, loss of PTCH function results in cancer formation.

HISTORY

Patients with basal cell nevus syndrome have a characteristic facies, with frontal bossing, broad nasal root, and hypertelorism. The basal cell epitheliomas begin to appear on exposed areas in childhood or early adolescence and continue to appear throughout life; there may be thousands of skin cancers. Basal cell nevus syndrome is often picked up by dentists or oral surgeons because of the mandibular bone cysts (odontogenic keratocysts of the jaw).

PHYSICAL EXAMINATION

Skin Findings

TYPE Papules, nodules (BCCs, Fig. 16-10A).
COLOR Flesh colored, brown.
SIZE 1 to 10 cm.
DISTRIBUTION Face, neck, trunk, axillae, usually sparing the scalp and extremities.
PALMOPLANTAR Palmar pits (50%).

General Findings

SKELETAL Mandibular jaw cysts, defective dentition, bifid or splayed ribs, pectus excavatum, short fourth metacarpals, scoliosis and kyphosis.

TABLE 16-4 Diagnostic Criteria for Basal Cell Nevus Syndrome

Major Diagnostic Criteria	>2 Basal cell carcinomas, or 1 BCC before age 20 Odontogenic keratocysts of the jaw ≥3 palmar or plantar pits Calcification of the falx cerebri Bifid, fused, or splayed ribs First-degree relative with Basal Cell Nevus Syndrome
Minor Diagnostic Criteria	Macrocephaly Cleft lip or palate, frontal bossing, coarse facies, or hypertelorism Skeletal deformities (pectus deformities or syndactyly) Vertebral anomalies or sella turcica bridging anomalies Ovarian fibroma Medulloblastoma

Clinical diagnosis is made by the presence of two major criteria or one major and two minor criteria.

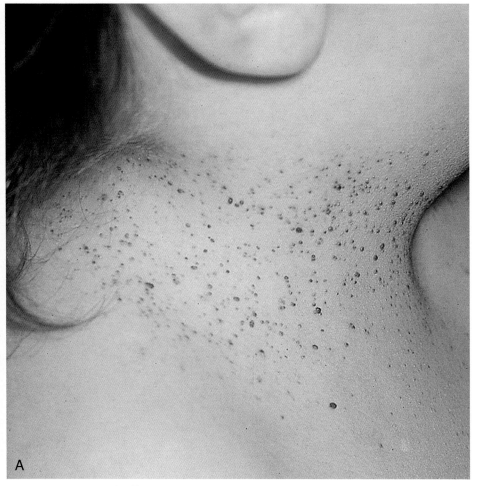

A

FIGURE 16-10 A: Basal cell nevus syndrome Numerous basal cell epitheliomas on the neck of a child. *(continued)*

OCULAR Strabismus, hypertelorism, dystopia canthorum, and congenital blindness.
CENTRAL NERVOUS SYSTEM Agenesis of the corpus callosum, medulloblastoma (Fig. 16-10B), mental retardation are rare. Calcification of the falx cerebri is often seen.
INTERNAL NEOPLASMS Fibrosarcoma of the jaw, ovarian fibromas, teratomas, and cystadenomas.

LABORATORY EXAMINATIONS

DERMATOPATHOLOGY Basal cell carcinomas: Solid, adenoid, cystic, keratotic, superficial, and fibrosing types.
IMAGING Lamellar calcification of the falx cerebri is seen.

DIFFERENTIAL DIAGNOSIS

Dermatologically, the multiple basal cell carcinomas may lead to confusion with XP.

COURSE AND PROGNOSIS

The prognosis for individuals with basal cell nevus syndrome is good. Those patients who develop medulloblastomas or aggressive deep epitheliomas are severely affected. The large number of skin cancers creates a lifetime problem of vigilance on the part of the patient and the physician. The multiple excisions can cause considerable scarring.

MANAGEMENT

Patients with basal cell nevus syndrome should be followed closely with regular skin examinations and counseled in sunscreen use and sun avoidance. Because of their propensity for enlargement, the basal cell epitheliomas should be treated with topical 5-FU, 5-aminolevulinic acid photodynamic therapy, electrodessication/curettage, surgical excision, cryotherapy, or topical imiquimod. Radiation should be avoided owing to patients' sensitivity to ionizing radiation. Vismodegib, a novel inhibitor of the SMO receptor, can be used for the management of large refractory basal cell carcinomas and may have a role in long-term maintenance use for individuals with basal cell nevus syndrome.

For infants and children, screening MRIs can be performed to rule out medulloblastoma and radiographs can be performed to detect skeletal and jaw anomalies. Odontogenic cysts, if detected, should be removed because they can deteriorate jawbones aggressively.

Genetic counseling and support groups are also helpful.

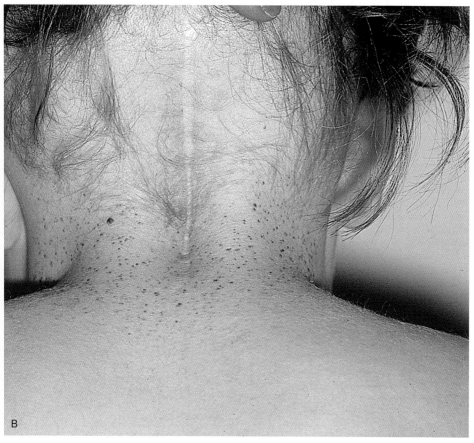

B

FIGURE 16-10 *(Continued)* **B: Basal cell nevus syndrome** Scar from surgical removal of a medulloblastoma on the same child.

ERYTHROPOIETIC PROTOPORPHYRIA

Erythropoietic protoporphyria (EPP) is the most common inherited metabolic disorder of heme biosynthesis. It is characterized by acute sunburn-like photosensitivity that begins in childhood.

SYNONYM Erythrohepatic protoporphyria.

EPIDEMIOLOGY

AGE 2 to 5 years.
GENDER M = F.
INCIDENCE 10/100,000 individuals.
GENETICS Affected individuals are usually compound heterozygotes, with one defect in chromosome 18q21.3 and one null copy of the gene; AD and X-linked cases are also reported.
ETIOLOGY Typically, an inherited gene mutation of ferrochelatase in one parent allele, with a specific intronic polymorphism (IVS3–48T/C) of the other parent allele leads to 25% decrease in ferrochelatase activity. X-linked cases are due to mutations in the delta-aminolevulinic acid synthase (ALAS2) gene.

PATHOPHYSIOLOGY

The specific enzyme defect typically occurs at the step in porphyrin metabolism in which protoporphyrin is converted to heme by the enzyme ferrochelatase. This leads to an accumulation of protoporphyrin, which absorbs 400 to 410 nm light intensely. The excited porphyrins create reactive oxygen molecules, which cause lipid peroxidation, clinically manifesting as edema and burning.

HISTORY

Stinging and itching may occur within a few minutes of sunlight exposure; erythema and edema appear after 1 to 8 hours. Affected children may choose to not go out in the direct sunlight after a few painful episodes. Symptoms may also occur when exposed to sunlight streaming through window glass or rarely when exposed to high intensity visible light.

PHYSICAL EXAMINATION

Skin Findings

TYPE Macules, plaques, edema, urticaria, vesicles, bullae, scarring (Fig. 16-11).
DISTRIBUTION Nose, dorsa of hands, tips of ears.

General Findings

HEMATOLOGIC Anemia with hypersplenism (rare).
GASTROINTESTINAL Cholelithiasis (protoporphyrin-containing stones), biliary colic, cholestasis, hepatic cirrhosis (10–15%), hepatic failure.

LABORATORY EXAMINATIONS

PORPHYRIN STUDIES Increased protoporphyrin in RBCs, plasma, and stools, but none excreted in the urine. Decreased activity of the enzyme ferrochelatase in the bone marrow, liver, and skin fibroblasts.
LIVER FUNCTION Abnormal LFTs. Liver biopsy has demonstrated portal and periportal fibrosis and deposits of brown pigment in hepatocytes and Kupffer cells; with electron microscopy, needle-like crystals have been observed. Hepatic failure caused by cirrhosis and portal hypertension.
FLUORESCENT ERYTHROCYTES RBCs in a blood smear exhibit a characteristic transient fluorescence when examined with a fluorescent microscope at 400 nm radiation.

DERMATOPATHOLOGY

SKIN BIOPSY Marked eosinophilic homogenization and thickening of the blood vessels in the papillary dermis and an accumulation of an amorphous, hyaline-like basophilic substance in and around blood vessels.
RADIOGRAPHY Gallstones may be present.

DIFFERENTIAL DIAGNOSIS

EPP must be differentiated from the other porphyrias that have deficiencies of other enzymes in the heme biosynthesis pathway. In EPP, there is photosensitivity but no rash, only an exaggerated sunburn response that appears much earlier than ordinary sunburn erythema. In addition, the skin changes can occur from UV that penetrates window glass. Finally, there are virtually no photosensitivity disorders in which the symptoms appear so rapidly (minutes) after exposure to sunlight. Porphyrin examination establishes the diagnosis with elevated free protoporphyrin levels in the RBCs and in the stool (but not urine, distinguishing it from the other more uncommon porphyrias). The fecal protoporphyrin is most consistently elevated.

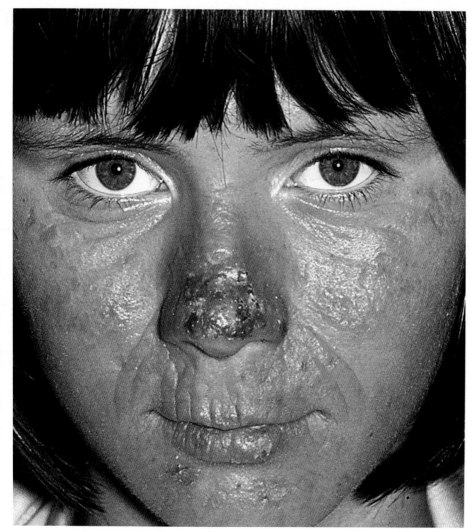

FIGURE 16-11 Erythropoietic protoporphyria Fifteen-year-old with deep wrinkling and waxy thickening of the upper lip and cheeks. (Reproduced with permission from TB Fitzpatrick et al., *Color Atlas and Synopsis of Clinical Dermatology*. 4th ed. New York, NY: McGraw-Hill; 2001.)

COURSE AND PROGNOSIS

EPP manifests in early childhood and persists throughout life, but the photosensitivity may become less apparent in late adulthood.

MANAGEMENT

Currently, there is no enzyme replacement, or gene therapy, for the basic metabolic abnormality in EPP. Management consists of early recognition, diagnosis, treatment with sunscreen (titanium and zinc oxide block 400 nm best), sun avoidance, and sun-protective clothing. Experimental trials of afamelanotide—a synthetic melanocyte stimulating hormone—are underway to increase skin pigmentation in EPP as a means of decreasing photosensitivity. Oral cysteine supplementation may help suppress the production of reactive oxygen species. Systemic β-carotene can ameliorate the photosensitivity but does not completely eliminate the problem. Nevertheless, many patients can participate in outdoor sports.

ATAXIA-TELANGIECTASIA

Ataxia-telangiectasia is a rare AR syndrome characterized by progressive cerebellar ataxia, oculocutaneous telangiectasias, recurrent respiratory tract infections, and an increased susceptibility to lymphoreticular malignancies.

SYNONYM Louis–Bar syndrome.

EPIDEMIOLOGY

AGE Telangiectasias: 3 to 5 years; ataxia may precede the skin findings.
GENDER M = F.
INCIDENCE Homozygotes > 1:40,000 births, gene frequency 1:100 (1% of the population are heterozygous trait carriers).
GENETICS AR, mapped to chromosome 11q22–23.

PATHOPHYSIOLOGY

Ataxia-telangiectasia is caused by a mutation in the *ATM* gene located on chromosome 11q22. ATM functions to respond to chromosomal strand breakage by phosphorylating the p53 protein, a tumor suppressor gene. Chromosomal instability is seen in the cells of patients with ataxia-telangiectasia as they lack appropriate function of this tumor suppressor.

HISTORY

Ataxia-telangiectasia patients initially present with ataxia shortly after learning to walk. The skin findings appear from ages 3 to 5 years with fine symmetric telangiectasias on the bulbar conjunctiva that subsequently involve the face, trunk, and extremities. With aging and continued sun exposure, the skin becomes sclerotic and acquires a mottled pattern of hypo- and hyperpigmentation.

PHYSICAL EXAMINATION

Skin Findings

TYPE Telangiectasias, sclerosis, follicular hyperkeratosis.
COLOR Red, brown, mottled hypo- and hyperpigmentation.
DISTRIBUTION Telangiectasia on the bulbar conjunctiva (Fig. 16-12A), eyelids, ears (Fig. 16-12B), malar areas, neck, V of chest, antecubital/popliteal fossa, dorsal aspects of hands and feet. Sclerodermatous changes on the face (sad mask-like facies), arms, and hands.
HAIR Diffuse graying, hirsutism of arms/legs (Fig. 16-13).
OTHER Diffuse dry skin, eczematous and seborrheic dermatitis.

General Findings

NEUROLOGIC Ataxia, clumsiness, intellectual deficit (30%), choreoathetosis, drooling, peculiar ocular movements, sad mask-like facies, stooped posture, drooping shoulders, head sunk/tilt, peripheral neuropathy, spinal muscular atrophy.
PULMONARY Pulmonary infection, rhinitis, bronchitis, pneumonias, and bronchiectasis (75–80%).
IMMUNOLOGIC Impaired humoral responses (IgA, IgE deficiency) and cell-mediated immunity (lymphopenia, impaired lymphocyte transformation). Structural anomalies of thymus and lymph nodes.
NEOPLASMS Lymphoreticular malignancy (Hodgkin lymphoma, lymphosarcoma, reticular cell sarcoma, leukemia), other neoplastic disorders (ovarian dysgerminoma, medulloblastoma, GI carcinoma) (15%).

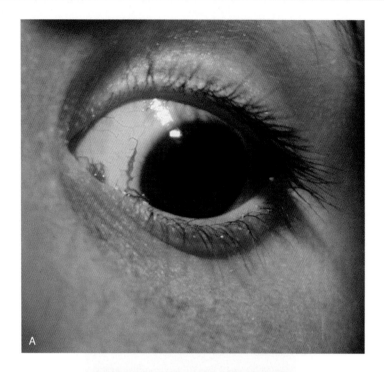

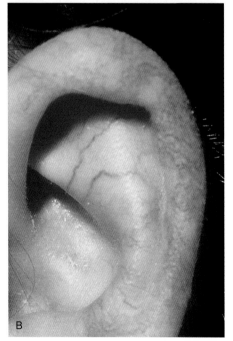

FIGURE 16-12 Ataxia-telangiectasia A: Telangiectasia on the bulbar conjunctiva. **B:** Telangiectasia on the ear of the same child.

DIFFERENTIAL DIAGNOSIS

Ataxia-telangiectasia may be confused with spider angiomas, angioma serpiginosum, hereditary hemorrhagic telangiectasia (Osler–Weber–Rendu disease), generalized essential telangiectasia, and telangiectasia macularis eruptiva perstans. Other ataxic disorders with which it may be confused include Friedrich's ataxia or an ataxic variant of cerebral palsy.

LABORATORY EXAMINATIONS

DERMATOPATHOLOGY Dilated blood vessels of the subpapillary plexus in telangiectatic areas. **SEROLOGY** Elevated levels of serum α-fetoprotein; very low levels of serum IgA. **CHEMISTRY** Glucose intolerance, elevated hepatic enzymes.

COURSE AND PROGNOSIS

Patients with ataxia-telangiectasia have a poor prognosis. Death usually occurs in late child-hood or early adolescence from bronchiectasis and respiratory failure secondary to recurrent sinopulmonary infections. Lymphoreticular malignancies occur in 15% of patients. Individuals who survive beyond adolescence develop severe neurologic morbidity, are confined to wheelchairs, and are unable to walk without assistance.

MANAGEMENT

Treatment for ataxia-telangiectasia is supportive. Antibiotics are used for infection, respiratory therapy is used for bronchiectasis, physical therapy is used for contractures, and sunscreens/sun avoidance minimize actinic damage. Genetic counseling is necessary and prenatal diagnosis is available (by the measurement of α-fetoprotein in amniotic fluid and by increased spontaneous chromosomal breakages of amniocytes).

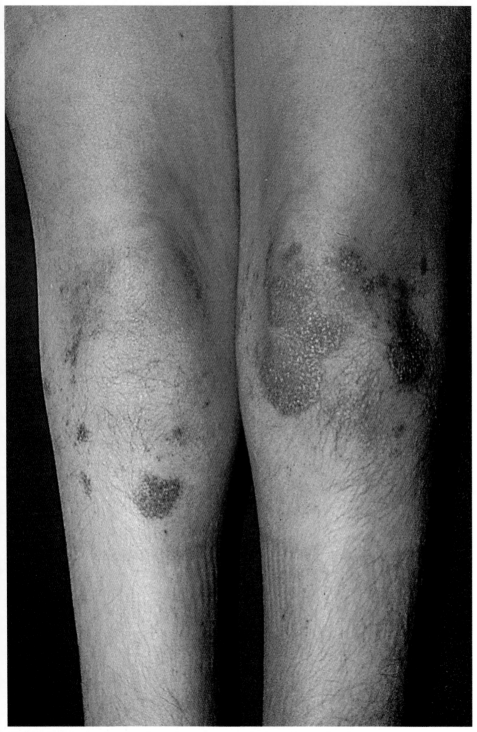

FIGURE 16-13 Ataxia-telangiectasia Hirsutism on the lower legs and ecchymoses secondary to ataxia and numerous falls.

BLOOM SYNDROME

Bloom syndrome is a rare AR disease characterized by photosensitivity, telangiectasias, and severe intrauterine and postnatal growth retardation.

SYNONYMS Congenital telangiectatic erythema; Bloom–Torre–Machacek syndrome.

EPIDEMIOLOGY

AGE 2 to 3 weeks of life.
GENDER M (80% of affected children) > F.
INCIDENCE Rare in general population. Gene mutation in up to 1% of Ashkenazi Jews, with 1/50,000 incidence in this population.
GENETICS AR mutation in the *BLM* gene.

PATHOPHYSIOLOGY

Bloom syndrome has been mapped to chromosome 15q26.1, and the *BLM* gene mutation impairs DNA helicase function. This results in an elevated frequency of chromosomal abnormalities and an increased rate of sister chromatid exchanges, chromosomal breakage, and rearrangements.

HISTORY

Affected infants are born at term with reduced body weight and size. In infancy, a facial rash becomes prominent after exposure to light. The photosensitivity gradually resolves but the erythema, telangiectasias, mottled pigmentation, and scarring persist. Systemic symptoms include an abnormal facies, growth retardation, respiratory and gastrointestinal (GI) tract infections, and sterility.

PHYSICAL EXAMINATION

Skin Findings

TYPE Macular erythema (Fig. 16-14), telangiectasia, bullae, scarring, café au lait macules (50%).
COLOR Red, red to brown, hyper- and hypopigmentation.
DISTRIBUTION Malar (nose, ears), dorsa of hands. Sparing trunk, buttocks, and lower extremities.

General Findings

ABNORMAL FACIES Narrow prominent nose, hypoplastic malar area, receding chin.
SKELETAL Dolichocephaly, polydactyly, clubbed feet.
OTHER Infections of the respiratory/GI tract, diabetes, neoplastic disease (leukemia, lymphoma, and GI adenocarcinoma). Normal intellectual and sexual development, but infertility is common.

DIFFERENTIAL DIAGNOSIS

The differential diagnosis for Bloom syndrome includes LE, Rothmund–Thomson syndrome, dyskeratosis congenita, hereditary acrokeratotic poikiloderma, Kindler's syndrome, Fanconi anemia, and XP.

LABORATORY EXAMINATIONS

DERMATOPATHOLOGY Skin biopsy reveals flattening of the epidermis, hydropic degeneration of the basal layer, and dilated capillaries in the upper dermis.
KARYOTYPE Increased chromatid exchange, chromosomal breakage and rearrangements.
IMMUNOLOGY Decreased IgA, IgM, IgG.

COURSE AND PROGNOSIS

Patients with Bloom syndrome have a shortened life span because of fatal respiratory or GI tract infections and neoplastic disease. Approximately 20% of patients will develop neoplasms, half of them before the age of 20 years. With increasing age, photosensitivity resolves and resistance to infection becomes more normal.

MANAGEMENT

There is no specific treatment for Bloom syndrome. Management includes sun avoidance, regular use of sunscreens and antibiotics for the management of patients with respiratory or GI infections. Patients with Bloom syndrome should also have symptomatic therapy, routine follow-up, and genetic counseling.

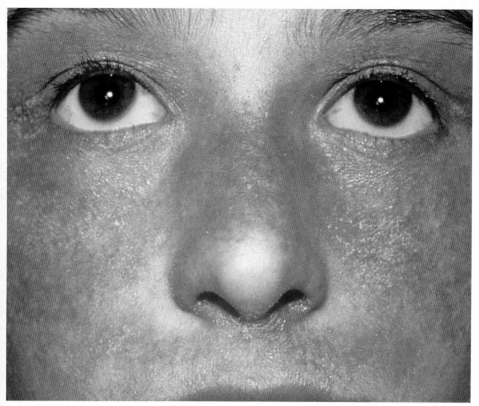

FIGURE 16-14 Bloom syndrome Facial erythema and desquamation after sun exposure in a patient with Bloom syndrome.

ROTHMUND–THOMSON SYNDROME

Rothmund–Thomson syndrome is a rare AR disorder characterized by photosensitivity, skin atrophy, mottled pigmentation, and telangiectasia, in association with juvenile cataracts, short stature, ectodermal changes, and hypogonadism.

SYNONYMS Hereditary poikiloderma congenitale, poikiloderma atrophicans.

EPIDEMIOLOGY

AGE Birth to 6 months old.
GENDER M > F, 2:1.
INCIDENCE Rare, 300 cases to date.
GENETICS AR inheritance.

PATHOPHYSIOLOGY

Rothmund–Thomson syndrome has been mapped to chromosome 8q24.3, the *RECQL4* gene. This gene encodes for the protein RECQL4 helicase, and mutations in the gene leads to dysfunctional DNA repair.

HISTORY

Skin changes are present at or by 6 months of age. One-third of patients have photosensitivity and exhibit bullae formation after UVR exposure. However, the poikiloderma changes of the skin are diffuse on both sun-exposed and unexposed skin. Systemically, patients characteristically have short stature, abnormal facies, amenorrhea in females, undescended testes in males, and blindness.

PHYSICAL EXAMINATION

Skin Findings

TYPE Macular erythema, telangiectasia (Fig. 16-15), bullae, vesicles, scarring.
COLOR Pink red, hyper- and hypopigmentation, poikiloderma.
DISTRIBUTION Cheeks (Fig. 16-16), chin, ears, forehead, extensor arms, legs, and buttocks. Verrucous hyperkeratoses on the hands, feet, knees, and elbows. Cutaneous squamous cell carcinomas (5%).
HAIR Partial/Total alopecia of scalp/eyebrows (50%). Sparse pubic/axillary hair. Premature graying of hair.
NAILS Rough, ridged, heaped-up, small, or atrophic.

General Findings

FACIES Triangular face, saddle nose, frontal bossing, wide forehead, narrow chin.
OCULAR Cataracts (75% onset before age 7 years).
SKELETAL Short stature, absence/hypoplasia/dysplasia of long bones, absence/shortening of digits, cleft hand/foot, asymmetric feet, osteoporosis, osteosarcoma (30%).
DENTAL Microdontia, failure of teeth to erupt.

DIFFERENTIAL DIAGNOSIS

Rothmund–Thomson syndrome must be differentiated from other photosensitive dermatoses, such as Bloom syndrome, dyskeratosis congenita, hereditary acrokeratotic poikiloderma, Kindler's syndrome, Fanconi anemia, and XP.

LABORATORY EXAMINATIONS

DERMATOPATHOLOGY Flattening and thinning of the epidermis, with basal layer vacuolization, pigment incontinence with melanophages, and sclerotic collagen in the papillary dermis with loss of dermal papillae.
RADIOLOGY X-ray of pelvic and long bones shows cystic spaces, osteoporosis, and sclerotic areas.

COURSE AND PROGNOSIS

Patients with Rothmund–Thomson syndrome have a normal life span and their photosensitivity decreases with age. Hyperkeratotic lesions of the extremities may transform into SCCs. There have also been multiple case reports of osteosarcoma in Rothmund–Thomson patients.

MANAGEMENT

There is no specific treatment for Rothmund–Thomson syndrome. Preventive measures include sunscreen use, sun avoidance, routine dermatologic examinations for precancerous keratoses/skin cancers, and genetic counseling.

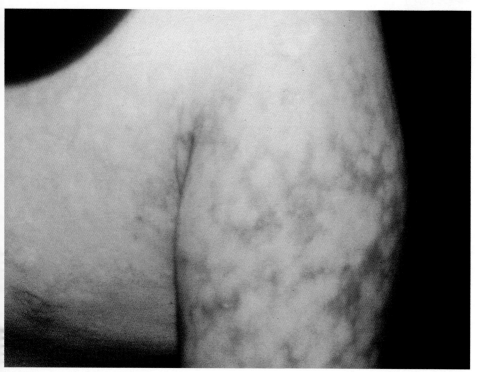

FIGURE 16-15 Rothmund–Thomson syndrome Reticulated pattern of telangiectasia on the arm of a child.

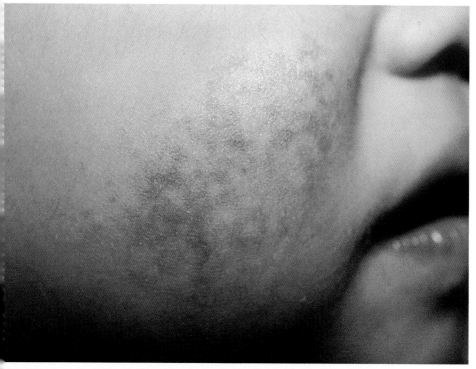

FIGURE 16-16 Rothmund–Thomson syndrome Erythema and poikiloderma on the cheek of a child.

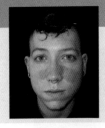

AUTOIMMUNE CONNECTIVE TISSUE DISEASES

JUVENILE RHEUMATOID ARTHRITIS

Juvenile rheumatoid arthritis (JRA) is a generalized systemic disease of unknown etiology characterized by a transient macular, papular, or urticarial rash and ensuing fever, lymphadenopathy (LAD), hepatosplenomegaly (HSM), anemia, and arthralgia.

INSIGHT There are four classical evanescent eruptions: (1) urticaria, (2) erythema marginatum (of acute rheumatic fever), (3) the rash of Still's disease, and (4) serum sickness.

CLASSIFICATION

JRA has three major types:

1. Systemic onset (15%): Still's disease, fevers, rash, LAD, HSM, serositis, polyarthritis
2. Polyarticular (35%): Five or more joints: hands, feet > knees/wrists/ankles
3. Oligo-/Pauciarticular (50%): Four or fewer joints: knees > ankles

SYNONYMS Still's disease, juvenile idiopathic arthritis, juvenile chronic arthritis.

EPIDEMIOLOGY

AGE Peaks: 1 to 4 years; adolescence.
GENDER Systemic JRA: M = F. Others: F > M, 2:1.
PREVALENCE 1/1,000.
GENETICS Polymorphisms for the genes encoding tumor necrosis factor-α (TNF-α), migratory inhibitory factor, interleukin-6 (IL-6), interleukin-10 (IL-10), and TAP genes (transporter of antigenic peptides) have been detected in this patient population. Several HLA alleles have also been associated with the subtypes of JRA, with the strongest genetic associations seen in early-onset pauciarticular JRA.
ETIOLOGY Unknown.

PATHOPHYSIOLOGY

Cytokines TNF-α, migratory inhibitory factor, and IL-6 parallel the fever spikes, but the pathogenesis of JRA is still not understood.

JRA tends to be precipitated by emotional, infectious, or surgical stress.

HISTORY

The onset of JRA may be sudden or insidious, depending on the age of the patient (the younger the patient, the more severe the systemic manifestations on average). Cutaneous eruptions occur in 90% of patients and may be the initial presentation. The rash of JRA is evanescent and can be macular or urticarial. Systemically, there may be associated fever, adenopathy, splenomegaly, anemia, and arthralgias.

PHYSICAL EXAMINATION

Skin Findings

TYPE Macules, papules, urticarial plaques (Fig. 17-1).
SIZE 2–6 mm to 8–9 cm.
COLOR Salmon pink to red, with a zone of pallor (Fig. 17-2).
DISTRIBUTION Areas of trauma/heat: axilla, waist, olecranon process/ulnar forearm, dorsal hands, knees, ears, scapula, sacrum, buttocks, and heels.
OTHER Palms and soles: thenar and hypothenar eminences may be erythematous. Periungual telangiectasias (5% of patients). Spindling fingers (50%, spindle-shaped deformity of fingers because proximal interphalangeal involvement > distal interphalangeal involvement).
GENERAL FINDINGS Fever > 38.98°C, LAD, HSM.
MUSCULOSKELETAL Arthralgias/arthritis: single joint (knees > ankles/hips > hands), symmetric polyarthritis joints, motion limitation (knees: 90%, fingers: 75%, wrists/ankles: 66%); dactylitis (sausage-appearing swollen digits).
SEROSITIS Pericarditis, pleuritis, or peritonitis.
OTHER Myocarditis, uveitis, CNS involvement.

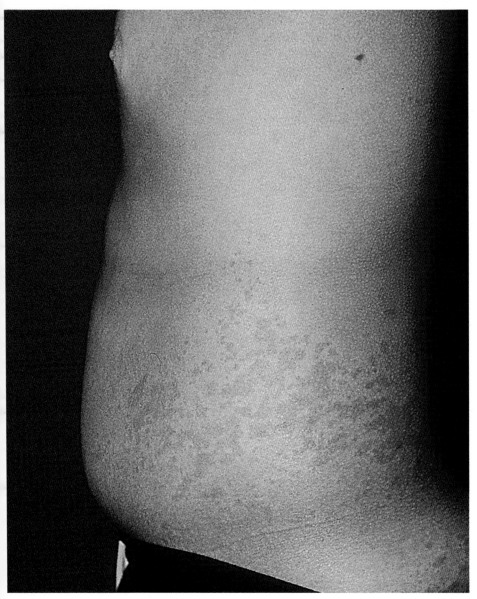

FIGURE 17-1 Juvenile rheumatoid arthritis Transient macular rash on the body characteristic of juvenile rheumatoid arthritis.

DIFFERENTIAL DIAGNOSIS

The diagnosis of JRA is made based on clinical characteristics and history of arthritis lasting for more than 6 weeks, with appropriate studies to exclude other causes such as other autoimmune diseases, other causes of periodic fever, urticaria, rheumatic fever, hypersensitivity reactions, systemic lupus erythematosus (SLE), granuloma annulare, sarcoid, and other granulomatous diseases.

LABORATORY EXAMINATIONS

DERMATOPATHOLOGY Edematous collagen fibers, perivascular infiltrate with neutrophils, plasma cells, and histiocytes.

HEMATOLOGY Leukocytosis, anemia, positive rheumatoid factor (80%), elevated erythrocyte sedimentation rate (ESR), low titer ANA positivity, hypoalbuminemia, hyperglobulinemia.

RADIOLOGY Joint destruction in late disease.

COURSE AND PROGNOSIS

The course and prognosis of JRA are variable. The younger the age of onset, the more prominent the systemic manifestations. The rash typically precedes the systemic symptoms by up to 3 years. The disease may end after a few months and never recur, or it may recur after months or years of remission. The disease typically improves by puberty and 85% of patients achieve remission; early treatment may expedite resolution and minimize long-term sequelae. Only 10% have residual severe crippling arthritis which may be associated with a positive rheumatoid factor.

MANAGEMENT

For active disease, symptoms can be relieved with aspirin, nonsteroidal anti-inflammatory drugs (NSAIDs, such as indomethacin or naproxen), hydroxychloroquine, and systemic steroids. Anti-TNF drugs (infliximab, etanercept, and adalimumab) have been used, but are less helpful in systemic-onset JRA. For severe cases that are resistant to other therapies, or have crippling deformities, iridocyclitis, or vasculitis, systemic corticosteroids, methotrexate, azathioprine, leflunomide, mycophenolate mofetil, chlorambucil, thalidomide, intravenous immunoglobulin, cyclophosphamide, IL-1/IL-6 receptor antagonists (anakinra, tocilizumab) have been used. For structural correction of severe deformities, surgery is a last resort.

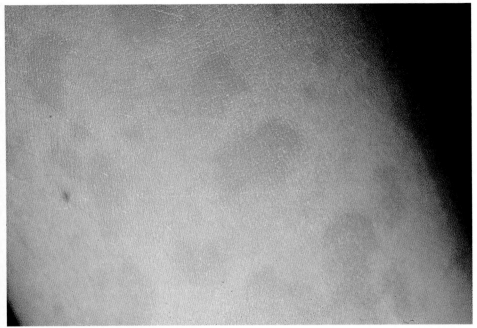

FIGURE 17-2 Juvenile rheumatoid arthritis Faint erythematous, urticarial plaques on the torso of a child.

ACUTE CUTANEOUS LUPUS ERYTHEMATOSUS

Acute cutaneous lupus erythematosus (ACLE) is the most common cutaneous presentation associated with SLE (Table 17-1). SLE is a serious multisystem disease involving connective tissue and blood vessels; the clinical manifestations include fever (90%); skin lesions (85%); arthritis; and renal, cardiac, and pulmonary disease.

 INSIGHT While any organ system may be affected by systemic lupus, the presence of cutaneous lupus erythematosus does not automatically indicate internal organ involvement.

EPIDEMIOLOGY

AGE 25% younger than 20 years, peaks: 11 to 13 years, 30 to 40 years.
GENDER Prepubertal: F > M for all ages.
INCIDENCE Prepubertal: rare; adults: 4 in 1,000.
RACE African American, Asian, Latin American >> Caucasian.
GENETICS Family history (<5%) suggests a hereditary component, though environmental factors are believed to play a strong role.

PATHOPHYSIOLOGY

SLE is antibody-mediated, and the trigger for autoantibody production may be multifactorial (genetics, viral or bacterial infection, host tissue response/susceptibility). The production of autoantibodies generates immune complexes targeting body tissues and results in host injury that is non-organ specific, and may differ from person to person.

HISTORY

Up to 80% of patients with SLE have ACLE (malar rash, discoid lesions, photosensitivity, or atrophy), and in 25% of patients, the skin is the first presenting symptom.

PHYSICAL EXAMINATION

Skin Findings

TYPE Macules, scale, erosions, atrophic plaques.
COLOR Pink, red, hypo- or hyperpigmentation.
SHAPE Round or oval.
DISTRIBUTION Localized "butterfly" rash on face in light-exposed areas (Fig. 17-3), forearms, dorsa of hands.
HAIR Patchy or diffuse alopecia.
MUCOUS MEMBRANE Ulcers, purpuric necrotic lesions on palate (80%), buccal mucosa, or gums (Fig. 17-4).
OTHER Periungual telangiectasias and palmar erythema are also seen.

General Findings

LYMPHADENOPATHY (LAD) 50%.
MUSCULOSKELETAL Arthralgia or arthritis (15%).
RENAL Proteinuria, cellular casts (up to 50%).
CARDIAC Pericarditis (up to 20%).
PULMONARY Pleuritis, pneumonitis (up to 20%).

TABLE 17-1 Type of Cutaneous Lupus

Acute Cutaneous Lupus Erythematosus (ACLE)—Highly associated with SLE
Subacute Cutaneous LE (SCLE)—Variably associated with SLE
Chronic Cutaneous LE—Rarely associated with SLE
Discoid LE—Uncommonly associated with SLE
LE tumidus
Lupus panniculitis
Chilblain lupus
Other variants (bullous, TEN-like, lupus/lichen planus overlap, etc.)

SLE, systemic lupus erythematosus.

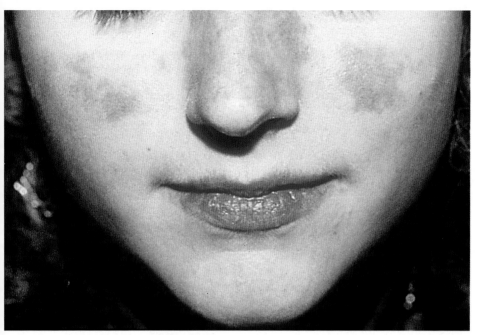

FIGURE 17-3 Systemic lupus erythematosus Erythematous, edematous plaques in a "butterfly distribution" on the face.

GASTROINTESTINAL Arteritis, peritonitis, hepatomegaly (30%), splenomegaly (20%).
NEUROLOGIC Peripheral neuropathy (14%), CNS disease (10%), seizures, or psychosis (14%).
HEMATOLOGIC Anemia, leukopenia, lymphopenia, thrombocytopenia, elevated ESR.

LABORATORY EXAMINATIONS

DERMATOPATHOLOGY Epidermal atrophy, liquefaction degeneration of the dermoepidermal junction, edema of the dermis, dermal inflammatory infiltrate (lymphocytes), and fibrinoid degeneration of the connective tissue and walls of the blood vessels.
OTHER ORGANS Fibrinoid degeneration of connective tissue and walls of the blood vessels associated with an inflammatory infiltrate of plasma cells and lymphocytes.
IMMUNOFLUORESCENCE The lupus band test (direct immunofluorescence) demonstrates IgG, IgM, and C1q granular/globular in a band-like pattern along the dermoepidermal junction. This is positive in lesional skin (90%), sun-exposed areas (80%), and non–sun-exposed areas (50%).
SEROLOGIC Antinuclear antibody (ANA) test positive (>95%), peripheral pattern of nuclear fluorescence and antidouble-stranded DNA antibodies are highly correlated with ACLE.

DIFFERENTIAL DIAGNOSIS

ACLE can be confused with sunburn, rosacea, drug-induced photosensitivity, eczema, or seborrheic dermatitis. The diagnosis of SLE can be made if four of the following criteria are present based on the American College of Rheumatology criteria:

1. Malar rash (butterfly appearance)
2. Discoid rash
3. Photosensitivity
4. Oral ulcers
5. Arthritis
6. Serositis (pleuritis or pericarditis)
7. Renal complications (proteinuria or cellular casts)
8. Neurologic disorder (seizures or psychosis)
9. Hematologic disorder (anemia, leukopenia, thrombocytopenia)
10. Immunologic disorder [+lupus erythematosus (LE) prep, anti-DNA, anti-Sm, false + RPR]
11. ANA (90% of patients have a titer of $\geq 1{:}32$)

An additional classification system proposed by the Systemic Lupus International Collaborating Clinics in 2012 broadens the diagnostic algorithm for lupus to include 17 possible clinical and immunologic criteria for making the diagnosis.

COURSE AND PROGNOSIS

SLE is a lifelong controllable disease with a survival rate of >90%. Mortality is secondary to renal failure, CNS lupus, cardiac failure, or infection.

MANAGEMENT

ACLE responds best to sun protection and sun avoidance. Topical management includes short courses of high-potency topical or intralesional steroids, calcineurin inhibitors (tacrolimus or pimecrolimus), and retinoids. SLE responds to NSAIDs and salicylates for mild disease (arthritis). More severe disease responds to systemic antimalarials (hydroxychloroquine, chloroquine, quinacrine). The indications for systemic steroids (prednisone, methylprednisolone) include CNS involvement, renal involvement, severely ill patients without CNS involvement, and hemolytic crisis. Antimalarial-resistant disease may require azathioprine, cyclophosphamide, retinoids, thalidomide, mycophenolate mofetil, dapsone, clofazimine, sulfasalazine, or immune response modifiers (rituximab).

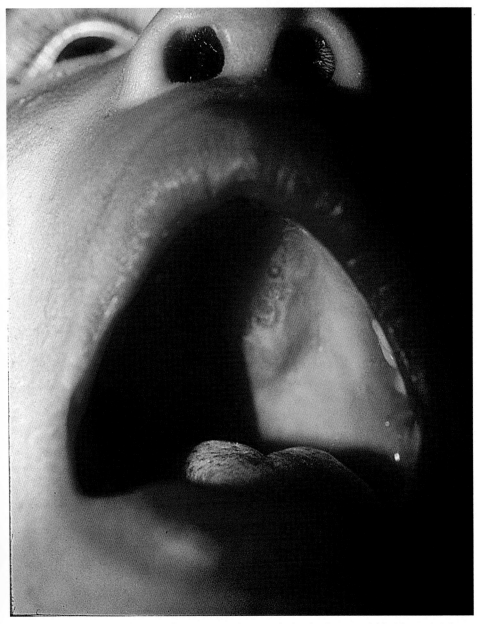

FIGURE 17-4 **Systemic lupus erythematosus** Ulcers on the hard palate in a child with systemic lupus erythematosus.

DISCOID LUPUS ERYTHEMATOSUS

Discoid lupus erythematosus (DLE) is a form of chronic cutaneous LE most commonly seen by dermatologists, but is rarely associated with SLE (Table 17-1).

 INSIGHT Discoid lupus frequently involves the conchal bowl of the ear; lesions present there are highly suggestive of discoid lupus.

EPIDEMIOLOGY

AGE All ages, peak: 20 to 40 years.
GENDER F > M, 3:1.
PREVALENCE 85% of chronic LE.
RACE African American > Asian, Latin American, Caucasian.

PATHOPHYSIOLOGY

DLE is antibody-mediated, and the trigger for autoantibody production may be multifactorial (genetics, infection, UV radiation, smoking).

HISTORY

Discoid lesions are chronic and recurrent, most commonly seen in photodistributed areas, but can be widespread on the body. The lesions spread centrifugally and may merge. Resolution of the active lesion results in atrophy, dyspigmentation, and scarring leading to permanent disfigurement.

PHYSICAL EXAMINATION

Skin Findings

TYPE Papules, plaques, scale, crust, scars (Fig. 17-5).
COLOR Pink, red, hypo- or hyperpigmentation.
SHAPE Round or oval.
PALPATION Indurated, atrophic.
DISTRIBUTION Face, scalp, ears, V-area of the upper chest > generalized, forearms.
HAIR Follicular plugging with perifollicular scale, patchy or diffuse scarring alopecia (Fig. 17-6).
MUCOUS MEMBRANE Discoid lesions on lips, nasal mucosa, conjunctivae, genitalia.

General Findings

MUSCULOSKELETAL Arthralgia or arthritis.

LABORATORY EXAMINATIONS

DERMATOPATHOLOGY Hyperkeratosis, atrophy of the epidermis, vacuolar changes in the basal cell layer, thickening of the basement membrane, follicular plugging, pigment incontinence, a perivascular lymphocytic infiltrate, and increased mucin in the dermis.
IMMUNOFLUORESCENCE The lupus band test (direct immunofluorescence) is positive in 90% of DLE patients.
SEROLOGIC ANA-positive (20%), SS-A (anti-Ro) autoantibodies (up to 5%), anti-dsDNA or anti-Sm antibodies (<5%) usually indicate SLE. Up to 15% of individuals with DLE eventually develop SLE.
OTHER Cytopenia, elevated ESR, positive rheumatoid factor, decreased complement levels, proteinuria.

DIFFERENTIAL DIAGNOSIS

DLE can be confused with prurigo nodularis, psoriasis, drug-induced photosensitivity, lichen planus, granuloma annulare, rosacea, sarcoid, eczema, or seborrheic dermatitis.

COURSE AND PROGNOSIS

Typically, DLE is limited to the skin and there is no systemic involvement. However, a discoid rash is one of the American College of Rheumatology eleven diagnostic criteria for SLE and up to 15% of patients with generalized DLE will get SLE. Rarely, squamous cell carcinomas can develop in chronic lesions of DLE.

MANAGEMENT

DLE management is targeted at controlling lesions and minimizing scarring. DLE responds best to sun protection, sun avoidance, and smoking cessation. Topical management includes short courses of high-potency topical or intralesional steroids, calcineurin inhibitors (tacrolimus or pimecrolimus), and retinoids. More severe disease responds to antimalarials (hydroxychloroquine, chloroquine, quinacrine). Antimalarial-resistant disease may require methotrexate, mycophenolate mofetil, azathioprine, or thalidomide. Scarring can be cosmetically covered with make-up or wigs.

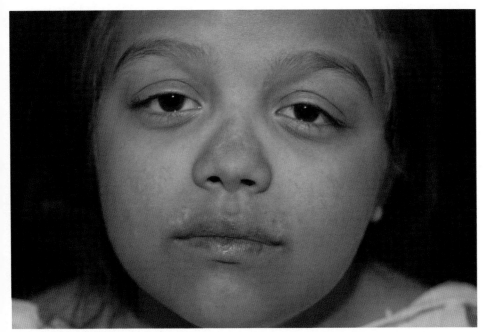

FIGURE 17-5 Discoid lupus erythematosus Atrophic hypopigmented scars on the face of a child with discoid lupus erythematosus.

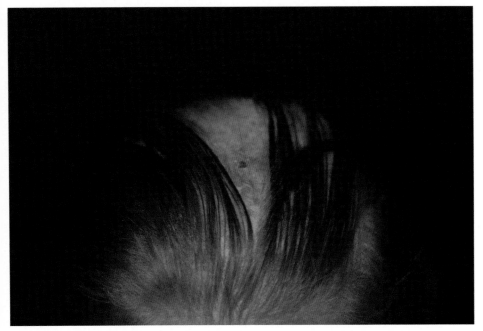

FIGURE 17-6 Discoid lupus erythematosus Scarring alopecia on the scalp of a child with DLE.

DERMATOMYOSITIS

Dermatomyositis (DM) is a systemic disease characterized by violaceous (heliotrope) inflammatory changes of the eyelids and periorbital area; erythema of the face, neck, and upper trunk; and flat-topped violaceous papules over the knuckles (Gottron's papules) associated systemically with polymyositis.

CLINICAL SPECTRUM Ranges from DM with only cutaneous inflammation (DM sine myositis or amyopathic DM) to polymyositis with only muscle inflammation (hypomyopathic myositis).
SYNONYMS Idiopathic inflammatory dermatomyopathies.

EPIDEMIOLOGY

AGE 25% of patients are children: peak 10 to 15 years. Adults: peak 40 to 50 years, up to 20% have an associated malignancy.
GENDER Children: F > M, 2:1. Adults: F > M, 5:1.
INCIDENCE 2 to 4 cases/million children.
ETIOLOGY Immune mediated with triggers such as infection, drug, or malignancy (in adults).
GENETICS Increased frequency of HLA-B8 and HLA-DQA1 in children and HLA-B14 in adults suggests a genetic predisposition exists. Juvenile DM may be associated with polymorphisms in the gene for TNF-α and interleukin-1 receptor antagonist as well.

PATHOPHYSIOLOGY

DM is an immune-mediated process triggered by external factors (infection, drug, or malignancy) in genetically predisposed individuals. There is often a seasonal predilection of cases in the spring and summer, suggesting an infectious trigger may be present. Systemically, acute and chronic inflammation of striated muscle accompanied by segmental necrosis of myofibers results in progressive muscle weakness.

HISTORY

In juvenile DM there is frequently a history of a preceding viral illness followed by fever, muscle weakness, fatigue, and rash. Unlike adult DM, juvenile DM has a decreased rate of associated malignancies and the mortality is low. However, the risk of cutaneous calcinosis—abnormal calcium deposition in the skin—is higher in juvenile DM.

PHYSICAL EXAMINATION

Skin Findings

TYPE Macules, scale, papules (Gottron's), atrophy, ulcers, scars.
COLOR Reddish-purple heliotrope. Poikiloderma (hypo- and hyperpigmentation, telangiectasia, and atrophy). Pink-to-purple colored papules over the joints of the dorsal hands (Gottron's papules), elbows, and knees (Gottron's sign).
DISTRIBUTION Photodistributed: eyes, malar area (Fig. 17-7), extensor surfaces, neck, upper chest, and nape of neck.
HANDS Gottron's papules—dorsa of knuckles (sparing interarticular areas, Fig. 17-8).
NAILFOLDS Periungual telangiectasias, "ragged" cuticles.
MUCOUS MEMBRANES Vivid red hue on gum line, ulceration, white plaques on tongue and mucosa.
OTHER Calcinosis cutis.

General Findings

MUSCULOSKELETAL Proximal/limb girdle muscle weakness > facial/bulbar, pharyngeal, esophageal muscle weakness. Muscle tenderness and atrophy.
PULMONARY (30%) Interstitial fibrosis, acute respiratory disease syndrome.
CARDIAC Rhythm disturbances, conduction defects.

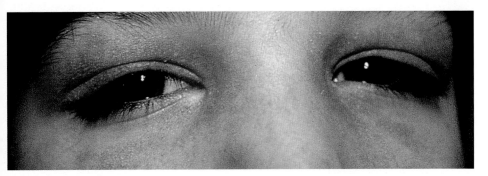

FIGURE 17-7 Dermatomyositis Violaceous periorbital rash characteristic of dermatomyositis.

DIFFERENTIAL DIAGNOSIS

The differential diagnosis for DM includes LE, mixed connective tissue disease (MCTD), psoriasis, allergic contact dermatitis, photodrug eruption, eczema, steroid myopathy, trichinosis, and toxoplasmosis.

The diagnosis of DM can be made on clinical grounds in individuals who present with classic physical examination findings cutaneous lesions and proximal muscle weakness as well as consistent clinical history. Additional laboratory findings which may be useful for individuals with skin findings but atypical or partially consistent presentations include the following:

1. Proximal muscle weakness
2. Elevated serum "muscle enzyme" levels: creatine kinase and/or aldolase
3. Diagnostic muscle biopsy
4. Characteristic electromyographic changes

LABORATORY EXAMINATIONS

DERMATOPATHOLOGY Flattening of epidermis, hydropic degeneration of basal cell layer, edema of upper dermis, scattered inflammatory infiltrate, PAS-positive fibrinoid deposits at dermoepidermal junction and around upper dermal capillaries, and an accumulation of acid mucopolysaccharides in dermis.

MUSCLE BIOPSY Muscle biopsy of deltoid, supraspinatus, gluteus, quadriceps will show segmental necrosis within muscle fibers with loss of cross-striations; waxy/coagulative type of eosinophilic staining; ± regenerating fibers; inflammatory cells, histiocytes, macrophages, lymphocytes, plasma cells. Vasculitis may also be seen.

MRI Magnetic resonance imaging may demonstrate areas of myositis in active inflammatory myopathies. These changes are not specific to DM or polymyositis and may be seen in other primary muscle disease processes.

CHEMISTRY Elevated creatine phosphokinase most specific for muscle disease; also aldolase, glutamic oxaloacetic transaminase, and lactic dehydrogenase may be elevated. Autoantibodies including ANA are detected in up to 80% of individuals with DM.

URINE Elevated 24-hour creatinine excretion (>200 mg/24 hours).

ELECTROMYOGRAM Increased irritability on insertion of electrodes, spontaneous fibrillations, pseudomyotonic discharges, positive sharp waves; excludes neuromyopathy. With evidence of denervation, suspect coexisting tumor.

ELECTROCARDIOGRAM Myocarditis; atrial, ventricular irritability, atrioventricular block.

X-RAY OF CHEST ± Interstitial fibrosis, confirmed with pulmonary function testing.

COURSE AND PROGNOSIS

Dermatitis and polymyositis usually are detected at the same time; however, skin or muscle involvement can occur initially, followed at some time by the other. Juvenile DM, unlike adult DM, is rarely associated with Raynaud's phenomenon, malignancies, or mortality. In children, roughly 33% of patients will have monocyclic disease with spontaneous remission in 1 to 2 years, 33% of patients will have polycyclic disease with 1 to 2 relapses, and 33% of patients will have chronic persistent symptoms for more than 2 years after diagnosis despite treatment.

MANAGEMENT

DM management includes sun protection and sun avoidance. Cutaneous lesions can be treated with topical steroids or calcineurin inhibitors. Systemic disease responds to NSAIDs, salicylates, systemic corticosteroids (prednisone or methylprednisolone). In most cases of DM with both skin and muscle involvement, immunosuppressive drugs (azathioprine, methotrexate, cyclosporine) are necessary early on in treatment. For refractory disease, possible therapies include plasmapheresis, hydroxychloroquine, systemic retinoids, mycophenolate mofetil, dapsone, thalidomide, intravenous immunoglobulin, chlorambucil, systemic tacrolimus, sirolimus, infliximab, or rituximab.

In the acute stages, children may need hospitalization to monitor for palatorespiratory muscle involvement with myositis. In such cases, adequate respiration and prevention of aspiration is needed.

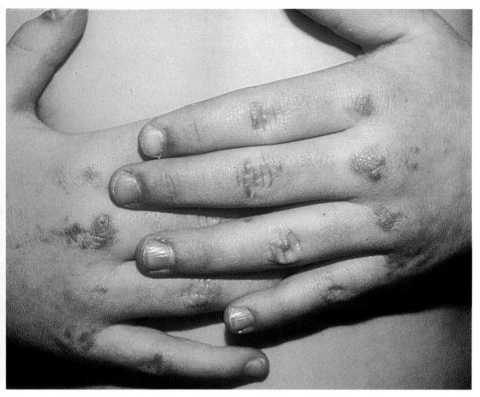

FIGURE 17-8 Dermatomyositis Gottron's papules on the dorsa of the knuckles.

MORPHEA (LOCALIZED SCLERODERMA)

Morphea is a localized cutaneous sclerosis characterized by early violaceous-colored plaques later evolving to ivory-colored sclerotic areas, which may be solitary, linear, or generalized.

 INSIGHT An important, though much less-frequent, presentation of morphea is bruise-like patches; the patients are often evaluated for bleeding disorders before they are referred to dermatology.

SYNONYMS Circumscribed scleroderma, linear scleroderma, scleroderma en coup de sabre.

EPIDEMIOLOGY

AGE 20% onset before 18 years. Average age onset: 7 years.
INCIDENCE 2 to 3/100,000.
GENDER F > M, 2:1.
ETIOLOGY Unknown. Lichen sclerosus may be somehow related.

PATHOPHYSIOLOGY

The pathogenesis of morphea is unknown. The primary event might be a local trigger occurring within the skin, which leads to focal, asymmetric inflammation and sclerosis of the skin. Vascular disruption is also postulated to play a role in the development of morphea. One possible trigger is thought to be infection related to *Borrelia* species in Western Europe.

HISTORY

The onset of morphea is insidious with erythematous violaceous plaques that slowly evolve into firm, waxy, ivory-colored, or postinflammatory hyperpigmented sclerotic areas.

PHYSICAL EXAMINATION

Skin Findings

TYPE Plaques, scar.
SIZE 2 to 15 cm.
COLOR Red, purplish, ivory; hyperpigmented (Fig. 17-9).
SHAPE Round or oval.
PALPATION Indurated, hard. May be hypoesthetic.
ARRANGEMENT Usually multiple, bilateral, asymmetric.
DISTRIBUTION Trunk, breasts, abdomen, limbs, face, genitalia > axillae, perineum, areola.

HAIR Follicles obliterated, scarring alopecia.
NAILS Nail dystrophy.

General Findings

MUSCULOSKELETAL (11%) Flexion contractures, underlying muscle, fascia, bone involvement.
OTHER "Coup de sabre" is used to describe linear morphea on the forehead. Parry–Romberg syndrome is a related condition with hemiatrophy of face (Fig. 17-10). Both can have neurologic (4%) and/or ocular (2%) complications.

DIFFERENTIAL DIAGNOSIS

The differential diagnosis for morphea includes progressive systemic sclerosis (SSc), lichen sclerosus et atrophicus, eosinophilic fasciitis, eosinophilia–myalgia syndrome associated with L-tryptophan ingestion, and acrodermatitis chronica atrophicans.

LABORATORY EXAMINATIONS

DERMATOPATHOLOGY Swelling and degeneration of homogenous, eosinophilic collagen fibrils, mild perivascular, and dermal–subcutis infiltrate; dermal appendages progressively disappear.
SEROLOGY ANA-positive, increased antibodies to ssDNA, topoisomerase IIa, phospholipid, fibrillin 1, and histone.

COURSE AND PROGNOSIS

Morphea lesions in children tend to progress from 3 to 5 years, and then stop. In less than 10% of patients, the scarring can lead to contractures, handicaps, or growth retardation.

MANAGEMENT

For morphea, physical therapy is warranted for lesions overlying joints, which may impede mobility. Topical and intralesional steroids are of limited use. Topical calcipotriol has been tried with mixed results. Early use of systemic anti-inflammatory medications such as systemic steroids and methotrexate may halt early progression. Severe cases may respond to psoralen plus ultraviolet A (PUVA), UVA1 phototherapy, antimalarials, phenytoin, penicillamine, sulfasalazine, cyclosporine, colchicine, or systemic calcipotriol.

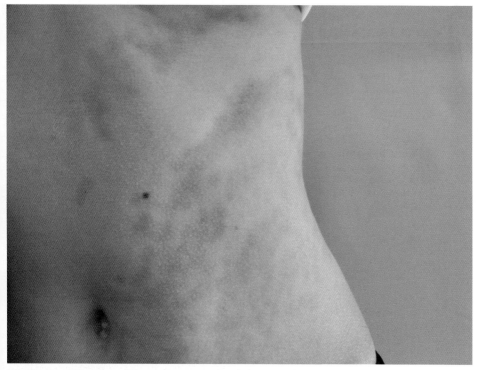

FIGURE 17-9 Morphea Sclerotic hyperpigmented plaque on the anterior torso of a child.

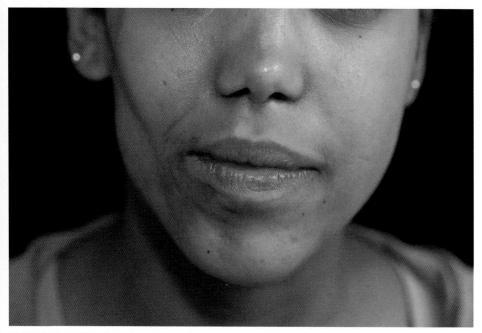

FIGURE 17-10 Morphea Hyperpigmentation and loss of subcutaneous tissue resulting in facial asymmetry.

SYSTEMIC SCLEROSIS

SSc is a rare, severe autoimmune disorder characterized by sclerotic changes of the skin and internal organs.

CLASSIFICATION

1. Limited cutaneous SSc is characterized by fibrotic changes of the fingers, hands, and face. Includes CREST (Calcinosis cutis, Raynaud's, Esophageal dysfunction, Sclerodactyly, Telangiectasia) syndrome.
2. Diffuse cutaneous SSc: Fibrotic changes of the fingers, hands, arms, trunk, face, and lower extremities.

SYNONYMS Progressive systemic sclerosis, systemic scleroderma.

EPIDEMIOLOGY

AGE All ages. Peak: 30 to 50 years.
GENDER F > M, 4:1.
INCIDENCE 20/million.
RACE Black > white.
GENETICS A 15-fold increase in first-degree relatives.

PATHOPHYSIOLOGY

The pathogenesis of SSc is unknown. The primary event might be autoimmune endothelial cell injury in blood vessels. Early in the course of the disease, target organ edema occurs followed by fibrosis; the cutaneous capillaries are reduced in number and the remaining vessels dilate and proliferate, becoming visible telangiectasias. Fibrosis is also present because of overproduction of collagen by fibroblasts.

HISTORY

Raynaud's phenomenon with pain/tingling of the fingertips/toes is usually the first sign of SSc. Patients with SSc have a characteristic tightening of the facial features producing a pinched-nose, pursed-lip appearance (Fig. 17-11). Systemic involvement leads to migratory polyarthritis, heartburn, dysphagia, constipation, diarrhea, abdominal bloating, malabsorption, weight loss, exertional dyspnea, and dry cough.

PHYSICAL EXAMINATION

Skin Findings

TYPE Macules, edematous plaques, ulcerations.
COLOR Triphasic: pallor, cyanosis, rubor. Hypo- or hyperpigmentation, sometimes giving a "salt and pepper" appearance.
FINGERS Sclerodactyly, flexion contractures (Fig. 17-12), bony resorption, periungual telangiectasia, cutaneous calcifications (Fig. 17-13), and digital ulceration. Early on in the disease, puffiness of the digits may be seen.
FACE Mask-like, thinning of lips, small mouth, radial perioral furrowing, small sharp nose.
PALPATION Indurated, stiff, smooth, hardened, bound down. Leathery crepitation over joints.
DISTRIBUTION Fingers, hands, upper extremities, trunk, face, lower extremities.
HAIR Thinning/complete loss of hair on distal extremities. Loss of sweat glands with anhidrosis.
NAILS Nails grow clawlike over shortened distal phalanges.
OTHER Mat-like telangiectasia on face, neck, upper trunk, hands, lips, oral mucous membranes, gastrointestinal (GI) tract.
MUCOUS MEMBRANES Sclerosis of sublingual ligament, induration of gums, tongue.

General Findings

LUNG Interstitial lung disease, pulmonary fibrosis, pulmonary artery hypertension.
CARDIAC Congestive heart failure.
RENAL Hypertensive renal disease.
GASTROINTESTINAL Esophageal reflux, dysphagia, constipation, diarrhea, malabsorption.
MUSCULOSKELETAL Carpal tunnel syndrome, muscle weakness.

DIFFERENTIAL DIAGNOSIS

Other sclerotic entities that need to be considered in the differential diagnosis of SSc include scleredema, scleromyxedema, MCTD, eosinophilic fasciitis, LE, DM, morphea, chronic graft-versus-host disease, lichen sclerosus et atrophicus, polyvinyl chloride exposure, and adverse drug reaction (pentazocine, bleomycin, taxanes).

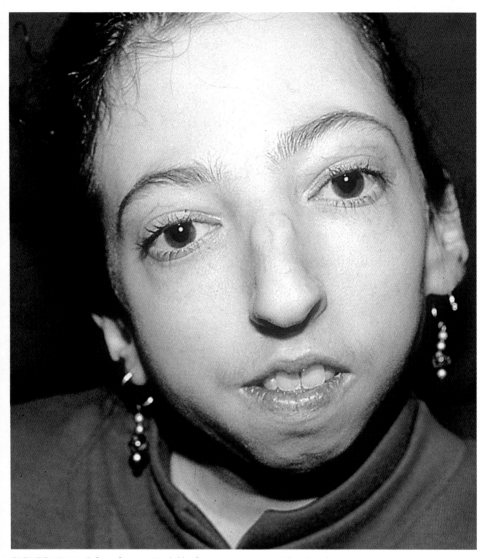

FIGURE 17-11 Scleroderma Mask-like facies in a patient with scleroderma.

LABORATORY EXAMINATIONS

DERMATOPATHOLOGY A mild cellular infiltrate around dermal blood vessels, eccrine coils, subcutaneous tissue, effacement of the rete ridges; paucity of blood vessels, thickening and hyalinization of vessel walls, narrowing of lumen; atrophied dermal appendages; calcium deposits; and compact, homogenized collagen.

SEROLOGY ANA-positive, nucleolar, discrete speckled pattern. Diffuse cutaneous SSc: anti-topoisomerase I (Scl 70), anti-RNA-polymerase I and III. Limited cutaneous SSc: anticentromere antibodies.

COURSE AND PROGNOSIS

The course for diffuse SSc is characterized by slow, relentless progression of skin and/or visceral sclerosis; 80% of patients die within 10 years after the onset of symptoms. With angiotensin-converting enzyme inhibitors for the management of renal crisis, the leading cause of death in SSc is now cardiac and pulmonary dysfunction. Spontaneous remissions do occur. CREST syndrome progresses more slowly and has a more favorable prognosis.

MANAGEMENT

The treatment of SSc is primarily focused on internal organ disease. For polyarthritis, salicylates and NSAIDs are helpful. For Raynaud's phenomenon, calcium channel blockers (nifedipine), angiotensin II receptor blockers (losartan), and intravenous prostaglandin E1 (alprostadil) can improve circulation. For renal disease, angiotensin-converting enzyme inhibitors have been life-saving. For GI involvement, small frequent meals, head elevation in bed, antacids, and prokinetic agents can help. For pulmonary disease, cyclophosphamide, mycophenolate mofetil, azathioprine, chlorambucil, 5-fluorouracil, cyclosporine, systemic steroids, prostacyclin analogs (epoprostenol, treprostinil), and endothelin receptor antagonists (sildenafil, sitaxsentan) have been used.

Cutaneous SSc can be managed with avoidance of vasospastic agents (cold, stress, fatigue, smoking), and minimizing trauma. Warm gloves, socks, and clothing are critical for individuals with SSc who have Raynaud's phenomenon. For cutaneous ulcers, occlusive wet dressings, enzyme-debriding agents (collagenase), and topical growth factors (PDGF) can be helpful. For severe cases, systemic therapeutic modalities such as minocycline, methotrexate, corticosteroids, extracorporeal photophoresis, intravenous immunoglobulins, calcipotriol, D-penicillamine, colchicine, potassium P-aminobenzoate, psoralen ultraviolet A, and UVA1 have been tried with varied results.

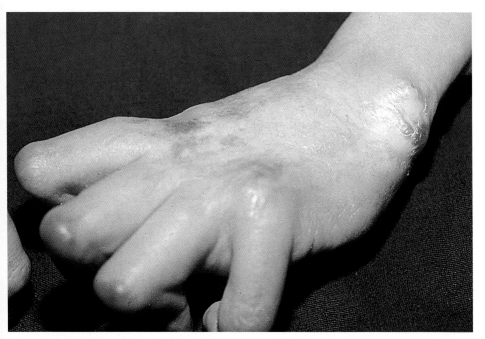

FIGURE 17-12 Scleroderma Debilitating joint contractures of the hands.

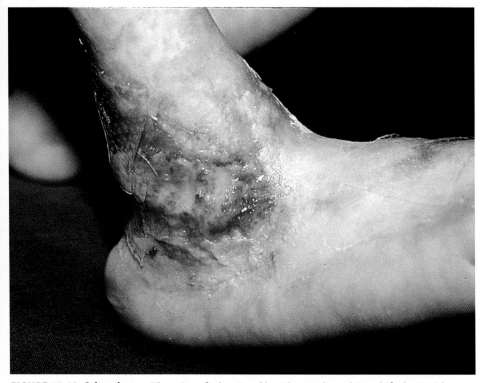

FIGURE 17-13 Scleroderma Ulceration of sclerotic ankle with extruding white calcified material.

MIXED CONNECTIVE TISSUE DISEASE

MCTD is a rare, autoimmune disease characterized by U1RNP-positive antibodies, Raynaud's phenomenon, dactylitis, low-grade fever, and arthritis.

 INSIGHT The clinical spectrum of the disease represents an overlap of features of systemic lupus erythematosus, systemic sclerosis, and polymyositis.

SYNONYMS Undifferentiated connective tissue disease, Sharp's syndrome.

EPIDEMIOLOGY

AGE All ages. Peak: 20 to 30 years.
GENDER F > M, upward of 16:1.
INCIDENCE Least common autoimmune connective tissue disease.
GENETICS HLA-DR4 and HLA-DR2.

PATHOPHYSIOLOGY

The exact pathogenesis of MCTD is unknown, but involves the production of autoantibodies against U1RNP more than in patients with lupus, scleroderma, or DM.

HISTORY

Raynaud's phenomenon with pain/tingling of the fingertips and dactylitis (sausage digits) are usually the first clinical sign of MCTD. The hands and fingers become tight and may ulcerate with, or without, calcinosis cutis. Sclerodermoid or poikilodermatous areas of the upper trunk and proximal extremities may evolve.

PHYSICAL EXAMINATION

Skin Findings

TYPE Macules, plaques, ulcerations.
COLOR Red, purple; hypo- or hyperpigmented.
DISTRIBUTION Fingers (dactylitis, bony resorption, periungual telangiectasia, cutaneous calcifications; Fig. 17-14), hands > upper extremities, upper trunk. Acute flares: malar face (Fig. 17-15).

General Findings

MUSCULOSKELETAL (85%) Polyarthritis.
GASTROINTESTINAL (75%) Esophageal dysmotility, reflux esophagitis, dysphagia.
PULMONARY Pulmonary hypertension.

DIFFERENTIAL DIAGNOSIS

Other sclerotic entities that need to be considered in the differential diagnosis of MCTD include scleroderma, LE, DM, other overlap syndromes, morphea, chronic graft-versus-host disease, and lichen sclerosus et atrophicus.

LABORATORY EXAMINATIONS

DERMATOPATHOLOGY Vasculopathy or small and medium blood vessels, interface dermatitis, dermal fibrosis.
SEROLOGY ANA-positive, high titers of U1RNP antibodies.

COURSE AND PROGNOSIS

The course for MCTD is characterized by slow, relentless progression of skin and pulmonary disease. Over time, some MCTD patients may develop classic systemic LE or scleroderma. A common complication from the arthritis in MCTD is Jaccoud's arthropathy from periarticular disease and ligament laxity. The major cause of death in patients with MCTD results from pulmonary hypertension.

MANAGEMENT

The treatment of MCTD is primarily focused on targeted organ involvement. For polyarthritis, salicylates and NSAIDs are helpful. For Raynaud's phenomenon, calcium channel blockers (nifedipine) can improve circulation. For GI involvement, small frequent meals, head elevation in bed, antacids, and prokinetic agents can help. For pulmonary disease, cyclophosphamide, mycophenolate mofetil, azathioprine, methotrexate, cyclosporine, plasmapheresis, and autologous peripheral stem cell transplantation have been used as experimental treatments.

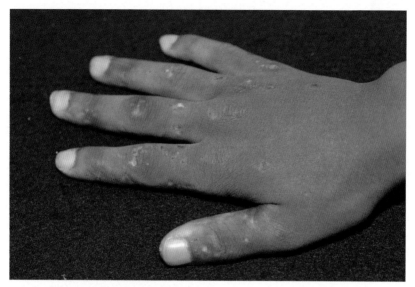

FIGURE 17-14 Mixed connective tissue disease Atrophic, sclerotic plaques on the hand of a child with mixed connective tissue disease.

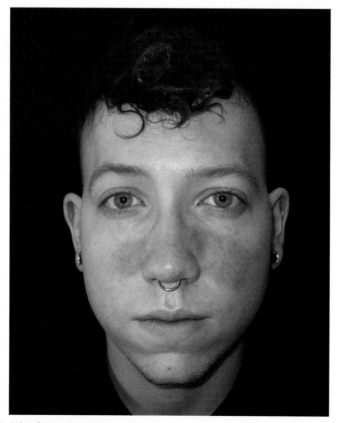

FIGURE 17-15 Mixed connective tissue disease Erythematous plaques on the cheeks of an adolescent with MCTD.

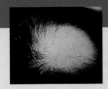

ENDOCRINE DISORDERS AND THE SKIN

ACANTHOSIS NIGRICANS

Acanthosis nigricans (AN) is a diffuse, velvety thickening and hyperpigmentation of the skin, chiefly in axillae and other body folds, which may be related to hereditary factors, associated endocrine disorders, obesity, drug administration, and, in one rare form, malignancy.

CLASSIFICATION

Type 1—Hereditary Benign AN: No associated endocrine disorder.

Type 2—Benign AN: Associated with insulin resistance (IR), impaired glucose tolerance, IR diabetes mellitus (DM), hyperandrogenism, acromegaly, gigantism, Cushing's disease, growth hormone, hypogonadism, Addison's disease, hypothyroidism, polycystic ovary syndrome, or total lipodystrophy.

Type 3—Pseudo-AN: Obesity-induced IR, darker skin types.

Type 4—Drug-induced AN: Nicotinic acid, oral contraceptives, insulin, or other exogenous hormone treatments.

Type 5—Malignant AN Paraneoplastic, usually adenocarcinoma; less commonly, lymphoma.

EPIDEMIOLOGY

AGE Any age. Peak: puberty to adulthood.
GENDER M = F.
INCIDENCE Up to 19% of the population. Incidence thought to be rising with increased obesity and diabetes in both pediatric and adult populations.
RACE African Americans > Hispanics, Native Americans > Caucasians, Asians.

PATHOPHYSIOLOGY

Epidermal changes of AN are likely caused by triggers that stimulate keratinocyte and fibroblast proliferation. In benign AN, the trigger is likely insulin or an insulin-like growth factor. In malignant AN, the trigger is likely the tumor or tumor secretions. Growth receptors that have been implicated in the development of AN include fibroblast growth factor receptor (FGFR), insulin-like growth factor receptor-1 (IGFR1), and epidermal growth factor receptor (EGFR).

HISTORY

AN has an asymptomatic, insidious onset. The first visible change is darkening of pigmentation which gradually progresses to velvety plaques that may be pruritic.

PHYSICAL EXAMINATION

Skin Findings

TYPE Plaque.
COLOR Dark brown to black, hyperpigmented, skin appears dirty. Longstanding lesions may show hyperlinearity of skin markings.
PALPATION Velvety, rugose, mammillated.
DISTRIBUTION Posterior neck > axillae (Fig. 18-1), groin > antecubital, knuckles, submammary, umbilicus, areola. Usually symmetric.
MUCOUS MEMBRANES Oral, nasal, laryngeal, and esophagus: velvety texture with delicate furrows.
NAILS Leukonychia, hyperkeratosis.
OTHER Skin tags in same areas, likely due to similar growth-factor stimulation.

General Findings

OCULAR Papillomatous lesions on the eyelids and conjunctiva.
BENIGN AN Obesity or underlying endocrine disorder.
MALIGNANT AN Underlying malignancy most commonly gastric adenocarcinoma (70%).

DIFFERENTIAL DIAGNOSIS

AN can be confused with confluent and reticulated papillomatosis of Gougerot and Carteaud (CARP), terra firma-forme dermatosis, hypertrichosis, Becker's nevus, epidermal nevus, hemochromatosis, Addison's disease, or pellagra.

LABORATORY EXAMINATIONS

DERMATOPATHOLOGY Papillomatosis, hyperkeratosis; epidermis thrown into irregular folds, showing varying degrees of acanthosis.

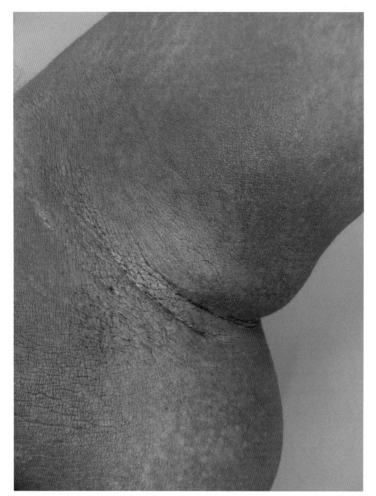

FIGURE 18-1 Acanthosis nigricans Hyperpigmented velvety plaque in the axilla of an adolescent.

COURSE AND PROGNOSIS

Type 1: Accentuated at puberty, and, at times, regresses when older.

Type 2: Prognosis related to severity of IR. AN may regress subsequent to treatment of the IR state.

Type 3: AN may regress subsequent to significant weight loss.

Type 4: Resolves when causative drug is discontinued.

Type 5: Poor prognosis, since the underlying malignancy is often aggressive. Adults with new-onset AN have an average survival time of 2 years.

MANAGEMENT

Treatment of AN should include a careful workup to exclude any underlying endocrine disorder. In children, AN is very rarely a sign of an underlying malignancy. Correction of any underlying disorder (obesity, endocrine disease) improves the skin condition. Cosmetically, AN is difficult to treat, but some improvement may be gained with topical keratolytics (retinoic acid, salicylic acid, or urea) or topical vitamin D analogs (calcipotriene). In severe cases, systemic retinoids (acitretin, isotretinoin), metformin, dietary fish oil, dermabrasion, and laser therapy have reported successes. In adults, malignant AN may respond to cyproheptadine because it may inhibit the release of tumor products.

NECROBIOSIS LIPOIDICA

Necrobiosis lipoidica (NL) is a cutaneous disorder characterized by distinctive, sharply circumscribed, red–brown plaques with palpable rims and yellow–brown atrophic centers occurring on the lower legs. It is frequently associated with DM.

SYNONYM Necrobiosis lipoidica diabeticorum (NLD).

EPIDEMIOLOGY

AGE Any age, peak: 25 to 30 years. Seen earlier in juvenile diabetic patients.
GENDER F > M, 3:1.
INCIDENCE <1% of patients with diabetes.
ETIOLOGY 65% patients with diabetes. Predilection for posttraumatic sites.

PATHOPHYSIOLOGY

NL is a granulomatous inflammatory reaction caused by alterations in collagen. The exact cause is unknown, but in DM, NL is thought to be secondary to diabetic microangiopathy. In non-DM cases, the trigger may be posttraumatic, postinflammatory, metabolic, or vasculitic antibody-mediated. A possible association with underlying inflammatory thyroid disease has also been suggested.

HISTORY

NL skin lesions evolve slowly and enlarge over months to years. The skin lesions are typically asymptomatic, but ulcerated lesions are painful. Diabetes may or may not be present at the time of onset of lesions and is present in up to 65% of NL patients.

PHYSICAL EXAMINATION

Skin Findings

TYPE Papules, plaques, ulcers.
SIZE 1 to 3 mm up to several centimeters.
COLOR Brownish-red border; yellow atrophic shiny center (Fig. 18-2).
SHAPE Serpiginous, annular, irregularly irregular.
ARRANGEMENT Often symmetrical.
DISTRIBUTION DISTAL Legs and feet (80%) > arms, trunk, face, and scalp.
OTHER Decreased sensation, hypohidrosis, and alopecia.

LABORATORY EXAMINATIONS

DERMATOPATHOLOGY Interstitial and pali-saded granulomas with reduced intradermal nerves, thickened blood vessel walls, and endothelial cell swelling in the dermis. Granulomas consist of histiocytes, multi-nucleated lymphocytes, plasma cells, and eosinophils.
IMMUNOFLUORESCENCE IgM, IgA, C3, and fibrinogen in the walls of small blood vessels.

DIFFERENTIAL DIAGNOSIS

NL can be confused with xanthomas, xantho-granuloma, sarcoidosis, rheumatoid nodules, stasis dermatitis, injection granulomas, and granuloma annulare (GA).

COURSE AND PROGNOSIS

The lesions are indolent and can enlarge to involve large areas of the skin surface unless treated. Up to 65% of NL patients have clinical DM, but the severity of NL is not directly proportional to diabetic severity or control. NL is chronic with variable scarring; rarely, squamous cell carcinomas have been reported within lesions.

MANAGEMENT

Most patients are troubled more by the clinical appearance of the lesions rather than the symptoms. Because localized trauma can precipitate NL, elastic support stockings and leg rest may be helpful. Lesions can be improved with topical or intralesional steroids. Antiplatelet aggregation therapy (aspirin, dipyridamole, pentoxifylline, stanozolol, inositol nicotinate, nicofuranose), TNF agents (etanercept, infliximab), thalidomide, topical bovine collagen, topical GM–CSF, cyclosporine, PUVA or UVA, mycophenolate mofetil, ticlopidine, nicotinamide, clofazimine, local heparin injections, surgical grafting, and laser therapy all have cases of reported success. Screening for DM is warranted if systemic symptoms are present. Diligent wound care is especially important for sites of ulceration in NL as these can prove challenging to heal and serve as a nidus for chronic cutaneous infection.

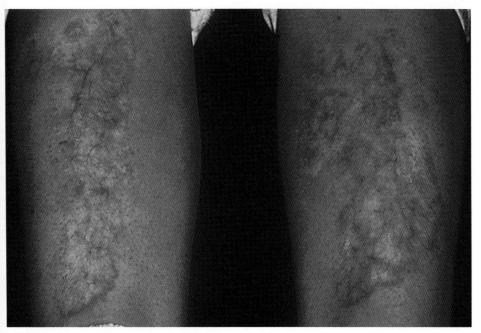

FIGURE 18-2 Necrobiosis lipoidica diabeticorum Well-demarcated yellow–orange plaques on the bilateral shins of a young female diabetic patient.

GRANULOMA ANNULARE

GA is a self-limited dermatosis of unclear etiology, clinically characterized by dermal papules arranged in an annular configuration commonly on the dorsa of the hands, feet, elbows, and knees.

 INSIGHT Annular lesions are frequently misdiagnosed as "ringworm" and treated as such. For an annular lesion that is not scaly, GA must be considered.

CLASSIFICATION

GA can be classified into several clinical variants:

1. Localized GA (most common): Solitary annular plaques on the extremities of young people.
2. Generalized GA (15%): Numerous papules on trunk/extremities in patients younger than 10 years or 30 to 60 years old.
3. Subcutaneous GA: Occurs in children younger than 6 years. Nodules on pretibial area (75%), hands, buttocks, scalp.
4. Perforating GA (5%): Occurs in children. Papules with crusting/ulceration on dorsal hands/fingers.

SYNONYM Pseudorheumatoid nodule.

EPIDEMIOLOGY

AGE Children, young adults, 67% in those who are younger than 30 years. Localized GA more common in pediatric population.
GENDER Female-to-male ratio of 2:1.
GENETICS Familial cases reported. HLA-Bw35, HLA-A29, HLA-B8 associated in small series.

PATHOPHYSIOLOGY

GA has been reported to follow insect bites, trauma, viral infections (EBV, VZV, HIV), sun exposure, PUVA therapy, tuberculin skin test, and malignancy. Generalized GA may be associated with DM. It is thought that GA may be an immune-mediated necrobiotic inflammation of collagen and elastin fibers, a T_H1 reaction-eliciting matrix degeneration or an abnormality of tissue monocytes.

HISTORY

The solitary skin lesions appear sporadically, are asymptomatic, and most self-resolve in a few months to years. Individual lesions often expand centrifugally outward. More generalized GA can persist for years and have a more recalcitrant course, improving in the winter and worsening in the summer.

PHYSICAL EXAMINATION

Skin Lesions

TYPE Papules, plaques, nodules.
SIZE 1 to 5 cm.
COLOR Flesh-colored, pink to violaceous.
ARRANGEMENT Annular (Fig. 18-3) or arciform.
DISTRIBUTION Dorsal upper extremities > lower extremities > trunk.

DIFFERENTIAL DIAGNOSIS

The differential diagnosis for GA is broad since it has several different clinical manifestations. The list includes lichen planus, tinea corporis, psoriasis, papular sarcoid, annular erythema, subacute lupus erythematosus (SCLE), erythema multiforme, erythema chronicum migrans, NL, rheumatoid nodule, xanthomas, eruptive histiocytomas, pityriasis lichenoides et varioliformis acuta (PLEVA), cutaneous T-cell lymphoma (CTCL), elastosis perforans serpiginosa, and perforating collagenosis.

LABORATORY EXAMINATIONS

DERMATOPATHOLOGY Early GA: Interstitial pattern with histiocytes scattered between collagen fibers. Later GA: Palisading granulomas in the upper/mid reticular dermis with a central zone of necrobiotic collagen surrounded by histiocytes, lymphocytes, and a few giant cells. Rare cases of sarcoidal GA are also described.

COURSE AND PROGNOSIS

Since solitary lesions of GA are asymptomatic and 50% spontaneously resolve by 2 years, reassurance is all that is needed. Recurrences can happen. Disseminated GA has a more recalcitrant course, but is uncommonly seen in children. Up to 21% of patients with generalized GA may have DM, though data examining this association are evolving. Similarly, an association between GA and dyslipidemia may exist but deserves further study.

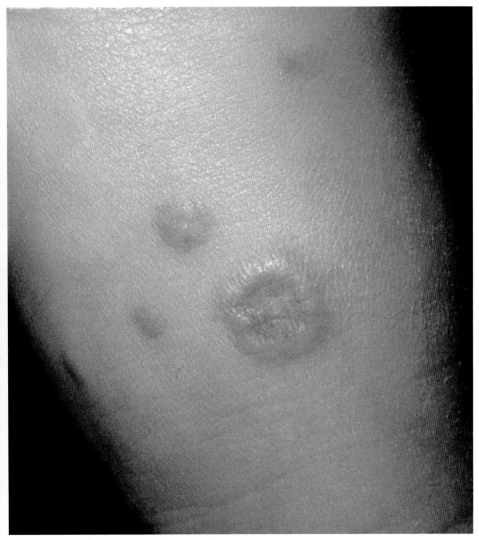

FIGURE 18-3 Granuloma annulare Erythematous papules in an annular configuration on the leg of a child.

MANAGEMENT

The skin lesions are typically asymptomatic and will eventually self-resolve, thus treatment is unnecessary. Symptomatic or extensive lesions can be treated with topical/intralesional steroids, tacrolimus, pimecrolimus, or cryotherapy.

Generalized GA may need more aggressive management with PUVA, UVA1, isotretinoin, dapsone, systemic steroids, pentoxifylline, hydroxychloroquine, cyclosporine, fumaric esters, γ-IFN, potassium iodide, nicotinamide, or laser therapy.

ALOPECIA AREATA

Alopecia areata (AA) is an autoimmune-mediated nonscarring loss of scalp hair in round or oval patches without any visible inflammation. Alopecia totalis is the loss of all the scalp hair and alopecia universalis is the loss of the scalp and all body hair.

 INSIGHT Although it is a relatively rare finding, if hair adjacent to an area of alopecia are gray or white suggesting pigment loss, the diagnosis is almost certainly AA.

EPIDEMIOLOGY

AGE Children are frequently affected; 60% of patients present before age 20 years.
GENDER M = F.
INCIDENCE 1 per 1,000; lifetime risk up to 2% of the population.
GENETICS One in five AA patients have positive family history for AA.
ETIOLOGY Genetic and environmental factors. HLA-DQB1, HLA-DRB1 associated in small series.

PATHOPHYSIOLOGY

AA is thought to be an autoimmune disease of T cells directed against follicular antigens. It may be associated with other autoimmune disorders such as vitiligo, IBD, atopy, polyendocrinopathy syndrome type 1, and thyroid disease (Hashimoto's disease). Stress (e.g., life crises) reportedly precipitates some cases of AA. Genetic studies have suggested dysregulation in genes related to T cell function. CTLA4, IL-2RA, and IL-2 may also play an etiologic role in AA.

HISTORY

Patients usually report abrupt hair loss and will present with an asymptomatic bald spot on the scalp. More spots may appear and severe cases can lead to loss of all the scalp and/or body hair. Most cases of localized areas in the scalp slowly regrow hair over a period of weeks to months.

PHYSICAL EXAMINATION

Skin Lesions

TYPE Nonscarring macules, patches (Fig. 18-4).
SHAPE Round to oval.
SIZE 1 cm to several centimeters.

DISTRIBUTION Localized (AA), regional (alopecia totalis), generalized (alopecia universalis).
SITES OF PREDILECTION Scalp, eyebrows, eyelashes, pubic hair, beard.
HAIR Proximally tapered short "exclamation point hairs" (Fig. 18-5).
NAILS "Hammered brass" pitting (Fig. 18-6), with pits often in a grid-like arrangement. Trachyonychia, brittle nails, onycholysis, and koilonychia also seen.

DIFFERENTIAL DIAGNOSIS

The differential diagnosis of AA includes telogen effluvium, trichotillomania, traction alopecia, androgenetic alopecia, secondary syphilis ("moth-eaten" appearance in beard or scalp), or tinea capitis.

LABORATORY EXAMINATIONS

DERMATOPATHOLOGY Peribulbar lymphocytic infiltrate, miniaturized hairs with fibrous tracts, and pigment incontinence. There is also a decreased anagen-to-telogen ratio.

COURSE AND PROGNOSIS

In the majority of patients, hair will regrow in less than 1 year without treatment. Total alopecia is rare. Recurrences of alopecia, however, are frequent and 7% to 10% of cases can have a chronic form of the condition. Repeated attacks, nail changes, and total alopecia before puberty are poor prognostic signs.

MANAGEMENT

No treatment changes the course of AA, but some palliative options include topical, intralesional, or systemic steroids; topical irritants (anthralin, tazarotene, azelaic acid); topical minoxidil; topical immunotherapy (diphenylcyclopropenone or squaric acid); PUVA; laser; photodynamic therapy; systemic cyclosporine or methotrexate. Prolonged regimens of various systemic immunosuppressive agents may show some benefit for hair regrowth in some patients. Reported success using the janus kinase (JAK) inhibitor class of medications for treating AA has led to clinical trials examining their efficacy.

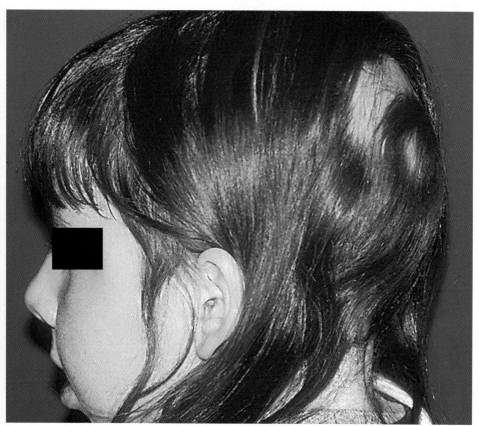

FIGURE 18-4 Alopecia areata, scalp Sudden onset of well-circumscribed areas of nonscarring alopecia in an otherwise healthy child.

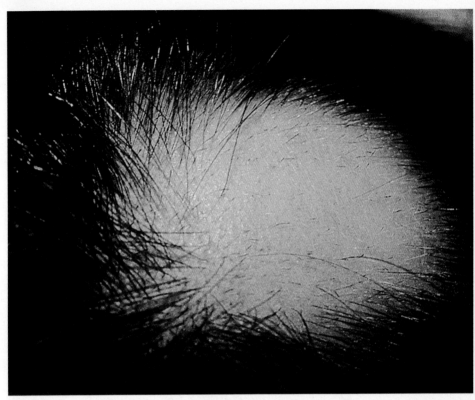

FIGURE 18-5 Alopecia areata, scalp Oval area of nonscarring alopecia on the scalp with evidence of "exclamation point hairs" (short hairs that taper proximally).

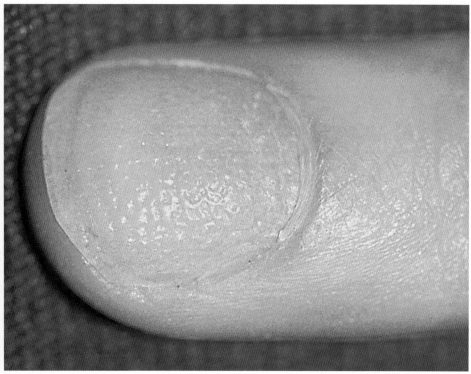

FIGURE 18-6 Alopecia areata, nails Pitting in organized transverse rows giving the nail a "hammered brass" appearance.

CONFLUENT AND RETICULATED PAPILLOMATOSIS OF GOUGEROT AND CARTEAUD

Confluent and reticulated papillomatosis of Gougerot and Carteaud (CARP) is a benign chronic, relapsing rash characterized by elevated, hyperpigmented scaly plaques that begin on the upper trunk, coalesce, and spread slowly with a reticulated pattern over the body.

 INSIGHT A helpful way to conceptualize this sesquipedalian entity is to place it between acanthosis nigricans and tinea versicolor; clinically, it has features reminiscent of both but not quite right for either one.

SYNONYMS Atrophie brilliante, papillomatose pigmentée innominée, erythrokeratodermia papillaris et reticularis, parakeratose brilliante, pigmented reticular dermatosis of the flexures.

EPIDEMIOLOGY

AGE Adolescence, average age of onset: 18 to 20 years.
GENDER F > M, 2:1 except in Japan M > F.
INCIDENCE Rare.
RACE Darker skin types > lighter skin types.
FAMILY Several cases affecting multiple family members.
ETIOLOGY Abnormal keratinocyte maturation and differentiation.

PATHOPHYSIOLOGY

CARP may represent an endocrine abnormality, an atypical response to an infection, a disorder of keratinization, or a hereditary disorder. CRP lesions show elevated keratin production of the skin and increased skin turnover. Hormones seem to play a role since the onset of the rash is associated with puberty, and at times with abnormal glucose tolerance, thyroid problems, menstrual problems, Cushing's disease, obesity, or hirsutism. In some cases, yeast (*Malassezia, Pityrosporum ovale, Pityrosporum orbiculare*) or bacteria (actinomycete *Dietzia*) have been isolated and thought to play a pathogenic role.

HISTORY

Patients with CARP usually report an asymptomatic or mildly pruritic rash that slowly spreads upper trunk to the rest of the body. CARP typically is chronic with relapses, but responds well to therapies.

PHYSICAL EXAMINATION

Skin Lesions

TYPE Papules, plaques, scale.
COLOR Gray, brown, blue.
SHAPE Round to oval, coalescing, reticulated (Fig. 18-7).
SIZE 1 mm to 1 cm.
PALPATION Elevated, warty.
DISTRIBUTION Neck, upper trunk > breasts, armpits, abdomen > shoulders, pubic area, gluteal cleft, face.

DIFFERENTIAL DIAGNOSIS

The differential diagnosis of CARP includes tinea versicolor, AN, verrucae, Darier disease, seborrheic keratoses, epidermal nevus syndrome, pityriasis rubra pilaris, or erythrokeratodermia variabilis.

LABORATORY EXAMINATIONS

DERMATOPATHOLOGY Compact hyperkeratosis (± yeast forms), decreased granular cell layer, papillomatosis, mild perivascular infiltrate.
WOOD'S LAMP Yellow fluorescence if yeast organisms are present.

COURSE AND PROGNOSIS

CARP is a benign skin disorder that results in cosmetic dyspigmentation which can be distressing to the patient. The condition is chronic with exacerbations and remissions. In some cases, after spreading slowly for a few years, the lesions remain permanently unchanged and cause no symptoms.

MANAGEMENT

Several therapies have been used in an attempt to clear CARP and prevent it from recurring. Systemic antibiotics (minocycline, tetracyclines, macrolides, or cephalosporins) show the most improvement. Topical antifungal agents (ketoconazole shampoo, antifungal creams), topical calcipotriol, topical or systemic retinoids are sometimes effective. Weight loss may also be helpful.

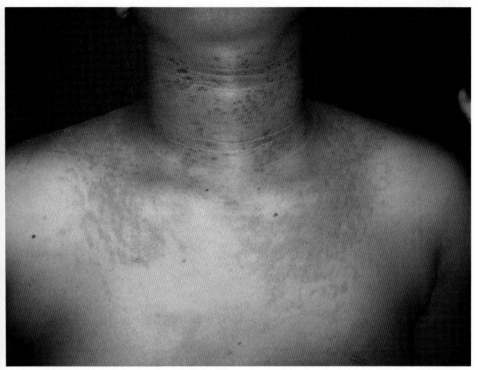

FIGURE 18-7 Confluent and reticulated papillomatosis of Gougerot and Carteaud Scaly hyperpigmented coalescing plaques on the anterior chest.

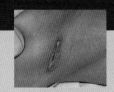

SKIN SIGNS OF RETICULOENDOTHELIAL DISEASE

HISTIOCYTOSIS

The disorders of xanthohistiocytic proliferation involving histiocytes, foam cells, and mixed inflammatory cells are divided into Langerhans cell histiocytosis (LCH) and non-Langerhans cell histiocytosis (non-LCH).

LANGERHANS CELL HISTIOCYTOSIS

LCH is an idiopathic spectrum of disorders characterized by a clonal proliferation of abnormal cells phenotypically similar to Langerhans cells of the skin. Clinically, LCH is characterized by lytic bony lesions and cutaneous findings that range from soft tissue swelling to eczema- and seborrheic dermatitis-like skin changes and ulceration.

INSIGHT Histiocytosis can be extremely difficult to diagnose. In infants with diaper rash that will not heal, particularly if there are erosions in the folds or petechiae/purpura, histiocytosis should be considered.

SYNONYMS Class I histiocytosis, nonlipid reticuloendotheliosis, eosinophilic granulomatosis. Previously termed Histiocytosis X.

CLASSIFICATION

In recent years, a concerted effort has been made to aggregate subforms of the disease under the single disease term LCH, given overlap in clinical and pathophysiologic feature. Prior classification approaches distinguished between the following overlapping subtypes, which we present for historical reference:

1. Letterer–Siwe disease: an aggressive form of LCH with diffuse skin and organ infiltration and thrombocytopenia
2. Hand–Schüller–Christian disease: LCH with lytic skull lesions, exophthalmos, and diabetes insipidus
3. Eosinophilic granuloma: single osteolytic bony lesion ± skin/soft tissue lesion
4. Hashimoto–Pritzker disease: congenital self-healing reticulohistiocytosis.

Given the rarity of the disease, we encourage the single term LCH to encompass the spectrum of disease.

EPIDEMIOLOGY

AGE Any age, most common 1 to 3 years.
GENDER M > F, 2:1.
INCIDENCE Rare, 3 to 5/million children.
GENETICS Familial case reports. Mutations in the BRAF oncogene have been seen in a large percentage of LCH lesions.

PATHOPHYSIOLOGY

The proliferating Langerhans-like cell appears to be primarily responsible for the clinical manifestation of LCH. The stimulus for the proliferation may be a disturbance of intracellular lipid metabolism, a reactive response to infection (possible viral), a primary immunologic disorder of the host, or an inherited neoplastic disorder. Gene expression studies have demonstrated upregulation of factors associated with T-cell recruitment and stimulation in LCH, as well as growth factors including TGF-β.

HISTORY

LCH has a broad clinical spectrum, but in the most aggressive form, the infant appears systemically ill with a generalized skin eruption (seborrhea, petechiae, and purpura) followed by fever, anemia, thrombocytopenia, adenopathy, hepatosplenomegaly, and/or skeletal lesions, demonstrating multisystem involvement. Conversely, in cases of single-system LCH, the affected individual may be asymptomatic.

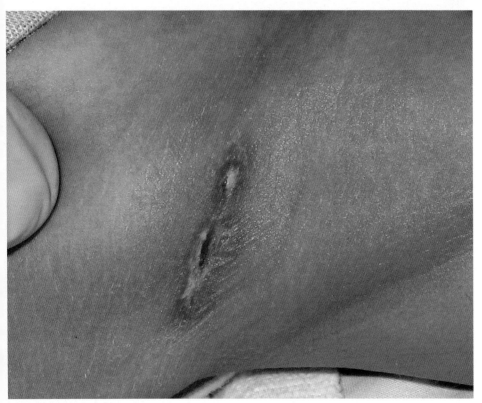

FIGURE 19-1 Histiocytosis X Erythematous plaques with ulceration and maceration in the axilla of an infant.

PHYSICAL EXAMINATION

Skin Findings

TYPE Papules, plaques, vesicles, scale, petechiae, purpura, ulceration, necrosis.
COLOR Pink, flesh-colored.
SIZE 1 to 2 mm up to 1 cm in size.
DISTRIBUTION Flexural areas: neck, axillae (Fig. 19-1), and perineum > trunk (Fig. 19-2).

General Findings

FEVER Lymphadenopathy (LAD). Ill appearance.
PULMONARY 10% of patients. Infiltrative disease of the lung upper and midzones, pneumothorax. Persistent cough.
LIVER Hepatosplenomegaly, transaminitis, clotting factor abnormalities.

BONE 75% of patients. Osteolytic lesions: calvarium, sphenoid bone, sella turcica, mandible, long bones of upper extremities (UEs), vertebrae.
OTHER Otitis media, diabetes insipidus/exophthalmos/bony lesions in previously classified Hand–Schüller–Christian variant.

DIFFERENTIAL DIAGNOSIS

The differential diagnosis of LCH based on skin manifestations is broad given the multiple cutaneous morphologies. The differential includes seborrhea, candidiasis, Darier disease, leukemia, lymphoma, multiple myeloma, urticaria pigmentosa (UP), mycosis fungoides (MF), and non-LCH.

LABORATORY EXAMINATIONS

HISTOPATHOLOGY Proliferation of Langerhans-like cells with distinct morphologic (pale eosinophilic cytoplasm, a kidney-shaped nucleus), ultrastructural (Birbeck granules), and immune-histochemical markers [CD1a$^+$, langerin (CD207)$^+$, ATPase$^+$, S-100$^+$, α-D-mannosidase$^+$, peanut agglutinin$^+$].

RADIOGRAPHIC FINDINGS Osteolytic lesion in calvarium, femur, rib, sphenoid, sella turcica, mandible, long bones of UEs. Chest: diffuse interstitial fibrosis in lung upper and midzones, pneumothorax; high-resolution chest CT demonstrates parenchymal cysts and nodules predominantly in the mid and upper lung zones.

COURSE AND PROGNOSIS

The prognosis of LCH varies according to the extent of systemic involvement. Patients with single-system, unicentric disease have a relatively benign course with excellent prognosis. Patients older than 2 years at the time of diagnosis, without involvement of the hematopoietic system, liver, lungs, or spleen, have 100% probability of survival. However, given the possibility for disease reactivation, close follow-up is recommended (see Management below).

Patients with systemic involvement have a higher mortality rate, especially children diagnosed before age 2 years with liver, lungs, spleen, or hematopoietic involvement. Even with aggressive treatment, mortality ranges up to 66% in this population if there is not early response to treatment. Of note, patients with leukemia (acute lymphoblastic leukemia or acute nonlymphoblastic leukemia) or solid tumors may have an increased incidence of LCH and vice versa.

MANAGEMENT

The management and treatment of LCH is dependent upon the severity and extent of involvement. Mild skin-only LCH can be treated with topical steroids, antibacterial agents, psoralen ultraviolet A (PUVA), topical nitrogen mustard. Diffuse skin disease has been treated with oral methotrexate or oral thalidomide. Localized bony lesions can be treated with nonsteroidal anti-inflammatory drugs (NSAIDs), intralesional steroids, curette with or without bony chip packing, or low-dose (300–600 rads) irradiation. Systemic chemotherapy may be warranted depending on the site of single bony lesions.

Multisystem LCH can be systemically treated with corticosteroids, vinblastine, methotrexate, or epipodophyllotoxin (etoposide). Failure to respond to treatment after 6 weeks of these drugs is a poor prognostic indicator. Even in responsive patients, there is a high (58%) rate of LCH reactivity. Reactive disease can be treated with additional chemotherapy regimens, etanercept, cyclosporine, 2-chloro-deoxyadenosine, or imatinib mesylate. Finally, in recalcitrant cases, bone marrow, stem cell liver or lung transplantation may be necessary. Given the rarity of the disease, enrolment in a clinical trial may provide patients with access to the latest therapeutic approaches and insights to the disease.

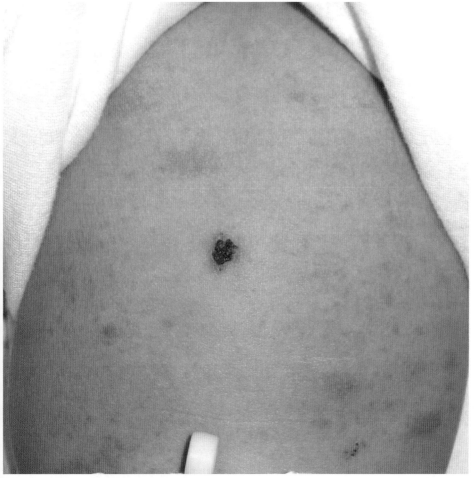

FIGURE 19-2 Langerhans cell histiocytosis Erythematous papules and a crusted, purpuric plaque on the abdomen of an infant.

NON-LANGERHANS CELL HISTIOCYTOSIS

Non-LCH encompasses a spectrum of disorders with a benign, cutaneous self-resolving proliferation of mononuclear phagocytes other than Langerhans cells. Clinical forms include juvenile xanthogranulomas (JXGs), benign cephalic histiocytosis, generalized eruptive histiocytosis, and indeterminate cell histiocytosis, which may represent different expressions of the same pathologic process. Rare forms in the adult population include Erdheim Chester disease, Rosai Dorfman disease, and multicentric reticulohistiocytosis.
SYNONYM Non-X histiocytosis.

JUVENILE XANTHOGRANULOMA

JXGs are common, benign, self-healing lesions of infancy and childhood characterized by one or several red to yellow papules and nodules on the skin and rarely in other organs.

SYNONYM Nevoxanthoendothelioma (a misnomer).

EPIDEMIOLOGY

AGE Birth (15%) to before age 1 year (75%).
GENDER M > F, 1.5:1.
INCIDENCE Most common form histiocytosis.
ETIOLOGY Unclear. Possibly reactive granuloma to unknown cause.

PATHOPHYSIOLOGY

The exact pathophysiology is unknown. Postulated mechanisms include a histiocytic proliferation to unknown traumatic or infectious stimulus.

HISTORY

Asymptomatic cutaneous JXGs are present at or soon after birth, may proliferate in number and size for 1 to 2 years, and then both cutaneous and visceral lesions involute spontaneously within 3 to 6 years.

PHYSICAL EXAMINATION

Skin Findings

TYPE Papules to nodules.
COLOR Red–brown (Fig. 19-3), transitioning to yellow quickly.
SIZE 2 to 20 mm in diameter.
SHAPE Round to ovoid.
NUMBER Solitary or multiple (can be hundreds; Fig. 19-4).
PALPATION Firm or rubbery.
DISTRIBUTION Face, scalp, neck > upper trunk > UEs > lower extremities > mucous membranes.

General Findings

OCULAR Ocular JXG (0.5%).
OTHER Rarely associated with systemic lesions (lungs, bones, kidneys, pericardium, colon, ovaries, testes), café au lait macules, Neurofibromatosis-1, juvenile myelomonocytic leukemia.

DIFFERENTIAL DIAGNOSIS

The differential for JXG includes UP, benign cephalic histiocytosis, generalized eruptive histiocytosis, self-healing reticulohistiocytosis, xanthomas, histiocytosis X, and nevi.

LABORATORY EXAMINATIONS

DERMATOPATHOLOGY Monomorphous, non–lipid-containing histiocytic infiltrate, may have foamy cells, foreign body giant cells, and Touton giant cells in the superficial dermis and periphery of the infiltrate. Fat stains are positive. Electron microscopy shows histiocytes with comma-shaped bodies, lipid vacuoles, cholesterol clefts, and myeloid bodies. Immunohistochemical stains are CD34+, CD163+, HAM56+, CD68+, factor XIIIa+. S100 and CD1a – markers of Langerhans cells – are negative.

COURSE AND PROGNOSIS

JXG skin lesions are often present at birth or during the first 9 months of life, run a benign course, often increasing in number until age 1 to 1.5 years, and then spontaneously involute. Rarely, systemic lesions involving the eyes, lung, pericardium, meninges, liver, spleen, and testes also occur. The patient's general health is not affected and development progresses normally.

Ocular JXGs are the most worrisome because of complications such as glaucoma, hemorrhage, and blindness. In rare instances, JXG may be associated with neurofibromatosis 1, and these patients have an increased risk of juvenile myelomonocytic leukemia.

MANAGEMENT

No treatment is necessary for the cutaneous lesions because they will involute without intervention. Ocular lesions may require

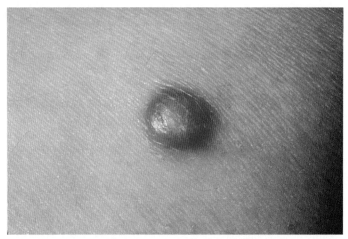

FIGURE 19-3 Juvenile xanthogranuloma Solitary red-brown nodule on the arm of a small child.

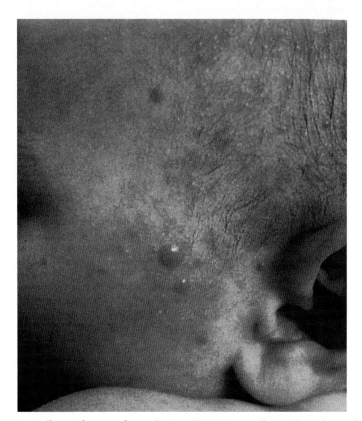

FIGURE 19-4 Juvenile xanthogranuloma Scattered 3- to 7-mm yellow-red papules on the face of a child with generalized lesions.

radiation and/or topical or systemic steroids to avert complications of glaucoma, hemorrhage, or blindness. Rare cases of systemic JXGs will also spontaneously involute, but severe symptomatic cases can be treated with systemic chemotherapy, radiotherapy, corticosteroids, or cyclosporine.

MASTOCYTOSIS SYNDROMES

The mastocytosis syndromes are a spectrum of clinical disorders associated with a proliferation of mast cells within the skin and, rarely, other organs (the liver, spleen, and lymph nodes).

CLASSIFICATION

Childhood cutaneous mastocytosis is distinct from adult mastocytosis and has three clinical forms:

1. Solitary mastocytoma (20%): individual lesion(s) typically on distal extremities
2. UP: generalized lesions over trunk
3. Diffuse cutaneous mastocytosis: erythrodermic infant with a boggy or doughy skin

An additional form of cutaneous mastocytosis (telangiectasia macularis eruptiva perstans) is also described (most often in adults and very rarely in children).

SYNONYMS Bullous mastocytoma, bullous UP, bullous mastocytosis.

EPIDEMIOLOGY

AGE By age 2 years (55%), 2 to 15 years (10%).
GENDER M = F.
INCIDENCE 1 in 8,000 children.
PREVALENCE Estimated 1/10,000 prevalence.
GENETICS Reported familial cases, but majority are sporadic.

PATHOPHYSIOLOGY

Alterations in the receptor tyrosine kinase KIT (CD117) structure and activity have been implicated in adult mastocytosis and some cases of extensive skin/systemic childhood mastocytosis, with gain of function mutations often present. Other mast cell growth promoting mechanisms (such as increased soluble stem cell factor) are likely responsible for the majority of childhood mastocytosis syndromes. Mast cell concentrations are 150-fold higher in childhood mastocytomas and 40-fold higher in childhood UP than normal skin. Mast cell activity is also higher. Degranulated mast cells release vasoactive substances such as histamine [leading to urticaria and gastrointestinal (GI)] symptoms], prostaglandin D_2 (leading to flushing, cardiac and GI symptoms), heparin, and neutral protease/acid hydrolases.

HISTORY

In children, mastocytosis typically begins before age 2 with one to many scattered cutaneous lesions. The lesions may be flat or slightly raised but have a tendency to become red and form an urticarial wheal or bulla with gentle rubbing, exercise, hot baths, or histamine-releasing drugs (NSAIDs, alcohol, dextran, polymyxin B, morphine, codeine). Children rarely have systemic symptoms, but with extensive cutaneous involvement, a flushing episode may be accompanied by headache, diarrhea, wheezing, or syncope. Diffuse cutaneous mastocytosis presents as a diffusely erythrodermic infant with a boggy or doughy appearance.

PHYSICAL EXAMINATION

Skin Findings

TYPE Macule/papule, urticarial wheals/ plaques or bullae when gently stroked (Darier's sign; Fig. 19-5).
COLOR Reddish-brown hyperpigmented color.
SIZE 1 mm to several centimeters.
NUMBER Solitary lesions or multiple (hundreds; Fig. 19-6).
DISTRIBUTION Trunk, extremities, neck > scalp, face, palms, soles, mucous membranes (Fig. 19-7).

DIFFERENTIAL DIAGNOSIS

The differential diagnosis for mastocytosis includes urticaria, insect bites, bullous impetigo, viral infection, lentigines, café au lait macules, JXG, nevi, linear IgA disease, and other autoimmune bullous dermatoses.

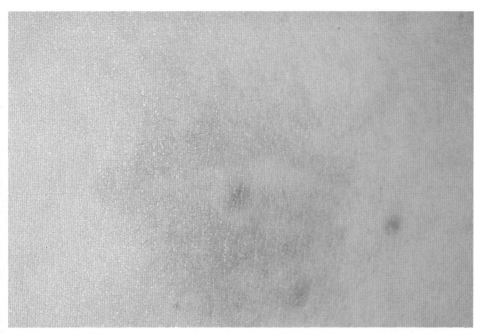

FIGURE 19-5 Solitary mastocytoma, Darier's sign Reddish-brown macules that urticate with mild trauma indicative of mastocytosis.

LABORATORY EXAMINATIONS

DERMATOPATHOLOGY Accumulation of mast cells in the dermis. Mast cell infiltrates may be sparse (spindle-shaped mast cells), dense (cube-shaped mast cells), interstitial, or nodular. Toluidine blue, Giemsa and Leder stains, or immunohistochemical stains for tryptase, chymase, carboxypeptidase A3, and CD117 (KIT) can help identify tissue mast cells.

SERUM α-Tryptase levels are elevated in symptomatic or asymptomatic patients with systemic mastocytosis. β-Tryptase (mature tryptase) is elevated in patients with anaphylaxis related or unrelated to mastocytosis. Total (α- and β-) serum tryptase levels can be correlated with the extent of mast cell disease in patients. More than 75 ng/mL total serum tryptase indicates definite systemic involvement, whereas only 50% of patients with levels between 20 and 75 ng/mL have systemic disease. If the total serum tryptase level is above 20 ng/mL on at least two occasions, systemic mastocytosis should be suspected.

URINE Patients with systemic mastocytosis or extensive cutaneous involvement may have increased 24-hour urinary histamine or histamine metabolite excretion. Of note, foods with high histamine content (spinach, eggplant, cheese, red wine) will artificially elevate urinary histamine.

BONE MARROW BIOPSY In bone marrow biopsies of children with UP, 18% can have mast cell infiltration.

COURSE AND PROGNOSIS

When seen in children younger than 10 years, all forms of mastocytosis have a good prognosis. Most childhood disease has limited cutaneous involvement; 50% of cases spontaneously remit by adolescence and another 25% of cases resolve by adulthood. Systemic involvement appears to affect <5% of children with mastocytosis. This percentage is much higher in adults with mastocytosis and their prognosis is much worse. When systemic involvement occurs, mast cells infiltrate the bones, liver, spleen, and lymph nodes. The presence of mast cells in the peripheral blood of patients with mastocytosis is a poor prognostic sign.

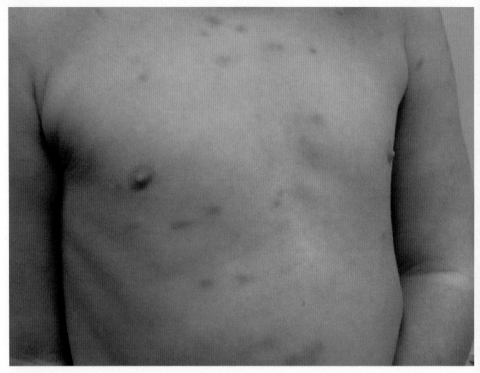

FIGURE 19-6 Mastocytosis, urticaria pigmentosa Numerous scattered red-brown macules on the body of a child.

MANAGEMENT

Solitary mastocytosis and UP cutaneous lesions self-resolve and need no treatment. Moderate sunlight exposure can help diffuse skin lesions resolve. Patients with numerous lesions or diffuse cutaneous mastocytosis should be counseled to avoid potential mast cell degranulating agents including aspirin, NSAIDs, codeine, opiates, procaine, alcohol, polymyxin B sulfate, radiographic dyes, ketorolac, scopolamine, systemic lidocaine, D-tubocurarine, metocurine, etomidate, thiopental, succinylcholine hydrochloride, enflurane, isoflurane, gallamine, decamethonium, and pancuronium. Hot baths, vigorous rubbing after baths or showers, tight clothing, and extremes of temperature may also potentiate mast cell degranulation.

Antihistamines may be helpful in mastocytosis. Second-generation H_1-blockers (cetirizine, loratadine, and fexofenadine) may work better than first-generation H_1-blockers (diphenhydramine, hydroxyzine HCl). Ketotifen fumarate or doxepin can be potent H_1-blockers used in conjunction with H_2-blockers. H_2-blockers (cimetidine, ranitidine, famotidine, or nizatidine) can be used in combination with H_1-blockers, particularly for controlling abdominal symptoms in cases of systemic mastocytosis.

Other medications that have been helpful for mastocytosis include oral cromolyn sodium, montelukast, zafirlukast, zileuton, PUVA, topical, intralesional or systemic steroids, cyclosporine, or interferon-α-2b.

Symptomatic patients with mastocytosis should carry an epinephrine pen because severe allergic reactions with anaphylaxis and hypotension can occur. Additional diagnostic evaluation should be performed in patients with evidence of further organ system involvement, such as GI bleeding, abdominal pain, enlarged liver or spleen, bone pain, or blood abnormalities.

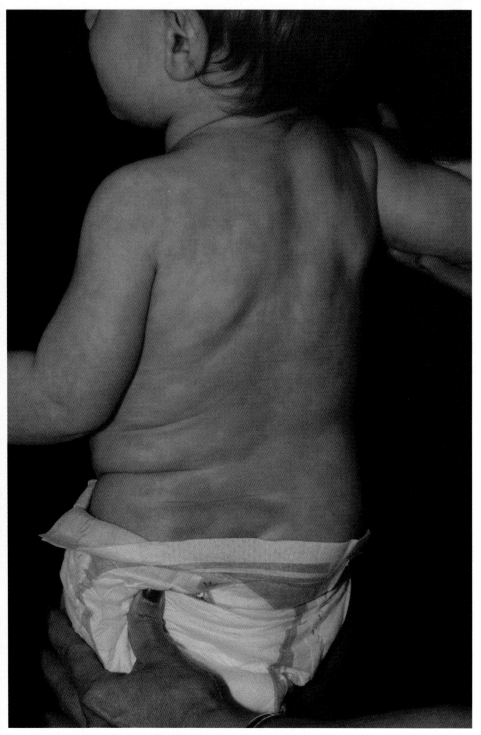

FIGURE 19-7 Diffuse cutaneous mastocytosis Large confluent orange-brown plaques on the body of a child.

LYMPHOMATOID PAPULOSIS

Lymphomatoid papulosis (LyP) is a recurrent self-healing papulovesicular dermatosis of the trunk and extremities with histologic features of lymphocytic atypia, but a low risk of malignant transformation.

CLASSIFICATION

LyP is part of a spectrum of CD30 (Ki-1)-positive cutaneous lymphoproliferative diseases (CD30⁺ lymphoproliferative disorders), including LyP, primary cutaneous anaplastic large cell lymphoma (pcALCL), and borderline CD30⁺ lesions.
SYNONYMS Macaulay disease, lymphoproliferative disorder.

EPIDEMIOLOGY

AGE Any age. Peak: 50 years.
GENDER M > F among childhood cases.
INCIDENCE 1 to 2/million.
RACE Blacks less frequently affected.
ETIOLOGY Unclear. Possible activated T cells responding to external or internal stimuli or an indolent skin T-cell malignancy held in check by the host immune system.

PATHOPHYSIOLOGY

The pathophysiology of LyP is unknown. CD30 signaling is important for the growth and survival of lymphoid cells; thus, accumulated genetic defects may have a role in the development of LyP. Cellular expression of Bcl-2, an antiapoptotic factor, may also stimulate the development of the CD30⁺ cells. Clinically, LyP spontaneously regresses, and Bax (a proapoptotic protein) or FADD (Fas-associating protein with death domain) may mediate the apoptosis of tumor cells.

HISTORY

LyP begins as asymptomatic or mildly pruritic macules and papules that appear in crops within 1 to 4 weeks. Ulceration may occur. Lesions typically resolve within 2 to 8 weeks or may recur and persist for decades. Constitutional symptoms (low-grade fever, malaise, night sweats) rarely occur.

PHYSICAL EXAMINATION

Skin Findings

TYPE Papules, vesiculopapules, scale, crust, ulcers, scars.

COLOR Red-brown, hemorrhagic, hypo- or hyperpigmented (Fig. 19-8).
SIZE 2 to 30 mm in diameter.
DISTRIBUTION Trunk, proximal extremities > hands, feet, scalp.
MUCOUS MEMBRANES Oral, genital mucosa rarely affected.

General Findings

LYMPHADENOPATHY (LAD) Regional or generalized LAD may be present.

DIFFERENTIAL DIAGNOSIS

The differential for LyP includes folliculitis, insect bites, LCH, milia, miliaria, scabies, pityriasis lichenoides et varioliformis acuta, cutaneous Hodgkin lymphoma, or cutaneous T-cell lymphoma (CTCL).

LABORATORY EXAMINATIONS

DERMATOPATHOLOGY Dense mixed cell infiltrate with a wedge- or band-like distribution on the upper dermis. The infiltrate is composed of histiocytes, eosinophils, plasma cells, and strikingly atypical lymphocytes with convoluted nuclei. According to the principal morphologic type, LyP is classified into three types: type A, which consists of large atypical lymphocytes with multinucleated variants and cells resembling Sternberg–Reed cells; type B, composed of cerebriform lymphocytes similar to cells in CTCL; and type C, with sheets of anaplastic large cells indistinguishable from ALCL.
IMMUNOHISTOLOGY Dominant cells in LyP express CD30 (Ki-1) antigen. Tumor cells may express CD56, TIA-1, granzyme B, or CXCR3. Clonality in LyP is controversial.

COURSE AND PROGNOSIS

In 90% of childhood LyP cases, the lesions usually resolve after 3 to 8 weeks or may have a slightly prolonged course. Crops of lesions may recur. Ten to twenty percent of adult patients may progress to malignant lymphoma (ALCL, Hodgkin disease, or MF) but no patients with LyP die of the disease. Development of nodules or tumors may be a useful clinical sign for malignant transformation of the disease

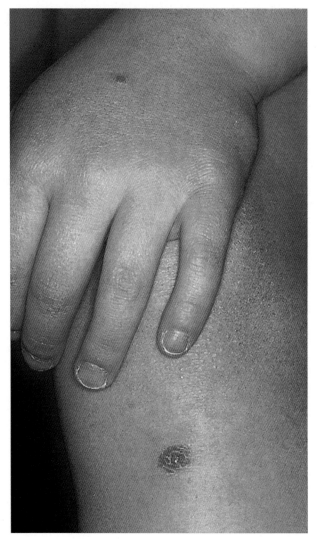

FIGURE 19-8 Lymphomatoid papulosis Few scattered red-brown papules and nodules on the extremities of a young otherwise healthy child.

and patients with such lesions should have a systemic workup.

MANAGEMENT

No treatments have been proven to be consistently effective. Many childhood cases resolve spontaneously or with sunlight exposure. Symptomatic, pruritic lesions can be treated with topical steroids or phototherapy. Because of the risk of malignant transformation, especially in adults, careful long-term follow-up is recommended.

For more severe or refractory and extensive disease in adults, both topical and systemic treatments have been tried. Topical treatments include carmustine, nitrogen mustard, imiquimod, and intralesional interferon. Systemic treatments such as steroids, antibiotics (tetracycline, erythromycin), sulfones, PUVA, UVA-1, electron beam, excimer laser, low-dose methotrexate, acyclovir, retinoids, chlorambucil, cyclophosphamide, cyclosporine, and dapsone have been reportedly effective.

CUTANEOUS T-CELL LYMPHOMA

CTCL applies to T-cell lymphoma, which first manifests in the skin and slowly progresses to lymph nodes and internal organs.

SYNONYMS MF (technically a subtype of CTCL), large plaque parapsoriasis.

EPIDEMIOLOGY

AGE All ages. Peak: 50 to 70 years.
GENDER M > F, 2:1.
RACE African American > Caucasian.
INCIDENCE Incidence 5/million. Causes 1% of deaths from lymphoma (about 200 deaths/year in the United States). Accounts for 4% of all non-Hodgkin Lymphoma in the United States.
ETIOLOGY Unknown. Chemical, physical, and microbial irritants may lead to an accumulation of mutations in oncogenes, suppressor genes, and signal-transducing genes.

PATHOPHYSIOLOGY

The pathophysiology of CTCL is unknown. Genetic instability followed by T-cell proliferation may produce numerous clonal chromosomal aberrations. Alteration in systemic cytokine expression may drive the pathogenesis of CTCL, or may reflect a response to the malignancy.

HISTORY

Skin symptoms are the presenting symptom of CTCL and often last for months to years with nonspecific diagnoses such as psoriasis, nummular dermatitis, or eczema. The skin lesions wax and wane and are asymptomatic or mildly pruritic. Systemically, the patient feels well until the skin becomes diffusely involved (erythrodermic CTCL), significant populations of circulating lymphoma cells develop (Sézary syndrome), or visceral organs become involved, in which case fever and B symptoms are likely.

PHYSICAL EXAMINATION

Skin Findings

TYPE Plaques, scale, "infiltrated" (Fig. 19-9), nodules, tumors, ulcers.
COLOR Red, pink, purple.
SHAPE Round, oval, arciform, annular, concentric, or bizarre configurations.
SIZE >3 cm.

ARRANGEMENT Discrete plaques, nodules, and tumors, or diffuse erythroderma (Sézary syndrome) and palmoplantar keratoderma.
DISTRIBUTION Buttocks, sun-protected areas > exposed areas.

General Findings

LYMPHADENOPATHY/HEPATOSPLENOMEGALY In late disease, LAD and/or splenomegaly may be present.
SÉZARY SYNDROME Leukemic form of CTCL consisting of (1) erythroderma, (2) LAD, (3) elevated WBC (>20,000) with a high proportion of so-called Sézary cells, (4) hair loss, and (5) intense pruritus.

DIFFERENTIAL DIAGNOSIS

In the early stages, the diagnosis of CTCL is difficult to recognize and may be mistaken for refractory psoriasis, eczema, contact dermatitis, irritant dermatitis, tinea corporis, or poikiloderma atrophicans vasculare.

LABORATORY EXAMINATIONS

Repeated and multiple (three) biopsies are often necessary.
DERMATOPATHOLOGY Dermal band-like, patchy infiltrate of atypical lymphocytes extending to skin appendages. Epidermal T cells with hyperchromatic, irregularly shaped nuclei and mitoses may be present. Intraepidermal collections of atypical cells (Pautrier microabscesses) are highly characteristic. Monoclonal antibody techniques identify most atypical cells as helper/inducer T cells. A dominant T-cell clone can be demonstrated by flow cytometry or polymerase chain reaction.

COURSE AND PROGNOSIS

Children typically live for 10 to 15 years before CTCL ever progresses to any worrisome degree.

MANAGEMENT

Children with CTCL need conservative symptomatic treatment with sunlight exposure, antipruritic creams or topical steroids, and routine long-term follow-up.

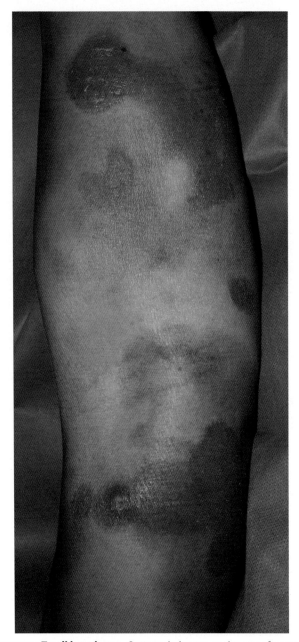

FIGURE 19-9 Cutaneous T-cell lymphoma Scattered plaques on the arm of a young adult.

For histologically proven plaque-stage CTCL, treatment possibilities include PUVA, topical nitrogen mustard, topical carmustine, bexarotene gel, tazarotene gel, total skin electron beam therapy, radiotherapy, interferon, bexarotene, methotrexate, etoposide, interferon-α, interleukin-2, receptor-targeted cytotoxic fusion proteins, alemtuzumab, or extracorporeal photopheresis. Additional experimental agents are continuing to be studied in multiple clinical trials.

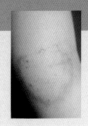

SECTION 20

CUTANEOUS BACTERIAL INFECTIONS

IMPETIGO

Impetigo is a common superficial infection of the skin characterized by honey-colored crusts or bullae, typically caused by *Staphylococcus aureus,* sometimes caused by *Streptococcus pyogenes,* or both.

INSIGHT Bacterial resistance such as community-acquired methicillin-resistant *Staphylococcus aureus* (MRSA) is becoming more prevalent; thus, treatment of infections must take evolving resistance patterns into account.

SYNONYMS Bullous impetigo, blistering distal dactylitis, impetigo contagiosa.

EPIDEMIOLOGY

AGE Preschool children, young adults.
GENDER M = F.
INCIDENCE Common; up to 10% of dermatology visits.
SEASON Peak summer and fall.
ETIOLOGY Bullous impetigo is most often caused by *Staphylococcus aureus* phage group II strains which produce exfoliative toxin A or B. Vesiculopustular impetigo is often caused by *Staphylococcus aureus* or group A β-hemolytic *Streptococcus* species.
PREDISPOSING FACTORS Colonization of the skin and/or nares of the patient or patient's family members, warm temperatures, high humidity, poor hygiene, atopic diathesis, skin trauma.

PATHOPHYSIOLOGY

Crusted impetigo is caused by *S. aureus* or occasionally *S. pyogenes* at sites of skin trauma. Bullous impetigo is caused by an *S. aureus* exfoliative toxin A, which binds to desmoglein 1, cleaving its extracellular domain, resulting in an intraepidermal blister.

HISTORY

The skin lesions begin as erythematous areas, which may progress to superficial vesicles and bullae that rupture and form honey-colored crusts. The skin lesions are contagious and spread by person-to-person contact or fomites. Systemic symptoms are rare but can include fever and lymphadenopathy.

PHYSICAL EXAMINATION

Skin Findings

TYPE Macules, vesicles, bullae, crusts, and erosions (Fig. 20-1).
COLOR Pink, yellow "stuck-on" crusts. Pustules may appear whitish-yellow.
SIZE 1 to 3 cm.
SHAPE Round or oval.
ARRANGEMENT Discrete, confluent, or satellite lesions from autoinoculation.
DISTRIBUTION Face, arms, legs, buttocks, distal fingers (Fig. 20-2), toes.

DIFFERENTIAL DIAGNOSIS

In the early vesicular stage, impetigo may simulate varicella, herpes simplex, or candidiasis. The bullous stage may be confused with bullous insect bites, autoimmune bullous dermatoses, adverse drug reactions, or burns. The crusted stage may resemble eczematous dermatoses or tinea infections.

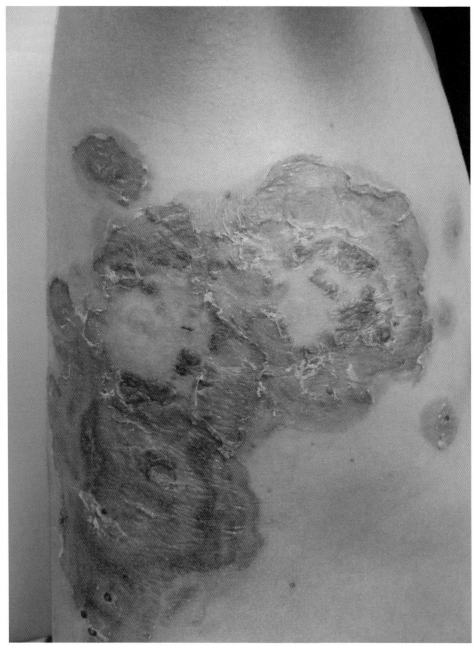

FIGURE 20-1 **Impetigo, bullous** Blisters and honey-colored crusts on the torso of a young child.

LABORATORY EXAMINATIONS

DERMATOPATHOLOGY Acantholytic cleft in the stratum granulosum with leukocytes; may also show scattered gram-positive cocci. Bacteria can be seen within the blister cavity of bullous lesions.

BACTERIAL CULTURE Group A streptococci and sometimes a mixed culture of streptococci and *S. aureus* can be cultured from lesions or nasopharynx. Use of a moistened culture swab to dissolve crusts may be necessary to isolate the pathogens.

COURSE AND PROGNOSIS

Impetigo is a benign but recurrent and contagious condition. Untreated, it can persist for 3 to 6 weeks and continue to spread. Once treatment is initiated, the clinical response is swift and effective. In 5% of cases of β-hemolytic *S. pyogenes* impetigo (serotypes 1, 4, 12, 25, and 49), acute glomerulonephritis can ensue.

MANAGEMENT

Preventive measures include antibacterial soaps, washes, and maintaining good hygiene.

For uncomplicated cases of impetigo, topical treatment is effective. Topical mupirocin, retapamulin, or fusidic acid ointments are highly effective in eliminating both *S. aureus* and *Streptococcus*. If bacterial nasal colonization is suspected or identified, the lower inner third of the nares should be treated to eradicate a chronic carriage state. All close household and/or family members should be treated at the same time because asymptomatic nasal carriage of the pathogenic bacteria can occur.

Systemic antibiotic therapy may be considered for moderate or refractory cases. The prevalence of MRSA has increased over the last decades; thus, traditional penicillin no longer seems as effective as β-lactamase-resistant penicillins (dicloxacillin), macrolides (erythromycin, clarithromycin), or cephalosporins. The risk of poststreptococcal glomerulonephritis is not decreased by administration of systemic antibiotics.

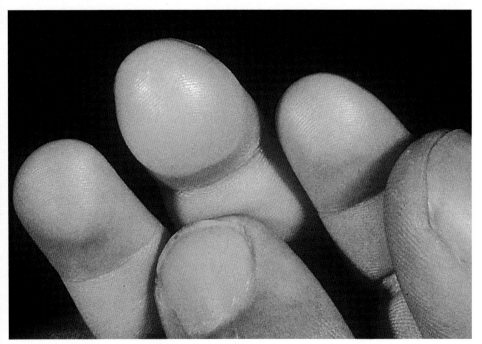

FIGURE 20-2 Blistering distal dactylitis Tense fluid-filled blister on the fingertip of a young boy with *S. aureus* nasal carriage. (Slide used with permission from Dr. Lisa M. Cohen.)

ECTHYMA

Ecthyma is a deep or ulcerative bacterial infection of the skin characterized by ulcers, typically occurring on the buttocks or legs of children.

SYNONYMS Ecthyma minor, ecthyma major.

EPIDEMIOLOGY

AGE Children, adolescents, elderly.
GENDER M = F.
INCIDENCE Common.
ETIOLOGY Group A streptococci or *S. aureus*, or both.

PATHOPHYSIOLOGY

Skin bacteria grow in excoriations, insect bites, and sites of trauma, particularly in susceptible individuals like young children, persons with lymphedematous limbs, poor hygiene, or immunosuppression. The extension of bacteria into the dermis results in the deeper lesions of ecthyma in contrast to the superficial lesions of impetigo.

HISTORY

Lesions begin as excoriations or insect bites with superinfection leading to saucer-shaped ulcers with a raised margin and a "punched out" appearance. The lesions are pruritic and tender and heal slowly, usually with scar formation. Systemic symptoms and bacteremia are rarely seen.

PHYSICAL EXAMINATION

Skin Findings

TYPE Vesicle, pustule, ulcer, scar (Fig. 20-3).
COLOR Purple, yellowish-gray crust.
SIZE 0.5 to 3.0 cm.

SHAPE Round or oval with a "punched out" appearance.
PALPATION Indurated, tender.
DISTRIBUTION Ankles; dorsa of feet, thighs, buttocks.

DIFFERENTIAL DIAGNOSIS

Ecthyma can be confused with ecthyma gangrenosum and other ulcers such as from vasculitis.

LABORATORY EXAMINATIONS

Skin Culture

Group A streptococci, staphylococci.

COURSE AND PROGNOSIS

Lesions persist for weeks and are slow to heal. They often heal with a resultant scar. Bacteremia is rarely seen, thus cellulitis and osteomyelitis are uncommon.

MANAGEMENT

Ecthyma should be treated with warm soaks to remove crusts. Systemic antibiotic therapy may be considered for moderate or refractory cases. The prevalence of MRSA has increased over the last decades; β-lactamase-resistant penicillins (dicloxacillin), macrolides (erythromycin, clarithromycin), or cephalosporins may be considered first-line agents for streptococcal infections, with trimethoprim-sulfamethoxazole, clindamycin, or tetracyclines (in appropriate age groups) useful for MRSA.

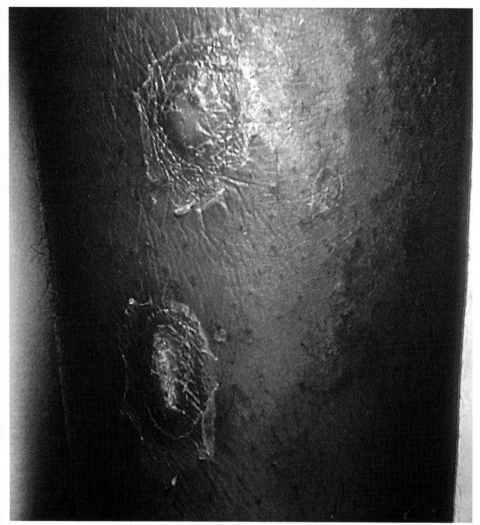

FIGURE 20-3 Ecthyma Crusted nodules on the leg of a child.

FOLLICULITIS

Folliculitis is a superficial or deep inflammation (often bacterial) of hair follicles. Different types occur on different regions of the body (Table 20-1).

SYNONYMS Bockhart's impetigo; sycosis barbae.

EPIDEMIOLOGY

AGE All ages.
INCIDENCE Common.
ETIOLOGY Bacterial: *S. aureus* most common.

PATHOPHYSIOLOGY

Folliculitis occurs when there is inflammation or infection of the hair follicle. The cause is most often bacterial (*S. aureus, Pseudomonas*) especially in skin that is occluded, macerated, or wet. It can be exacerbated by shaving, plucking or waxing hair, hot/humid weather, topical steroids, tar, or mineral oils.

HISTORY

Folliculitis begins with inflammation of the follicular ostium that may be symptomatic or pruritic. Deep-seated inflammation of the hair follicle may be more tender (see Furuncle). Systemic symptoms are not typically present.

PHYSICAL EXAMINATION

Skin Findings

TYPE Papules, pustules.
COLOR Pink, red, yellow, gray.
SIZE 1 to 5 mm.
ARRANGEMENT Confined to the ostium of the hair follicles (Fig. 20-4).
DISTRIBUTION Scalp, face, chest, back, buttocks, extremities.

LABORATORY EXAMINATIONS

GRAM STAIN Gram-positive cocci.
CULTURE *S. aureus* >> *Candida albicans, Pseudomonas aeruginosa* > Streptococcus, Proteus, or *Staphylococcus epidermidis*.

DIFFERENTIAL DIAGNOSIS

The differential diagnosis for folliculitis includes acne, rosacea, keratosis pilaris, flat warts, molluscum contagiosum, tinea barbae, tinea corporis, and pustular miliaria.

MANAGEMENT

In the treatment of folliculitis, occlusive agents or precipitants (clothes, topical oils, etc.) should be removed.

For uncomplicated cases, folliculitis can be managed with antibacterial soaps and washes (benzoyl peroxide, chlorhexidine, or triclosan). For localized disease, topical antibiotics (mupirocin, bacitracin, erythromycin, or clindamycin) are highly effective. If bacterial nasal colonization is suspected or identified, the lower inner third of the nares should be treated to eradicate a chronic carriage state. All close household and/or family members should be treated at the same time because asymptomatic nasal carriage of the pathogenic bacteria can occur. Dilute bleach baths may also be useful for bacterial decolonization and prevention of recurrent folliculitis.

Systemic antibiotic therapy may be considered for moderate-to-severe, refractory, widespread, or recurrent cases. Despite rising bacterial-resistance rates, folliculitis continues to be responsive to β-lactam antibiotics (penicillins, cephalosporins), macrolides (erythromycin, clarithromycin), and lincosamides (clindamycin).

TABLE 20-1 Types of Folliculitis

Location	Synonym	Etiology
Neck	Acne keloidalis nuchae, folliculitis keloidalis nuchae	*Staphylococcus aureus*, ingrown hairs, curly hairs
Back	Periporitis suppurativa	*Candida albicans*
Buttocks, body	Hot tub folliculitis, whirlpool folliculitis, pseudomonas folliculitis	*Pseudomonas aeruginosa* acquired from hot tubs
Face	Folliculitis barbae, sycosis barbae, pseudofolliculitis barbae	*Staphylococcus aureus*, ingrown hairs

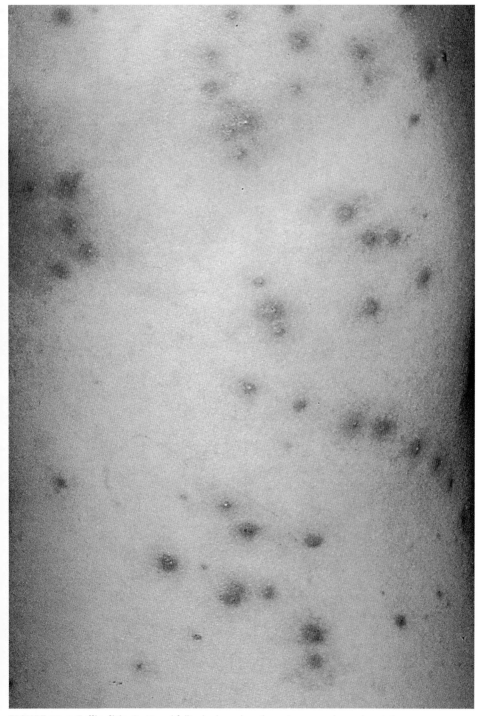

FIGURE 20-4 Folliculitis Scattered follicular-based erythematous papules and pustules.

FURUNCLES AND CARBUNCLES

Furuncle is an acute, deep-seated, red, hot, tender inflammatory nodule that frequently evolves from a folliculitis. A carbuncle is a large lesion of coalescing furuncles.

SYNONYMS Boils, abscesses.

EPIDEMIOLOGY

AGE Adolescents and young adults.
GENDER M > F.
INCIDENCE Common.
ETIOLOGY *S. aureus* most common. Anaerobic bacteria in the anogenital region.

PATHOPHYSIOLOGY

Furuncles are inflammatory areas of pus involving the entire hair follicle and surrounding tissue. A contiguous collection of furuncles makes a carbuncle. The predisposing factor for both include chronic staphylococcal carrier state in nares, axillae or perineum, friction of collars or belts, obesity, poor hygiene, bactericidal defects (e.g., in chronic granulomatous disease), defects in chemotaxis, and in hyperimmunoglobulin E (IgE) syndrome, diabetes mellitus.

HISTORY

Furuncles result from folliculitis that becomes deeper and larger from friction or maceration. They begin as enlarging tender, red nodules that become painful, fluctuant, and then rupture. With numerous furuncles that coalesce, carbuncles can ensue. Systemic symptoms are rare but can include low-grade fever and malaise. Occasionally, lymphadenopathy or peripheral leukocytosis may also occur with widespread lesions.

PHYSICAL EXAMINATION

Skin Findings

TYPE Nodules, pustules, ulcers, scars.
COLOR Bright red (Fig. 20-5).

PALPATION Indurated, firm, tender.
ARRANGEMENT Scattered, discrete.
DISTRIBUTION Hair follicles and in areas subject to friction and sweating: neck, scalp, face, axillae, buttocks, thighs, and perineum.

LABORATORY EXAMINATION

DERMATOPATHOLOGY Subcutaneous dense neutrophilic infiltrate with a suppurative reaction around the hair follicle below the infundibulum, perifollicular necrosis, and fibrinoid debris.
SKIN CULTURE Incision and drainage of lesions for Gram stain, culture, and antibiotic sensitivity studies with identification of the bacteria (*S. aureus* >> anaerobic bacteria).
BLOOD CULTURE In rare cases with fever and/or constitutional symptoms; if blood culture is positive, systemic antibiotics may be necessary.

DIFFERENTIAL DIAGNOSIS

Furuncles and carbuncles can sometime be confused with ruptured cysts, hidradenitis suppurativa, or acne.

COURSE AND PROGNOSIS

Furuncles and carbuncles resolve, but some need incision, drainage, and systemic antibiotic treatment. Some patients are subject to recurrent furunculosis and these patients and their family members need to be treated simultaneously and aggressively to eradicate recurrences. At times, furunculosis is complicated by bacteremia and possible hematogenous seeding of heart valves, joints, spine, long bones, and viscera (especially kidneys).

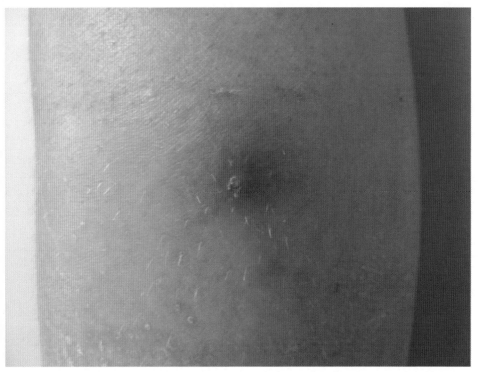

FIGURE 20-5 Furuncle Deep-seated, tender furuncle on the leg of a teenage girl.

MANAGEMENT

Simple furunculosis is treated by local application of heat, such as with warm compresses. Fluctuant lesions may require incision and drainage, particularly for carbuncles. No systemic antibiotics are needed except in patients with systemic symptoms, patients with furunculosis in the perinasal or periauricular regions, or in patients with immunosuppression or other significant comorbidities.

Furunculosis with surrounding cellulitis or with fever should be treated with systemic antibiotics. Most cases of folliculitis continue to be responsive to b-lactam antibiotics (penicillins, cephalosporins), macrolides (erythromycin, clarithromycin), and lincosamides (clindamycin), but consideration should be given to the increasing prevalence of MRSA and consideration of empiric antibiotics with MRSA coverage (e.g., trimethoprim-sulfamethoxazole, clindamycin) or for refractory disease.

Recurrent furunculosis may be difficult to control. This may be related to persistent staphylococci in the nares, perineum, and body folds. Effective control can sometimes be obtained with frequent showers (not baths), antibacterial soaps, and washes (benzoyl peroxide, chlorhexidine, or triclosan); topical mupirocin antibiotic ointment for skin lesions and nasal passages is effective in eliminating *S. aureus*. Dilute bleach baths are also effective for reducing bacterial colonization. All close household and/or family members should be treated at the same time because asymptomatic nasal carriage of the pathogenic bacteria can occur. Systemic antibiotics at lower doses on a daily basis prophylactically may be needed to avoid relapses for particularly refractory cases.

CELLULITIS

Cellulitis is an acute, spreading infection of dermal and subcutaneous tissues, characterized by a red, hot, tender area of skin, often at the site of bacterial entry.

 INSIGHT Bilateral or multifocal cellulitis is exceedingly rare; in all such cases, other possible diagnoses should be considered, with allergic contact dermatitis at the top of the list.

EPIDEMIOLOGY

AGE Children younger than 3 years; adults 45 to 65 years.
GENDER M > F.
INCIDENCE Common, up to 3/100 individuals.
ETIOLOGY Bacterial: Group A streptococci, or *S. aureus*. Less commonly, *Haemophilus influenza*, pneumococci, or *Neisseria meningitidis*.

PATHOPHYSIOLOGY

Break in the skin from puncture, laceration, abrasion, surgical site, underlying dermatosis (tinea pedis, atopic dermatitis), or impaired circulation (lymphedema, peripheral vascular disease, diabetes) allows bacterial entry and proliferation in the soft tissues with a marked inflammatory response. In children, *H. influenzae* enters through the middle ear or nasal mucosa, though less common in vaccinated children.

HISTORY

Cellulitis occurs 1 to 3 days after a break in the skin (wound, trauma) as a red, tender, hot swelling of the skin and underlying tissues. Rarely bullae may develop. Systemic symptoms such as malaise, anorexia, fever, chills can co-occur or precede skin changes; an associated bacteremia may be present.

PHYSICAL EXAMINATION

Skin Findings

TYPE Plaque, edema, bullae.
COLOR Red, purple (*H. influenzae*).
SIZE Few to several centimeters.
PALPATION Firm, hot, tender.
DISTRIBUTION Children: cheek, periorbital area (Fig. 20-6), head, neck. Adults: extremities.

General Findings

LYMPHADENOPATHY Can be enlarged and tender regionally.

DIFFERENTIAL DIAGNOSIS

The differential diagnosis of cellulitis includes atopic dermatitis, contact dermatitis, urticaria, erysipelas, impetigo, insect bites, vaccination reactions, fixed drug eruptions, annular erythema, stasis dermatitis, superficial thrombophlebitis or deep vein thrombosis, and panniculitis.

LABORATORY EXAMINATIONS

DERMATOPATHOLOGY Dermal inflammation with lymphocytes and neutrophils. Edema of the lymphatics and blood vessels. Special stains for organisms can be performed, but are only positive in the minority of cases.
COMPLETE BLOOD COUNT White cell count and sedimentation rate may be elevated.
SKIN CULTURES Cultures of the skin can be aspirated or biopsied at the leading edge of inflammation. Positive cultures are obtained in only up to 40% of cases.
BLOOD CULTURES Positive bacterial cultures are obtained in fewer than 25% of cases.

COURSE AND PROGNOSIS

The prognosis for cellulitis is good if early detection and treatment is initiated. Complications are rare, but include acute glomerulonephritis (*Streptococcus*), lymphadenitis, and subacute bacterial endocarditis. Facial, orbital, and periorbital cellulitis require special attention, early recognition, and systemic treatment because of the risk of serious visual impairment in untreated cases.

MANAGEMENT

Identifying the organism that is causing the cellulitis can aid in choosing the correct antibiotic coverage. Mild cases of staphylococcal and streptococcal cellulitis can be treated on an outpatient basis with a 10-day course of oral antibiotics with good gram-positive coverage. For severe refractory cases, facial and/or periorbital cellulitis, hospitalization and intravenous (IV) antibiotics may be necessary. For cases of purulent cellulitis, empiric coverage of MRSA is warranted given the increased prevalence of this organism.

For cellulitis affecting an extremity, supportive measures such as elevation and compression to relieve swelling are useful.

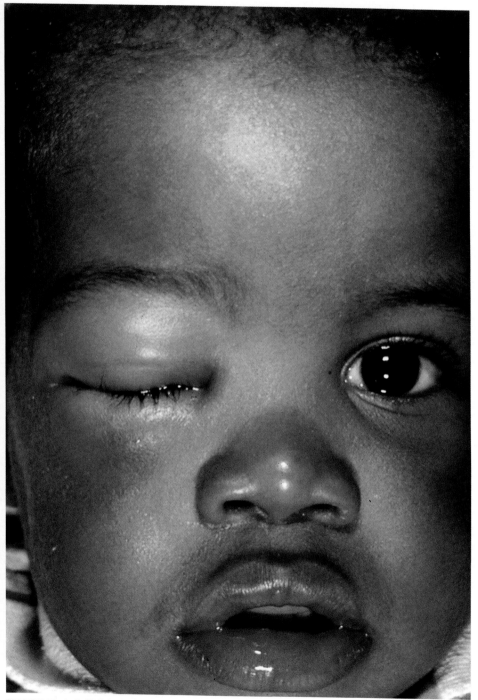

FIGURE 20-6 **Cellulitis, *H. influenzae*** Two-year-old with a right periorbital cellulitis. (Reproduced with permission from Fitzpatrick TB, Wolff K, and Johnson RA. *Color Atlas and Synopsis of Clinical Dermatology.* 3rd ed. New York, NY: McGraw-Hill; 1997.)

ERYSIPELAS

Erysipelas is a dermal and lymphatic infection of the skin most often caused by group A β-hemolytic streptococci.

SYNONYM St. Anthony's fire.

EPIDEMIOLOGY

AGE Young children. Elderly.
GENDER Children: M > F. Elderly: F > M.
INCIDENCE Uncommon.
SEASON Increased in summer.
ETIOLOGY Group A streptococci > groups G, B, C, or D streptococci, *S. aureus, Streptococcus pneumoniae, Klebsiella pneumoniae, Yersinia enterocolitica, H. influenzae* type B.

PATHOGENESIS

Group A streptococci enters the dermis and lymphatics from an external break in the skin or pharynx, or, less likely, through internal hematogenous spread.

HISTORY

Two to five days after a break in the skin, a red, hot, tender well-demarcated erythematous plaque begins to form and enlarge around the inoculation site. Fever, chills, malaise, nausea, lymphadenopathy, and lymphatic streaking may be present and may precede the skin changes.

PHYSICAL EXAMINATION

Skin Findings

TYPE Plaques > bullae, necrosis. Sharply demarcated borders.
COLOR Bright red (Fig. 20-7).
PALPATION Firm, hot, tender.
DISTRIBUTION Bridge of nose, cheeks, face, scalp, lower extremities.

General Findings

FEVER Malaise, nausea.
LYMPHADENOPATHY With, or without, lymphatic streaking.

DIFFERENTIAL DIAGNOSIS

Erysipelas can be confused with cellulitis, lupus, sunburn, contact dermatitis, urticaria, or dermatomyositis.

LABORATORY EXAMINATIONS

DERMATOPATHOLOGY Edema of the dermis and a dermal neutrophilic infiltrate. Special stains, direct immunofluorescence, and latex agglutination tests can detect streptococci within biopsy specimens.
SKIN CULTURE Tissue or wound swab cultures may grow organism.
BLOOD CULTURE Positive in only 5% of cases.
OTHER Anti-DNase B and antistreptolysin O titers are good indicators of streptococcal infections. Peripheral leukocytosis may also be present.

COURSE AND PROGNOSIS

Once identified and treated, erysipelas has a good prognosis. Complications are rare, occurring in patients with underlying disease (lymphedema, chronic cutaneous ulcers).

MANAGEMENT

The treatment of choice for streptococcal erysipelas is a 10- to 14-day course of penicillin. Penicillin-allergic individuals can be treated with macrolides (erythromycin, clarithromycin) but macrolide-resistant *S. pyogenes* strains have been reported.

Refractory or recurrent cases of erysipelas may require hospitalization and IV or intramuscular antibiotics. Patients with local circulatory problems (lymphedema) and recurrent erysipelas may need daily prophylactic penicillin.

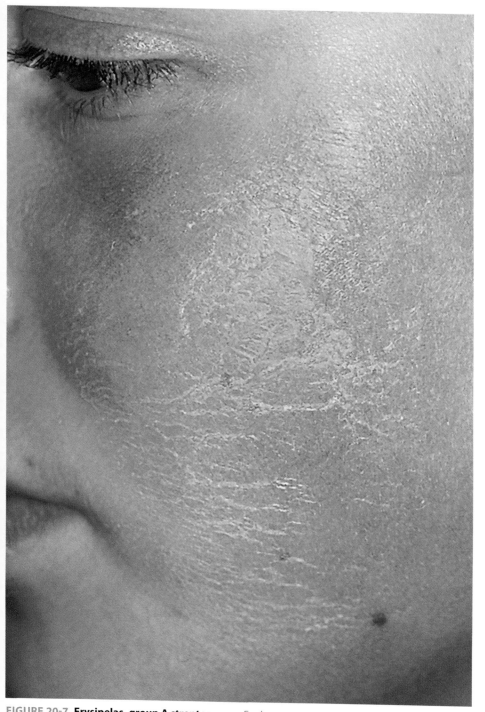

FIGURE 20-7 **Erysipelas, group A streptococcus** Erythematous warm, tender plaque on the cheek.

PERIANAL STREPTOCOCCAL INFECTION

Perianal streptococcal infection is characterized by bright red perianal dermatitis that leads to pruritus, pain, fissures, and can lead to behavioral defecation disorders.

SYNONYMS Perianal streptococcal cellulitis, streptococcal perianal disease.

EPIDEMIOLOGY

AGE Children younger than 4 years.
GENDER M > F.
INCIDENCE Uncommon.
ETIOLOGY Group A streptococci.

PATHOPHYSIOLOGY

Perianal streptococcal dermatitis may be precipitated by group A streptococcal pharyngitis or act as the infectious precipitant for a flare of guttate or recurrent psoriasis.

HISTORY

Perianal streptococcal infection typically presents as well-demarcated bright red perianal erythema extending 2 to 3 cm around the anus with itching or pain. No systemic symptoms are usually present.

PHYSICAL EXAMINATION

Skin Findings

TYPE Plaque.
COLOR Bright red.
SIZE Few to several centimeters.
DISTRIBUTION Perianal area (Fig. 20-8).

DIFFERENTIAL DIAGNOSIS

Perianal streptococcal infection can be clinically confused with psoriasis, candidiasis, contact dermatitis, seborrheic dermatitis, atopic dermatitis, pinworm infection, inflammatory bowel disease, early Kawasaki's disease, or sexual abuse.

LABORATORY EXAMINATIONS

SKIN CULTURE Perianal area will grow β-hemolytic streptococcus.

COURSE AND PROGNOSIS

Perianal streptococcal infection has a good prognosis when properly treated, but relapses (seen in up to 40% of cases) occur requiring retreatment. Untreated cases can lead to perianal irritation or pruritus, perianal fissures, painful defecation, streaks of blood on the stool, soiling of undergarments, and behavioral defecating disabilities.

MANAGEMENT

The treatments for perianal streptococcal infection include a 10-day course of penicillin or 7-day course of oral cephalosporin. Penicillin-allergic individuals can be treated with macrolides (erythromycin, clarithromycin) but macrolide-resistant S. pyogenes strains have been reported.

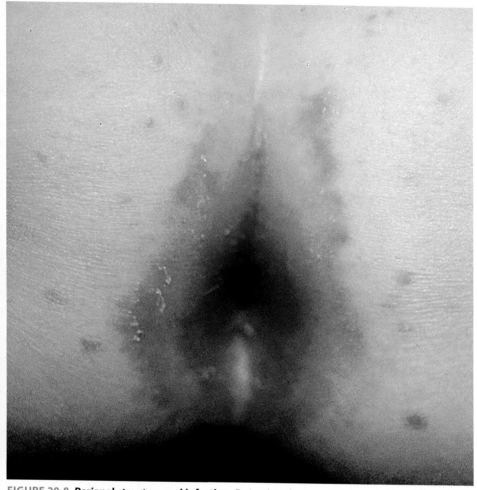

FIGURE 20-8 Perianal streptococcal infection Perianal erythema and fissures. A skin culture revealed β-hemolytic streptococcus.

SCARLET FEVER

Scarlet fever is a group A streptococcal infection of the tonsils, pharynx, or skin, associated with a characteristic toxin-mediated diffuse erythematous exanthem.

SYNONYMS Scarlatina, surgical scarlet.

EPIDEMIOLOGY

AGE 1 to 10 years.
INCIDENCE Uncommon.
SEASON Seen more commonly in late fall, winter, and early spring.
ETIOLOGY Group A β-hemolytic S. pyogenes. Uncommonly, exotoxin-producing S. aureus. Household members may be carriers.

PATHOPHYSIOLOGY

Group A streptococcal erythrogenic toxin (or pyrogenic exotoxins) types A, B, and C cause a delayed-type hypersensitivity reaction. Patients with prior exposure to the erythrogenic toxins have antitoxin immunity and may have a sore throat, but do not typically present with the rash. Since several erythrogenic strains of β-hemolytic streptococcus cause infection, it is theoretically possible to have a second episode of scarlet fever. Additionally, several strains of S. aureus can produce an exotoxin and simulate a scarlatiniform exanthem.

HISTORY

The rash of scarlet fever appears within 2 to 3 days after the onset of streptococcal tonsillitis or pharyngitis. Initial systemic symptoms can include fever, malaise, and a sore throat. The rash begins 12 to 48 hours later with punctate lesions (goose pimples), become confluently erythematous (i.e., scarlatiniform), and linear petechiae (Pastia's sign) can occur in body folds. The onset of the exanthem may rarely be delayed more than 48 hours after the onset of the tonsillitis or pharyngitis.

The exanthem fades within 4 to 5 days and is followed by brawny desquamation on the body and extremities (Fig. 20-9) and by sheet-like exfoliation on the palms and soles (Fig. 20-10). The face becomes flushed with perioral pallor. The tongue initially is white with scattered red swollen papillae (white strawberry tongue). By the fifth day, the hyperkeratotic membrane is sloughed and the lingular mucosa appears bright red (red strawberry tongue; Fig. 20-11).

PHYSICAL EXAMINATION

Skin Findings

TYPE Macules, papules, petechiae.
COLOR Pink, scarlet.
PALPATION Sandpaper texture to skin.
DISTRIBUTION Starts on chest, spreads to extremities, accentuated at pressure points/ body folds. Linear petechiae (Pastia's sign) in antecubital/axillary/inguinal folds.
MUCOUS MEMBRANES Pharynx and/or tonsils beefy red. Punctate erythema/petechiae on the soft palate.

General Findings

FEVER Malaise, headache, sore throat, vomiting.
LYMPHADENOPATHY Anterior cervical lymphadenitis.

DIFFERENTIAL DIAGNOSIS

Scarlet fever can be confused with staphylococcal infection, measles, rubella, toxic shock syndrome (TSS), staphylococcal scalded skin syndrome (SSSS), viral exanthems, and drug eruptions.

LABORATORY EXAMINATIONS

DERMATOPATHOLOGY Skin biopsy shows perivascular neutrophilic inflammation with dilated small blood and lymph vessels.
GRAM STAIN Reveals gram-positive cocci in pairs and chains.
BACTERIAL CULTURE Nose, throat culture will grow β-hemolytic streptococcus.
SEROLOGY Fourfold rise in antistreptolysin O titer, antihyaluronidase, antifibrinolysin, and anti-DNase B antibodies as markers of streptococcal infection.
COMPLETE BLOOD COUNT Elevated leukocyte count with left shift, eosinophilia, mild anemia.
OTHER May have mild albuminuria or hematuria.

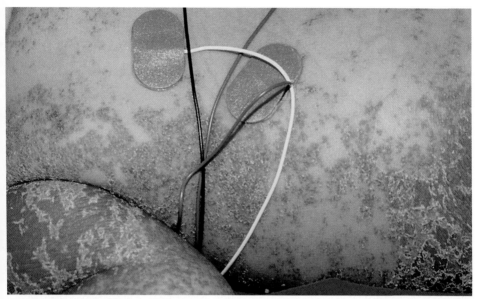

FIGURE 20-9 Scarlet fever, exanthem Brawny desquamation on the torso and extremities of a child.

COURSE AND PROGNOSIS

Uncomplicated scarlet fever has a good prognosis. As with all streptococcal diseases, worrisome sequelae such as otitis, mastoiditis, sinusitis, pneumonia, meningitis, arthritis, hepatitis, acute rheumatic fever, myocarditis, or acute glomerulonephritis can ensue. Peripheral eosinophilia may persist for 2 to 3 weeks after recovery.

MANAGEMENT

The treatment of choice for scarlet fever is a 10- to 14-day course of penicillin, which can also prevent the development of rheumatic fever. Clinical response can be expected in 24 to 48 hours. Penicillin-allergic individuals can be treated with macrolides (erythromycin, clarithromycin) but macrolide-resistant S. *pyogenes* strains have been reported.

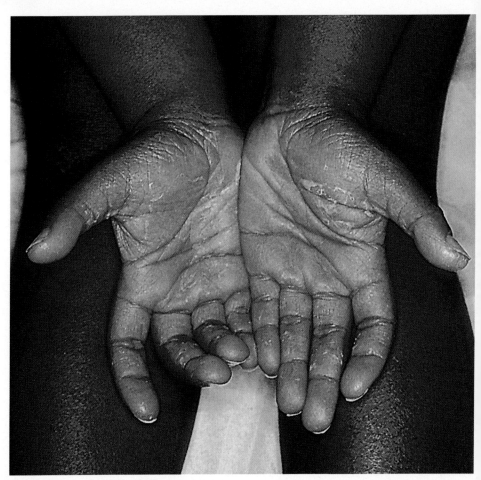

FIGURE 20-10 **Scarlet fever, late desquamation** Palmar desquamation on the hands of a child.

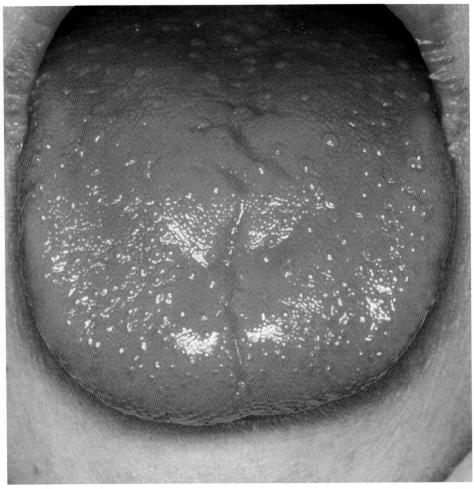

FIGURE 20-11 Scarlet fever, early exanthem Bright red tongue with prominent papillae on the fifth day after onset of group A streptococcal pharyngitis. (Reproduced with permission from Fitzpatrick TB, Johnson RA, Wolff K, et al. *Color Atlas and Synopsis of Clinical Dermatology*. 3rd ed. New York, NY: McGraw-Hill; 1997.)

STAPHYLOCOCCAL SCALDED SKIN SYNDROME

SSSS is a toxin-mediated epidermolytic disease characterized by erythema and widespread detachment of the superficial layers of the epidermis.

 INSIGHT Generally the affected skin is sterile; to find the staphylococcus, cultures of nasopharynx, conjunctiva, and perianal areas can be helpful.

SYNONYMS Pemphigus neonatorum, Ritter's disease.

EPIDEMIOLOGY

AGE Newborns, infants younger than 6 years.
GENDER M > F, 2:1.
ETIOLOGY *S. aureus* of phage group II (types 3A, 3C, 5S, or 71).

PATHOPHYSIOLOGY

SSSS is predominantly a disease of newborns and infants. After age 10, the majority of people are thought to have antistaphylococcal antibodies and a greater ability to localize and metabolize the staphylococcal exotoxin, thus, limiting widespread dissemination of the toxin. Individuals with renal failure, however, may be prone to exotoxin accumulation due to poor clearance.

In newborns and infants, *S. aureus* colonizes the nose, conjunctivae, or umbilical stump without causing a clinically apparent infection. Certain strains can produce exfoliative toxins (ETA: chromosomally encoded; ETB: plasmid encoded) that are transported hematogenously to the skin. The exfoliative toxins are serine proteases that bind human desmoglein 1 causing acantholysis and intraepidermal cleavage within the stratum granulosum. This leads to generalized sloughing of the superficial epidermis.

HISTORY

SSSS begins as fever, malaise, and erythema of the head and neck that progresses to a generalized scarlatiniform painful eruption. The child appears irritable and inconsolable. The skin then develops fluid bullae and exfoliates (giving the child a "scalded" appearance). Classically, the flexures are the first to exfoliate and in 1 to 2 days the skin is entirely sloughed. Scaling and desquamation continues for 3 to 5 days, then reepithelialization takes 10 to 14 days. Eventually, if properly treated, the skin will heal without scarring due to the very superficial nature of the skin split.

PHYSICAL EXAMINATION

Skin Findings

TYPE Macules, papules, bullae, desquamation (Fig. 20-12).
COLOR Pink to red.
PALPATION Lateral pressure causes shears off superficial epidermis (Nikolsky's sign).
DISTRIBUTION Begins face, neck, axillae, groins; generalized in 24 to 48 hours.
MUCOUS MEMBRANES Usually uninvolved.

General Findings

FEVER Malaise, irritability, inconsolability.

DIFFERENTIAL DIAGNOSIS

The differential diagnosis for SSSS includes sunburn, Kawasaki's disease, bullous impetigo, viral exanthema, TSS, graft-versus-host disease, toxic epidermal necrolysis, erythema multiforme, or other bullous diseases.

LABORATORY EXAMINATIONS

DERMATOPATHOLOGY Cleavage at the stratum granulosum, no inflammatory cells, no organisms. Frozen sections on a "jelly roll" (taken by rolling the sloughed skin on the wooden or plastic end of a cotton-tipped swab) will demonstrate cleavage of the skin at the level of the stratum granulosum for a faster diagnosis of SSSS. Latex agglutination, double immunodiffusion, or enzyme-linked immunosorbent assay (ELISA) can identify SSSS toxins.
GRAM STAIN Gram stain of infected source (i.e., umbilical stump, nose, pharynx, conjunctiva, feces, etc.) will show gram-positive cocci.

COURSE AND PROGNOSIS

Following adequate antibiotic treatment, the superficially denuded areas of SSSS heal without scarring in 3 to 5 days following full-body desquamation of the superficial epidermis. The mortality rate is 3% for children, 50% in adults, and nearly 100% in adults with underlying disease (chronic renal insufficiency or immunosuppression).

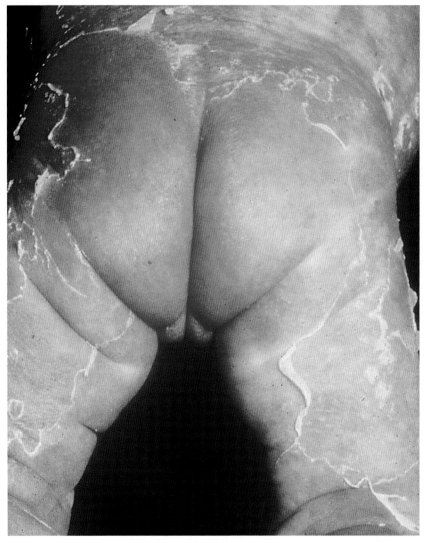

FIGURE 20-12 Staphylococcal scalded skin syndrome Diffuse sheet-like desquamation of the entire body.

MANAGEMENT

Treatment for SSSS is dependent on early recognition and prompt identification of the primary infectious source. Once the infectious source of S. *aureus* is cleared, the production of toxin is stopped. The treatment of choice is β-lactamase-resistant antibiotics, such as dicloxacillin, cloxacillin, or cephalexin, for a minimum of 7 days.

Topical care includes gentle cleansing baths and compresses, topical emollients (hydrated petrolatum, silver sulfadiazine), or antibiotic ointments (mupirocin) to decrease tenderness and pruritus. Identification and treatment of asymptomatic carriers at the same time is important to eradicate further spread.

In seriously affected newborns, hospitalization, isolation from other neonates, and treatment with IV oxacillin may be needed. IV fluid hydration may also be required to ensure individuals with extensive skin involvement are able to keep up with insensible losses.

TOXIC SHOCK SYNDROME

TSS is an acute exotoxin-mediated illness caused by *S. aureus* and characterized by rapid onset of fever, generalized skin and mucosal erythema, hypotension, and multisystem failure, sometimes leading to shock.

SYNONYM Staphylococcal scarlet fever.

EPIDEMIOLOGY

AGE 15 to 35 years. Less often in children or elderly.
GENDER M = F, except females only affected by tampon-associated TSS.
RACE White > black.
INCIDENCE Uncommon.
ETIOLOGY *S. aureus*-producing TSS exotoxin-1 (TSST-1). Most strains are MSSA, though cases of MRSA TSS have been reported.

PATHOPHYSIOLOGY

Up to half of TSS cases are in women using highly absorptive vaginal tampons during menses. Other TSS cases are seen with surgical wounds, vaginal contraceptive devices, postpartum infections, deep abscesses, nasal packings, postoperative infections, insulin pump infusion sites, and so on.

TSS is caused by *S. aureus* colonization and the subsequent production of TSST-1. TSST-1 is directly toxic to multiple organs; it impairs clearance of endogenous endotoxins and acts as a superantigen to mediate damage. Thus, TSST-1 leads to a decrease in vasomotor tone, leakage of intravascular fluid, hypotension, and end-organ failure.

In newborns, a transient TSS-like eruption may appear, termed neonatal TSS-like exanthematous disease. This self-resolving eruption is typically mild and self-limited given the immature immune system of neonates and the inability to mount a robust T-cell–mediated inflammation.

HISTORY

TSS starts with high fever and systemic symptoms, which may include myalgias, muscle tenderness, hypotension, headache, confusion, disorientation, pharyngitis, seizures, vomiting, diarrhea, or dyspnea. The skin is diffusely red and painful and the patient appears severely ill.

PHYSICAL EXAMINATION

Skin Findings

TYPE Maculopapular rash, edema, bullae, desquamation (Fig. 20-13A and B).

COLOR Bright red.
DISTRIBUTION Generalized. Often starts on the trunk and spreads diffusely. Patients may become erythrodermic.
SITES OF PREDILECTION Edema is most marked on face, hands, feet.
MUCOUS MEMBRANES Bulbar conjunctiva injections, subconjunctival hemorrhages (Fig. 20-13C). Tongue strawberry red. Ulcerations may be present.
NAILS May be shed or develop Beau's lines.
HAIR Telogen effluvium (loss of hair) may be seen 2 to 6 months later.

General Findings

FEVER Malaise, myalgia, vomiting, diarrhea, hypotension, and shock.

DIFFERENTIAL DIAGNOSIS

The differential diagnosis of TSS includes SSSS, scarlet fever, erythema multiforme, toxic epidermal necrolysis, drug reaction, viral infection, Kawasaki's disease, Rocky Mountain spotted fever, other bacterial infections, urticaria, or juvenile rheumatoid arthritis.

The Centers for Disease Control and Prevention has set a list of criteria for the diagnosis of TSS. Four of the following criteria plus desquamation or five of the following criteria without desquamation must be present:

1. Fever > 38.9°C (102°F).
2. Rash (diffuse erythema and edema).
3. Desquamation 1 to 2 weeks after acute episode.
4. Hypotension.
5. Involvement of three or more organ systems: gastrointestinal, muscles, mucous membranes, kidney, liver, hematologic, or central nervous system.
6. Negative blood and cerebrospinal fluid (CSF) cultures; negative serologic tests for Rocky Mountain spotted fever, leptospirosis, and measles.

LABORATORY EXAMINATIONS

DERMATOPATHOLOGY Confluent epidermal necrosis, vacuolar changes at the dermal–epidermal junction, and a superficial and interstitial inflammatory infiltrate.

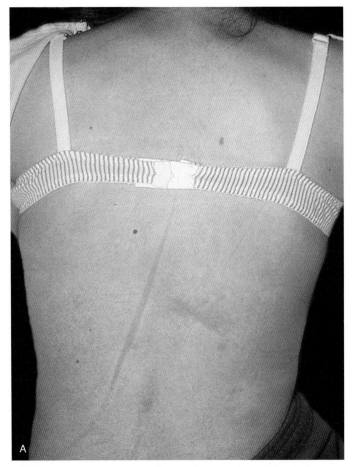

FIGURE 20-13 Toxic shock syndrome A: Diffuse erythema and a maculopapular eruption on the back of a young woman with toxic shock syndrome. *(continued)*

GRAM STAIN Vaginal swabs will show leukocytes and gram-positive cocci in clusters in cases of tampon-associated TSS.

BACTERIAL CULTURES Affected sites (vagina, throat, nose, conjunctiva, blood, or stool) will grow *S. aureus*.

COURSE AND PROGNOSIS

Untreated TSS has a high morbidity and mortality rate. Complications include decreased renal function, prolonged weakness, protracted myalgias, vocal cord paralysis, upper extremity paresthesias, carpal tunnel syndrome, arthralgias, amenorrhea, and gangrene. Treating TSS reduces the mortality rate from 15% to 3%, and deaths are secondary to refractory hypotension, respiratory distress, cardiac arrhythmias, cardiomyopathy, encephalopathy, metabolic acidosis, liver necrosis, or disseminated intravascular coagulation.

MANAGEMENT

Cases usually require hospitalization in an intensive care unit to manage hypotension (with fluids and vasopressors), electrolytes, metabolic and nutritional support. Foreign bodies (tampons, nasal packing, surgical meshes) should be removed and the area should be irrigated to reduce bacterial overgrowth. The patient should be started on β-lactamase-resistant antibiotics such as dicloxacillin, cloxacillin, or cephalexin. Antibiotics that suppress protein production and thus toxin formation, such as clindamycin, rifampin, or fluoroquinolones, may be useful. Intravenous immunoglobulin (IVIg) may also have a role in the neutralization of exotoxin.

FIGURE 20-13 *(Continued)* **B:** Close up of the bright red papular rash coalescing into a confluent plaque.

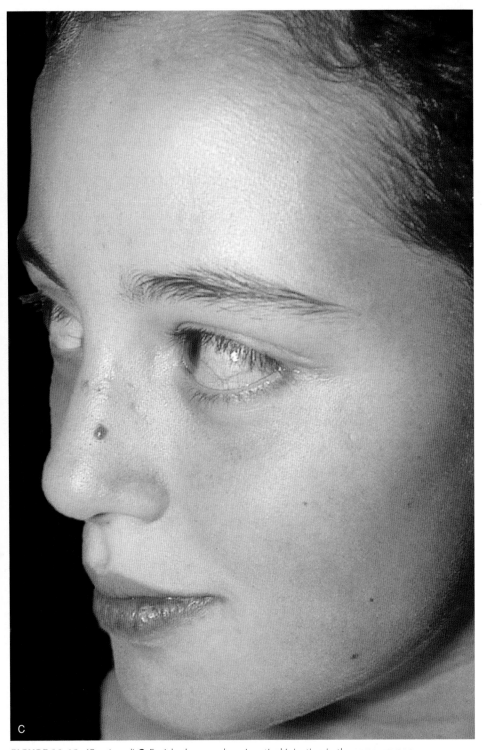

FIGURE 20-13 *(Continued)* **C:** Facial edema and conjunctival injection in the same woman.

ERYTHRASMA

Erythrasma is a superficial, localized bacterial infection caused by *Corynebacterium minutissimum* affecting the intertriginous areas of the toes, groin, or axillae.

ETYMOLOGY Greek: "red spot" disease.

EPIDEMIOLOGY

AGE 5 to 14 years. More common in adults.
GENDER M = F.
INCIDENCE Uncommon.
PREDISPOSING FACTORS May coexist with tinea cruris or tinea pedis.
ETIOLOGY *C. minutissimum.*

PATHOPHYSIOLOGY

Erythrasma is a *C. minutissimum* overgrowth in the stratum corneum of warm, moist intertriginous areas of the skin. Predisposing factors include diabetes, warm humid climate, poor hygiene, hyperhidrosis, obesity, advanced age, and immunocompromised states.

HISTORY

Erythrasma begins in body folds such as the web spaces between the toes, the groin, or the axillae. It tends to be chronic for months or years with symptoms of pruritus or pain from maceration. Systemic symptoms are not present.

PHYSICAL EXAMINATION

Skin Findings

TYPE Macules, patches, plaques, scale.
COLOR Red or brownish-red.
ARRANGEMENT Scattered discrete lesions coalescing into confluent patches.
DISTRIBUTION Toe web spaces (Fig. 20-14), groin, axilla, intergluteal fold.

DIFFERENTIAL DIAGNOSIS

Erythrasma is often confused with a dermatophyte infection (i.e., tinea pedis, tinea cruris), seborrheic dermatitis, candidal infection, or intertrigo.

LABORATORY EXAMINATIONS

GRAM STAIN Gram-positive rods and filaments.
WOOD'S LAMP Fluoresces a characteristic coral red color owing to the production of porphyrins by the corynebacterial organisms.

COURSE AND PROGNOSIS

Erythrasma tends to be a chronic condition persisting for months to years if untreated. There are only minor skin symptoms of pruritus or maceration and no systemic symptoms. Relapses after treatment are common, typically about 6 months later.

MANAGEMENT

Erythrasma can be controlled and prevented with antibacterial soaps and washes and less restrictive clothing. Effective topical therapies include 10% to 20% aluminum chloride, erythromycin, clindamycin, or miconazole creams.

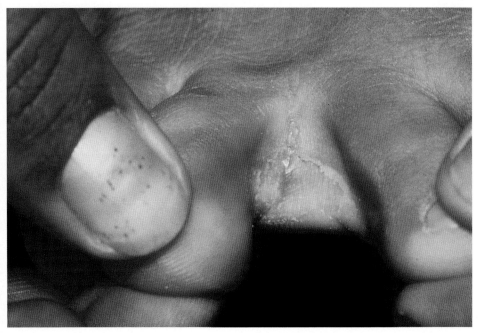

FIGURE 20-14 **Erythrasma** Scale and maceration in the toe web spaces that fluoresces with Wood's lamp.

MENINGOCOCCEMIA

Meningococcemia is a severe bacterial septicemia characterized by fever, petechial or purpuric lesions, hypotension, and signs of meningitis associated with high morbidity and mortality.

SYNONYM Waterhouse–Friderichsen syndrome.

EPIDEMIOLOGY

AGE 6 months to 1 year and young adults.
GENDER M > F, 3:1.
INCIDENCE Uncommon.
RISK GROUPS Asplenic patients or complement deficiency (C5, C6, C7, or C8), properdin deficiency, or Ig deficiency.
ETIOLOGY N. meningitidis, a gram-negative diplococcus that seeds the blood from the nasopharynx (carrier rate: 5–15%). Strains A, B, C, Y, and W-135 are most implicated in human disease.
TRANSMISSION Person-to-person inhalation of droplets of nasopharyngeal secretions.
SEASON Winter, spring.
GEOGRAPHY Worldwide. Occurs in epidemics or sporadically.

PATHOPHYSIOLOGY

The primary focus of N. meningitidis is usually a subclinical nasopharynx infection. Transmission is by respiratory droplets with an incubation period of 2 to 10 days. In most people, infection leads to a lifelong carrier state.

When meningococcemia does occur, hematogenous dissemination of the diplococcus seeds the skin and meninges, especially in the presence of a concurrent viral illness or tobacco smoke. Bacterial-derived endotoxin is thought to be involved in causing hypotension and vascular collapse. Meningococci are found within endothelial and polymorphonuclear cells leading to local endothelial damage, thrombosis, and necrosis of the vessel walls. Edema and infarction of overlying skin, with extravasation of red blood cells, is responsible for the characteristic macular, papular, petechial, hemorrhagic, and bullous lesions. Similar vascular lesions occur in the meninges and in other tissues.

The frequency of hemorrhagic cutaneous manifestations in meningococcal infections, compared to infections with other gram-negative organisms, may be owing to increased potency and/or unique properties of meningococcal endotoxins for the dermal reaction. Chronic meningococcemia is rarely seen in children but during periodic fevers, rash, and joint manifestations, meningococci can be isolated from the blood. It is thought that an unusual host–parasite relationship is central to this persistent infection. In fulminant meningococcemia, disseminated intravascular coagulation can be seen.

HISTORY

Acute meningococcemia may present as a flu-like illness with spiking fevers, chills, arthralgias, and myalgias. Hemorrhagic skin lesions and profound hypotension may be evident within a few hours of onset. Younger children may manifest with progressive symptoms more rapidly than older children. Chronic meningococcemia manifests as intermittent fevers, rashes, myalgias, arthralgias, headaches, and anorexia.

PHYSICAL EXAMINATION

Skin Findings

TYPE Macules, petechiae, urticaria, purpura, ecchymoses, necrosis (Fig. 20-15).
COLOR Pink, red with pale grayish center.
DISTRIBUTION Trunk, extremities > face, palms, and soles.
MUCOUS MEMBRANES Petechiae on conjunctiva and other mucous membranes.

General Findings

HIGH FEVER Acutely ill with marked prostration tachypnea, tachycardia, hypotension.
CNS 50% to 88% develop meningitis, meningeal irritation, altered consciousness.
OTHER Rarely, septic arthritis, purulent pericarditis, bacterial endocarditis, adrenal hemorrhage (Waterhouse–Friderichsen syndrome).

DIFFERENTIAL DIAGNOSIS

Meningococcemia can mimic other acute bacteremias and endocarditis, acute hypersensitivity vasculitis, enteroviral infections, Rocky Mountain spotted fever, TSS, purpura fulminans, Sweet's syndrome, Henoch–Schönlein purpura, typhoid fever, erythema multiforme, or gonococcemia.

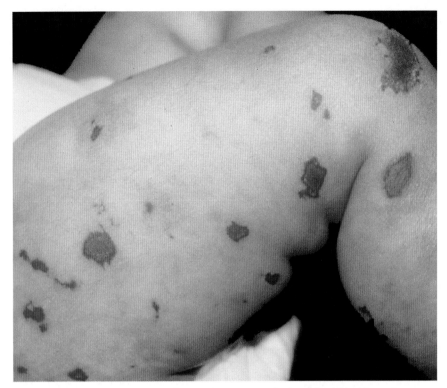

FIGURE 20-15 Meningococcemia Stellate necrotic areas on the legs of a child with meningococcemia.

LABORATORY EXAMINATIONS

DERMATOPATHOLOGY Leukocytoclastic vasculitis, thrombosis, and meningococcal organisms may be demonstrated in the lumina of vessels, within thrombi in perivascular spaces, or in the cytoplasm of endothelial cells.

GRAM STAIN Skin lesion stains for gram-negative diplococci in up to 85% of cases.

CULTURES Blood, skin, CSF, synovial, and pericardial cultures have low sensitivity.

LATEX AGGLUTINATION A, B, C, Y, and W-135 antigens in CSF and urine have high specificity, but low sensitivity.

POLYMERASE CHAIN REACTION Polymerase chain reaction of skin specimens is more sensitive and specific than blood or CSF.

COURSE AND PROGNOSIS

Meningococcemia, if undiagnosed and untreated, ends fatally. Adequately treated, recovery rate for meningitis or meningococcemia is >90%. Mortality for severe disease or Waterhouse–Friderichsen syndrome remains high. Prognosis is poor when late symptoms or purpura and ecchymosis are present at time of diagnosis.

MANAGEMENT

Prompt recognition and treatment of acute meningococcemia is critical. The treatment of choice is high-dose IV penicillin. For penicillin-allergic individuals, IV chloramphenicol is recommended. In areas of high penicillin resistance, third-generation cephalosporin is effective. Chronic meningococcemia is treated with lower doses of the same antibiotics. All contacts (family, day care, hospital) should be treated prophylactically with rifampin or ciprofloxacin (the latter to be avoided in areas where ciprofloxacin resistance has been previously encountered).

A vaccine that protects against serotypes A, C, Y, and W-135 is available and routinely given to children between ages 11 and 18 years and to individuals at high risk for infection (students, military, etc.). Additional meningococcal vaccines approved in recent years for infants as young as 2 months and a combined meningococcal-Haemophilus vaccine for infants as young as 6 weeks are also available for children at high risk of meningococcemia.

GONOCOCCEMIA

Gonococcemia is a severe bacterial infection caused by *Neisseria gonorrhoeae* in the bloodstream characterized by fever, chills, scanty acral pustules, and septic polyarthritis.

SYNONYMS Disseminated gonococcal infection, gonococcal arthritis–dermatitis syndrome.

EPIDEMIOLOGY

AGE Females: 15 to 19 years. Males: 20 to 24 years.
GENDER F > M.
RACE Whites > blacks.
INCIDENCE 600,000 cases of gonococcal infection in the United States annually, second most common sexually transmitted disease after chlamydia.
ETIOLOGY *N. gonorrhoeae,* a gram-negative diplococcus.

PATHOPHYSIOLOGY

Gonococcus is sexually transmitted from a primary mucosal site, such as endocervix, urethra, pharynx, or rectum. Up to 3% of patients with untreated mucosal gonococcal infection develop bacteremia caused by host factors (menses, pregnancy, complement deficiency, human immunodeficiency virus, systemic lupus erythematosus), which lead to infection of the skin, joints, and other organs. Most signs and symptoms of gonococcemia are manifestations of immune complex formation and deposition.

HISTORY

Gonorrhea is a sexually transmitted mucosal infection that begins with fever, anorexia, malaise, and shaking chills. Three to twenty-one days later, erythematous and hemorrhagic papules occur over distal joints with systemic migratory polyarthralgias.

PHYSICAL EXAMINATION

Skin Findings

TYPE Macules, papules, pustules (Fig. 20-16A), hemorrhagic bullae or pustules.
COLOR Erythematous to purple to black.
SIZE 1 to 5 mm.
DISTRIBUTION Acral, arms > legs, joints of hands or feet (Fig. 20-16B).
MUCOUS MEMBRANES Oropharynx, urethra, anorectum, or endometrium asymptomatically colonized with *N. gonorrhoeae.*

General Findings

FEVER 38°C or higher.
OTHER Rare tenosynovitis, septic arthritis, ± infection at other sites/organs, perihepatitis (Fitz–Hugh–Curtis syndrome), myopericarditis, endocarditis, meningitis, pneumonitis, adult respiratory distress syndrome, or osteomyelitis.

DIFFERENTIAL DIAGNOSIS

Gonococcemia can be confused with other bacteremias, meningococcemia, endocarditis, infectious arthritis, Lyme disease, infectious tenosynovitis, Reiter's syndrome, psoriatic arthritis, syphilis, or systemic lupus erythematosus.

LABORATORY EXAMINATIONS

DERMATOPATHOLOGY Perivascular neutrophilic infiltrate and neutrophils in pustules in the epidermis. Immunofluorescence of skin lesion biopsy or skin smear shows *N. gonorrhoeae* in up to 60% of cases.
GRAM STAIN OR BACTERIAL CULTURE Mucosal sites (pharynx, urethra, cervix, or rectum) yield 80% to 90% positive cultures. Skin biopsy, joint fluid, blood only has a 10% chance of positive culture.
POLYMERASE CHAIN REACTION (NUCLEIC ACID AMPLIFICATION TEST) 79% sensitivity and 96% specificity, performed on urethral specimens or first-void urine specimen; it is a noninvasive, rapid test and the first preferred test. However, polymerase chain reaction cannot report antibiotic sensitivities; therefore, they do not eliminate the need for culture.
SEROLOGY Latex agglutination, ELISA, immunoprecipitation, and complement fixation tests have a low sensitivity and specificity; thus, these tests are not routinely used for diagnosis of gonococcemia.
OTHER Elevated WBC and ESR.

COURSE AND PROGNOSIS

Untreated skin and joint lesions of gonococcemia often gradually resolve. Severe untreated complications of gonococcemia include osteomyelitis, meningitis, endocarditis, adult respiratory distress syndrome, and fatal septic shock.

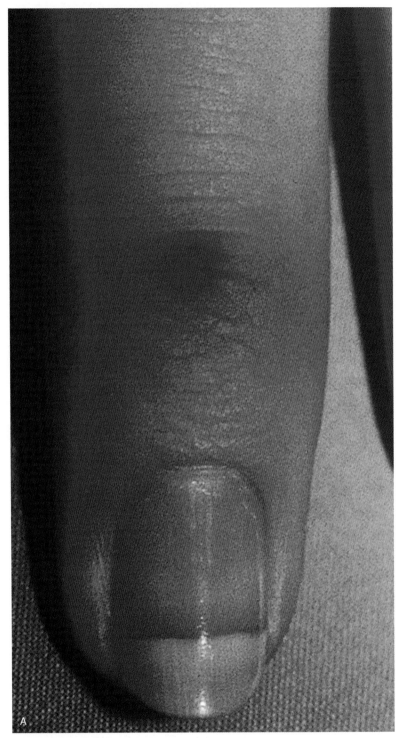

FIGURE 20-16 Gonococcemia A: Hemorrhagic macule over the joint of a young patient infected with gonococcus. *(continued)*

MANAGEMENT

Hospitalization is recommended for initial therapy, especially for patients who cannot reliably comply with treatment, have uncertain diagnoses, or have purulent synovial effusions or other complications. Patients should be examined for clinical evidence of endocarditis or meningitis. Recommended regimens include a third-generation cephalosporin (ceftriaxone) until *N. gonorrhoeae* susceptibilities are obtained and a single dose of oral azithromycin for dual gonococcal coverage. Then patients can be treated with penicillin G or ampicillin.

An alternative regimen for patients allergic to β-lactam drugs is spectinomycin. Treatment should last for at least 7 days or up to 14 days in cases of purulent arthritis. Reliable patients with uncomplicated disease may be discharged after 24 to 48 hours to complete the therapy with oral antibiotics.

The Centers for Disease Control and Prevention recommend that all patients with gonorrheal infection be also treated for presumed coinfection with *Chlamydia trachomatis*. This treatment can be easily accomplished with a tetracycline antibiotic (e.g., doxycycline) or a macrolide antibiotic (e.g., azithromycin).

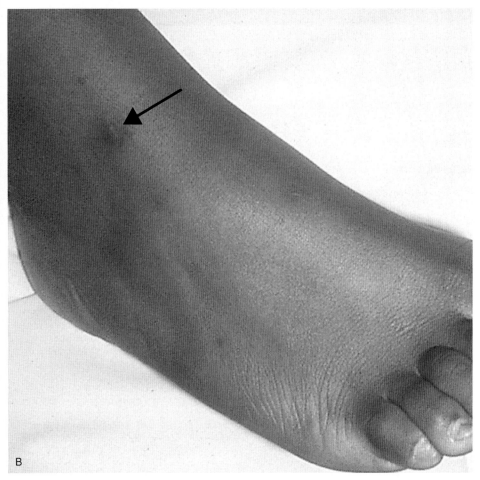

B

FIGURE 20-16 *(Continued)* **Gonococcemia B:** Hemorrhagic papule on the foot of a young patient infected with gonococcus.

CAT SCRATCH DISEASE

Cat scratch disease is a benign, self-limited zoonotic infection characterized by skin or conjunctival lesion(s) following cat scratches or contact with a cat and subsequent chronic tender regional lymphadenopathy.

SYNONYMS Cat scratch fever, benign lymphoreticulosis, inoculation lymphoreticulosis, subacute regional lymphadenitis, English-Wear infection.

EPIDEMIOLOGY

AGE Younger than 21 years. Median age: 15 years with highest incidence in children <10 years old.
GENDER M = F.
INCIDENCE 22,000 cases in the United States annually.
ETIOLOGY *Bartonella henselae.*
SEASON Fall, winter.

PATHOPHYSIOLOGY

Transmission of *B. henselae* infection in cats occurs with high efficiency via flea vectors (*Ctenocephalides felis*). Cat scratch disease in humans has a transmission history of kitten or cat contact (scratch, bite, lick) in 90% of cases.

HISTORY

Seven to twelve days after cat contact (typically a kitten younger than age 6 months), red papules develop at the scratch site. Systemically, mild fever, malaise, chills, general aching, and nausea may be present. One to four weeks later, chronic lymphadenitis and regional lymphadenopathy can be found and can last 2 to 5 months or longer if fibrosis occurs.

PHYSICAL EXAMINATION

Skin Findings

TYPE Papule, vesicle, or pustule.
COLOR Flesh colored to pink to red.
SIZE 5 to 15 mm.
PALPATION Firm, hot, tender to touch.
DISTRIBUTION Primary lesion on exposed skin of head, neck, or extremities.
MUCOUS MEMBRANE 3-mm yellow granulation on palpable conjunctiva with preauricular/cervical lymphadenopathy (5%, oculoglandular syndrome of Parinaud).

OTHER Urticaria (<5%), maculopapular/vesiculopapular lesions, erythema nodosum, or annular erythema.

General Findings

FEVER Malaise, fatigue, weakness, headache.
LYMPHADENOPATHY Regional lymphadenopathy: solitary, erythematous, moderately tender, mobile, may suppurate (Fig. 20-17). Most commonly axillary location.
OTHER Less commonly encephalitis, pneumonitis (15%), thrombocytopenia, osteomyelitis (15%), hepatitis, or abscesses in liver or spleen.

DIFFERENTIAL DIAGNOSIS

The differential diagnosis of cat scratch disease includes suppurative bacterial lymphadenitis, atypical mycobacteria, sporotrichosis, tularemia, toxoplasmosis, infectious mononucleosis, tumors, sarcoidosis, lymphogranuloma venereum, and coccidioidomycosis.

LABORATORY EXAMINATIONS

DERMATOPATHOLOGY Affected lymph nodes will show central necrosis surrounded by necrobiosis and palisaded histiocytes; multinucleated giant cells and eosinophils may also be seen. Warthin–Starry stain may demonstrate the gram-negative bacillus. Fluorescent antibody tests and antibody titers to *B. henselae* are usually high during the first few weeks after the onset of lymphadenopathy.

COURSE AND PROGNOSIS

In immunocompetent hosts, cat scratch disease is a benign, self-limited disease characterized by tender regional lymphadenitis that has a good prognosis and usually resolves in 2 to 4 months. In rare cases, cat scratch disease may persist longer.

In immunosuppressed patients, a more severe and complicated disease course with encephalitis, pneumonitis, thrombocytopenia, osteomyelitis, hepatitis, abscesses in liver or spleen may occur.

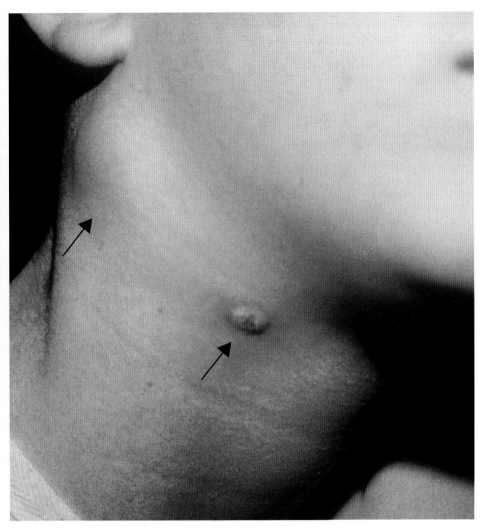

FIGURE 20-17 **Cat scratch disease** Suppurative nodule in a child with cat scratch exposure, with adjacent enlarged lymph node.

MANAGEMENT

Cat scratch disease is self-limited and seems unresponsive to antibiotics; thus, needle aspiration of suppurative nodes and supportive care (analgesics) will give symptomatic relief. Doxycycline plus rifampin and single-agent azithromycin have been used and, if started early in the disease, may be of slight benefit. Evidence from randomized controlled trials demonstrates a 5-day course of azithromycin is effective in decreasing lymph node volume. Surgical removal of lymph nodes is rarely necessary. Of note, the disease is self-limited in the cat as well; thus, declawing or removing the animal is not necessary.

MYCOBACTERIAL INFECTIONS

LEPROSY (HANSEN'S DISEASE)

Leprosy is a chronic infection caused by *Mycobacterium leprae,* a bacillus that has a predilection for peripheral nerves and the skin. The clinical manifestations, course, and prognosis of leprosy depend on the patient's degree of immunity to *M. leprae.*

CLASSIFICATION

1. Tuberculoid (TT): high host T-cell resistance (Th1), 1 to 5 skin lesions, no bacilli
2. Borderline tuberculoid (BT): >5 larger skin lesions, peripheral nerve involvement
3. Borderline borderline (BB): both TT and LL, many skin lesions, many bacilli
4. Borderline lepromatous (BL): many skin lesions, leonine facies, late neural lesions
5. Lepromatous (LL): no host T cell (Th2), generalized disease, huge globi of bacilli

An indeterminate classification also exists for individuals without diagnostic features of one of the above groups.

EPIDEMIOLOGY

AGE Peaks: 10 to 15 years and 30 to 60 years.
GENDER M > F, 1.5:1.
PREVALENCE Worldwide: 219,000 cases in 2011.
ETIOLOGY *M. leprae,* a slender acid-fast bacillus (AFB) 3.0×0.5 μm.
GEOGRAPHY Africa, Southeast Asia, South/Central America. Endemic in Louisiana, Hawaii, and California.

PATHOPHYSIOLOGY

Leprosy is caused by *M. leprae* of the nasal, oral, or eroded skin of an infected person being transmitted to a susceptible host via nasal mucosa, open skin wound, or contaminated needle. Although humans are the main reservoir for *M. leprae,* armadillos (southern United States), monkeys, chimpanzees, and mice can harbor the organism.

M. leprae is an obligate intracellular parasite that targets macrophages and Schwann cells requiring cooler (<35°C) body sites (peripheral nerves, skin, nose, mucous membranes, bones, viscera) to grow. Depending on the host's level of cell-mediated immunity (lepromin test), the disease can progress [Th2 response, interleukin 4 (IL-4), IL-10], plateau, or resolve spontaneously (Th1 response, IL-2, IFN-γ).

HISTORY

The incubation period from the time of exposure can be anywhere from 4 to 10 years. Childhood leprosy begins with small hyperemic self-resolving macules that, after 18 to 24 months, disappear with a wrinkled, hypopigmented scar. There is a quiescent period until adolescence or adulthood when the more typical skin lesions and neural involvement becomes apparent.

PHYSICAL EXAMINATION

Skin Findings

TYPE Macules (TT) to papules, nodules, infiltrated plaques (LL).
COLOR Red or hypopigmented.
SIZE Few millimeters to several centimeters.
SHAPE Annular, oval, round (Fig. 20-18).
PALPATION Anesthetic or hypoesthetic infiltrated plaques.
DISTRIBUTION Face—"leonine" facies, trunk, buttocks, lower extremities.
MUCOUS MEMBRANES Tongue: nodules, plaques, fissures.
HAIR Absent in skin lesions.

General Findings

NERVES Enlarged peripheral nerves (facial, greater auricular, ulnar, radial, median, common peroneal or posterior tibial nerves; may be easily palpable), anesthesia of skin lesions, neuropathic changes (muscle atrophy), peripheral sensory neuropathy, vasomotor instability, or secretory disturbances.
EYES Dry eyes. Anterior chamber can be involved with resultant glaucoma and cataract formation (LL). Corneal damage and uveitis can also occur.
TESTES May be involved with resultant hypogonadism (LL).

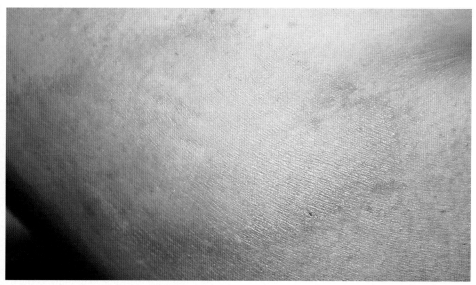

FIGURE 20-18 Borderline lepromatous leprosy Annular, anesthetic plaque in a child with leprosy.

DIFFERENTIAL DIAGNOSIS

The differential diagnosis of leprosy is broad given the wide spectrum of clinical disease. Leprosy can be mistaken for tinea corporis, pityriasis alba, tinea versicolor, seborrheic dermatitis, vasculitides, panniculitides lichen planus, scleroderma, cellulitis, vitiligo, morphea, granuloma annulare, drug reaction, sarcoidosis, leishmaniasis, syphilis, lupus erythematosus, annular erythema, cutaneous T-cell lymphoma, or cutaneous tuberculosis (TB).

LABORATORY EXAMINATIONS

DERMATOPATHOLOGY TT lesions will show perineural granuloma formation. Cutaneous nerves will be edematous. AFB will be sparse or absent. LL lesions will show an extensive cellular infiltrate of plasma cells, lymphocytes, and Virchow cells (macrophages are loaded with *M. leprae*) separated from the epidermis by a narrow zone of normal collagen (Unna band, or Grenz zone). Skin appendages are destroyed. POLYMERASE CHAIN REACTION PCR for detection of *M. leprae* DNA exists for tissue samples as a confirmatory test or in equivocal cases. SLIT SKIN SMEAR A small skin incision (from earlobes or skin lesions) is made and the site is scraped for tissue fluid and organisms visualized with Ziehl–Neelsen, Gram, Fite, Wade, Sudan III, Sudan IV, or methenamine silver stainings. Organisms will be found in 100% of LL cases, 75% of BT/BL cases, and only 5% of TL cases. Given more advanced diagnostic testing such as PCR, slit skin smears usually reserved less commonly performed.

LEPROMIN TEST (Mitsuda test) Intradermal injection of heat-killed *M. leprae*-positive (nodule forms at injection site 3–4 weeks later) in TT and BT leprosy.

COURSE AND PROGNOSIS

Leprosy is a disfiguring, socially stigmatizing disease whose treatment may be complicated by reactional phenomena triggered by antimicrobial drugs, pregnancy, other infections, or even mental distress.

1. *Lepra type 1 reactions:* The skin lesions become inflamed and painful with severe edema of the hands, feet, and face because of type IV delayed hypersensitivity reaction. Treatment of choice: prednisone.
2. *Lepra type 2 reactions (erythema nodosum leprosum):* Painful red nodules appear on the face and limbs and form abscesses or ulcerate. Postulated to be due to immune complex deposition with cutaneous and small vessel vasculitis. Treatment of choice: thalidomide.
3. *Lucio's reaction:* Irregularly shaped erythematous plaques appear and may ulcerate or become necrotic with thrombotic phenomena and vasculopathy. Treatment: corticosteroids and antimycobacterials. Poor prognosis.

After drug therapy, the main complications are neurologic: contractures of the hands and feet.

MANAGEMENT

WHO recommends multidrug therapy based on patient age and number of bacilli. The United States National Hansen's Disease Program (NHDP) has separate treatment recommendations.

In children aging 5 to 14 years with paucibacillary single lesion leprosy, WHO recommendations call for one dose of rifampin, ofloxacin, and minocycline.

In children younger than 14 years with multibacillary disease, WHO recommends 12 to 18 months of sulfones (dapsone) if there is no G6PD deficiency. Because of dapsone resistance, rifampin should be given in conjunction with dapsone for 6 months for the treatment of TT and BT. Clofazimine should be added for treatment of BB, BL, and LL disease and continued for at least 2 years and until skin smears are negative.

The NHDP recommends 12 months of dapsone plus rifampicin for all children with TT or BT disease, and 24 months of treatment with dapsone plus rifampicin plus clofazimine for LL, BL, and BB disease.

After the first dose of medication, the patient is no longer infectious to others and after completion of the multidrug therapy, patients are considered cured. Relapses are uncommon and bacilli may still be found on the patients, but they are nonviable.

CUTANEOUS TUBERCULOSIS

Cutaneous TB is highly variable in its clinical presentation depending on the route of *Mycobacterium tuberculosis* inoculation and the host response.

 INSIGHT There has been a resurgence of TB worldwide because of human immunodeficiency virus, *Mycobacterium tuberculosis* resistance, increased immunosuppressive therapies, and increased human migration.

SYNONYMS Prosector's wart, lupus verrucosus, TB cutis colliquativa, TB cutis orificialis, TB luposa, TB cutis acuta generalisata, metastatic TB abscess.

CLASSIFICATION

Exogenous Infection

1. Tuberculous chancre: primary inoculation TB through skin/mucosa in nonimmune host.
2. TB verrucosa cutis: inoculation TB through skin/mucosa in previously exposed host.

Endogenous Spread

1. Scrofuloderma: skin TB from underlying TB focus (lymph node, bone).
2. Orificial TB: autoinoculation of skin/mucosa in setting of impaired immunity.
3. Lupus vulgaris: direct extension, spread, reinfection in delayed type hypersensitivity (DTH) T-cell-immune patient.
4. Miliary TB: hematogenous spread from lungs in low-immunity patient.
5. TB gumma: hematogenous spread during bacteremia and lowered resistance.

EPIDEMIOLOGY

AGE All ages.
INCIDENCE 300/100,000 in developing countries. 1% to 2% of all TB patients.
ETIOLOGY *M. tuberculosis* >> *Mycobacterium bovis*, Bacille Calmette–Guérin.
TRANSMISSION Exogenous, autoinoculation, or endogenous.

PATHOPHYSIOLOGY

TB is caused by the AFB *M. tuberculosis*. It spreads in saliva droplets via inhalation, ingestion, or direct inoculation. The host may be previously sensitized versus never exposed, which leads to different degrees of cell-mediated immunity and different clinical presentations. Lesions can occur from direct inoculation of the skin or mucosa (TB chancre, TB verrucosa cutis) from an exogenous source, or from an endogenous infection (scrofuloderma, miliary TB, TB gumma, orificial TB, lupus vulgaris). Finally, there are also skin immune reactions to *M. tuberculosis* called tuberculids.

HISTORY

The clinical presentation of *M. tuberculosis* depends upon the inoculation route, mode of spread, and host cellular immune response.

1. TB chancre develops 2 to 4 weeks after inoculation, starts as a papule, enlarges to a nodule, erodes to an ulcer, and heals spontaneously in 3 to 12 months.
2. TB verrucosa cutis begins as a wart-like papule, enlarges to a plaque, which may exude pus or keratinaceous debris, then heals spontaneously after several years.
3. Scrofuloderma begins as subcutaneous nodule from underlying lymph node or bone infection that drains with ulceration and sinus formation, healing with keloid scarring.
4. Orificial TB occurs near an orifice draining an active TB infection (pulmonary, intestinal, or anogenital). It begins as a papule that painfully ulcerates and will not heal spontaneously.
5. Lupus vulgaris begins as a plaque, ulcer, vegetating lesion, tumor, or papulonodular lesion in a DTH-sensitized host, which can persist for years and heals with scarring.
6. Miliary TB usually occurs in the setting of pulmonary TB and bacteremia. The skin lesions present as tiny papules or vesicles that heal with scarring.
7. TB gumma usually occurs with bacteremia. The skin lesions present as subcutaneous nodules that drain with ulceration and sinus formation, often on one of the extremities.

PHYSICAL EXAMINATION

Skin Findings

TYPE Macules, papules, ulcers (TB chancre; Fig. 20-19), crusts, plaques, nodules.
COLOR Red to reddish-brown.
DIASCOPY (i.e., glass slide applied with pressure on lesion) Reveals an "apple jelly" yellow-brown coloration.
DISTRIBUTION Exposed skin: hands, feet, head, and neck.

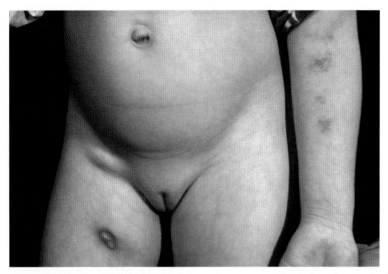

FIGURE 20-19 Cutaneous tuberculosis Primary inoculation site on the thigh with associated inguinal lymphadenopathy and a positive tuberculin test demonstrated on the arm. (Reproduced with permission from Fitzpatrick TB, Johnson RA, Wolff K, et al. *Color Atlas and Synopsis of Clinical Dermatology.* 4th ed. New York, NY: McGraw-Hill; 2001.)

DIFFERENTIAL DIAGNOSIS

The differential diagnosis of TB is broad given the wide spectrum of clinical disease. *M. tuberculosis* can be confused with syphilis, cat scratch disease, sporotrichosis, *Mycobacterium marinum,* deep fungal infection, sarcoidosis, warts, hypertrophic lichen planus, hidradenitis suppurativa, acne conglobata, herpes simplex virus, recurrent aphthous stomatitis, varicella, pityriasis lichenoides et varioliformis acuta, viral exanthems, lymphoma, lupus erythematous, leprosy, leishmaniasis, or panniculitis.

LABORATORY EXAMINATIONS

Dermatopathology

1. TB chancre: nonspecific inflammation with necrosis and bacilli, then Langerhans cells, lymphocytes, caseation necrosis, and no bacilli.
2. TB verrucosa cutis: pseudoepitheliomatous hyperplasia, microabscesses, sparse granulomatous foci, few bacilli.
3. Scrofuloderma: granulation tissue and caseation necrosis in deeper dermis with bacilli in pus.
4. Orificial TB: nonspecific inflammation and necrosis, bacilli easy to find.
5. Lupus vulgaris: well-developed tubercles, no visible bacilli.
6. Miliary TB/TB gumma: necrosis and abscesses with abundant bacilli.

CULTURE *M. tuberculosis* can be grown from all clinical forms of TB.

POLYMERASE CHAIN REACTION Detects *M. tuberculosis* DNA in tissue in all forms of TB.

SKIN TESTING Intradermal skin test converts from negative to positive in TB chancre; is negative in military TB and TB gumma; is positive in lupus vulgaris, scrofuloderma, and TB verrucosa cutis; and is variable in orificial TB.

COURSE AND PROGNOSIS

The course of cutaneous TB is variable.

1. A TB chancre heals spontaneously in 3 to 12 months.
2. TB verrucosa cutis heals spontaneously after several years.
3. Scrofuloderma heals slowly with keloid scarring.
4. Orificial TB results in an ulcer that is painful and will not heal spontaneously.
5. Lupus vulgaris lesions persist for years and heal with scarring.
6. Miliary TB/TB gumma heals slowly with scarring.

MANAGEMENT

The treatment for cutaneous TB is the same as for pulmonary TB. Isoniazid and rifampin, rifapentine, or rifabutin supplemented with ethambutol, streptomycin, or pyrazinamide can be used for 9 to 12 months and should continue for at least 2 months after resolution of cutaneous symptoms. Shorter courses can be attempted with a four-drug regimen, but the hallmark of treatment for cutaneous tuberculosis is multidrug therapy.

ATYPICAL MYCOBACTERIA: *MYCOBACTERIUM MARINUM*

Atypical mycobacteria are commonly found in water and soil and have low-grade pathogenicity. *M. marinum* infection follows traumatic inoculation in a fish tank (most common), swimming pool, or brackish water.

SYNONYMS Swimming pool granuloma, fish tank granuloma, infection by *Mycobacterium balnei*.

EPIDEMIOLOGY

AGE All ages.
GENDER M = F.
INCIDENCE Uncommon.
ETIOLOGY *M. marinum* in fresh water or salt-water fish.

PATHOPHYSIOLOGY

M. marinum infection occurs after traumatic inoculation through the skin and exposure to contaminated fish, fish tank, swimming pool, lake, or other aquatic environment.

HISTORY

Red papules appear at the site of inoculation. Over a period of 3 weeks, the papules grow to 1-cm nodules and break down into ulcers or plaques. They may remain as a single lesion or spread proximally along the course of the draining lymphatics (sporotrichoid spread). In immunocompetent hosts, systemic symptoms are absent.

PHYSICAL EXAMINATION

Skin Findings

TYPE Papule (Fig. 20-20), nodule, plaque, ulcer.
COLOR Red to reddish-brown.
SIZE 2 mm to 1 cm.
ARRANGEMENT Solitary lesion. Linear lesions in a "sporotrichoid pattern" following lymphatic drainage.
DISTRIBUTION Arms > legs.

General Findings

LYMPHADENOPATHY Regional lymphadenopathy.

DIFFERENTIAL DIAGNOSIS

The differential diagnosis for *M. marinum* infection includes warts, sporotrichosis, blastomycosis, *M. tuberculosis*, other non-tuberculous mycobacterial infection, leishmaniasis, syphilis, or foreign body reaction.

LABORATORY EXAMINATIONS

DERMATOPATHOLOGY Early lesions will show dermal inflammation with lymphocytes, neutrophils, and histiocytes. Older lesions show epithelial cells and Langerhans giant cells. AFB stain demonstrates *M. marinum* in only 50% of cases. Smears of exudates can also demonstrate AFB.
BACTERIAL CULTURE *M. marinum* will grow at 32°C in 2 to 4 weeks on Lowenstein–Jensen medium and is photochromogenic, differentiating it from the other atypical mycobacteria (i.e., *Mycobacterium ulcerans* or *Mycobacterium fortuitum*).
POLYMERASE CHAIN REACTION PCR of *M. marinum* DNA from biopsy samples can be used to confirm the diagnosis.

COURSE AND PROGNOSIS

M. marinum lesions tend to heal spontaneously in 1 to 2 years. Occasionally, deeper infections can be complicated by tenosynovitis, septic arthritis, or osteomyelitis. Immunocompromised hosts may have disseminated disease.

MANAGEMENT

For *M. marinum* treatment, antibiotic sensitivity testing should be performed and systemic minocycline, doxycycline, clarithromycin (+ rifampin), rifampin (+ ethambutol), trimethoprim-sulfamethoxazole, or ciprofloxacin is effective. Treatment duration should last for 2 months after resolution of cutaneous symptoms and for a minimum of 3 to 4 months. Surgery may be required if the lesions respond inadequately to antibiotic treatment.

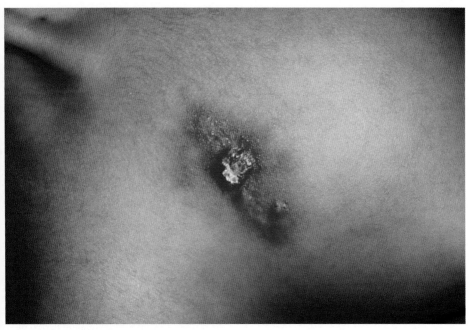

FIGURE 20-20 **Mycobacterial infection** Erythematous plaque with central pustule on the neck of a child exposed to *Mycobacterium marinum.*

LYME BORRELIOSIS

Lyme borreliosis is a spirochetal infectious disease transmitted to humans by the bite of an infected tick. Lyme disease, the syndrome occurring early in the infection, is characterized by a transient annular rash (erythema chronicum migrans, ECM), followed by late involvement of the joints, nervous system, and/or heart.

INSIGHT

The annular lesions of erythema migrans can range from 1 or 2 cm to tens of centimeters in size.

SYNONYMS Lyme disease, erythema migrans, Lyme arthritis.

EPIDEMIOLOGY

AGE Peaks: 5 to 9 years and 50 to 54 years.
GENDER Children: M > F. Adults: F > M.
INCIDENCE Common. In endemic areas, 5% to 10% of the population. 30,000 cases in the United States in 2012. Ninety percent of US cases between Maryland and Maine with rising incidence in New England states. Sweden: 69 cases/100,000, up to 130/100,000 in Austria.
RACE Whites > all other races.
ETIOLOGY The spirochete *Borrelia burgdorferi* is responsible for Lyme disease in the United States. *B. burgdorferi* also occurs in Europe, but the two dominant genospecies there are *B. burgdorferi garinii* and *B. burgdorferi afzelii*.
SEASON United States: Eighty percent summer in Midwestern and NE; spring in NW.
GEOGRAPHY The US northeast coast (Massachusetts, Rhode Island, Connecticut, New York, New Jersey, Pennsylvania, Delaware, Maryland), midwest (Minnesota, Wisconsin), and west (California, Oregon, Nevada, Utah). In Europe, Lyme borreliosis occurs widely throughout the continent and Great Britain. It also occurs in Australia, China, and Japan.

PATHOPHYSIOLOGY

B. burgdorferi is transmitted by the bite of deer ticks (*Ixodes scapularis* or *Ixodes dammini*) in eastern United States and Great Lakes region, black-legged ticks (*Ixodes pacificus*) in the western United States, *Ixodes ricinus* in Europe, and *Ixodes persulcatus* in Asia. *Borrelia* is transmitted to humans following biting and feeding of ticks or nymphs (Fig. 20-21).

Lyme borreliosis begins with the rash of erythema migrans, which occurs at the site of the tick bite soon after inoculation. The rash

persists for 2 to 3 weeks. Secondary lesions occur following hematogenous dissemination to the skin; up to one quarter of children with Lyme may show multiple erythema migrans lesions. The late joint manifestations appear to be mediated by immune-complex formation. Meningitis results from direct spirochete invasion of CSF. The pathogenesis of cranial and peripheral neuropathies in Lyme disease is unknown, but might also result from immune mechanisms.

HISTORY

An infected tick must be on a person 2 to 3 days to feed before passing on the infection. Lyme borreliosis has an incubation period of 1 to 36 days (median, 9 days) after the tick bite. Of note, only a small minority of Lyme borreliosis cases are aware of a preceding tick bite. Early Lyme disease is characterized by malaise, fatigue, lethargy, headaches, fever, chills, stiff neck, arthralgias, myalgias, backaches, anorexia, sore throat, nausea, dysesthesia, vomiting, abdominal pain, and photophobia; 75% of patients will have an associated ECM rash. Early Lyme disease symptoms disappear by 1 to 2 months. Late Lyme disease can occur in 15% of untreated cases after several weeks to months. Late sequelae include joint, neurologic, and cardiac complications.

PHYSICAL EXAMINATION

Skin Findings

TYPE Macule, papule, annular plaque.
COLOR Red to purple.
SIZE 2 cm to several centimeters (range 3–70 cm, median 15 cm in diameter).
NUMBER ECM: solitary lesion. Multiple secondary lesions develop in 25% of cases, resemble EM but are smaller, migrate less, and lack central induration (Fig. 20-22).
DISTRIBUTION Trunk and proximal extremities, axillary and inguinal areas.
MUCOUS MEMBRANES Red throat, conjunctivitis.

Late Skin Findings

LYMPHOCYTOMA CUTIS Infiltrative red-purple nodules from tick bite on the head,

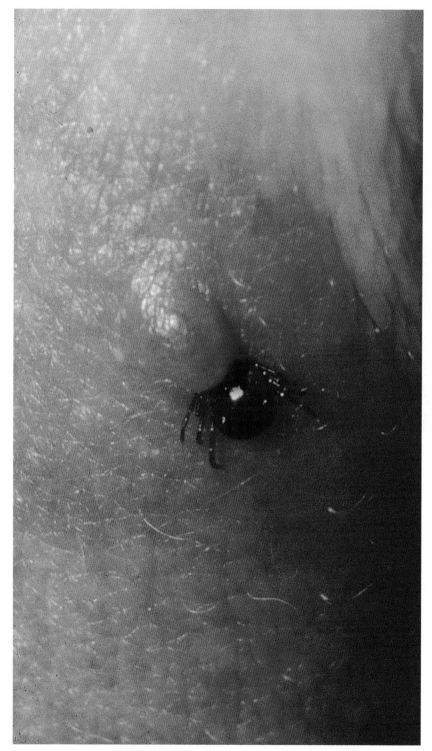

FIGURE 20-21 **Lyme borreliosis** A blood-distended nymph *Ixodes scapularis* feeding on human skin. Borrelia transmission usually occurs after prolonged attachment and feeding (36 hours).

especially ear lobes, nipples, scrotum, extremities; 3 to 5 cm in diameter; usually asymptomatic. May also be called cutaneous "pseudolymphoma."

ACRODERMATITIS CHRONICA ATROPHICANS Erythema on an extremity that slowly extends centrifugally over several months to years, leaving central areas of atrophy and fibrosis.

General Findings

FEVER Malaise, headache.

LYMPHADENOPATHY Regional lymphadenopathy.

EYES Conjunctivitis, keratitis, iritis, episcleritis, retrobulbar neuritis.

RHEUMATOLOGIC (60%) 4 to 6 weeks after the tick bite, arthralgias, tendonitis, oligoarthritis. Knee (89%), shoulder (9%), hip (9%), ankle (7%), and elbow (2%).

NEUROLOGIC (up to 20%) 1 to 6 weeks after the tick bite. Meningitis, encephalitis, sleep disturbances, difficulty concentrating, poor memory, irritability, emotional lability, dementia, cranial neuropathies (optic neuropathy, sixth nerve palsy, facial or Bell's palsy, eighth nerve deafness), sensory/motor radiculopathies (pain, dysesthesias, sensory loss, weakness, loss of reflexes).

CARDIAC (up to 10%) 4 weeks after tick bite. Atrioventricular block, myopericarditis, arrhythmias, cardiomyopathy, and left ventricular dysfunction.

OTHER Right upper quadrant tenderness, arthritis, hepatosplenomegaly, muscle tenderness, periorbital edema, and abdominal tenderness.

Variants

Lyme disease occurring in Europe is reportedly milder than in the United States, probably as a result of strain differences in *B. burgdorferi*. *B. garinii* is associated with neurologic disease while *B. afzelii* is associated with the dermatologic manifestation known as acrodermatitis chronica atrophicans.

DIFFERENTIAL DIAGNOSIS

The differential diagnosis of Lyme disease includes tinea corporis, herald patch of pityriasis rosea, insect (e.g., brown recluse spider) bite, cellulitis, urticaria, erythema multiforme, fixed drug eruption, fibromyalgia, gonococcal arthritis, gout, meningitis, lupus erythematosus, and secondary syphilis.

LABORATORY EXAMINATIONS

DERMATOPATHOLOGY Perivascular and interstitial lymphohistiocytic infiltrate containing plasma cells. Spirochetes can be demonstrated in up to 40% of skin biopsy specimens.

SEROLOGY Indirect immunofluorescence antibody and ELISA are used to detect antibodies to *B. burgdorferi*. Initial antibody response is with IgM antibodies followed by IgG. Early in Lyme disease, when only the rash has occurred, as few as 50% of patients have positive serologies; adequate treatment may block seroconversion. Individuals with multiple erythema migrans lesions tend to have higher rates of positive serology. Virtually all cases with late manifestations are seropositive with a titer > 1:256. Positive titers should be confirmed with a Western blot.

OTHER *Ixodes* ticks removed from patients can also be tested for the presence of *Borrelia* infection.

COURSE AND PROGNOSIS

The skin lesions in untreated early Lyme disease fade in a median time of 28 days. Both EM and secondary lesions can fade and recur for months. However, following adequate treatment, early lesions resolve within several days and late manifestations are prevented. Late manifestations identified early usually clear following antibiotic therapy; but a delay may result in permanent joint, neurologic, or cardiac disabilities.

MANAGEMENT

Education regarding disease prevention, especially in Lyme endemic areas, includes wearing long-sleeved shirts and tucking pants into socks or boot tops may help keep ticks from reaching the skin, and insect repellents (DEET, permethrin) applied to clothes and exposed skin can help reduce the risk of tick attachment.

Transmission of *B. burgdorferi* from an infected tick usually takes 2 to 3 days of tick attachment; thus, daily checks for ticks and prompt removal will prevent infection. A tick should be removed with fine-tipped tweezers by grasping the tick near the skin and pulling it off. Petroleum jelly, a hot match, or other home remedies are *not* recommended.

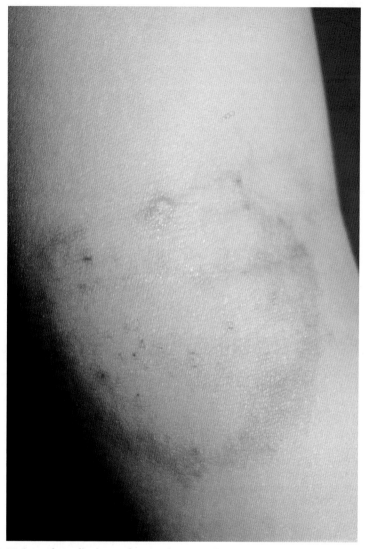

FIGURE 20-22 Lyme borreliosis, erythema migrans Solitary enlarging annular plaque on the leg at the site of an asymptomatic tick bite.

In children older than 8 years, in endemic areas, one dose of 200 mg of doxycycline within 72 hours of removing a tick can prevent the development of Lyme disease. If skin lesions are apparent, then 21 days of tetracycline, doxycycline, amoxicillin, or cefuroxime axetil is recommended. In children younger than 8 years, 21 days of cefuroxime axetil or amoxicillin and in penicillin-allergic patients, erythromycin is recommended.

Late Lyme disease, arthritis, and neurologic complications can be treated with 28 days of tetracycline, doxycycline, or amoxicillin, and IV ceftriaxone or chloramphenicol for 21 to 28 days if the first oral course is unsuccessful.

Of note, a vaccine, LYMErix, had been considered for individuals aged 15 to 70 with moderate to high risk, but is no longer available because of lack of interest.

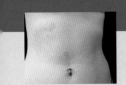
CUTANEOUS FUNGAL INFECTIONS

Cutaneous fungal infections are categorized as follows:

1. *Superficial:* infecting the stratum corneum, hair, and nails.

   The three major genera are *Trichophyton, Microsporum,* and *Epidermophyton.* The term "tinea" is used to denote fungal infection and is typically modified by body site (e.g., tinea capitis, tinea corporis).

   Candida is a normal inhabitant of the oropharynx and gastrointestinal tract. Moist, wet conditions favor *Candida* overgrowth and can lead to superficial infection of the skin or mucosal surfaces.

2. *Deep:* involving the dermis and subcutaneous tissues.

   Subcutaneous mycoses are the result of implantation and include chromoblastomycosis, mycetoma, sporotrichosis, basidiobolomycosis, and lobomycosis.

   Deep mycoses are the result of hematogenous spread or extension from an underlying structure. True pathogens infect hosts with normal immunity and include histoplasmosis, coccidioidomycosis, and paracoccidioidomycosis. Opportunistic pathogens infect immunocompromised hosts and include disseminated candidiasis and aspergillosis.

SUPERFICIAL DERMATOPHYTOSES

TINEA CAPITIS

Tinea capitis is a fungal infection (*Microsporum* or *Trichophyton*) of the scalp and hair characterized by follicular inflammation with painful, boggy nodules that drain pus and result in hair loss.

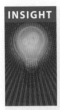

INSIGHT If there is any doubt about the diagnosis, a fungal culture of affected hairs and scale can be very helpful. If systemic treatment is given without improvement, the initial diagnosis is called into question, but culture after treatment is extremely low-yield.

SYNONYMS Scalp ringworm, tinea tonsurans, herpes tonsurans, hair ringworm.

EPIDEMIOLOGY

AGE Children: 2 to 10 years; rarely seen in infants or adults.
GENDER M > F, >2:1.
RACE Blacks > whites.
INCIDENCE Most common fungal infection in childhood. Up to 8% of the pediatric population affected.
ETIOLOGY *Trichophyton tonsurans* (90%) in the United States and West Europe > *Microsporum canis* > *M. audouinii* > *T. verrucosum.*

T. violaceum > *T. tonsurans* in Southeast Europe and North Africa.

HISTORY

Two to four days after exposure, scaly pruritic patches appear in the scalp with hair loss. Untreated, the lesions enlarge and boggy papular lesions may develop within the alopecic patches. Systemic symptoms may include cervical lymphadenopathy, malaise, or fever. Additionally, a systemic allergy to fungal elements can be seen (see "**Tinea and Id Reaction**").

PHYSICAL EXAMINATION

Skin Lesions

1. Ectothrix (infection on the outside of the hair shaft).
   a. **Gray patch ringworm.** Brittle hair; shafts break off 1 to 2 mm above the scalp surface. Broken hairs give patch a grayish appearance. Caused by *M. audouinii* and *M. canis* (Fig. 21-1).

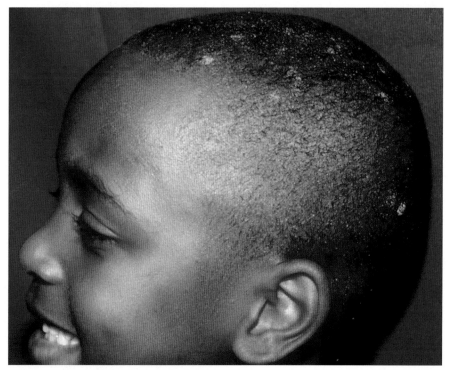

FIGURE 21-1 Tinea capitis, "gray patch" type Well-delineated scaly patches scattered on the scalp of a child with "ringworm."

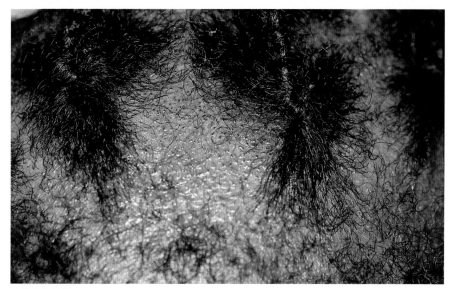

FIGURE 21-2 Tinea capitis, "black-dot" type Asymptomatic patch of alopecia on the frontal scalp of a 4-year-old child with a *Trichophyton tonsurans* infection. (Reproduced with permission from Fitzpatrick TB, Wolff K, Johnson RA. *Color Atlas and Synopsis of Clinical Dermatology.* 4th ed. New York, NY: McGraw-Hill; 2001.)

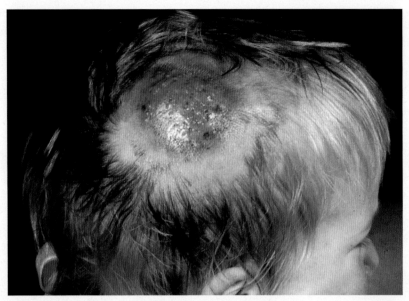

FIGURE 21-3 Tinea capitis, "kerion" type Large boggy, erythematous nodule on the scalp of a child. (Reproduced with permission from Fitzpatrick TB, Wolff K, Johnson RA. *Color Atlas and Synopsis of Clinical Dermatology*. 4th ed. New York, NY: McGraw-Hill; 2001.)

2. Endothrix (infection on the inside of the hair shaft).
   a. **Black dot ringworm.** Broken-off hair shafts flush with the level of the scalp give the appearance of black dots, caused by *T. tonsurans* and *T. violaceum* (Fig. 21-2). Easily spread via fomites.
   b. **Kerion.** Boggy, purulent, inflamed painful nodule drains pus. Hairs do not break but fall out easily. Heals with residual hair loss (Fig. 21-3).
   c. **Favus.** Scutula (yellowish crusts) are present on the scalp infected with *T. schoenleinii* (Fig. 21-4). Favus is endemic in Asia, the Middle East, and South Africa.

WOOD'S LAMP Wood's lamp reveals bright green hair shafts in scalp infections caused by *M. audouinii* and *M. canis*. *T. schoenleinii* fluorescence is grayish green. *T. tonsurans*, however, does not exhibit fluorescence.

LABORATORY EXAMINATIONS

DIRECT MICROSCOPIC EXAMINATION WITH 10% KOH Spores within (*T. tonsurans* and *T. violaceum*, Fig. 21-5) or surrounding (*Microsporum*) the hair shaft, consistent with endothrix or ectothrix tinea capitis, respectively.
FUNGAL CULTURE Infected hair or scalp scale can be inoculated on Sabouraud's agar or other Dermatophyte Test Medium (DTM) and the causative organism can be identified in several weeks' time.

MANAGEMENT

Tinea capitis spreads on brushes, combs, towels, pillowcases, and hats. Children with scalp ringworm should not share these items. Tinea capitis can also be spread by close contact with infected children. The current recommendation is that infected children may attend school once treatment has begun.

Antifungal shampoos (ketoconazole 2% or selenium sulfide 2.5%) decrease shedding fungal elements and thus decrease spread of infection. Patients should be instructed to lather the shampoo and let it sit on the scalp for 5 to 10 minutes before rinsing 2 to 3 times per week. Household contacts can also shampoo daily or every other day until the patient is disease-free. Pets including cats and dogs are reservoirs of *M. canis* and veterinary treatment of household pets should be considered if they are suspected to be the source of infection or reinfection.

SYSTEMIC THERAPIES Topical treatments are not effective in treating the hair bulb; thus oral antifungal treatment is needed. Oral griseofulvin is the gold standard for tinea capitis in children, and refractory cases may need higher doses or fluconazole. Known side effects include headaches and gastrointestinal upset. Newer antifungal agents (itraconazole, terbinafine) are efficacious, but none of these agents have the long-term safety profile of griseofulvin.

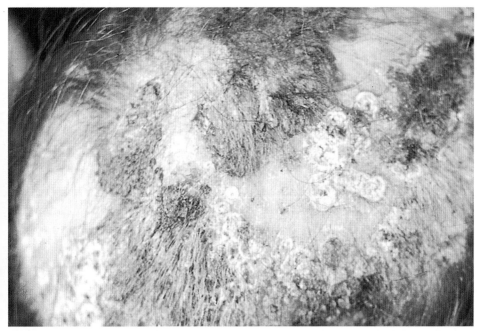

FIGURE 21-4 Tinea capitis, "favus" type Yellowish adherent crusts and scales called "scutula" on a child with a *Trichophyton schoenleinii* infection. (Reproduced with permission from Freedberg IM, Irwin M. *Dermatology in General Medicine.* 5th ed. New York, NY: McGraw-Hill; 1999.)

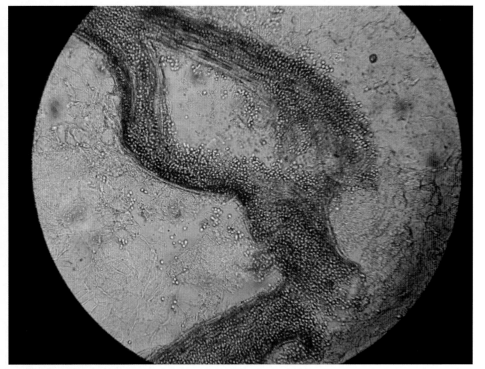

FIGURE 21-5 Tinea capitis, potassium hydroxide (KOH) preparation KOH preparation demonstrating spores in the hair shaft characteristic of an endothrix.

TINEA FACIEI

Tinea faciei is a superficial fungal infection on the face, characterized by a well-circumscribed erythematous enlarging plaque.

SYNONYMS Tinea faciale, tinea facialis, ringworm of the face.

EPIDEMIOLOGY

AGE Most common in children.
INCIDENCE Common.
ETIOLOGY *T. mentagrophytes*, *T. rubrum* > *M. audouinii*, *M. canis*.

PATHOPHYSIOLOGY

Tinea faciei is most commonly caused by a child's exposure to an infected animal, especially puppies or kittens. By hugging or playing with the animal, the dermatophyte is transferred by fur to skin contact.

HISTORY

An asymptomatic papule slowly enlarges to a plaque. The lesion is asymptomatic or mildly pruritic. Multiple discrete lesions may be present. No systemic symptoms are present.

PHYSICAL EXAMINATION

Skin Findings

TYPE Macule, plaque, scale (Fig. 21-6).
COLOR Pink to red, hyperpigmentation.
DISTRIBUTION Any area of face; cheeks are most common.

DIFFERENTIAL DIAGNOSIS

Tinea faciei is the most commonly misdiagnosed fungal infection. It is often mistaken for seborrheic dermatitis, contact dermatitis, erythema chronicum migrans, lupus erythematosus, polymorphic light eruption, or a photoinduced drug eruption.

LABORATORY EXAMINATIONS

KOH Examination of scraping shows hyphae. Scrapings from patients who have used topical antifungals may be falsely negative. Patients who have used topical corticosteroids show massive numbers of hyphae.
FUNGAL CULTURE Skin scrapings taken from the area and inoculated on Sabouraud's agar or other DTM media will grow the causative dermatophyte in a few weeks.

MANAGEMENT

For the treatment of tinea faciei, topical antifungals such as substituted pyridine (ciclopirox), naphthiomates (tolnaftate), imidazoles (clotrimazole, econazole, miconazole, ketoconazole, oxiconazole), allylamines (terbinafine, naftifine) are effective if applied BID at least 2 cm beyond the advancing edge of the skin lesion until the lesion clears (typically 6 weeks). It is recommended to continue the topical medication for one more week after clinical clearing to ensure clinical cure.

Affected household members or pets should also be treated. In severe refractory or recurrent cases, systemic fluconazole, griseofulvin, itraconazole, or terbinafine may be necessary.

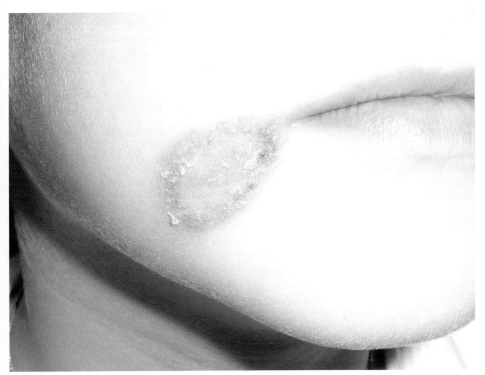

FIGURE 21-6 Tinea faciei Sharply marginated, enlarging plaque with a raised annular border on the face of a child.

TINEA CORPORIS

Tinea corporis is a superficial fungal infection characterized by scaling papular lesions occurring in an annular arrangement with peripheral enlargement and central clearing on the trunk, limbs, or face.

SYNONYMS "Ringworm," tinea corporis gladiatorum.

EPIDEMIOLOGY

AGE All ages.
INCIDENCE Common.
ETIOLOGY *T. rubrum* > *T. mentagrophytes* > *M. canis* > *M. audouinii.*

PATHOPHYSIOLOGY

Tinea corporis can result from human-to-human, animal-to-human, or soil-to-human spread. Kittens and puppies are an important risk factor in the transmission of organisms, as are gymnasiums, crowded housing, locker rooms, wrestling, outdoor occupations, and immunosuppressive states.

HISTORY

One to three weeks after inoculation, the infection spreads centrifugally resulting in annular scaly plaques with pustules at the active border. Lesions may be asymptomatic, pruritic, or with a burning sensation. Systemic symptoms are not present.

PHYSICAL EXAMINATION

Skin Findings

TYPE Plaques with or without pustules or vesicles.
SIZE 1 to 10 cm.
COLOR Pink to red.
ARRANGEMENT Enlargement, central clearing, annular configuration (Fig. 21-7).

DISTRIBUTION Exposed skin of forearm, neck most common; found on all locations on trunk.

DIFFERENTIAL DIAGNOSIS

Tinea corporis is often mistaken for annular erythemas, psoriasis, contact dermatitis, eczema, pityriasis rosea, seborrhea, granuloma annulare, or lupus erythematosus.

LABORATORY EXAMINATIONS

KOH Scales from the edge demonstrate hyphae, arthrospores, or budding yeasts. The type of dermatophyte cannot be determined, but rather its presence or absence.
FUNGAL CULTURE Skin lesion scrapings can be inoculated on Sabouraud's agar or other media, and dermatophyte types will grow and can be identified in a matter of weeks.

MANAGEMENT

For the treatment of tinea corporis, topical antifungals such as substituted pyridine (ciclopirox), naphthiomates (tolnaftate), imidazoles (clotrimazole, econazole, miconazole, ketoconazole, oxiconazole), and allylamines (terbinafine, naftifine) are effective if applied BID at least 2 cm beyond the advancing edge of the skin lesion until the lesion clears (typically 6 weeks). It is recommended to continue the topical medication for one more week after clinical clearing to ensure clinical cure. Affected household members or pets should also be treated.

In severe refractory or recurrent cases, systemic fluconazole, griseofulvin, itraconazole or terbinafine may be necessary.

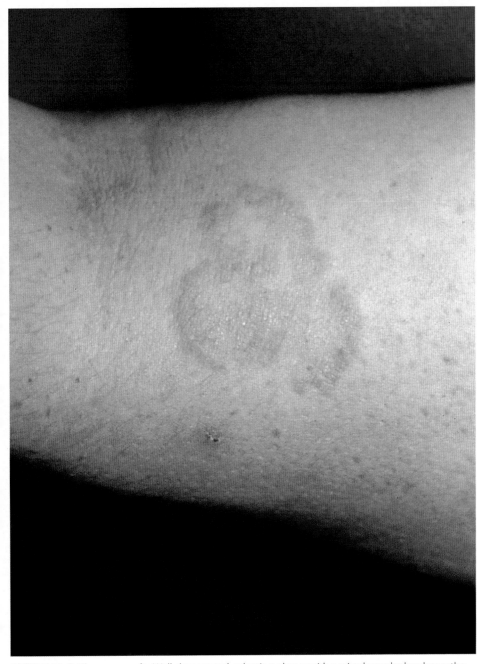

FIGURE 21-7 Tinea corporis Well-demarcated enlarging plaque with a raised annular border on the forearm.

TINEA CRURIS

Tinea cruris is a subacute or chronic fungal infection of the upper thigh or groin area, usually caused by *Epidermophyton floccosum, T. rubrum,* or *T. mentagrophytes.*

SYNONYM Jock itch.

EPIDEMIOLOGY

AGE Adolescents and young adults.
GENDER M > F.
ETIOLOGY *T. rubrum* > *T. mentagrophytes* > *E. floccosum.*

PATHOPHYSIOLOGY

Most patients with tinea cruris have concomitant tinea pedis. The fungal infection on the feet typically precedes the groin infection. The fungal elements are spread when underclothes are dragged over the infected feet up to the groin area. Other predisposing factors include warm, humid environment, tight clothing, obesity, diabetes, and immunosuppression.

HISTORY

Often seen in athletes, tinea cruris begins as erythema and mild pruritus in the groin area. Occlusive, wet clothing (tight clothes, exercise outfits, bathing suits) aggravates the condition.

PHYSICAL EXAMINATION

Skin Findings

TYPE Plaques, papules, scale, pustules.
COLOR Dull red to brown.
DISTRIBUTION Bilateral intertriginous areas, upper thighs, and buttock (Fig. 21-8). Scrotum is rarely involved (in contrast to candidiasis).

DIFFERENTIAL DIAGNOSIS

The differential diagnosis for tinea cruris includes candidiasis, erythrasma, intertrigo, seborrheic dermatitis, psoriasis, irritant dermatitis, and contact dermatitis.

LABORATORY EXAMINATIONS

KOH Scrapings will show hyphae, arthrospores, or budding yeasts.
FUNGAL CULTURE Skin scrapings taken from the area and inoculated on Sabouraud's agar or other DTM media will grow causative dermatophyte in a few weeks.

MANAGEMENT

Measures to prevent tinea cruris include less occlusive clothing, shower shoes in public or home bathroom floor, antifungal foot powder, and concomitant treatment of tinea pedis (athlete's foot) if present. Patients should be instructed to put on their socks before their underwear to avoid dragging the fungal elements from the floor or their infected feet up to their groin area.

For the treatment of tinea cruris, topical antifungals such as substituted pyridine (ciclopirox), naphthiomates (tolnaftate), imidazoles (clotrimazole, econazole, miconazole, ketoconazole, oxiconazole), allylamines (terbinafine, naftifine) are effective if applied BID at least 2 cm beyond the advancing edge of the skin lesion until the lesion clears (typically 6 weeks). It is recommended to continue the topical medication for one more week after clinical clearing to ensure clinical cure.

In severe refractory or recurrent cases, systemic fluconazole, griseofulvin, itraconazole, or terbinafine may be necessary.

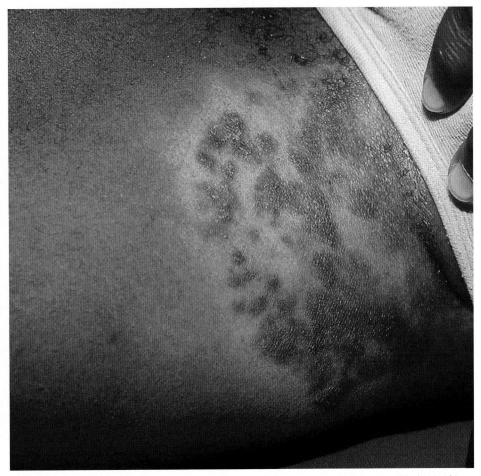

FIGURE 21-8 Tinea cruris Enlarging pruritic plaque in the groin area worsening on topical steroids.

TINEA PEDIS

Tinea pedis is an itchy, scaly fungal infection of the feet seen in adolescents or adults, but rarely in young children.

SYNONYM Athlete's foot.

EPIDEMIOLOGY

AGE Adolescents and adults; rare in children.
GENDER M = F.
INCIDENCE Most common fungal infection in adolescents and adults.
ETIOLOGY *T. rubrum, T. mentagrophytes* > *E. floccosum, T. tonsurans.*

PATHOPHYSIOLOGY

Tinea pedis is caused by *T. rubrum, T. mentagrophytes, E. floccosum,* or *T. tonsurans* growing in humid weather with occlusive footwear. The fungal organisms are likely contracted from going barefoot in locker rooms, gymnasiums, or public facilities, but host susceptibility also plays a role in that some people never get tinea pedis despite exposure and others always have recurrences despite treatment. Prevalence is more common with increasing age.

HISTORY

Tinea pedis usually begins as interdigital scaling and fissuring, especially between the fourth and fifth toes. It can then spread to affect both plantar aspects of the feet ("moccasin distribution") and palmar aspects of the hands. Inflammation and/or ulceration may be present. Also, a systemic autoeczematization response can be seen (see "**Tinea and Id Reaction**").

PHYSICAL EXAMINATION

Skin Findings

TYPE Scale, maceration, vesicles, bullae (Fig. 21-9).
COLOR Pink to red; opaque white scales.
DISTRIBUTION Webspace between third/fourth toes, plantar surface, especially arch.

DIFFERENTIAL DIAGNOSIS

Tinea pedis, although common in adolescents and adults, is **uncommon** in children. Most instances of "athlete's foot" in children are actually atopic dermatitis, contact dermatitis, psoriasis, juvenile plantar dermatosis, erythrasma, or a bacterial infection.

LABORATORY EXAMINATIONS

KOH Webspace or scaly areas reveal hyphae, arthrospores, or budding yeasts.
FUNGAL CULTURE Skin scrapings inoculated on Sabouraud's agar or DTM media will show fungal growth in a few weeks.

COURSE AND PROGNOSIS

Tinea pedis tends to be chronic and recurrent with exacerbations in hot weather or with exercise. Macerated skin may lead to lymphangitis or cellulitis.

MANAGEMENT

Tinea pedis is difficult to treat and is prone to recurrences. Acute episodes can be treated with open wet compresses (Burow's solution, 1:80 dilution) and topical antifungal creams such as substituted pyridine (ciclopirox), naphthiomates (tolnaftate), imidazoles (clotrimazole, econazole, miconazole, ketoconazole, oxiconazole), or allylamines (terbinafine, naftifine). They should be applied BID over both feet up to the ankles bilaterally until the lesions clear (typically 2–6 weeks). It is recommended to continue the topical medication for one more week after clinical clearing to ensure clinical cure. The addition of keratolytic creams (glycolic acid, lactic acid, or urea) can help reduce hyperkeratosis. Keeping the feet dry will help prevent relapses and can be achieved with open footwear or absorbent socks/antifungal foot powder.

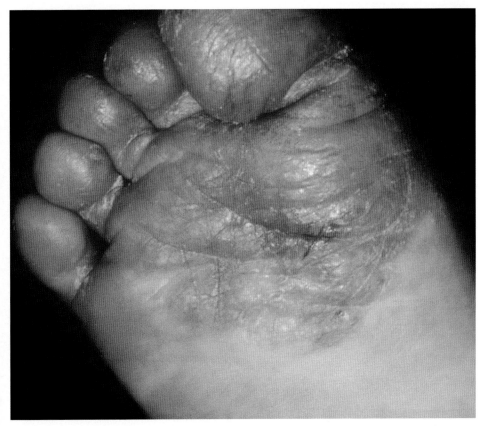

FIGURE 21-9 Tinea pedis Erythema, scale, and vesiculation on the plantar aspect of a child's foot. KOH scraping demonstrated hyphae.

TINEA MANUUM

Tinea manuum is a chronic dermatophytosis of the hand(s), often unilateral, and most commonly on the dominant hand. There is almost invariably a pre-existing tinea pedis, with or without nail involvement (onychomycosis).

SYNONYM Tinea manus.

EPIDEMIOLOGY

AGE Adolescents and adults. Uncommon in children.
GENDER M = F.
INCIDENCE Common.
ETIOLOGY *T. rubrum, T. mentagrophytes* > *E. floccosum.*

PATHOPHYSIOLOGY

Tinea manuum is a dermatophyte infection of the palm and interdigital spaces often seen in patients with concomitant moccasin-type tinea pedis, and is thought to spread from the feet.

HISTORY

Tinea manuum usually presents as unilateral (usually dominant hand) palmar scaling in an individual with chronic or intermittent pre-existing tinea pedis or onychomycosis. Like tinea pedis, it tends to have a chronic and relapsing course.

PHYSICAL EXAMINATION

Skin Findings

TYPE Papules, vesicles (Fig. 21-10).
COLOR Pink to red.
DISTRIBUTION Diffuse hyperkeratosis of the palms or patchy scaling on sides of fingers; 50% of patients have *unilateral* involvement. Associated nail involvement (tinea unguium) may be a helpful diagnostic clue.

DIFFERENTIAL DIAGNOSIS

Tinea manuum is often mistaken for psoriasis, lichen planus, allergic contact or irritant dermatitis, or dyshidrotic eczema.

LABORATORY EXAMINATIONS

KOH Scales taken from the advancing edge will show hyphae elements.
FUNGAL CULTURE Skin scrapings can be inoculated on Sabouraud's agar or DTM media and will grow the causative dermatophyte in several weeks' time.

COURSE AND PROGNOSIS

When combined with tinea capitis, onychomycosis, tinea pedis, or tinea corporis, tinea manuum may recur following treatment, and this can be a frustrating problem.

MANAGEMENT

Acute episodes of tinea manuum can be treated with open wet compresses (Burow's solution, 1:80 dilution) and topical antifungal creams such as substituted pyridine (ciclopirox), naphthiomates (tolnaftate), imidazoles (clotrimazole, econazole, miconazole, ketoconazole, oxiconazole), or allylamines (terbinafine, naftifine). It is recommended to continue the topical medication for one more week after clinical clearing to ensure clinical cure. Eradication of other concomitant tinea infections (e.g., tinea capitis, onychomycosis) needs to occur to prevent recurrences.

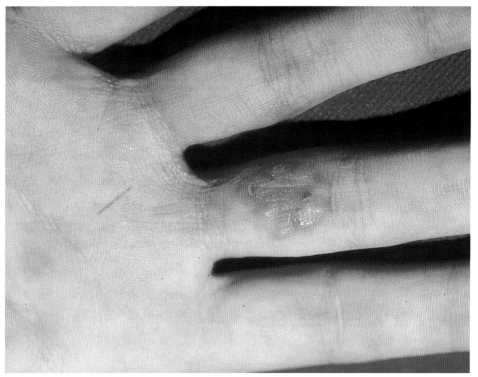

FIGURE 21-10 Tinea manuum Clustered erythematous papules on the hand of a child. KOH scraping demonstrated hyphae.

ONYCHOMYCOSIS

Onychomycosis is a common fungal infection of the toenails and/or fingernails.

SYNONYM Tinea unguium.

EPIDEMIOLOGY

AGE Adolescents and adults, rarely children.
GENDER M > F.
INCIDENCE Common.
ETIOLOGY *T. rubrum, T. mentagrophytes* >
E. floccosum.

PATHOPHYSIOLOGY

Onychomycosis is associated with tinea pedis
and trauma helps inoculate the nail with fungus. Host susceptibility to tinea pedis predis-
poses the patient to onychomycosis. However,
onychomycosis can also superinfect diseased
nails (psoriasis or eczema).

HISTORY

Onychomycosis typically is seen in individuals
with chronic tinea pedis or tinea manuum. The
onset is slow and insidious, and typically affects
the toenails more often than the fingernails. Topical treatments are of limited efficacy and oral regimens, while efficacious, do not prevent relapses.

PHYSICAL EXAMINATION

Nail Lesions

DISTAL SUBUNGUAL ONYCHOMYCOSIS Whitish-
yellow discoloration of the free nail edge with
separation of nail plate/nail bed and subungual
accumulation of debris.
WHITE SUPERFICIAL ONYCHOMYCOSIS White area
on the nail plate, occurs relatively commonly
in HIV-infected patients in both toenails and
fingernails.
PROXIMAL SUBUNGUAL ONYCHOMYCOSIS Rare.
Starts as whitish-brown area on the proximal
part of the nail plate. May enlarge to affect the
whole nail plate.

CANDIDA ONYCHOMYCOSIS Toenails/fingernails
in chronic mucocutaneous candidiasis (CMC)
are thickened, rough, furrowed, and eventually
disintegrate into a brittle mass.
DISTRIBUTION Infected nails coexist with
normal-appearing nails (Fig. 21-11). Toenails >
fingernails. Twenty nails involved in immunosuppressed patients (seen in chronic mucocutaneous
candidiasis and acrodermatitis enteropathica).

DIFFERENTIAL DIAGNOSIS

The differential diagnosis of onychomycosis
includes nail psoriasis, eczema, trauma, photoonycholysis, pachyonychia congenita, and other
inherited nail disorders.

LABORATORY EXAMINATIONS

KOH Examination of nail scrapings reveals
hyphae.
FUNGAL CULTURE Nail clippings taken and
inoculated on Sabouraud's agar or other DTM
media will grow the causative dermatophyte in
a few weeks.
DERMATOPATHOLOGY A PAS stain of an infected
nail clipping will reveal hyphae.

MANAGEMENT

Topical treatment for onychomycosis is of
limited efficacy, but topical preparations
(ciclopirox) are safer in children and with
chronic use can eliminate tinea pedis, which in
turn may clear onychomycosis slowly. Efficacy
of newer topical agents such as efinaconazole
has not been established in children.

Oral antifungals are the treatment of choice
in adolescents and adults. Oral griseofulvin
is slow and not as effective as oral fluconazole, itraconazole, or terbinafine for toenail
clearance, which have an 80% cure rate, but a
significant relapse rate. Old shoes should be
discarded; proper footwear, cotton socks, and
absorbent powders may be helpful.

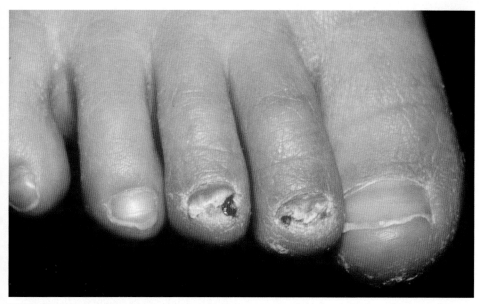

FIGURE 21-11 Onychomycosis Onycholysis of the second and third toenails. Fungal culture of the nail grew *Trichophyton rubrum*.

TINEA AND ID REACTION

An "id" reaction is a generalized acute cutaneous reaction to an infection (e.g., tinea) or inflammatory skin condition (e.g., contact dermatitis) characterized by a vesicular eruption on the trunk and extremities.

SYNONYMS Dermatophytid reaction, autoeczematization, autosensitization.

INSIGHT The word "id" comes from the Greek suffix **ides**, meaning "son or daughter of" and is not related to the psychoanalytic term.

EPIDEMIOLOGY

AGE Any age.
GENDER M = F.
INCIDENCE Up to 5% of tinea infections.
ETIOLOGY Unclear.

PATHOPHYSIOLOGY

The exact pathophysiology is poorly understood. An id reaction may be caused by an abnormal immune recognition of autologous skin antigens, increased stimulation of T cells, a lower irritation threshold, disseminated infectious antigen with a secondary response, or hematogenous cytokines.

HISTORY

An id reaction is an uncommon generalized vesicular eruption that appears after the primary focus of infection (tinea capitis, faciei, corporis, pedis, or manuum) has been present for a while and clearance has started. Symptomatically, the rash can be very pruritic and systemically the patients may have mild fever or lymphadenopathy. Id reactions may also be triggered by other sources in the absence of a superficial dermatophyte infection.

PHYSICAL EXAMINATION

Skin Findings

TYPE Diffuse papules and vesicles, edema (Fig. 21-12).
COLOR Pink to red.
SIZE 2 to 5 mm.
DISTRIBUTION Trunk, extremities (Fig. 21-13), face.

General Findings

FEVER
LAD Mild lymphadenopathy may be present.

DIFFERENTIAL DIAGNOSIS

An id reaction can be confused with a drug reaction, viral exanthem, dyshidrotic eczema, contact dermatitis, cutaneous T-cell lymphoma (CTCL), folliculitis, scabies, or generalized tinea infection.

LABORATORY EXAMINATIONS

DERMATOPATHOLOGY Epidermal spongiotic vesicles, a few dermal eosinophils.

COURSE AND PROGNOSIS

Once the primary infection or inflammatory condition has been cleared, the id reaction will self-resolve. Unfortunately, recurrences are common, especially if the primary source is not fully eradicated.

MANAGEMENT

Eradication of the primary infection or inflammatory condition is the best way to treat an id reaction. Symptomatic relief can be obtained with a short course of topical steroids, wet compresses, and systemic antihistamines (diphenhydramine, loratadine).

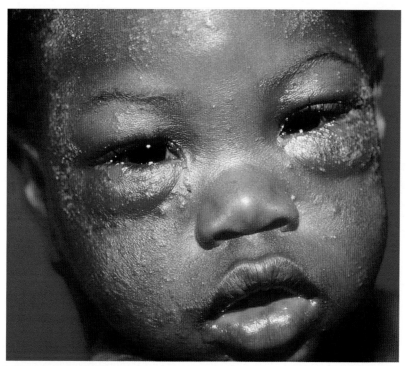

FIGURE 21-12 Tinea and id reaction Diffuse vesicular rash in a child being treated for tinea capitis.

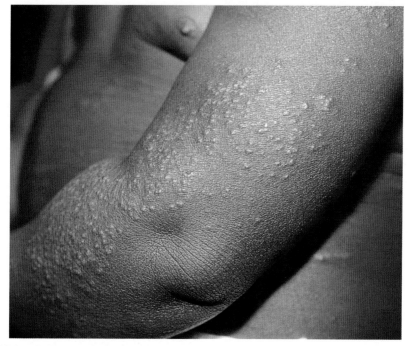

FIGURE 21-13 Tinea and id reaction Diffuse vesicular lesions on the arm of the same child shown in Figure 21-12.

SUPERFICIAL CANDIDIASIS

ORAL CANDIDIASIS

Oral candidiasis is characterized by the presence of painful, white, milk-like removable plaques on the oral mucosa.

SYNONYMS Moniliasis, thrush, mycotic stomatitis, *Candida* leukoplakia.

EPIDEMIOLOGY

AGE Newborns, 8 or 9 days old.
GENDER M = F.
INCIDENCE Common in newborns and infants, with risk factors including prematurity and low birth weight. Uncommon in adults: may be a marker for immunodeficiency or associated with oral/inhaled corticosteroid use.
ETIOLOGY *Candida albicans,* most commonly.

PATHOPHYSIOLOGY

Candida is present in the mouth and intestinal tract in up to 50% of the normal population and >20% of the genital tract in normal women. *Candida* is transmitted to the infant at the time of delivery during passage through the vaginal canal or during breastfeeding from colonized maternal skin.

HISTORY

In newborns and infants, the white curd-like plaques appear at day of life 8 to 9 and are usually asymptomatic. Mechanical removal with a dry gauze pad leaves an erythematous or bleeding mucosal surface.

PHYSICAL EXAMINATION

Mucous Membrane Findings

TYPE Plaques.
SIZE Few millimeters to several centimeters.

COLOR White to creamy.
PALPATION Plaques are friable and removable with dry gauze.
DISTRIBUTION Tongue, buccal mucosa, hard/soft palate, and pharynx (Fig. 21-14).

DIFFERENTIAL DIAGNOSIS

The differential diagnosis for oral candidiasis includes oral hairy leukoplakia, condyloma acuminatum, geographic tongue, hairy tongue, lichen planus, and a bite irritation.

LABORATORY EXAMINATIONS

KOH Scraping shows *Candida* pseudohyphae as well as budding yeast forms.
CULTURES Buccal or tongue plaques scraped and cultured will grow species of *Candida*.

COURSE AND PROGNOSIS

Oral candidiasis is benign and usually asymptomatic. It responds nicely to topical treatment, but may intermittently recur. In adults, chronic recurrent oral candidiasis may be a sign of immunosuppression or immunodeficiency.

MANAGEMENT

For mild cases, nystatin suspension can be used until clinical clearing is noted. Refractory or recurrent cases may require topical clotrimazole, systemic itraconazole, or fluconazole.

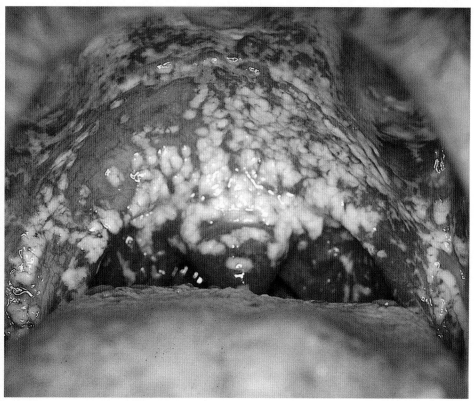

FIGURE 21-14 Oral candidiasis White plaques on the hard palate representing colonies of *Candida* that can be removed by rubbing the area with gauze. (Reproduced with permission from Fitzpatrick TB, Wolff K, Johnson RA. *Color Atlas and Synopsis of Clinical Dermatology*. 3rd ed. New York, NY: McGraw-Hill; 1997.)

CUTANEOUS CANDIDIASIS

Cutaneous candidiasis is a superficial infection occurring on moist cutaneous sites and mucosal surfaces; many patients have predisposing factors such as occluded moist skin sites, diabetes, antibiotic therapy, or alteration in systemic immunity.

CLASSIFICATION

1. **Intertrigo:**
   a. Body folds (neck, groin, intergluteal, axilla, inframammary).
   b. Webspaces: fingers, toes; may be associated with candidal paronychia; also termed "erosio interdigitalis blastomycetica."
2. **Genital:** balanoposthitis, balanitis, vulvitis.
3. **Occluded skin:** diaper (Fig. 21-15), surgical cast, immobilized patient, etc.
4. **Chronic mucocutaneous candidiasis:** rare immunologic (e.g., T-cell defects) or associated endocrinologic disorders (e.g., hypoparathyroidism, hypoadrenalism, hypothyroidism, diabetes, vitiligo) that lead to chronic mucosal, cutaneous, or nail *C. albicans* infections.

SYNONYMS Moniliasis, candidosis, erosio interdigitalis blastomycetica.

EPIDEMIOLOGY

AGE Any age. Infants (diaper area, mouth).
GENDER M = F.
INCIDENCE Common.
ETIOLOGY *C. albicans*; normal in oropharynx and GI tract, **not** on the skin.

PATHOPHYSIOLOGY

Abnormal *C. albicans* overgrowth on the skin can occur in the setting of diabetes, obesity, hyperhidrosis, heat, maceration, immunologic defects (depressed T-cell function), polyendocrinopathies, systemic antibacterial agents, systemic and topical corticosteroids, chronic debilitation (carcinoma, leukemia), and chemotherapy.

HISTORY

Areas of candida overgrowth tend to be moist and warm with frequent episodes of wetness (from sweating, water exposure). The lesions begin as pink, slightly pruritic areas that progress to red, macerated, sore, painful, irritated skin.

PHYSICAL EXAMINATION

Skin Findings

TYPE Papules, pustules, plaques, erosions.
COLOR Beefy red skin, white exudates.
DISTRIBUTION Body folds, webspaces between fingers (Fig. 21-16) and toes. Diaper distribution in newborns.

DIFFERENTIAL DIAGNOSIS

The differential diagnosis for candidiasis includes psoriasis, erythrasma, atopic dermatitis, an irritant dermatitis, seborrheic dermatitis, or other fungal infections.

LABORATORY EXAMINATIONS

KOH Gram stain or 10% KOH of skin scraping shows pseudohyphae and yeast forms.
FUNGAL CULTURE Skin scrapings inoculated on Sabouraud's agar will grow *Candida*.

COURSE AND PROGNOSIS

Unless a precipitating causative agent can be removed (a diaper, a surgical cast), most cases of candidiasis (intertrigo, CMC) are chronic and recurrent.

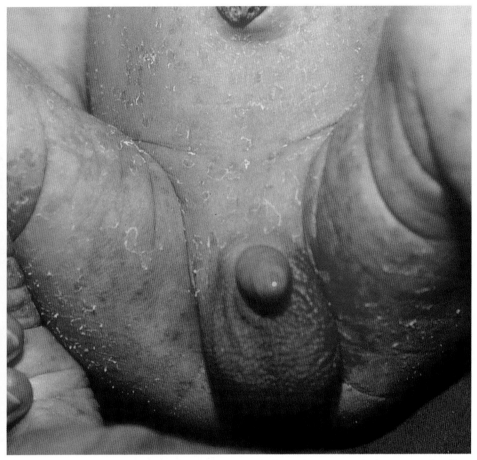

FIGURE 21-15 Candidiasis, diaper dermatitis *Candida* diaper dermatitis with characteristic "satellite pustules." (Slide used with permission from Dr. Karen Wiss.)

MANAGEMENT

Preventatively, keeping intertriginous areas dry and open to air as much as possible will help. Daily application of drying topical powders or antifungal creams can help. Useful topical antifungal preparations include polyenes (nystatin, amphotericin B), substituted pyridine (ciclopirox), imidazoles (clotrimazole, econazole, miconazole, ketoconazole, oxiconazole, or sulconazole). They should be applied BID to the affected areas until the lesion clears (typically 6 weeks). It is recommended to continue the topical medication for one more week after clinical clearing to ensure clinical cure. Topical antifungal with steroid combinations (1% clotrimazole + betamethasone dipropionate; nystatin + triamcinolone) are effective for *Candida* treatment, but have a strong steroid component and thus should be used sparingly for a limited time.

If extensive or resistant to topical treatment, oral antifungal treatment (fluconazole, ketoconazole, itraconazole) for 2 to 3 weeks may be needed. Side effects include nausea, vomiting, and LFT abnormalities.

For fluconazole-resistant candidiasis, amphotericin B may be necessary. Side effects include renal tubular acidosis, hypokalemia, hypomagnesemia, fever, chills, delirium, phlebitis, nausea, vomiting, hypotension, hypertension, renal failure, and bone marrow suppression.

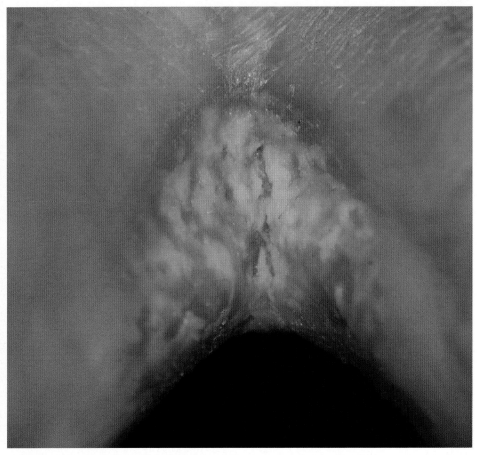

FIGURE 21-16 Candidiasis, interdigital Eroded and macerated area of candidal overgrowth in the webspace of the hand.

PITYRIASIS VERSICOLOR

Pityriasis versicolor is a common asymptomatic superficial fungal infection of the trunk, characterized by white or brown scaling macules and associated with the overgrowth of *Malassezia* species (formerly known as *Pityrosporum*).

SYNONYMS Tinea versicolor, dermatomycosis furfuracea, tinea flava.

EPIDEMIOLOGY

AGE Any age. Most common in young adults.
GENDER M = F.
INCIDENCE Common.
PREVALENCE Temperate zones: 2% of population during summer; tropical zones: 40% of the population. In athletes, rash may persist year round.
ETIOLOGY *Malassezia globosa, Malassezia furfur* (previously known as *P. ovale* or *P. orbiculare*).

PATHOPHYSIOLOGY

Malassezia are lipophilic yeast that are normal inhabitants of skin. Infections are not contagious, but an overgrowth of resident cutaneous yeast form under certain favorable conditions. Seborrheic dermatitis and *Pityrosporum* folliculitis are thought to be other cutaneous manifestations of *P. ovale* overgrowth, and all three conditions can be seen concomitantly. High humidity, sweat, sebum, occlusion, poor nutrition, pregnancy, topical steroids, and application of oils (e.g., cocoa butter, bath oil) on the skin can lead to *P. ovale* overgrowth. The pigmentary changes are caused by dicarboxylic acids (including azelaic acid) formed by enzymatic oxidation of fatty acids in skin surface lipids inhibiting tyrosinase in epidermal melanocytes and leading to hypopigmentation. Hyperpigmentation may also develop due to inflammation directed against the superficial infection.

HISTORY

The rash of pityriasis versicolor begins insidiously and spreads over months to years. It is typically asymptomatic or mildly pruritic. There are no systemic symptoms and the resultant blotchy pigmentation is what usually brings the patient into the office.

PHYSICAL EXAMINATION

Skin Findings

TYPE Macules, patches, scale.
COLOR Light skin: hyperpigmentation. Dark skin: hypopigmentation (Fig. 21-17).
SIZE 5 mm to several centimeters.
SHAPE Round or oval.
DISTRIBUTION Sebaceous areas: trunk, arms, neck, axillae, groin, thighs, genitalia. Rarely on the face.

DIFFERENTIAL DIAGNOSIS

The differential diagnosis for pityriasis versicolor includes vitiligo, pityriasis rosea, pityriasis alba, postinflammatory hypopigmentation, tinea corporis, seborrheic dermatitis, guttate psoriasis, secondary syphilis, and nummular eczema.

LABORATORY EXAMINATIONS

DERMATOPATHOLOGY Budding yeast and hyphae forms in the most superficial layers of the stratum corneum. PAS stain will stain *Malassezia* very bright pink.
KOH 10% KOH of skin scrapings will show filamentous hyphae and spores (a so-called spaghetti-and-meatballs appearance; Fig. 21-18).
WOOD'S LAMP Faint yellow-green fluorescence of scales may be detected.

COURSE AND PROGNOSIS

Pityriasis versicolor has a benign but chronic/relapsing course. Skin or systemic symptoms are rare, but the pigmentary changes can be very noticeable, persist for months and are cosmetically unappealing to the patient.

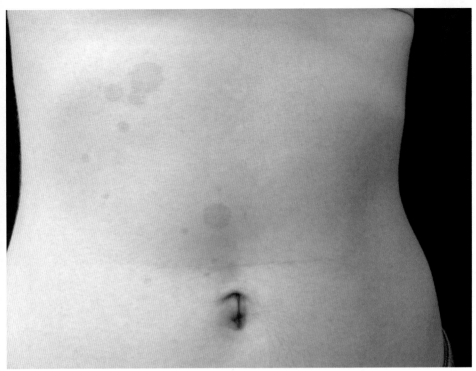

FIGURE 21-17 Pityriasis versicolor Scaly, hyperpigmented macules of pityriasis versicolor on the abdomen of a child.

MANAGEMENT

Pityriasis versicolor responds well to topical agents such as antimycotic shampoos (selenium sulfide 2.5%, ketoconazole 2%) which can be lathered on the body and left on for 15 minutes followed by a bath/shower twice weekly for 2 to 4 weeks. Imidazole creams (clotrimazole, econazole, miconazole, oxiconazole, sulconazole) can be used to small, localized areas for 1 to 2 weeks.

For chronic, recurrent, or severe involvement, oral antifungals (ketoconazole, fluconazole, itraconazole) may be warranted. Side effects include nausea, vomiting, and LFT abnormalities.

All patients should be counseled regarding likely recurrences and predisposing factors (sweat, topical oils). In athletes, prophylactic weekly shampoo with selenium sulfide may be helpful. Additionally, even when *Malassezia* are cleared, the pigmentary changes of pityriasis versicolor can persist for months and do not represent therapeutic failure.

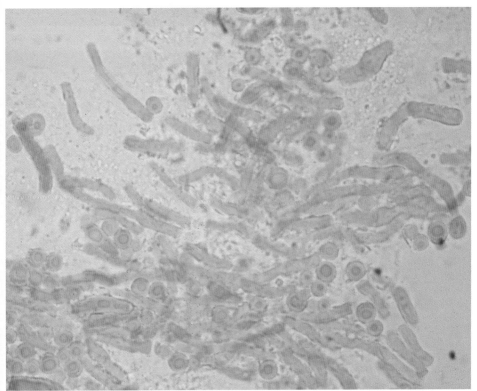

FIGURE 21-18 Pityriasis versicolor, potassium hydroxide (KOH) preparation KOH preparation demonstrating filamentous hyphae and spores, the "spaghetti and meatballs" appearance characteristic of pityriasis versicolor.

DEEP FUNGAL INFECTIONS

SPOROTRICHOSIS

Sporotrichosis is a deep fungal infection that follows accidental inoculation of the skin. It is characterized by ulceration and/or nodule formation at the inoculation site, followed by subcutaneous nodule formation along the course of lymphatic drainage.

CLASSIFICATION

1. **Lymphocutaneous sporotrichosis:** most common, seen in 25% of cases. Proximal to local cutaneous lesion, intervening lymphatics become indurated, nodular, thickened, with occasional ulcer formation.
2. **Fixed cutaneous sporotrichosis:** 20% of cases, subcutaneous papule at inoculation. The patient is previously sensitized to sporotrichosis; no lymphatic spread.
3. **Chancriform form of sporotrichosis:** rare, <8% of cases with associated lymphadenopathy proximally.
4. **Disseminated sporotrichosis:** <1% of cases. Hematogenous spread to lungs, liver, spleen, pancreas, thyroid, myocardium, or CNS in immunocompromised host.

SYNONYMS Sporotrichum infection, rose gardener's disease.

EPIDEMIOLOGY

AGE Any age. More common in adults.
GENDER M > F.
ETIOLOGY *Sporothrix schenckii*, a dimorphic fungus commonly found in soil, rose and barberry thorns, wood splinters, sphagnum moss, straw, and marsh hay.
GEOGRAPHY Ubiquitous, worldwide. More common in temperate and tropical zones; endemic in Central and South America.

PATHOPHYSIOLOGY

Commonly, sporotrichosis begins with a subcutaneous inoculation by a contaminated thorn, rock, glass, barb, splinter, cat scratch, or other sharp item. Following subcutaneous inoculation, *S. schenckii* grows locally and slowly spreads along the draining lymphatics. Secondary skin lesions develop along the lymphatic chain. Rarely inhalation, aspiration, or ingestion cause systemic infection.

HISTORY

Three days to 12 weeks after inoculation of the fungal organism, an asymptomatic or slightly painful nodule will appear at the inoculation site followed by erythematous nodule formation extended proximally along the path of lymphatic drainage.

PHYSICAL EXAMINATION

Skin Findings

TYPE Papules, nodules, ulcers (Fig. 21-19).
COLOR Pink, red.
SIZE 1 to 2 cm.
ARRANGEMENT Linear lymphocutaneous arrangement described as "sporotrichoid" spread (Fig. 21-20).
DISTRIBUTION Upper extremity > face, trunk.

DIFFERENTIAL DIAGNOSIS

The differential diagnosis for sporotrichosis includes tuberculosis, atypical mycobacterial infection (particularly *M. marinum)*, anthrax, tularemia, cat scratch disease, primary syphilis, leishmaniasis, herpes simplex virus infection, staphylococcal lymphangitis, histoplasmosis, coccidioidomycosis, blastomycosis, nocardiosis, and cryptococcosis.

LABORATORY EXAMINATIONS

DERMATOPATHOLOGY Granulomatous, Langerhans-type giant cells, pyogenic microabscesses. Organisms rare, difficult to visualize. Yeast, if visible, appear as 1 to 3 μm by 3 to 10 μm cigar-shaped forms and will stain with PAS or silver stains. Fluorescent antibody or PCR can help detect the *S. schenckii* organism *in vitro*.
CULTURE Organism isolated few days after culture of skin lesion aspirate.

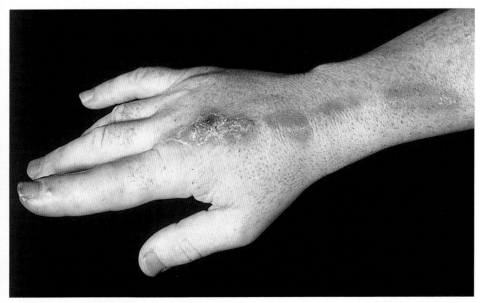

FIGURE 21-19 Sporotrichosis, sporotrichoid type Inoculation site on the dorsa of the hand with a linear arrangement of dermal and subcutaneous nodules extending along the lymphatic vessels on the arm. (Reproduced with permission from Fitzpatrick TB, Wolff K, and Johnson RA. *Color Atlas and Synopsis of Clinical Dermatology*. 4th ed. New York, NY: McGraw-Hill; 2001.)

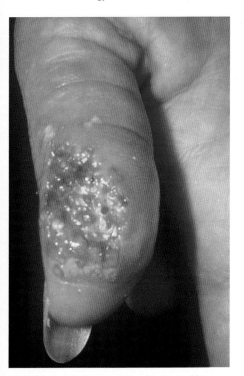

FIGURE 21-20 Sporotrichosis, chancriform An ulcerated nodule at the site of inoculation with sporotrichosis.

COURSE AND PROGNOSIS

Sporotrichosis shows little tendency to resolve spontaneously. The deep fungal infections respond well to systemic therapy, but relapses are possible.

MANAGEMENT

Topical therapy for sporotrichosis is not effective. Oral antifungal agents (fluconazole, ketoconazole, itraconazole) work, but should be taken 4 to 6 weeks beyond resolution of the lesions for a total course of 3 to 6 months. Side effects include nausea, vomiting, and LFT abnormalities. There has also been reported success with saturated solution of potassium iodide (oral SSKI), which enhances the host's immune system. It should also be given for 4 to 6 weeks beyond clinical resolution of cutaneous lesions. Side effects include iododerma, GI upset, and thyroid suppression.

For severe or systemic disease, especially in immunocompromised hosts, IV amphotericin B may be needed for 2 to 3 weeks. Side effects include renal tubular acidosis, hypokalemia, hypomagnesemia, fever, chills, delirium, phlebitis, nausea, vomiting, hypotension, hypertension, renal failure, and bone marrow suppression.

CRYPTOCOCCOSIS

Cryptococcosis is a deep fungal infection acquired by the inhalation of *Cryptococcus neoformans*, causing a primary pulmonary infection that can lead to hematogenous dissemination, and spread of infection to the CNS, kidneys, and/or skin.

SYNONYMS Torulosis, European blastomycosis.

EPIDEMIOLOGY

AGE All ages. Most commonly: 30 to 60 years.
GENDER M > F, 3:1.
INCIDENCE Rare.
ETIOLOGY *C. neoformans*, a yeast.
GEOGRAPHY Worldwide, ubiquitous. Europe, South America > United States. AIDS-associated cases highest in Sub-Saharan Africa.

PATHOPHYSIOLOGY

C. neoformans is an opportunistic pathogen that is accidentally inhaled from infected dust of avian feces (pigeons, parakeets, and canaries). Serotypes A, B, C, and D can cause disease in humans. After inhalation, *Cryptococcus* causes a pulmonary infection. Immunodeficient hosts may have a subsequent hematogenous dissemination of the organism to meninges, kidneys, and skin. Transplacental transmission is possible and *Cryptococcus* may also inhabit the female genital tract leading to inoculation of the infant as it passes through the birth canal.

HISTORY

Often, cryptococcal disease remains localized to the lungs with absent or minimal symptoms. In immunosuppressed individuals, hematogenous dissemination leads to CNS infection with headache (80%), mental confusion, and visual disturbances for months. Up to 30% of disseminated cases are associated with malignancy (usually Hodgkin's disease).

PHYSICAL EXAMINATION

Skin Findings

Seen in 15% of systemic cases.

TYPE Papules, pustules, plaques, nodules, ulcers (Fig. 21-21).
COLOR Pink to red, blue.
DISTRIBUTION Any site.
SITE OF PREDILECTION Face (especially around nose and mouth), scalp.

General Findings

CNS Headache, behavioral disturbances, seizures.
PULMONARY Cough, pneumonia, pleural effusions.
OTHER Hepatomegaly, splenomegaly, lymphadenopathy.

DIFFERENTIAL DIAGNOSIS

The differential diagnosis for *Cryptococcus* includes blastomycosis, histoplasmosis, molluscum contagiosum, HSV, and other bacterial or systemic fungal infections.

LABORATORY EXAMINATIONS

DERMATOPATHOLOGY Thick-walled organisms 5 by 20 μm in the skin biopsy. Methylene blue, alcian blue, or mucicarmine will brightly stain the polysaccharide capsule.
INDIRECT IMMUNOFLUORESCENCE Antibodies available to detect cryptococcal organism in body fluids of tissue specimens.
CULTURE *Cryptococcus* from body fluids or tissues can be grown on Sabouraud's agar.
CXR Pneumonia, infiltrates, nodules, abscesses, or pleural effusions may be present.

COURSE AND PROGNOSIS

Untreated, secondary cutaneous cryptococcosis is fatal in 80% of cases. Appropriate antifungal treatment leads to an 80% cure rate. A dramatic decrease in the incidence of *Cryptococcal* infection in the HIV population has been seen with the use of fluconazole and highly active antiretroviral therapy.

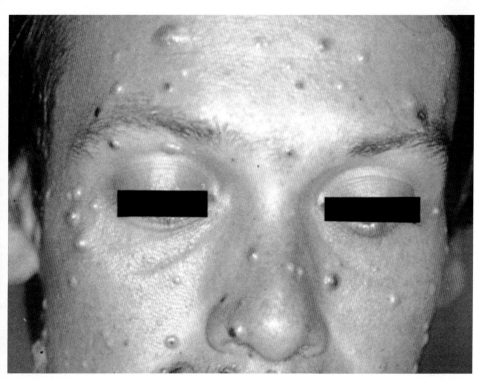

FIGURE 21-21 Cryptococcosis, disseminated Umbilicated nodules on the face of an HIV patient with disseminated cryptococcosis. (Reproduced with permission from Freedberg IM, Irwin M. *Dermatology in General Medicine.* 5th ed. New York, NY: McGraw-Hill; 1999.)

MANAGEMENT

Prevention of *Cryptococcus* in high-risk patients (on chemotherapy, high-dose steroids, neutropenia, HIV/AIDS) and antifungal prophylaxis (fluconazole, voriconazole, miconazole, ketoconazole, itraconazole) is recommended. The treatment of choice for *Cryptococcus* infection of a single site without involvement of the CNS or evidence of immu-nosuppression is daily fluconazole for 6 to 12 months. Amphotericin B for 2 months may be used for more severe disease. Side effects of amphotericin B include renal tubular acidosis, hypokalemia, hypomagnesemia, fever, chills, delirium, phlebitis, nausea, vomiting, hypo-tension, hypertension, renal failure, and bone marrow depression. For patients with CNS involvement or cryptococcemia, liposomal amphotericin B is recommended.

HISTOPLASMOSIS

Histoplasmosis is a common, highly infectious systemic fungal infection caused by *Histoplasma capsulatum* and characterized by an asymptomatic pulmonary infection that occasionally disseminates.

SYNONYMS Darling's disease, cave disease, Ohio Valley disease, reticuloendotheliosis.

EPIDEMIOLOGY

AGE All ages.
GENDER M = F.
INCIDENCE Common.
ETIOLOGY *H. capsulatum* exists in the soil in warm moist climates.
GEOGRAPHY Endemic in SE and central US with a predilection for Mississippi and Ohio River valleys.

PATHOPHYSIOLOGY

Birds, fowl, or bats are reservoirs for histoplasmosis. The feces of these animals contain the organism, thus their habitats (caves, chicken coops, construction sites) are high-risk areas for contracting the disease.

HISTORY

Humans acquire *H. capsulatum* by inhaling the aerosolized spores from contaminated soil. Histoplasmosis exists as self-limited, asymptomatic pulmonary infection in 75% of cases. Flu-like pulmonary symptoms (fever, malaise, cough, and chest pain) develop in 25% of cases and <1% of patients progress to disseminated histoplasmosis (fever, hepatosplenomegaly, anemia, and weight loss). Immunosuppression is a strong risk factor for disseminated disease. Cutaneous involvement may be due to disseminated disease or rarely through primary inoculation.

PHYSICAL EXAMINATION

Skin Findings

TYPE Papules, plaques, pustules (Fig. 21-22), nodules, abscesses, or ulcers.
COLOR Pink, red, purple.
DISTRIBUTION Any site, mucosa surface.

General Findings

FEVER
PULMONARY Cough, dyspnea, chest pain.
OTHER Hepatosplenomegaly and weight loss.

DIFFERENTIAL DIAGNOSIS

The differential diagnosis of histoplasmosis includes miliary tuberculosis, coccidioidomycosis, paracoccidioidomycosis, cryptococcosis, leishmaniasis, and lymphoma.

LABORATORY EXAMINATIONS

DERMATOPATHOLOGY Skin biopsy may show small intracellular yeast-like forms with a rim of clearing within histiocytes and giant cells (so-called "parasitized macrophages"). PAS or Gomori methenamine silver stains will make yeast more visible.
TOUCH PREPARATION Lesional skin touched to glass slide and stained with Giemsa stain will show *H. capsulatum.*
CULTURE Tissue or blood inoculated on Sabouraud's agar may grow *H. capsulatum.*
HISTOPLASMOSIS SKIN TEST In infants, a positive reaction 2 to 3 weeks after infection indicates active, current infection. In endemic populations, however, up to 90% of children and adults react positively, signifying past or present infection. Skin testing is more of a historic diagnostic methodology and may be of limited availability currently.
SEROLOGY Enzyme immunoassay, serologic immunodiffusion, agar gel precipitin test, yeast phase complement fixation, collodion, or latex particle agglutination can be performed on blood samples. Titers greater than 1:32 are highly suggestive of active histoplasmosis disease.
CXR Interstitial infiltrates and/or hilar adenopathy.

COURSE AND PROGNOSIS

In 99% of cases, asymptomatic pulmonary histoplasmosis is a benign and self-limited disease, and treatment is not necessary. In symptomatic or disseminated form, untreated histoplasmosis has a high mortality rate.

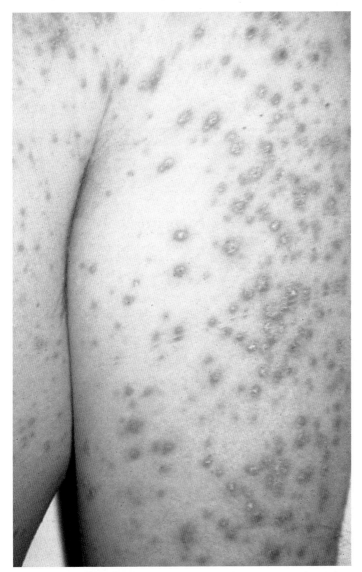

FIGURE 21-22 Histoplasmosis, disseminated Scattered erythematous papules and pustules in an HIV-infected individual with disseminated histoplasmosis. (Reproduced with permission from Fitzpatrick TB, Wolff K, Johnson RA. *Color Atlas and Synopsis of Clinical Dermatology*. 4th ed. New York, NY: McGraw-Hill; 2001.)

MANAGEMENT

If bird or bat droppings are to be cleared in an endemic area for *H. capsulatum,* protective equipment (respirators, goggles, and so forth) should be worn. Most cases of histoplasmosis do not require therapy. In severe systemic cases or disseminated disease, systemic antifungals (amphotericin B, itraconazole, voriconazole) may be necessary. Side effects include renal tubular acidosis, hypokalemia, hypomagnesemia, fever, chills, delirium, phlebitis, nausea, vomiting, hypotension, hypertension, renal failure, and bone marrow suppression.

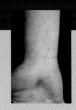

RICKETTSIAL INFECTION

ROCKY MOUNTAIN SPOTTED FEVER

Rocky Mountain spotted fever (RMSF), the most severe of the rickettsial infections, is characterized by sudden onset of fever, severe headache, myalgia, and a characteristic acral exanthem; it is associated with significant mortality particularly in children under age 4.

EPIDEMIOLOGY

AGE Any age
GENDER M > F.
RACE More common in Native Americans > whites, blacks
INCIDENCE Uncommon, though increasing. Highest incidence = 60 cases/million, southeastern U.S.
ETIOLOGY Caused by *Rickettsia rickettsii,* a gram-negative obligate intracellular bacterium.
SEASON April to September in the United States (95% of patients).
GEOGRAPHY Endemic in Virginia, North Carolina, South Carolina, Georgia, Kansas, Oklahoma, Texas, New York, northern Mexico, central, and South America.

PATHOPHYSIOLOGY

Occurs through bite of an infected tick or inoculation through abrasions contaminated with tick feces or tissue juices. The reservoirs and vectors are the wood tick (*Dermacentor andersoni)* in the western United States, the dog tick (*D. variabilis*) in the eastern and southern United States, and rarely the lone star tick (*Amblyomma americanum*) in the southern United States. Patients either live in or have recently visited an endemic area; *however, only ~62% may have knowledge of a recent tick bite.* Following inoculation, there is an initial local replication of the organism in endothelial cells followed by hematogenous dissemination. Focal infection of vascular smooth muscle causes a generalized vasculitis. Hypotension, local necrosis, gangrene, and DIC may follow. The classic petechial rash results from extravasated blood after vascular necrosis.

HISTORY

The typical incubation period for RMSF after tick exposure ranges from 5 to 7 days, but can be as short as 2 days or as long as 2 weeks. The rash, present in 90% of cases, begins on day 3 or 4 on the extremities and spreads proximally. By day 6 or 7, the rash is generalized. Systemic symptoms include abrupt onset of fever (94%); severe headache (94%); generalized myalgia, especially the back and leg muscles (87%); a sudden shaking rigor; photophobia; prostration; and nausea with occasional vomiting.

PHYSICAL EXAMINATION

Skin Findings

TYPE Petechial macule, papule, infarcts, gangrene.
COLOR Pink, deep red, violaceous (Fig. 22-1A).
SIZE 2 to 6 mm.
DISTRIBUTION Distal extremities, palms, soles to arms, thighs, trunk, face (Fig. 22-1B). Gangrene (4%) occurs in acral digits, extremities, ears, and prepuce.

General Findings

FEVER Up to 40°C.
RHEUMATOLOGIC Myalgias.
PULMONARY Cough, pneumonitis, lung infections, pulmonary edema, ARDS.
GI Nausea, abdominal pain, hepatosplenomegaly, GI hemorrhages.
RENAL Incontinence, oliguria, acute renal failure.
CNS Altered consciousness, headache, meningoencephalitis, stupor, coma.

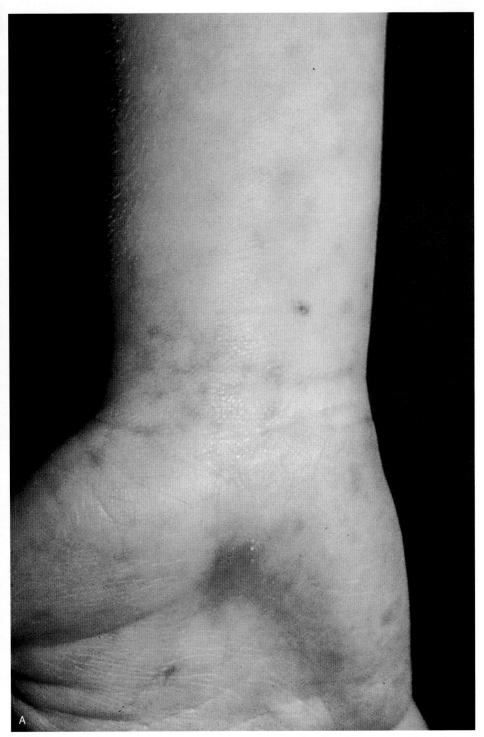

FIGURE 22-1 Rocky Mountain spotted fever A. Scattered pink, red, and purpuric macules and papules on the forearm of a child. *(continued)*

OTHER Hypotensive, deafness, middle ear/parotid gland infections, septic shock.

Variants

Spotless Fever (13%) No cutaneous manifestations. Higher mortality because diagnosis is missed.

Abdominal Syndrome Mimics acute abdomen, acute cholecystitis, acute appendicitis.

DIFFERENTIAL DIAGNOSIS

The differential diagnosis for RMSF includes meningococcemia, *Staphylococcus aureus* septicemia, other rickettsioses (ehrlichiosis, murine typhus, epidemic typhus, rickettsialpox), leptospirosis, typhoid fever, viral exanthem (measles, varicella, rubella, enterovirus, parvovirus, adenovirus), hemorrhagic fevers (Ebola, Marburg, Lassa), meningococcemia, chancroid, tularemia, syphilis, anthrax, ITP, drug reaction, or an immune–complex-mediated vasculitis.

LABORATORY EXAMINATIONS

DERMATOPATHOLOGY Necrotizing vasculitis. *Rickettsia* can at times be demonstrated within the endothelial cells.

DIRECT IMMUNOFLUORESCENCE Stains for *R. rickettsii* antigen within endothelial cells.

SEROLOGY Immunofluorescent antibody test can be used to measure both IgG and IgM antibodies against *R. rickettsii*. A fourfold rise in titer between acute and convalescent stages of the disease is diagnostic.

COURSE AND PROGNOSIS

Untreated, the fatality rate for RMSF is 20%. With adequate therapy, the mortality decreases to 3%. Severely affected patients may experience DIC, purpura fulminans, permanent cardiac, and/or neurologic sequelae. The most important prognostic factor is early diagnosis and treatment even if this means starting antibiotics before confirmatory study results are available.

MANAGEMENT

The drug of choice for RMSF in older children and adults is doxycycline, tetracycline, or chloramphenicol for 7 to 10 days. Chloramphenicol may be considered for treating pregnant women. In younger children, azithromycin or clarithromycin may be used to avoid the risks of dental staining from doxycycline or tetracycline; however, the tetracyclines remain the first-line treatment of choice.

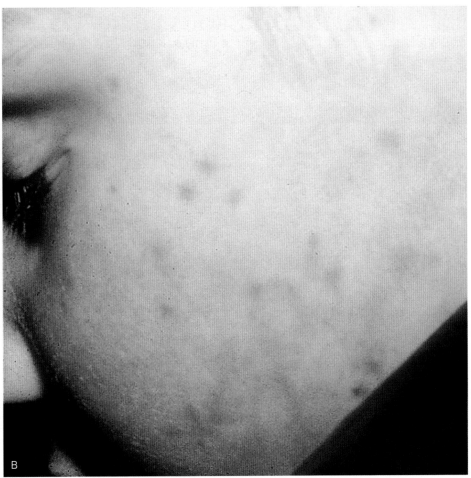

FIGURE 22-1 *(Continued)* **B.** Later face involvement of the rash is seen in the same child.

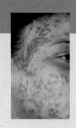

CUTANEOUS VIRAL INFECTIONS

HERPES SIMPLEX VIRUS

HERPETIC GINGIVOSTOMATITIS

Primary herpetic gingivostomatitis is caused by herpes simplex virus 1 (HSV-1) infection in children and characterized by painful vesicular lesions of the mouth.

INSIGHT

Any oral ulceration should be evaluated for herpes infection.

SYNONYMS Herpes, herpes simplex, cold sore, fever blister, herpes febrilis, herpes labialis.

EPIDEMIOLOGY

AGE 1 to 10 years. Peak incidence between 6 months and 5 years age.
GENDER M = F.
INCIDENCE 90% HSV-1 seropositive by age 10.
ETIOLOGY HSV-1 >> HSV-2.

PATHOPHYSIOLOGY

Transmission and primary infection of HSV occurs through close contact with a person shedding the virus at a peripheral site, mucosal surface, or through secretion. HSV is inactivated promptly at room temperature; thus, aerosolized or fomite spread is unlikely. Infection occurs via inoculation onto susceptible mucosal surface or breaks in skin. Subsequent to primary infection at the inoculation site, HSV ascends peripheral sensory nerves and enters the sensory or autonomic nerve root ganglia, where latency is established. Latency can occur after either symptomatic or asymptomatic primary infection.

HISTORY

Three to seven days after exposure, primary herpetic infections may be asymptomatic (the majority) or symptomatic with gingivostomatitis, high fever, sore throat, and lymphadenopathy. The pain may be so debilitating that hospitalization is necessary for intravenous (IV) hydration.

PHYSICAL EXAMINATION

Skin Findings

TYPE Plaque, vesicles, ulcerations (Fig. 23-1).
ARRANGEMENT Herpetiform (grouped) vesicles.
DISTRIBUTION Oral mucosa, oropharynx.

General Findings

FEVER, LAD.
OTHER Headache, fever, nuchal rigidity, ± positive HSV cerebrospinal fluid culture in severe disease.

DIFFERENTIAL DIAGNOSIS

The differential diagnosis for primary HSV gingivostomatitis includes aphthous stomatitis, hand-foot-and-mouth disease (HFMD), herpangina, erythema multiforme, or Behçet's disease, oral candidiasis, and chemotherapy mucositis.

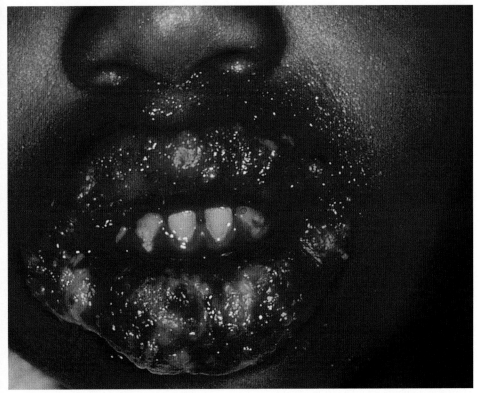

FIGURE 23-1 Herpetic gingivostomatitis Severe circumferential perioral erosions and ulcerations that prevent the child from being able to eat or drink.

LABORATORY EXAMINATIONS

TZANCK SMEAR Cells from the base of an intact vesicle are smeared thinly on a microscope slide, dried, stained with Wright's or Giemsa's stain, showing multinucleated giant keratinocytes (Fig. 23-2). Tzanck smear is positive in 75% of early cases, but does not differentiate HSV-1 from HSV-2 or varicella-zoster virus (VZV).

DIRECT IMMUNOFLUORESCENCE Cells from the base of an intact vesicle can be smeared on a glass slide and immunofluorescent antibodies can be used to stain specifically for the presence of HSV-1 or HSV-2.

DERMATOPATHOLOGY Ballooning and reticular epidermal degeneration, acanthosis, and intraepidermal vesicle formation. Intranuclear inclusion bodies, multinucleate giant keratinocytes, and multilocular vesicles may be present.

ELECTRON MICROSCOPY Can detect HSV particles.

VIRAL CULTURE HSV can be cultured in 2 to 5 days from early vesicular fluid or from scraping the base of an erosion.

POLYMERASE CHAIN REACTION Scrapings from the base of an erosion or patient serum can also be tested using real-time HSV PCR to diagnose and differentiate between HSV-1 and HSV-2. May be particularly useful in diagnosis of asymptomatic viral shedding.

SEROLOGY Primary HSV-1 infection can be documented by seroconversion.

COURSE AND PROGNOSIS

Episodes of primary herpetic gingivostomatitis are self-limited within 2 to 6 weeks but can range in severity from mild asymptomatic infection to severe debilitating disease requiring hospitalization.

MANAGEMENT

The treatment of choice for primary herpetic gingivostomatitis is oral or IV acyclovir and symptomatic measures. Initiation within the first 4 days of symptoms has been demonstrated to reduce symptom duration. Acetaminophen and 2% viscous lidocaine can be used for oral pain and IV fluids may be needed to prevent dehydration.

In older children, immunocompromised patients, or more refractory cases, oral valacyclovir or oral famciclovir may be used. Topical 1% penciclovir or 5% acyclovir ointment can be used in conjunction with oral therapy. Acyclovir-resistant HSV-1 requires IV foscarnet or topical cidofovir. Individuals with severe HSV gingivostomatitis and those with active secretions not yet on treatment should be placed on contact precautions and limit interaction with other children.

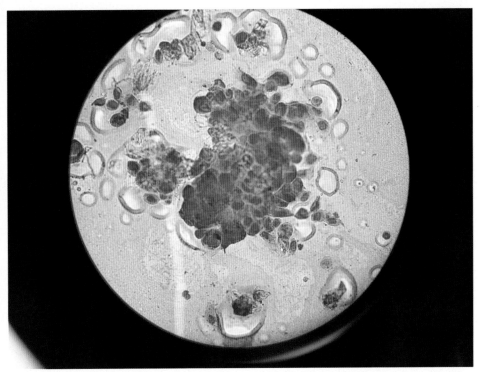

FIGURE 23-2 Herpetic infection, Tzanck smear Giemsa's stain of vesicle contents demonstrating multinucleated giant cells (fused virally infected keratinocytes) are indicative of a herpetic infection.

RECURRENT FACIAL–ORAL HERPES

Recurrent facial–oral herpes is a reactivation of latent herpetic infection caused by HSV-1 and characterized by grouped blisters, typically on the vermillion border.

SYNONYMS Cold sores, fever blisters, herpes, herpes simplex, herpes labialis.

EPIDEMIOLOGY

AGE Any age. Most common in young adults.
GENDER M = F.
PREVALENCE Common. One-third of population.
INCIDENCE 90% of population serologically positive for HSV-1 infection.
ETIOLOGY HSV-1 >> HSV-2.

PATHOPHYSIOLOGY

Herpes virus is transmitted by skin-to-skin, skin-to-mucosa, or mucosa-to-mucosa contact. Subsequent to the primary HSV-1 infection, HSV ascends the peripheral sensory nerves and enters the ganglion where latency is established. Recurrences occur at the same site each time and may be clinically asymptomatic or symptomatic.

Sunlight, stress, illness, or local trauma may precipitate blistering episodes.

HISTORY

Recurrent HSV-1 episodes are typically heralded by a prodrome of tingling, itching, or burning, which usually precedes any visible skin changes by 24 hours. The skin then flares with a small, localized crop of blisters followed by healing in 1 to 2 weeks. Systemic symptoms are usually absent.

PHYSICAL EXAMINATION

Skin Findings

TYPE Plaque, papules, vesicles, crust (Fig. 23-3).
COLOR Pink, red.
SIZE 1 to 2 mm.
ARRANGEMENT Herpetiform (i.e., grouped) vesicles.
DISTRIBUTION Vermillion border >> any other mucocutaneous site.

General Findings

LYMPHADENOPATHY Rarely present in immunocompetent individuals.

DIFFERENTIAL DIAGNOSIS

The differential diagnosis for recurrent facial–oral herpes includes varicella zoster, aphthous ulcers, and contact dermatitis.

LABORATORY EXAMINATIONS

TZANCK SMEAR Cells from the base of an intact vesicle are smeared thinly on a microscope slide, dried, stained with Wright's or Giemsa's stain, showing multinucleated giant keratinocytes (Fig. 23-2). Tzanck smear is positive in 75% of early cases, but does not differentiate HSV-1 from HSV-2 or VZV.
DIRECT IMMUNOFLUORESCENCE Cells from the base of an intact vesicle can be smeared on a glass slide and immunofluorescent antibodies can be used to stain specifically for the presence of HSV-1 or HSV-2.
DERMATOPATHOLOGY Ballooning and reticular epidermal degeneration, acanthosis, and intraepidermal vesicle formation. Intranuclear inclusion bodies, multinucleate giant keratinocytes, and multilocular vesicles may be present.
ELECTRON MICROSCOPY Can detect HSV particles.
VIRAL CULTURE HSV can be cultured in 2 to 5 days from early vesicular fluid or from scraping the base of an erosion.
SEROLOGY Recurrent HSV-1 infections can be detected by immunoglobulin M (IgM) and IgG antibody titers.
POLYMERASE CHAIN REACTION Scrapings from the base of an erosion or patient serum can also be tested using real-time HSV PCR to diagnose and differentiate between HSV-1 and HSV-2. May be particularly useful in diagnosis of asymptomatic viral shedding.

COURSE AND PROGNOSIS

Recurrent facial–oral herpetic outbreaks are localized, self-limited, typically number one to four per year, are milder, and have shorter duration than the primary infection. They tend to become less frequent as the individual gets older. Oral antiviral agents, if used early (during prodromal period), may abort or minimize symptoms.

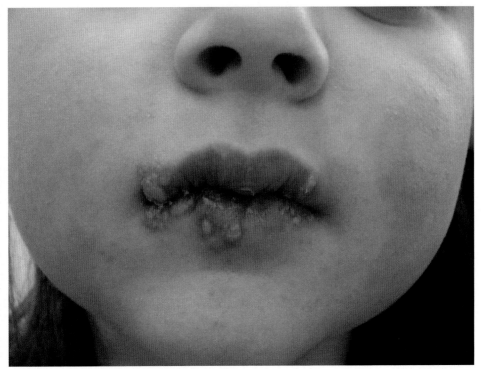

FIGURE 23-3 Recurrent facial–oral herpes Localized recurrent lesion that begins with vesicles and heals with crusting on the lower lip.

MANAGEMENT

In recurrent facial–oral herpes, patients who start oral antiviral therapy (acyclovir, valacyclovir, or famciclovir) at the beginning of the prodrome or within 2 days after onset of lesions may experience diminished symptoms and faster resolution. Topical 1% penciclovir or 5% acyclovir ointment can be used in conjunction with oral therapy. Impetiginized lesions may benefit from topical antibiotics (mupirocin). Acyclovir-resistant HSV requires IV foscarnet or topical cidofovir.

For individuals with multiple recurrences (six to eight or more annually), chronic suppressive therapy with one of the oral antiviral agents listed above may decrease viral shedding and prevent frequent recurrences.

ECZEMA HERPETICUM

Eczema herpeticum is a widespread HSV-type infection superimposed on diseased skin (most commonly atopic dermatitis). It is characterized by widespread vesicles and erosions, fever, and malaise and can be a severe, recurrent problem.

 INSIGHT An area of eczema that "just won't seem to heal" can be a sign of eczema herpeticum and should be evaluated for herpes infection.

SYNONYMS Kaposi's varicelliform eruption, pustulosis varioliformis acute, Kaposi–Juliusberg dermatitis.

EPIDEMIOLOGY

AGE Children > adults.
ETIOLOGY HSV-1, less commonly HSV-2.
RISK FACTORS Increased incidence in individuals with filaggrin mutation.

PATHOPHYSIOLOGY

On abnormal skin (atopic dermatitis >> Darier's disease, burns, pemphigus vulgaris, ichthyosis vulgaris), the barrier function of the skin is impaired and viral or bacterial superinfection can easily become widespread. In the case of eczema herpeticum, frequently a child with atopic dermatitis becomes inoculated with HSV-1 from a parent or other caregiver with a clinical or subclinical case of recurrent facial–oral herpes. The disease then becomes widespread because of the infant's uncontrolled scratching, autoinoculation, and impaired skin barrier function.

HISTORY

Herpetic skin lesions begin on inoculated, impaired skin and extend rapidly during primary infection. Systemic symptoms include fever, malaise, and irritability.

PHYSICAL EXAMINATION

Skin Findings

TYPE Vesicles, erosions (Fig. 23-4), pustules, crust (Fig. 23-5). Monomorphic appearance, may appear "punched-out."
DISTRIBUTION Common sites: face, neck, trunk.

General Findings

FEVER, LAD.

DIFFERENTIAL DIAGNOSIS

The differential diagnosis of eczema herpeticum includes varicella zoster with dissemination, disseminated (systemic) HSV infection, widespread bullous impetigo, staphylococcal folliculitis, pseudomonal (hot tub) folliculitis, and *Candida* folliculitis. A similar-appearing eruption may also be caused by coxsackie A16 virus (the virus responsible for HFMD).

LABORATORY EXAMINATIONS

TZANCK SMEAR Cells from the base of an intact vesicle are smeared thinly on a microscope slide, dried, stained with Wright's or Giemsa's stain, showing multinucleated giant keratinocytes (Fig. 23-2). Tzanck smear is positive in 75% of early cases, but does not differentiate HSV-1 from HSV-2 or VZV.
DIRECT IMMUNOFLUORESCENCE Cells from the base of an intact vesicle can be smeared on a glass slide and immunofluorescent antibodies can be used to stain specifically for the presence of HSV-1 or HSV-2.
DERMATOPATHOLOGY Ballooning and reticular epidermal degeneration, acanthosis, and intraepidermal vesicle formation. Intranuclear inclusion bodies, multinucleate giant keratinocytes, and multilocular vesicles may be present.
ELECTRON MICROSCOPY Can detect HSV particles.
CULTURE HSV-1 > HSV-2 can be cultured in 2 to 5 days from early vesicular fluid or from scraping the base of an erosion. Frequently, superinfection with *Staphylococcus aureus* or *Streptococcus pyogenes* is present.
SEROLOGY HSV infections can be detected by IgM and IgG antibody titers.
POLYMERASE CHAIN REACTION Scrapings from the base of an erosion or patient serum can also be tested using real-time HSV PCR to diagnose and differentiate between HSV-1 and HSV-2. May be particularly useful in diagnosis of asymptomatic viral shedding.

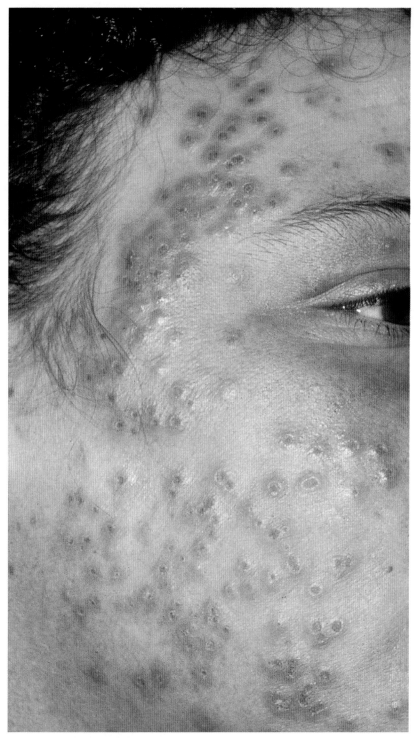

FIGURE 23-4 Eczema herpeticum Widespread punched-out lesions on a child with atopic dermatitis and superimposed herpes simplex infection.

COURSE AND PROGNOSIS

Eczema herpeticum self-resolves in 2 to 6 weeks. Recurrent episodes tend to be milder and not associated with as severe systemic symptoms as in the primary episode. The risk of systemic dissemination is possible, especially in immunocompromised patients.

MANAGEMENT

Eczema herpeticum may be considered a pediatric dermatologic emergency and early recognition can prevent significant sequelae. Preventative measures aimed at controlling the underlying chronic dermatosis (e.g., atopic dermatitis) will improve the skin's barrier function and prevent widespread cutaneous viral and bacterial infection.

Mild cases of eczema herpeticum can be managed on an outpatient basis with acyclovir, valacyclovir, or famciclovir. Topical 1% penciclovir or 5% acyclovir ointment can be used in conjunction with oral therapy. Impetiginized crusted lesions may benefit from topical antibiotics (mupirocin).

In more severe cases with high fever or marked prostration, hospitalization may be needed with IV acyclovir, antibiotics, IV fluids, and pain medications.

Acyclovir-resistant HSV eczema herpeticum requires IV foscarnet or topical cidofovir.

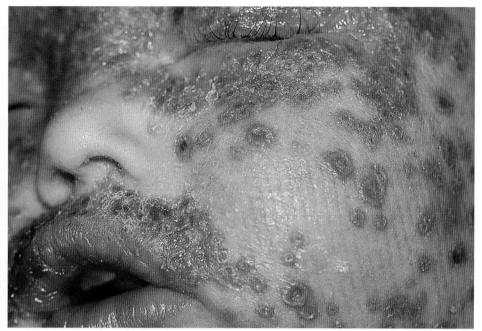

FIGURE 23-5 Eczema herpeticum Widespread crusted lesions on a child with atopic dermatitis kissed by a parent with active HSV-1 recurrent facial–oral herpes infection with resultant eczema herpeticum. Clinical picture is complicated by *Staphylococcus aureus* superinfection causing yellow-brown crusted appearance.

HERPETIC WHITLOW

Herpetic whitlow is a cutaneous herpetic infection of the distal fingertip, usually caused by recurrent HSV-1 or HSV-2, inadvertently inoculated onto the hand.

EPIDEMIOLOGY

AGE Children > adults.
GENDER M = F.
INCIDENCE Common.

PATHOPHYSIOLOGY

Herpetic whitlow is typically seen in physicians, dentists, dental hygienists, nurses, and children. HSV, from infected mucosa with clinical or subclinical herpes, gets inoculated onto a finger, and herpetic whitlow ensues. After the primary infection, the herpes virus becomes dormant in the nerve and can recur in the same location.

HISTORY

Two to eight days following exposure, painful vesicular lesions appear on the fingertips of the infected individual, often in association with swelling and surrounding erythema. Systemic symptoms are rare but can include fever and regional lymphadenopathy. Lesions take 1 to 3 weeks to resolve, and recurrences are possible.

PHYSICAL EXAMINATION

Skin Findings

TYPE Vesicles.
COLOR Whitish-red or blue (Fig. 23-6).
SIZE 2- to 4-mm vesicles.
ARRANGEMENT Herpetic (grouped vesicles).
DISTRIBUTION Distal fingertips.

DIFFERENTIAL DIAGNOSIS

The differential diagnosis of herpetic whitlow includes dyshidrotic eczema, contact dermatitis, orf, or other paronychial infection.

LABORATORY EXAMINATIONS

TZANCK SMEAR Cells from the base of an intact vesicle stained with Wright's or Giemsa's stain show multinucleated giant keratinocytes (Fig. 23-2). Tzanck smear is positive in 75% of early cases, but does not differentiate HSV-1 from HSV-2 or VZV.
DIRECT IMMUNOFLUORESCENCE Cells from the base of an intact vesicle can be smeared on a glass slide and immunofluorescent antibodies can be used to stain specifically for the presence of HSV-1 or HSV-2.
DERMATOPATHOLOGY Ballooning and reticular epidermal degeneration, acanthosis, and intraepidermal vesicle formation. Intranuclear inclusion bodies, multinucleate giant keratinocytes, and multilocular vesicles may be present.
ELECTRON MICROSCOPY Can detect HSV particles.
CULTURE HSV-1 > HSV-2 can be cultured in 2 to 5 days from early vesicular fluid or from scraping the base of an erosion.
SEROLOGY HSV infections can be detected by IgM and IgG antibody titers.
POLYMERASE CHAIN REACTION Scrapings from the base of an erosion or patient serum can also be tested using real-time HSV PCR to diagnose and differentiate between HSV-1 and HSV-2. May be particularly useful in diagnosis of asymptomatic viral shedding.

COURSE AND PROGNOSIS

Herpetic whitlow will self-resolve without treatment, but recurrences are possible.

MANAGEMENT

Much of the treatment of herpetic whitlow is symptomatic with analgesics for pain, topical penciclovir cream, or 5% acyclovir ointment. More severe or refractory cases may require treatment with oral acyclovir, valacyclovir, or famciclovir.

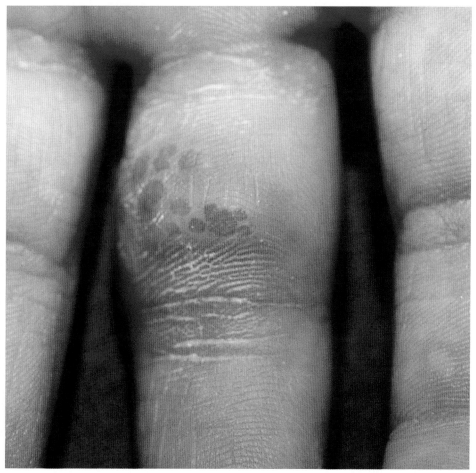

FIGURE 23-6 Herpetic whitlow Painful grouped red-blue vesicles on the middle finger of a child.

HERPES GLADIATORUM

Herpes gladiatorum is an infection seen primarily in contact sports players (e.g., wrestlers, rugby play-ers) who abrade their skin and come into direct contact with an active HSV infection.

SYNONYMS Scrumpox, herpes rugbiorum, wrestler's herpes, mat pox.

EPIDEMIOLOGY

AGE Any age.
GENDER M > F.
INCIDENCE Common, up to 67% of wrestlers/rugby players.
ETIOLOGY HSV-1 >> HSV-2.

PATHOPHYSIOLOGY

HSV-1 is transmitted during infected skin-to-skin exposure in rough contact sports. Of note, studies have shown negative oropharyngeal swabs for active mucosal HSV-1; thus, saliva seems not to be a major source of infection. The virus then becomes latent in the sensory nerve ganglia, and recurrences at the ectopic site are possible.

HISTORY

Two to eight days after contact, herpetic lesions can occur at atypical sites (head, trunk, extremities; sites of skin-to-skin contact during sports) and are often associated with edema, pain, and regional lymphadenopathy.

PHYSICAL EXAMINATION

Skin Findings

TYPE Grouped vesicles.
COLOR White, pink, red (Fig. 23-7).
SIZE 2 to 5 mm.
NUMBER One lesion >> multiple sites.
DISTRIBUTION Head (73%), trunk (28%), and extremities (42%).

General Findings

FEVER' Malaise and lymphadenopathy.

DIFFERENTIAL DIAGNOSIS

The differential diagnosis of herpes gladiato-rum includes contact dermatitis and varicella zoster.

LABORATORY EXAMINATIONS

TZANCK SMEAR Cells from the base of an intact vesicle stained with Wright's or Giemsa's stain show multinucleated giant keratinocytes (Fig. 23-2). Tzanck smear is positive in 75% of early cases, but does not differentiate HSV-1 from HSV-2 or VZV.
DIRECT IMMUNOFLUORESCENCE Cells from the base of an intact vesicle can be smeared on a glass slide and immunofluorescent antibodies can be used to stain specifically for the presence of HSV-1 or HSV-2.
DERMATOPATHOLOGY Ballooning and reticu-lar epidermal degeneration, acanthosis, and intraepidermal vesicle formation. Intranuclear inclusion bodies, multinucleate giant kera-tinocytes, and multilocular vesicles may be present.
ELECTRON MICROSCOPY Can detect HSV particles.
CULTURE HSV-1 > HSV-2 can be cultured in 2 to 5 days from early vesicular fluid or from scraping the base of an erosion.
SEROLOGY HSV infections can be detected by IgM and IgG antibody titers.
POLYMERASE CHAIN REACTION Scrapings from the base of an erosion or patient serum can also be tested using real-time HSV PCR to diagnose and differentiate between HSV-1 and HSV-2. May be particularly useful in diagnosis of asymptomatic viral shedding.

COURSE AND PROGNOSIS

The primary episode of herpes gladiatorum may last 2 to 6 weeks but does self-resolve. Recurrences are less painful and resolve more quickly.

MANAGEMENT

Wrestlers, rugby players, parents, and coaches need to be made aware of the transmission of HSV-1, and active lesions should be covered to prevent spread. Much of the treatment of herpes gladiatorum is symptomatic with analgesics for pain, topical penciclovir cream, or 5% acyclovir ointment. For crusted impe-tiginized lesions, a topical antibiotic should be added (mupirocin). More severe or refrac-tory herpes gladiatorum cases may require treatment with oral acyclovir, valacyclovir, or famciclovir. Athletes with active lesions should occlude the areas or avoid competing in events with skin-to-skin contact to mini-mize disease spread.

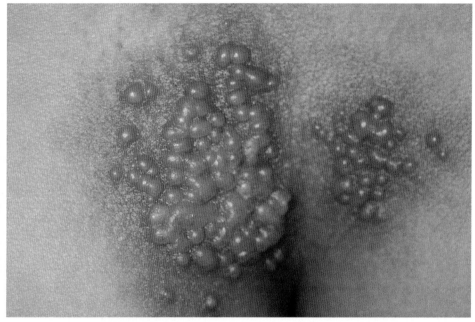

FIGURE 23-7 Herpes gladiatorum Localized recurrent lesion that begins with clustered vesicles on an erythematous base on the buttocks of an infant.

DISSEMINATED HERPES SIMPLEX INFECTION

Disseminated herpes simplex infection is a potentially fatal, systemic HSV infection, characterized by widespread mucocutaneous vesicles, pustules, erosions, and ulcerations. It is associated with signs of pneumonia, encephalitis, and hepatitis, as well as involvement of other organ systems. Disseminated HSV infection usually occurs in an immunocompromised host.

EPIDEMIOLOGY

AGE Any age.
INCIDENCE Uncommon, but increasing because of immunosuppressive therapies.
ETIOLOGY HSV-1 or HSV-2.

PATHOPHYSIOLOGY

Disseminated herpes typically occurs in immunocompromised states (organ transplantation, cancer chemotherapy, corticosteroid therapy), hematologic and lymphoreticular malignancies, and in the setting of severe malnutrition. Eighty percent of HSV seropositive transplant recipients and patients undergoing chemotherapy for hematologic malignancies will reactivate HSV. Following viremia, disseminated cutaneous or visceral HSV infection may follow.

HISTORY

Disseminated herpes simplex infection is typically seen in hospitalized patients with underlying disease. It presents as tender and painful mucocutaneous erosions with systemic fever, malaise, and organ involvement.

PHYSICAL EXAMINATION

Skin Findings

TYPE Vesicles, crusts, erosion, ulcers.
DISTRIBUTION Generalized, disseminated (Fig. 23-8).
MUCOUS MEMBRANES Oropharyngeal erosion, HSV tracheobronchitis with erosions.

General Findings

HSV pneumonitis, hepatitis, or encephalitis may be present.

DIFFERENTIAL DIAGNOSIS

The differential diagnosis of disseminated HSV includes eczema herpeticum, varicella, and cutaneous disseminated zoster.

LABORATORY EXAMINATIONS

TZANCK SMEAR Cells from infected mucocutaneous sites or infected body fluids stained with Wright's or Giemsa's stain show multinucleated giant keratinocytes (Fig. 23-2). Tzanck smear is positive in 75% of early cases, but does not differentiate HSV-1 from HSV-2 or VZV.
DIRECT IMMUNOFLUORESCENCE Cells from a mucocutaneous lesion or infected body fluids can be smeared on a glass slide and immunofluorescent antibodies can be used to stain specifically for the presence of HSV-1 or HSV-2.
DERMATOPATHOLOGY Ballooning and reticular epidermal degeneration, acanthosis, and intraepidermal vesicle formation. Intranuclear inclusion bodies, multinucleate giant keratinocytes, and multilocular vesicles may be present.
ELECTRON MICROSCOPY Can detect HSV particles.
CULTURE HSV-1 > HSV-2 can be cultured in 2 to 5 days from scraping the base of a mucocutaneous erosion or from infected body fluids.
SEROLOGY HSV infections can be detected by IgM and IgG antibody titers.
POLYMERASE CHAIN REACTION Scrapings from the base of an erosion or patient serum can also be tested using real-time HSV PCR to diagnose and differentiate between HSV-1 and HSV-2. May be particularly useful in diagnosis of asymptomatic viral shedding.

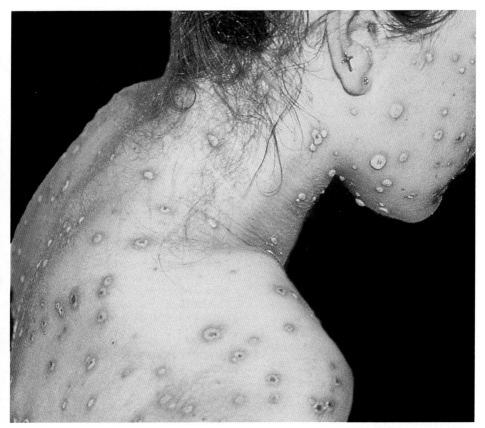

FIGURE 23-8 Disseminated herpes simplex virus Widespread vesicular lesions in an immunocompromised patient.

COURSE AND PROGNOSIS

When widespread, visceral dissemination of HSV may occur to liver, lungs, adrenals, gastrointestinal (GI) tract, and central nervous system. Severe cases can be complicated by disseminated intravascular coagulation. Untreated, the mortality rate of disseminated HSV with organ involvement approaches 70% and residual neurological defects are common.

MANAGEMENT

Early recognition and treatment are essential in the treatment of disseminated herpes which can be considered a dermatologic and medical emergency.

Prophylaxis with acyclovir is recommended for seropositive patients undergoing bone marrow transplantation; induction therapy for leukemia; and solid organ transplantation from the day of conditioning, induction, or transplantation lasting for 4 to 6 weeks. For disseminated HSV infection, systemic acyclovir, valacyclovir, or famciclovir is necessary. In more severe cases with high fever or marked prostration, hospitalization may be needed with IV acyclovir, antibiotics, fluids, and pain medications.

Acyclovir-resistant disseminated HSV requires IV foscarnet.

VARICELLA-ZOSTER VIRUS

VARICELLA

Varicella is a highly contagious primary infection caused by VZV, characterized by successive crops of pruritic vesicles that evolve to pustules and crusts, and can heal with scarring. The rash is often accompanied by constitutional symptoms such as fever and malaise.

SYNONYM Chickenpox.

INSIGHT The live attenuated VZV vaccine is 90% effective in preventing chickenpox and currently recommended for all children in the United States.

EPIDEMIOLOGY

AGE Before vaccine and in unvaccinated populations: 90% younger than 10 years.
GENDER M = F.
INCIDENCE Before vaccine: nearly universal in the United States. Common worldwide.
SEASON Winter, spring.
ETIOLOGY VZV, a herpesvirus.
GEOGRAPHY Worldwide.

PATHOPHYSIOLOGY

Varicella virus is highly contagious and spreads via airborne droplets between persons or, less commonly, through direct contact with the vesicle fluid. Patients are contagious several days before exanthem appears and until the last crop of vesicles crusts over. Varicella virus enters the host through the mucosa of upper respiratory tract and oropharynx, replicates in the lymph nodes, and causes primary viremia. VZV then replicates in organs with subsequent secondary viremia and dissemination of the virus to the skin and mucous membranes. Once crusted over, the skin lesions are no longer infectious.

Primary attack usually confers lifelong immunity. Second episodes of varicella have been documented but are rare. As with all herpesviruses, VZV enters a latent phase, residing in sensory ganglia, and reactivation of VZV later in life results in herpes zoster (shingles).

HISTORY

Varicella is usually transmitted by exposure to a sick contact at day care, school, an older sibling, or even an adult with zoster. The rash appears following an inoculation period of 14 days (range, 10–23 days), a mild prodrome of headache, general aches and pains, and malaise. Crops of vesicles with an erythematous base appear ("dewdrops on a rose petal") and crust over an 8- to 12-hour period. With subsequent crops, all stages of evolution may be noted simultaneously: papules, vesicles, pustules, crusts. The exanthem appears within 2 to 3 days (Fig. 23-9).

PHYSICAL EXAMINATION

Skin Findings

TYPE Vesicles (Fig. 23-10), pustules, crusts, scars.
COLOR Clear, white, yellow, red.
SIZE 2 to 5 mm.
NUMBER Few to >100 lesions.
DISTRIBUTION Face, scalp, then trunk, extremities. Palms/soles spared.
MUCOUS MEMBRANES Vesicles or erosions on palate, nasal mucosa, conjunctivae, GI, genitourinary, or respiratory tract.

General Findings

FEVER Low grade.

DIFFERENTIAL DIAGNOSIS

The differential diagnosis of varicella includes disseminated HSV infection, cutaneous dissemination of zoster, eczema herpeticum, Coxsackie virus, enteric cytopathic human orphan virus, pityriasis lichenoides et varioliformis acuta, rickettsialpox, drug eruption, contact dermatitis, insect bites, scabies, bullous impetigo, and historically, smallpox.

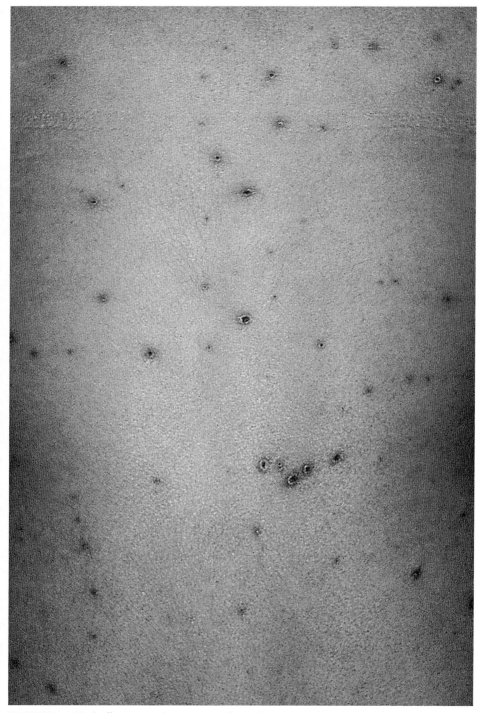

FIGURE 23-9 Varicella Scattered papules, vesicles, and crusts noted simultaneously in a patient with varicella.

LABORATORY EXAMINATIONS

TZANCK PREPARATION Cytology of scraping from fluid or base of vesicle or pustule shows both giant and multinucleated giant epidermal cells. Tzanck test does not differentiate HSV from VZV.

ELECTRON MICROSCOPY VZV particles can be seen but cannot be distinguished from HSV.

CULTURES Isolation of virus from skin lesions is possible, but VZV takes longer and is much more difficult to culture than HSV.

SEROLOGY Seroconversion is documented by a fourfold or greater rise in VZV titers.

POLYMERASE CHAIN REACTION Scrapings from the base of an erosion, patient serum, or CSF can also be tested using real-time PCR to diagnose VZV with high specificity and sensitivity.

COURSE AND PROGNOSIS

The symptoms and rash of varicella typically last for 1 to 3 weeks. The primary infection should confer lifelong immunity. If the primary infection occurs at an early age when maternal antibodies are still present, a patient may have a second episode of varicella later in life owing to incomplete immunity. Varicella in children is a self-limited, benign, but itching and painful eruption. In older or immunocompromised individuals, varicella may have a more severe clinical course, with a higher rate of respiratory or systemic complications.

Neonatal varicella, with infection acquired during the first 10 days of life, is also associated with a high mortality.

MANAGEMENT

Varicella is a self-limited cutaneous eruption in immunocompetent children, and treatment usually consists of supportive care with anti-pyretics, antihistamines, and antipruritic agents (oatmeal baths, calamine lotion). Acyclovir administered within the first 24 to 72 hours of the exanthem can lessen the severity of the outbreak, but higher doses are needed because VZV is not as sensitive to the systemic antivirals as HSV. In cases complicated by pneumonitis, encephalitis, or varicella occurring in an immunocompromised host, IV acyclovir is recommended. Varicella-zoster immune globulin administration may also be helpful, particularly as postexposure prophylaxis for neonates whose mothers demonstrate evidence of varicella in the peripartum period.

Prevention of primary varicella is now the strategic approach in the United States:

1. Varicella-zoster immune globulin administration is indicated for individuals with leukemia, lymphoma, cellular immune deficiency, or on immunosuppressive treatment within the first 96 hours following significant exposure to VZV.
2. VZV vaccine (live attenuated virus, Oka strain) given at age 12 months and 4 to 6 years is now recommended for all immunocompetent children. Studies indicate the vaccine is 90% effective in preventing primary varicella, and the severity is decreased in those who do contract the disease.

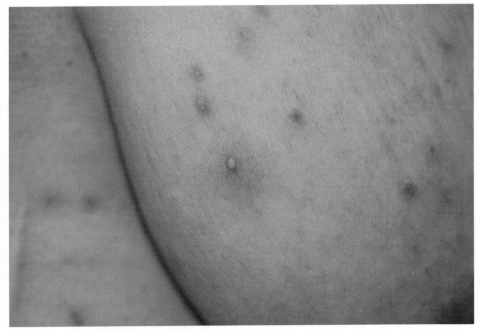

FIGURE 23-10 Varicella Thin-walled vesicle on an erythematous base likened to a "dewdrop on a rose petal" characteristic of varicella infection.

HERPES ZOSTER

Herpes zoster is a reactivation of VZV and is characterized by localized unilateral pain with a vesicular eruption limited to a dermatome innervated by a corresponding sensory ganglion.

SYNONYMS Shingles; zoster.

EPIDEMIOLOGY

AGE Any age, typically older than 50 years.
GENDER M = F.
INCIDENCE Before VZV vaccine: 300,000 cases annually in the United States. Estimated up to 32% of US population will experience herpes zoster during their lifetime.

PATHOPHYSIOLOGY

VZV, during the course of primary varicella infection (chickenpox), ascends along the sensory nerves and establishes latency in the ganglia. Humoral and cellular immunity to VZV established with primary infection persists, and when this immunity ebbs, viral replication within the ganglia occurs. The virus then travels down the sensory nerve, resulting in dermatomal pain and skin lesions (shingles). As the neuritis precedes the skin involvement, pain or paresthesias appear before the skin lesions are visible.

Zoster in children is seen in immuno-compromised settings (lymphoproliferative disorders, chemotherapy) or in children who contracted primary varicella younger than age 6 months. Zoster vesicular fluid is contagious and susceptible contacts can contract primary varicella (chickenpox), but not zoster (shingles).

HISTORY

Pain, tenderness, and paresthesia (itching, tingling, burning) in the involved dermatome precede the eruption by 3 to 5 days. Rarely, "zoster sine herpete" (zoster without rash) can occur with just the pain as a clinical manifestation. Systemic symptoms (headache, malaise, fever, fatigue) occur in up to 20% of zoster patients.

PHYSICAL EXAMINATION

Skin Findings

TYPE Papules (24 hours), vesicles bullae (48 hours), pustules (96 hours), crusts (7 to 10 days).

COLOR Clear vesicles, red base.
SIZE 2 to 5 mm.
ARRANGEMENT Dermatomal (Fig. 23-11). Few stray lesions outside of dermatome, usually occurring in adjacent dermatomes.
DISTRIBUTION Thoracic (50%), trigeminal (20%), lumbosacral/cervical (20%).
MUCOUS MEMBRANES Vesicles/erosions in mouth, genitalia, bladder.

General Findings

FEVER, LAD Regional nodes enlarged and tender.
NEUROLOGIC Sensory or motor nerve changes.
OPHTHALMIC (7%) Nasociliary branch: vesicles on the tip of the nose (Hutchinson's sign), conjunctivitis, keratitis, scleritis, or iritis.

DIFFERENTIAL DIAGNOSIS

The prodromal pain of herpes zoster can mimic cardiac or pleural disease, an acute abdomen, or vertebral disease. The rash of zoster must be distinguished from HSV and contact dermatitis.

LABORATORY EXAMINATIONS

TZANCK PREPARATION Cytology of scraping from fluid or base of vesicle or pustule shows both giant and multinucleated giant epidermal cells. Tzanck test does not differentiate HSV from VZV.
ELECTRON MICROSCOPY VZV particles can be seen but cannot be distinguished from HSV.
CULTURES Isolation of virus from skin lesions is possible, but VZV takes longer and is much more difficult to culture than HSV.
SEROLOGY VZV titers should be four times higher in acute versus convalescent serum.
POLYMERASE CHAIN REACTION Scrapings from the base of an erosion, patient serum, or CSF can also be tested using real-time PCR to diagnose VZV with high specificity and sensitivity.

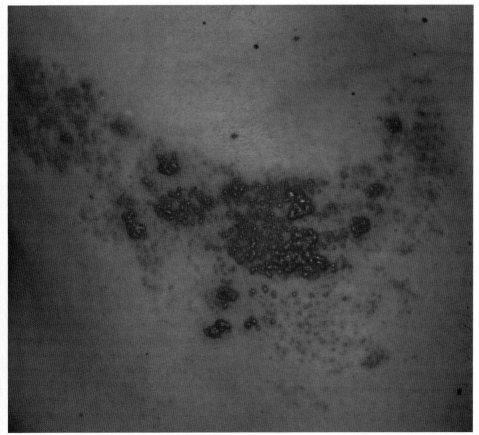

FIGURE 23-11 Herpes zoster Grouped vesicles on an erythematous base in a dermatomal distribution on the torso of an adolescent.

COURSE AND PROGNOSIS

The rash of zoster is self-limited. The risk of postherpetic neuralgia is around 20% to 40% in adult patients, but less common in children. The highest incidence of postherpetic neuralgia is in ophthalmic zoster (involvement of the V1 branch of the trigeminal nerve). Ophthalmic zoster can lead to keratitis and blindness; thus, aggressive treatment should be pursued.

Disseminated zoster (10%), defined by 20 or more lesions outside the affected or adjacent dermatome is usually only seen in immunosuppressed individuals. Motor paralysis occurs in 5% of patients with disseminated zoster, especially when the cranial nerves are affected.

MANAGEMENT

Zoster is a self-limited cutaneous eruption in children, and treatment usually consists of supportive care with antihistamines and antipruritic agents (oatmeal baths, calamine lotion). Oral acyclovir lessens the severity of outbreak and duration of postherpetic neuralgia, but higher doses are needed because VZV is not as sensitive to the systemic antivirals as HSV. In severe disseminated VZV, ophthalmic VZV, or zoster in the setting of immunosuppression, systemic acyclovir is recommended.

Although rare in children, postherpetic neuralgia can be treated with topical capsaicin, analgesics, EMLA cream, lidocaine patches, narcotics, nerve blocks, biofeedback, tricyclic antidepressants, gabapentin, and pregabalin. To decrease the incidence of postherpetic neuralgia in adults, the varicella zoster vaccine consisting of live attenuated virus is approved for susceptible persons older than 50 years and recommended for all individuals over age 60.

HUMAN PAPILLOMAVIRUS

Warts are discrete benign epithelial proliferations caused by human papillomavirus (HPV). There are more than 200 types of HPV, causing different clinical manifestations, depending on the anatomical location and immune status of the host. Verruca vulgaris (a common wart) is caused by HPV types 2, 4, 7, 27, and 29. Verruca plana (flat warts) are caused by HPV types 3, 10, 28, and 41. Verruca plantaris (plantar warts) are caused by HPV types 1, 2, and 4. Condyloma acuminatum (anogenital warts) are caused by HPV types 6, 11 (low risk for oncogenic potential), types 16, 18, 31, 33, and 45 (high risk for cervical cancer).

VERRUCA VULGARIS

Verruca vulgaris are benign keratotic papules typically located on the hands, fingers, and knees of children.

SYNONYM Common wart.

EPIDEMIOLOGY

AGE School children, incidence decreases after age 25 years.
GENDER M = F.
PREVALENCE Common, 20% of schoolchildren.
ETIOLOGY HPV types 1, 2, 4 > types 7, 27, 29.

PATHOPHYSIOLOGY

HPV enters the skin through minor abrasions or macerated areas, and targets the basal keratinocytes where productive infection and induction of hyperproliferation occurs. HPVs have evolved mechanisms to evade immune surveillance; thus, the host immune response may be slow and the warts may take years to eradicate.

HISTORY

Common wart contagion occurs in groups—small (home) or large (school gymnasium)—directly by person-to-person skin contact or indirectly through contaminated surfaces (public showers, swimming pools). Nail biters or cuticle pickers are more prone to periungual lesions. Primary lesions typically are inoculated on the hands, fingers, and knees. Autoinoculation to other sites, especially the face, is possible.

PHYSICAL EXAMINATION

Skin Findings

TYPE Papules (Fig. 23-12), cleft, filiform nodules.
COLOR Flesh color with red dots (thrombosing capillary loops).
SIZE 1 to 10 mm.
SHAPE Round, polycyclic.
ARRANGEMENT Isolated lesion, scattered discrete lesions.
DISTRIBUTION Sites of trauma—hands, fingers, knees.
NAILS Nailfold/matrix involvement can cause onychodystrophy.

DIFFERENTIAL DIAGNOSIS

The differential diagnosis of common warts includes nevi, acne, molluscum, seborrheic keratoses, keratoacanthomas, angiokeratomas, acrochordon, and pyogenic granulomas.

LABORATORY EXAMINATIONS

DERMATOPATHOLOGY Well-circumscribed "church spire" papillomatosis heaped with ortho- and parakeratosis, acanthosis, hypergranulosis, and koilocytosis.

COURSE AND PROGNOSIS

Warts are slow-growing, but evade the host immune response and are resistant to heat and desiccation. Thus, spontaneous resolution may take months to years.

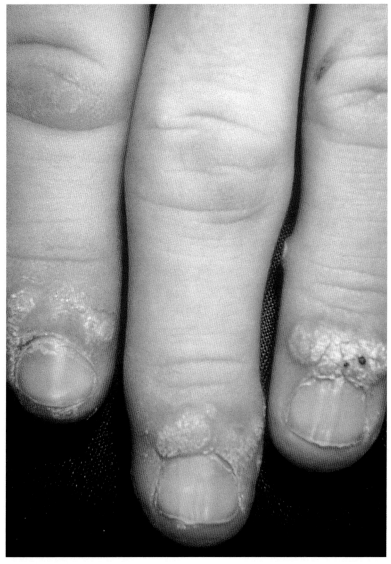

FIGURE 23-12 **Verruca vulgaris** Verrucous papules on the periungual region of a child's fingers.

MANAGEMENT

In asymptomatic children, warts will often self-resolve within 2 years without treatment. Since there are no antivirals specific for HPV, management of common warts focuses on the destruction of visible lesions or induction of cytotoxicity against infected cells. Thus, enlarging or spreading lesions can be targeted with destructive therapies, such as, trichloro-acetic/salicylic/squaric/lactic acid, curettage, cryotherapy, electrosurgery, scalpel excision, or laser surgery. Remission rates are nearly 80% with repeated wart treatments, but recurrences are frequent in approximately 40% of cases.

Other reported attempts to stimulate host cellular immunity to HPV include treatment with topical imiquimod, topical canthari-din, topical retinoids, topical 5-FU, topical diphenylcyclopropenone, duct tape occlusion, hot-water immersion (113°F for 30 minutes three times per week), hypnosis, oral cimeti-dine, intralesional *Candida* or *Trichophyton*, and intralesional bleomycin.

VERRUCA PLANA

Verruca plana are flat-topped, 2- to 5-mm papules, typically scattered on the face, arms, and legs of children.

SYNONYM Flat wart.

EPIDEMIOLOGY

AGE Young children, can also be seen in adults.
GENDER M = F.
INCIDENCE Common.
ETIOLOGY HPV types 2, 3, and 10 >> 1 and 11.

PATHOPHYSIOLOGY

HPV enters the skin through minor abrasions or macerated areas, and targets the basal keratinocytes where productive infection and induction of hyperproliferation occurs. HPVs have evolved mechanisms to evade immune surveillance; thus, the host immune response may be slow and flat warts may take years to clear.

HISTORY

Flat wart contagion occurs directly by person-to-person skin contact or indirectly through contaminated surfaces (razors). In adolescents and adults, shaving can spread the lesions.

PHYSICAL EXAMINATION

Skin Findings

TYPE Flat-topped papules (Fig. 23-13).
COLOR Skin-colored or light brown.
SIZE 1 to 5 mm.
SHAPE Round, oval, polygonal.
ARRANGEMENT Linear lesions (inoculation of virus by scratching).
NUMBER Few to hundreds.
DISTRIBUTION Face, dorsa of hands, shins.

DIFFERENTIAL DIAGNOSIS

The differential diagnosis of flat warts includes lichen planus, nevi, and seborrheic keratoses.

LABORATORY EXAMINATIONS

DERMATOPATHOLOGY Orthokeratosis, parakeratosis, acanthosis, hypergranulosis, and vacuolization of cells in the granular layer and upper malpighian layers. A surrounding immune response may signal imminent resolution or clearance.

COURSE AND PROGNOSIS

Flat warts eventually spontaneously resolve with time.

MANAGEMENT

In asymptomatic children, flat warts will often self-resolve within 2 years without treatment. Since there are no antivirals specific for HPV, management of flat warts focuses on the destruction of visible lesions or induction of cytotoxicity against infected cells. Thus, enlarging or spreading lesions can be targeted with destructive therapies, such as trichloroacetic/salicylic/squaric/lactic acid, curettage, cryotherapy, electrosurgery, scalpel excision, or laser surgery.

Other reported attempts to stimulate host cellular immunity to HPV include treatment with topical imiquimod, topical cantharidin, topical retinoids, topical 5-FU, topical diphenylcyclopropenone, duct tape occlusion, hot-water immersion (113°F for 30 minutes three times per week), hypnosis, oral cimetidine, and intralesional *Candida* or *Trichophyton*.

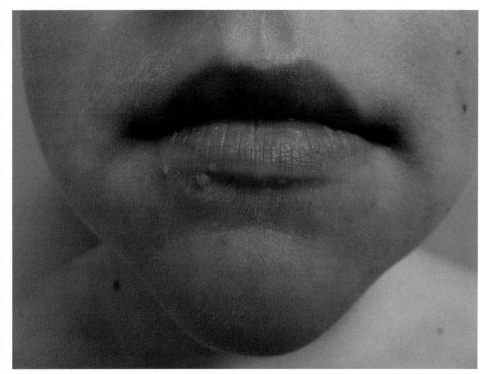

FIGURE 23-13 Verruca plana Scattered flat-topped papules increasing in number around a child's mouth.

VERRUCA PLANTARIS

Verruca plantaris are keratotic lesions located on the plantar aspect of the feet. They tend to be painful HPV-associated lesions that are more refractory to treatment.

SYNONYM Plantar wart.

EPIDEMIOLOGY

AGE Any age, typically 5 to 25 years.
GENDER M = F.
INCIDENCE Common.
ETIOLOGY HPV 1, 2, and 4.

PATHOPHYSIOLOGY

HPV enters the skin through minor abrasions or macerated areas, and targets the basal keratinocytes where productive infection and induction of hyperproliferation occurs. HPVs have evolved mechanisms to evade immune surveillance; thus, the host immune response may be slow and plantar warts may take years to clear.

HISTORY

Plantar wart contagion occurs directly by person-to-person skin contact or indirectly through contaminated surfaces (gymnasium floors, public showers, swimming pools). Trauma is a factor, because the lesions often occur on sites of pressure, and the wart is often painful to the host.

PHYSICAL EXAMINATION

Skin Findings

TYPE Papule, plaque (Fig. 23-14).
COLOR Skin-colored with red dots (thrombosed capillary loops).
PALPATION Tenderness may be marked, especially in certain acute types.
DISTRIBUTION Plantar pressure points: heads of metatarsal, heels, and toes.

DIFFERENTIAL DIAGNOSIS

The differential diagnosis of plantar warts includes corns, calluses, punctuate porokeratosis, poromas, hyperhidrotic pitting, or scars.

LABORATORY EXAMINATIONS

DERMATOPATHOLOGY Papillomatosis, ortho- and parakeratosis, acanthosis, hypergranulosis, and koilocytosis.

COURSE AND PROGNOSIS

Untreated, 50% of plantar warts self-resolve within 2 years. Others persist and can become quite large and/or painful.

MANAGEMENT

In asymptomatic children, plantar warts will often self-resolve within 2 years without treatment. Since there are no antivirals specific for HPV, management of plantar warts focuses on the destruction of visible lesions or induction of cytotoxicity against infected cells. Thus, enlarging or spreading lesions can be targeted with destructive therapies, such as, trichloroacetic/salicylic/squaric/lactic acid, curettage, cryotherapy, electrosurgery, scalpel excision, or laser surgery.

Other reported attempts to stimulate host cellular immunity to HPV include treatment with topical imiquimod, topical retinoids, topical cantharidin, topical 5-FU, topical diphenylcyclopropenone, duct tape occlusion, hot-water immersion (113°F for 30 minutes three times per week), hypnosis, oral cimetidine, and intralesional *Candida* or *Trichophyton*.

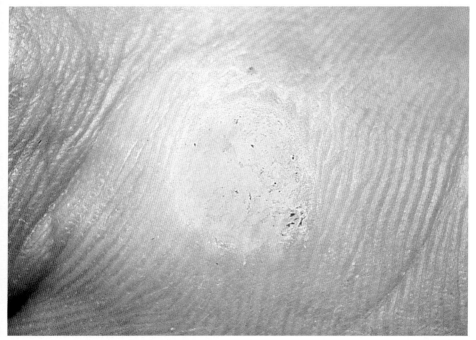

FIGURE 23-14 Verruca plantaris Rough keratotic plaque with pinpoint red dots representing dilated blood vessels characteristic of a plantar wart.

CONDYLOMA ACUMINATUM

Condylomas are soft, skin-colored, fleshy warts occurring on mucocutaneous junctions and intertriginous areas, resulting from an infection by HPV.

SYNONYMS Genital acuminate or venereal wart, verruca acuminata.

EPIDEMIOLOGY

AGE Sexually active young adults. Can be seen in infants and toddlers due to neonatal passage following maternal-child transmission during vaginal birth.
GENDER F ≥ M.
ETIOLOGY HPV types 6, 11 >> types 16, 18, 31, 33.
PREVALENCE Common, 20 million people in the United States; up to 20% to 40% of young women.
INCIDENCE Increasing in the past two decades. Incidence decreasing in vaccinated populations.

PATHOPHYSIOLOGY

Genital warts are highly contagious and are typically transmitted sexually by mucosa-to-mucosa contact. In infants, HPV may be acquired during delivery. In prepubertal children, the presence of condyloma in the anogenital area in the absence of other skin warts should alert one to the possibility of sexual abuse. Nonvenereal transmission is more likely if there are (1) no other signs of sexual abuse, (2) the lesions are distant from the anus or introitus, or (3) warts are present in close contacts (e.g., mother's hands).

HISTORY

Condyloma can appear weeks to years after exposure and can spread with irritation of trauma. Subclinical infections are much more common than visible genital warts leading to asymptomatic shedding and increased sexual transmission. Behavioral risk factors for genital warts include sexual intercourse at an early age, numbers of sexual partners, and partner's number of partners.

PHYSICAL FINDINGS

Skin Findings

TYPE Papules, plaques (Fig. 23-15).
COLOR Flesh-colored, pink, brown, white.
SIZE 1 mm to several millimeters.
PALPATION Soft.

SHAPE May be filiform or sessile.
ARRANGEMENT May be solitary. Grouped into grape-like or cauliflower-like clusters.
DISTRIBUTION External genitalia, perineum, perianal/buttock area.

DIFFERENTIAL DIAGNOSIS

The differential diagnosis of condyloma includes condylomata lata (syphilis), intraepithelial neoplasia, bowenoid papulosis, squamous cell carcinoma, molluscum contagiosum, lichen nitidus, lichen planus, normal sebaceous glands, pearly penile papules, folliculitis, moles, seborrheic keratoses, skin tags, pilar cyst, and scabies.

LABORATORY EXAMINATIONS

DERMATOPATHOLOGY Epidermal acanthosis, pseudoepitheliomatous hyperplasia.
ACETOWHITENING Gauze with 5% acetic acid makes warts appear as tiny white papules.

COURSE AND PROGNOSIS

Condyloma may clear spontaneously but tend to recur even after appropriate therapy, because of persistence of latent HPV in normal-appearing perilesional skin. The major significance of HPV infection is their oncogenicity later in life. HPV types 16, 18, 31, and 33 are the major etiological factors for cervical carcinoma in women. The importance of routine Pap test must be stressed to women with history of genital warts and anal Pap testing should be considered in populations at high risk for anal carcinoma (e.g., men who have sex with men).

Additionally, genital warts can be transmitted perinatally to the infant.

MANAGEMENT

Condylomas are often difficult to treat, recurrences are frequent (25–67%), and it is unclear whether treatment reduces the transmission rate to sexual partners. Since there are no antivirals specific for HPV, management of genital warts focuses on the destruction of visible lesions or induction of cytotoxicity against infected cells. Thus, lesions can be targeted with destructive therapies, such as podophyllotoxin,

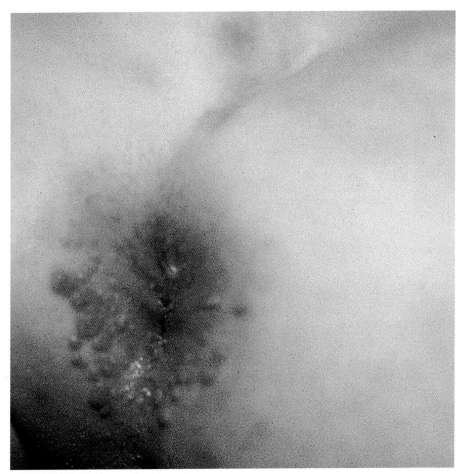

FIGURE 23-15 Condyloma acuminatum Perianal verrucous papules in a child. The perianal location should alert one to the possibility of sexual abuse, but often these warts occur through non-venereal transmission..

podophyllin, cryotherapy, trichloroacetic/ salicylic/squaric/lactic acid, interferons, cidofovir, topical sinecatechins, curettage, electrosurgery, scalpel excision, or laser vaporization.

Other reported attempts to stimulate host cellular immunity to HPV include treatment with topical imiquimod, topical retinoids, topical cantharidin, topical 5-FU, topical diphenylcyclopropenone, oral cimetidine, and intralesional *Candida* or *Trichophyton*.

Anogenital condyloma in prepubertal children should alert the physician to the possibility of child abuse. Fortunately, most instances are nonvenereal in transmission caused by autoinoculation (concomitant warts on the child's hands) or spread from close family members (changing diapers).

Prevention of condyloma is now the strategic approach in the United States. HPV virus-like particle vaccines are approved for prophylactic vaccination. A quadrivalent vaccine (Gardasil) for HPV types 6, 11, 16, and 18 or a bivalent vaccine (Cervarix) for HPV types 16 and 18 are recommended for all prepubertal girls prior to the onset of sexual activity (preferentially younger than 12 years). Studies indicate the vaccine is 90% effective in preventing the HPV types listed for at least 5 years. These vaccines have been demonstrated to reduce the incidence of condylomata acuminata and will hopefully decrease the incidence of cervical cancer from these HPV types in the coming years.

POXVIRUS

MOLLUSCUM CONTAGIOSUM

Molluscum contagiosum is a common, benign self-limited viral infection of childhood, characterized by discrete, umbilicated papules.

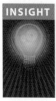 **INSIGHT** Although not as contagious as the name would suggest, molluscum can spread and persist for many years in some individuals; one method of transmission seems to be via water or fomites in pools and baths.

EPIDEMIOLOGY

AGE Children 3 to 16 years.
GENDER M > F.
INCIDENCE Common.

PATHOPHYSIOLOGY

In children, molluscum is spread via swimming pools, hot tubs, bath water, skin-to-skin contact, or fomites. In adults, genitally located lesions are likely to spread sexually. Molluscum is also seen in increased incidence in persons with atopic dermatitis or immunosuppressed individuals.

HISTORY

Molluscum lesions appear anywhere from 14 days to 6 months after exposure and self-resolve in a few months. The lesions are asymptomatic or mildly pruritic and can look inflamed with or without a surrounding area of dermatitis prior to spontaneous involution. Systemic symptoms are absent.

PHYSICAL EXAMINATION

Skin Findings

TYPE Papules, nodules.
COLOR Pearly white or flesh-colored.
SIZE 2 to 5 mm.
SHAPE Round, oval, hemispherical, umbilicated (Fig. 23-16).

NUMBER Isolated single lesion or multiple scattered discrete lesions.
DISTRIBUTION Axillae (Fig. 23-17), antecubital and crural folds.

DIFFERENTIAL DIAGNOSIS

The differential diagnosis of molluscum contagiosum includes nevi, warts, acne, appendageal tumors, condyloma, juvenile xanthogranuloma, papular granuloma annulare, pyogenic granuloma, histoplasmosis, cryptococcosis, or basal cell carcinoma.

LABORATORY EXAMINATION

DERMATOPATHOLOGY Molluscum bodies: epithelial cells with large eosinophilic intracytoplasmic inclusions (Henderson–Patterson bodies).
GIEMSA'S STAIN A simple skin scrape of the central core reveals molluscum bodies.

COURSE AND PROGNOSIS

Molluscum is asymptomatic in children and self-resolves with time.

MANAGEMENT

Since molluscum self-resolves, treatment is reserved for enlarging or spreading lesions, or those that are cosmetically disfiguring. In children, topical cantharidin is a safe and effective therapy, which is relatively painless and nontraumatic. Other treatment approaches include curettage, cryotherapy, topical retinoids, imiquimod, podophyllotoxin, topical keratolytics, topical cidofovir, tape stripping, and laser therapy.

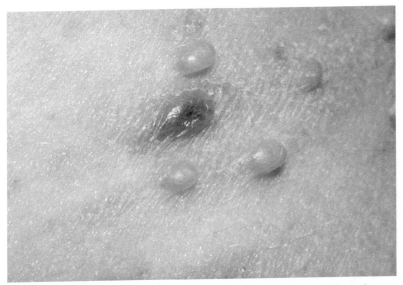

FIGURE 23-16 Molluscum contagiosum Close-up of dome-shaped umbilicated papules.

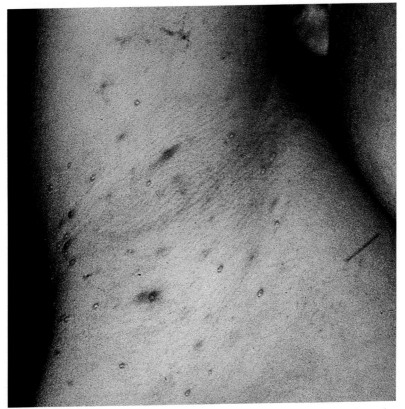

FIGURE 23-17 Molluscum contagiosum Scattered umbilicated dome-shaped papules in the axillary region of a child.

EPSTEIN–BARR VIRUS

INFECTIOUS MONONUCLEOSIS

Infectious mononucleosis is a contagious viral disease caused by the Epstein–Barr virus (EBV) and characterized by fever, malaise, tonsillitis, hepatosplenomegaly (HSM), lymphadenopathy, ± rash. The disease is notorious for its association with debilitating fatigue.

INSIGHT The Epstein–Barr Virus (HHV-4) has been linked with several rare diseases, including hydroa vacciniforme, oral hairy leukoplakia, Burkitt's lymphoma, and nasopharyngeal carcinoma, but is most commonly encountered clinically as infectious mononucleosis.

SYNONYMS Mono, EBV infection, human herpesvirus 4 (HHV-4), kissing disease.

EPIDEMIOLOGY

AGE All ages, adolescents, 13 to 25 years.
GENDER M = F.
INCIDENCE Common, 45 cases/100,000.
ETIOLOGY EBV.

PATHOPHYSIOLOGY

EBV is spread via saliva or blood during viremia phase. The virus preferentially infects human mucosal cells and B lymphocytes. Active viral replication leads to the infectious mononucleosis syndrome. The host eventually mounts an immune response and terminates viral replication in the oropharynx.

HISTORY

Infectious mononucleosis begins 30 to 50 days after exposure with fever, malaise, and sore throat. Marked tonsillitis and associated cervical lymphadenopathy ensue. HSM is common; 10% to 15% of patients will have a generalized exanthem (macular or papular), 50% of patients will have periorbital edema, 25% of patients have an associated enanthem (petechiae on the palate). Chronic debilitating fatigue is often a hallmark of this disease. Nausea and/or GI distress are often present.

PHYSICAL EXAMINATION

Skin Findings

TYPE Macules, papules, vesicles, edema, urticaria, purpura.

COLOR Bright pink or red.
SIZE 1 to 5 mm.
DISTRIBUTION Trunk, upper extremities to face, forearms, periorbital edema.
MUCOUS MEMBRANES Petechiae at the junction of the soft and hard palate, marked membranous tonsillitis (Fig. 23-18).

General Findings

FEVER (101°F–104°F).
LYMPHADENOPATHY Malaise, fatigue, HSM.

DIFFERENTIAL DIAGNOSIS

The differential diagnosis for infectious mononucleosis includes group A streptococcal infection, viral hepatitis, cytomegalovirus infection, human immunodeficiency virus infection, toxoplasmosis, lymphoma, or drug eruption.

LABORATORY EXAMINATIONS

DERMATOPATHOLOGY Nonspecific perivascular lymphocytic infiltrate.
MONOSPOT TEST A rapid slide test of the patient's blood for the presence of EBV IgM heterophile antibodies can be false negative, especially in children younger than 4 years old.
SEROLOGY Three serologic antibody tests may be helpful in staging EBV infection. During the acute primary infection, IgG and IgM antibodies to the EBV viral capsid antigen (VCA) are positive, but the EBNA IgG is negative. During a past persistent infection, VCA IgGs and EBNA IgGs are positive, but the VCA IgM is negative. An assay to measure circulating EBV DNA levels is also available.
COMPLETE BLOOD COUNT Absolute lymphocytosis—with predominantly atypical lymphocytes—is common.
LIVER FUNCTION TESTS Elevations in alanine and aspartate aminotransferases (ALT, AST) are seen in the vast majority of patients with infectious mononucleosis.

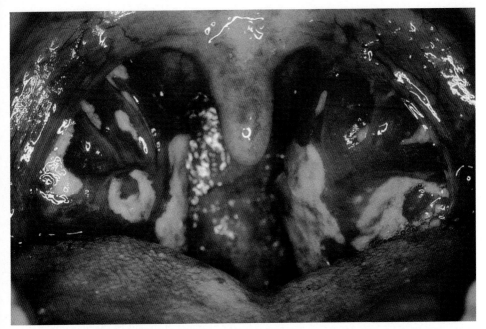

FIGURE 23-18 Infectious mononucleosis Marked white exudate on the tonsils of a child with infectious mononucleosis.

COURSE AND PROGNOSIS

Infectious mononucleosis in children can be mild and asymptomatic. In adolescents, the disease tends to be more severe and thus easier to recognize. Most cases of infectious mononucleosis self-resolve in 10 to 20 days, although the fatigue may last longer. The most severe complication is splenomegaly with the risk of splenic rupture in 0.2% or significant oropharyngeal swelling that leads to airway obstruction. In rare instances, a more chronic form of the disease has been seen, with relapses and chronic fatigue.

MANAGEMENT

Infectious mononucleosis will self-resolve with supportive measures. If the tonsillitis is severe, hospitalization and corticosteroids may be necessary to avoid airway obstruction. In up to 25% of cases, a concurrent β-hemolytic strep throat is present and should be treated with erythromycin.

It should be noted that ampicillin, penicillin, cephalosporins, or amoxicillin given to patients with infectious mononucleosis can cause a copper-colored generalized skin reaction. IgM and IgG antibodies to EBV are responsible for this reaction as opposed to a true IgE-mediated hypersensitivity to the antibiotics. Since this is not a true drug allergy, the patient can use these antibiotics in the future without problems.

For adolescents participating in contact sports, a minimum of 3 weeks avoidance after diagnosis is recommended to limit the low but serious risk of splenic rupture.

HUMAN PARVOVIRUS B19

ERYTHEMA INFECTIOSUM

Erythema infectiosum is a childhood exanthem caused by parvovirus B19 and characterized by a "slapped-cheek" appearance on the face followed by a lacy reticulated rash on the body.

SYNONYMS Fifth disease, "slapped cheek" disease.

EPIDEMIOLOGY

AGE All ages. School-aged children 3 to 12 years.
GENDER F > M.
INCIDENCE Common, 80% of adults are sero-positive for parvovirus.
SEASON Late winter, early spring.
EPIDEMICS Every 6 years on average, lasting for 3 to 6 months.
ETIOLOGY Human parvovirus B19.

PATHOPHYSIOLOGY

Parvovirus B19 is spread via aerosolized respiratory droplets during the viremic stage, blood products, or vertically from a mother to her fetus. B19 has an affinity for erythrocytes precursors and binds to the erythrocyte P antigen (globoside).

HISTORY

Erythema infectiosum begins 4 to 14 days after exposure with fever, malaise, headache, chills, arthritis, and arthralgias. During the period of B19 viremia, reticulocytopenia occurs which is inconsequential to a normal host, but can lead to an aplastic crisis, pancytopenia, fetal hydrops, or intrauterine demise in at-risk populations. On day 3 to 4, a slapped-cheek appearance on the face occurs as the viremia resolves. One to four days later, a lacy reticulated rash appears on the trunk and extremities that waxes and wanes, exacerbated by sunlight or overheating. The body rash may last 1 to 3 weeks and pruritus may be present.

PHYSICAL EXAMINATION

Skin Findings

TYPE Plaques, macules, papules.
COLOR Pink to red.
SHAPE Round to oral.
DISTRIBUTION Slapped cheeks (Fig. 23-19); lacy reticulated rash on extensor surfaces of extremities, trunk, neck (Fig. 23-20).
MUCOUS MEMBRANES ±Enanthem.

General Findings

RHEUMATOLOGIC (10%) Arthritis; arthralgias of hands, wrists, knees, ankles.

DIFFERENTIAL DIAGNOSIS

The differential diagnosis of erythema infectiosum includes rubella, measles, scarlet fever, exanthem subitum, juvenile inflammatory arthritis, enteroviral infections, or drug reactions.

LABORATORY EXAMINATIONS

DERMATOPATHOLOGY Nonspecific lymphocytic infiltrate.
SEROLOGY Blood may show anti-B19 IgM antibodies (indicating infection within previous 2–4 months) or IgG seroconversion. Nucleic acid hybridization and polymerase chain reaction assays are also available but persistent low levels of viremia following infection resolution—or clearance of viremia by the time immune-mediated symptoms develop—may limit their utility relative to serology.

COURSE AND PROGNOSIS

By the time the slapped cheek and lacy body rash are present, the viremia has resolved. The rash slowly resolves over 1 to 3 weeks and can recur or seem to flare with temperature fluctuations, sunlight, or friction. Rarely, there may be an associated arthritis (10%), but this is seen more commonly in adults (60%). In persons with chronic anemias (sickle cell anemia, hereditary spherocytosis, thalassemia, pyruvate kinase deficiency, or autoimmune hemolytic anemia), parvovirus B19 may induce an aplastic crisis with worsening anemia. Similarly, pregnant women have a chance of infection with parvoviral B19 exposure if never previously infected. The virus is able to affect erythrocyte precursor cells in the developing fetus, especially before 20 weeks' gestation, leading to hydrops fetalis or intrauterine demise in 5%.

MANAGEMENT

Erythema infectiosum is self-limited in healthy children, and thus no treatment is necessary. Nonsteroidal anti-inflammatory drugs can be used for arthralgias, if present. By the time the rash is noted, the viremia is over; thus, children are no longer contagious and can resume normal activities.

At-risk patients with aplastic crisis may need a blood transfusion. Pregnant women with documented B19 infection should undergo serial ultrasounds and *in utero* fetal transfusions if necessary.

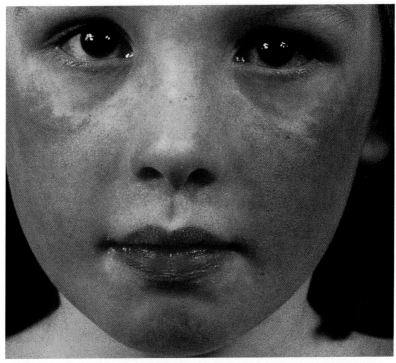

FIGURE 23-19 **Erythema infectiosum** "Slapped-cheek" appearance in a child with parvovirus B19 infection.

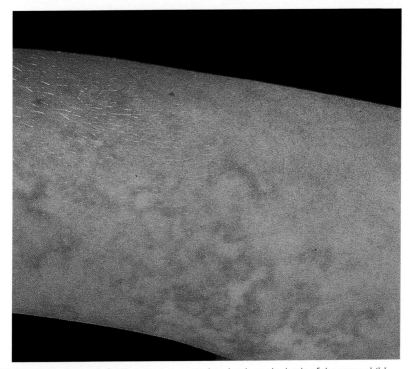

FIGURE 23-20 **Erythema infectiosum** Lacy reticulated rash on the body of the same child.

HUMAN HERPESVIRUS 6 AND 7

EXANTHEM SUBITUM

Exanthem subitum is a common, benign rash caused by HHV 6 and 7, characterized by fever and followed by rash in an otherwise well-appearing child.

SYNONYMS Roseola infantum, sixth disease.

EPIDEMIOLOGY

AGE Infants, toddlers: 6 months to 3 years.
GENDER M = F.
INCIDENCE Common, 90% of infants younger than age 1 month have HHV-6 antibodies (likely passive maternal transplacental transfer). The infants then become seronegative for HHV-6, making them susceptible to infection, and by age 3, 90% of children are seropositive again for HHV-6 antibodies. Seropositivity for HHV-7 seems to occur at a later age.
SEASON Spring.
ETIOLOGY HHV-6 >> HHV-7.

PATHOPHYSIOLOGY

HHV-6 and 7 are spread via asymptomatic viral shedding in respiratory secretions. HHV-6 and 7 target CD4$^+$ T-cell lymphocytes where they actively replicate and cause viremia. As with all HHVs, latency is eventually established, with HHV-6 and 7 dormant in the salivary glands or peripheral mononuclear cells.

HISTORY

HHV-6 and 7 have an incubation period of 9 to 10 days, followed by 3 to 5 days of fever and subsequent rash in a well-appearing infant (Fig. 23-21).

PHYSICAL EXAMINATION

Skin Findings

TYPE Macules, papules, edema.
COLOR Rose pink.
SIZE 2 to 3 mm.
DISTRIBUTION Trunk (Fig. 23-22), neck, extremities, periorbital edema.
MUCOUS MEMBRANES Papules on soft palate (Nagayama's spots), uvula, palatoglossal ulcers.

General Findings

FEVER 104°F to 105°F, rapid defervescence. Lymphadenopathy.
NEUROLOGIC Bulging fontanelle, encephalitis/encephalopathy/meningitis, seizures.

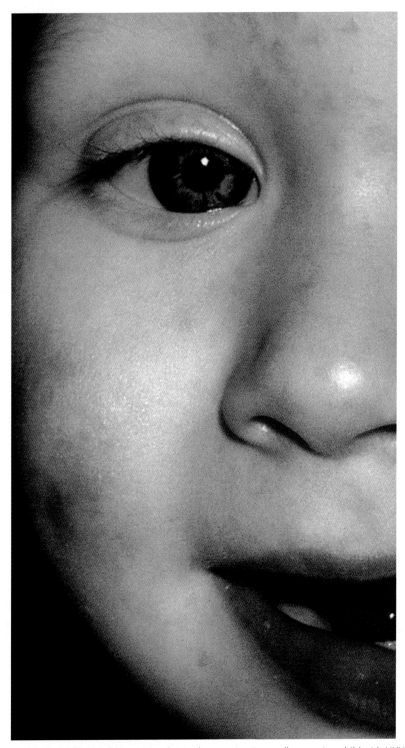

FIGURE 23-21 Exanthem subitum Maculopapular eruption in a well-appearing child with HHV-6 infection.

DIFFERENTIAL DIAGNOSIS

The differential diagnosis includes enterovirus, adenovirus, parainfluenza, measles, rubella, scarlet fever, erythema infectiosum, Kawasaki disease, and other viral exanthems.

LABORATORY EXAMINATIONS

SEROLOGY IgM; four times rise in IgG, polymerase chain reaction, immunofluorescence; cultures are available.
OTHER Mild leukopenia with relative lymphocytosis.

COURSE AND PROGNOSIS

Exanthem subitum is self-limited, and infection confers lifelong immunity.

MANAGEMENT

No treatment besides symptomatic fever management (antipyretics, fluids) is necessary, because most children have a mild, benign self-limited course.

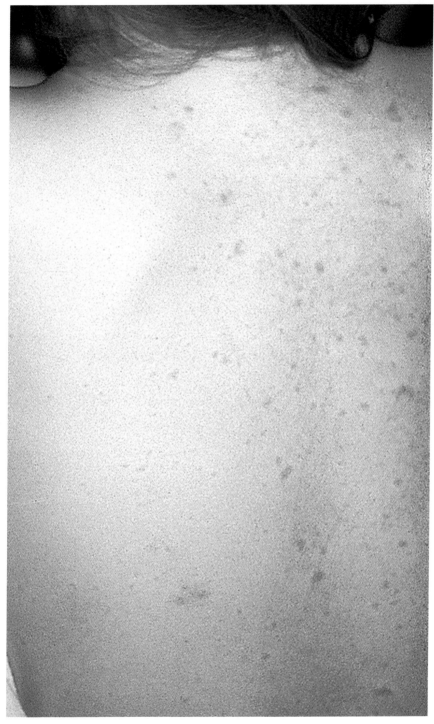

FIGURE 23-22 Exanthem subitum Maculopapular rash on the body of the same child.

MEASLES VIRUS

MEASLES

Measles is a highly contagious childhood viral infection characterized by fever, coryza, cough, conjunctivitis, pathognomonic enanthem (Koplik's spots), and an exanthem. It can be complicated by significant morbidity and mortality.

SYNONYMS Rubeola, morbilli.

 INSIGHT The term "morbilliform"—often used to describe a rash composed of pink macules and papules such as a drug-induced eruption—refers to an eruption that is measles-like in appearance.

EPIDEMIOLOGY

AGE Before immunization: ages 5 to 9 years. Now: younger than 15 months or older than 10 years.
GENDER M = F.
INCIDENCE United States: 1989 epidemic: 27,000 cases. Postvaccination: 2014: >600 cases. Current outbreaks in the United States occur in unimmunized preschool-age children, school-age persons immunized at early age, and imported cases. Most outbreaks have been linked to primary or secondary schools, colleges, universities, amusement parks, and day care centers.
SEASON Late winter to early spring.
EPIDEMICS Prior to widespread use of vaccine, epidemics occurred every 2 to 3 years. Incidence rising in population clusters associated with nonvaccination.
GEOGRAPHY Worldwide.
ETIOLOGY Measles virus, a paramyxovirus.

PATHOPHYSIOLOGY

Measles is spread by respiratory droplets aerosolized by sneezing and coughing. Infected persons are contagious from several days before onset of rash up to 5 days after lesions appear. The attack rate for susceptible contacts exceeds 90% to 100%. Measles virus enters cells of the respiratory tract; replicates locally; spreads to local lymph nodes; and disseminates hematogenously to skin, mucous membranes, and organs.

HISTORY

Ten to fifteen days after exposure, a prodrome of coryza and a hacking, bark-like cough; photophobia; malaise; and fever may be present. An enanthem (Koplik's spots) appears, then an exanthem beginning behind the ears/hairline spreads downward and gradually transitions from red to tan-brown.

PHYSICAL EXAMINATION

Skin Findings

TYPE Macules, papules. Periorbital edema.
COLOR Red fading to yellow tan.
ARRANGEMENT Lesions become confluent on face, neck, and shoulders (Fig. 23-23).
DISTRIBUTION Forehead, hairline, behind ears; spreads to face, trunk (Fig. 23-24).
MUCOUS MEMBRANES Koplik's spots: cluster of tiny bluish-white papules with an erythematous areola (Fig. 23-25). Bulbar conjunctivae: conjunctivitis.

General Findings

FEVER, LAD.

DIFFERENTIAL DIAGNOSIS

The differential diagnosis of measles includes enterovirus, EBV, Kawasaki's disease, parvovirus, HHV-6, secondary syphilis, scarlet fever, and morbilliform drug eruption.

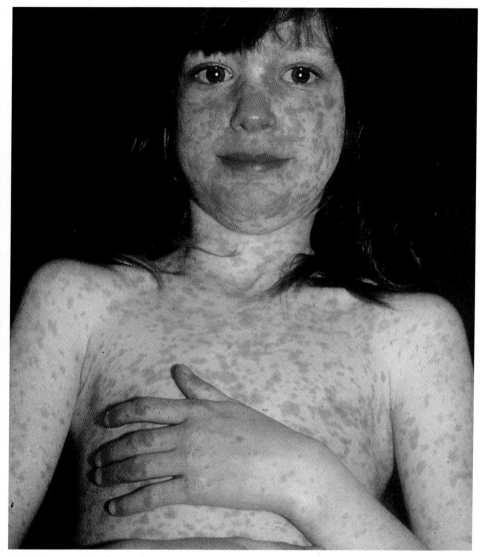

FIGURE 23-23 Measles Erythematous coalescing macules on face and trunk of a child with measles.

LABORATORY EXAMINATIONS

DERMATOPATHOLOGY Superficial perivascular lymphocytic infiltrate, spongiosis, and dyskeratosis. Multinucleated giant cells with intracytoplasmic inclusions may be seen in secretions or on biopsies of mucosal tissue.

SEROLOGY Four times rise in measles titer between acute and convalescent sera; immunofluorescence; or viral culture from blood, urine, pharyngeal secretions.

HEMATOLOGY Leukocytosis with lymphopenia.

COURSE AND PROGNOSIS

Measles is self-limited but can be complicated by pneumonia, otitis media, laryngitis, encephalitis, myocarditis, and/or pericarditis.

MANAGEMENT

Currently, in the United States, prophylactic immunization with the live attenuated measles vaccine is recommended for all children first between ages 12 and 15 months and again between 4 and 6 years.

For measles treatment, no specific antiviral therapy is used, but high-dose vitamin A does seem to decrease the morbidity and mortality of the infection. Otherwise, symptomatic treatment and respiratory isolation are recommended.

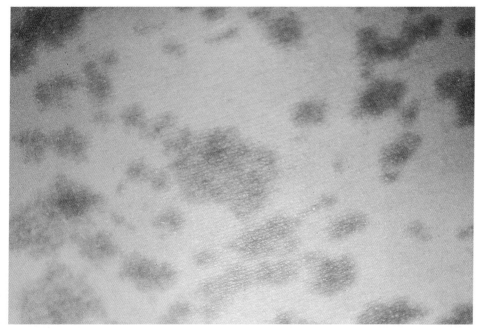

FIGURE 23-24 Measles Close-up view of erythematous macules coalescing into plaques.

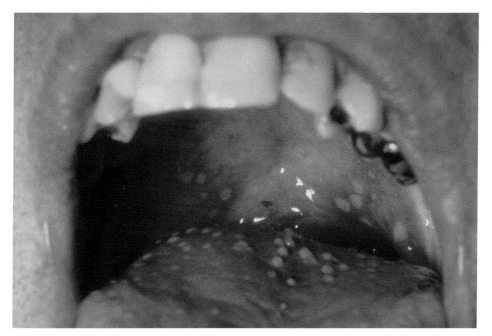

FIGURE 23-25 Measles White spots (Koplik's spots) on the hard palate of a person with measles.

RUBELLA VIRUS

RUBELLA

Rubella is a mild, self-limited childhood infection manifested by characteristic exanthem and lymphadenopathy. However, it can be associated with significant disease when transmitted to a fetus *in utero*, including miscarriage, stillbirth, or malformations.

SYNONYMS German measles, three-day measles.

EPIDEMIOLOGY

AGE Before immunization: younger than 15 years. Now: young adults.
GENDER M = F.
INCIDENCE After the vaccine was developed (1969), the incidence of rubella has decreased by 98%.
SEASON Spring.
EPIDEMICS Before vaccination: every 6 to 9 years. Recent outbreak in Japan in 2013 with >15,000 cases.
GEOGRAPHY Worldwide.
ETIOLOGY Rubella virus, an RNA virus of the Togaviridae family.

PATHOPHYSIOLOGY

Rubella virus is spread by inhalation of aerosolized respiratory droplets and is moderately contagious. The period of infectivity is from the end of the incubation period to the disappearance of the rash. A viremia ensues, followed by the exanthem, which is thought to be caused by the antigen–antibody complexes deposited in the skin.

HISTORY

Fourteen to twenty-one days after exposure to the rubella virus, a prodrome of anorexia, malaise, conjunctivitis, headache, low-grade fever, and mild upper respiratory tract symptoms may be present. Asymptomatic infection is common and can be seen in 80% cases. One to five days after the prodrome, the exanthem of rubella begins with macules and papules on the face that spread downward. Lymphadenopathy, arthritis, and arthralgias may be present. Adults have more severe symptoms than children.

PHYSICAL EXAMINATION

Skin Findings

TYPE Macules, papules.
COLOR Pink.
ARRANGEMENT Truncal lesions form confluent scarlatiniform eruption (Fig. 23-26).
DISTRIBUTION Forehead, face (Fig. 23-27), trunk, extremities.
MUCOUS MEMBRANES Petechiae on soft palate, uvula (Forchheimer's sign; Fig. 23-28).

General Findings

LYMPHADENOPATHY Postauricular, suboccipital, and posterior cervical lymph nodes enlarged.
RHEUMATOLOGIC Arthritis, arthralgias.
OTHER Splenomegaly, hepatitis, myocarditis, pericarditis, anemia, encephalitis, thrombocytopenia.

DIFFERENTIAL DIAGNOSIS

The differential diagnosis includes other viral infections (enteroviral infections, reoviruses, EBV, adenoviruses, measles), parvovirus B19, scarlet fever, or drug eruption.

LABORATORY EXAMINATIONS

DERMATOPATHOLOGY Superficial perivascular infiltrate with atypical lymphocytes.
SEROLOGY IgM; four times rise in IgG titers; virus cultured from throat, joint fluid aspirate.
HEMATOLOGY Leukopenia and neutropenia.

COURSE AND PROGNOSIS

In most people, infection with rubella is mild and self-limited. However, when rubella occurs in a nonimmune pregnant woman during the first trimester, congenital rubella syndrome can occur. Half of the infants who acquire rubella during the first trimester of intrauterine life will show clinical signs of damage: congenital heart defects (patent ductus arteriosus, ventricular septal defect), cataracts, microphthalmia, deafness, microcephaly, and hydrocephaly.

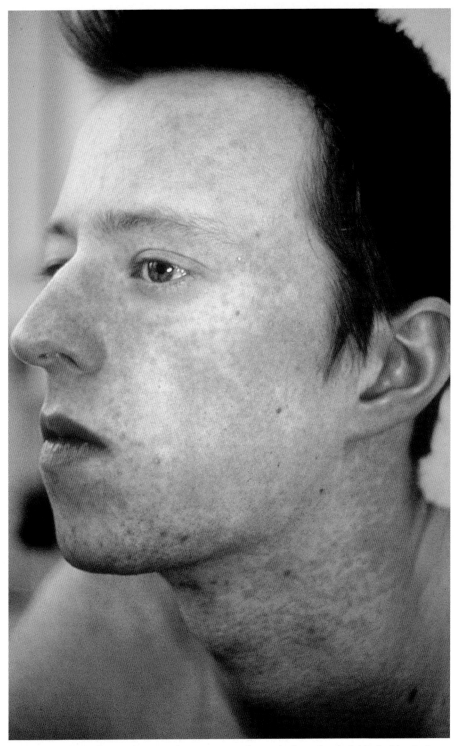

FIGURE 23-26 Rubella Confluent erythematous macules on the face of an individual with rubella.

MANAGEMENT

Rubella is preventable by immunization with a live attenuated vaccine between ages 12 and 15 months, then again between ages 4 and 6 years. If antirubella antibody titers are negative in young women, another immunization dose should be given. Otherwise, symptomatic treat- ment (antihistamines, antipruritics) for rubella is all that is needed. Infected children should be kept home from school for 5 days after the onset of the rash and pregnant women need to document immunity or avoid exposures, especially during the first trimester. If rubella occurs during pregnancy, prenatal counseling is recommended.

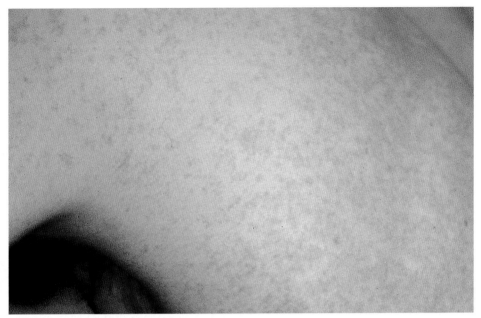

FIGURE 23-27 Rubella Rash spreading from face to trunk of the same individual.

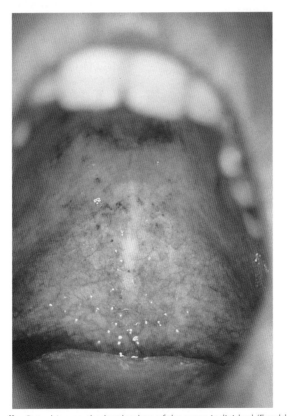

FIGURE 23-28 Rubella Petechiae on the hard palate of the same individual (Forchheimer's sign).

COXSACKIE VIRUS

HAND-FOOT-AND-MOUTH DISEASE

HFMD is an enteroviral infection characterized by fever, ulcerative oral lesions, and vesicular eruption of the palms and soles.

EPIDEMIOLOGY

AGE Children younger than 10 years.
GENDER M = F.
SEASON Warmer months.
EPIDEMICS Outbreak every 3 years, in temperate climates.
ETIOLOGY Coxsackie A16, enterovirus 71 > Coxsackie A6 > Coxsackie A4 to A7, A9, A10, B2, and B5.

PATHOPHYSIOLOGY

HFMD is highly contagious and spreads by oral–oral and fecal–oral routes. Enterovirus in the GI tract (buccal mucosa, ileum) spreads to lymph nodes, and 72 hours later, viremia occurs with seeding of the oral mucosa and skin, causing vesicle formation.

HISTORY

Three to six days after exposure, HFMD causes a prodrome of fever, malaise, abdominal pain, and respiratory symptoms. Frequently, painful oral lesions erupt leading to refusal to eat, and tender palmar and plantar lesions appear.

PHYSICAL EXAMINATION

Skin Findings

TYPE Macules, papules, vesicles, ulcers, crust over.
COLOR Pink to red.
SIZE 2 to 8 mm.
SHAPE Round, oval, football-shaped.
DISTRIBUTION Sides of fingers (Fig. 23-29), toes, palms, soles (Fig. 23-30).
MUCOUS MEMBRANES Oral ulcers on hard palate, tongue, buccal mucosa (Fig. 23-31).

General Findings

FEVER Severe malaise, diarrhea, and joint pains.

LABORATORY EXAMINATIONS

DERMATOPATHOLOGY Intraepidermal vesicle with neutrophils, mononuclear cells, and proteinaceous eosinophilic material, dermal perivascular mixed-cell infiltrate.
ELECTRON MICROSCOPY Intracytoplasmic particles in a crystalline array.
SEROLOGY Acute serum: neutralizing antibodies may be detected but disappear rapidly. Convalescent serum: elevated titers of complement-fixing antibodies.
POLYMERASE CHAIN REACTION/CULTURE Virus detected from vesicles, throat washings, stool specimens.

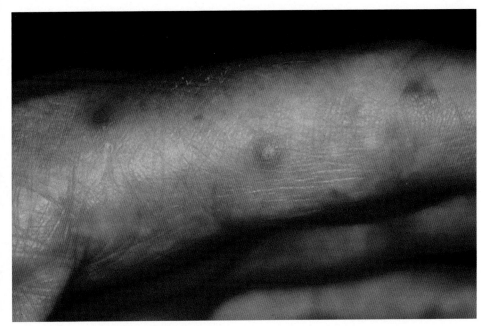

FIGURE 23-29 Hand-foot-and-mouth disease Vesicular lesions on the sides of the fingers of a patient with hand-foot-and-mouth disease.

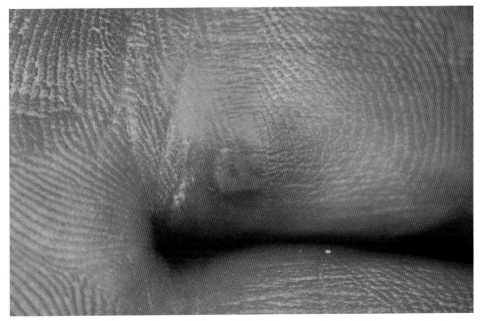

FIGURE 23-30 Hand-foot-and-mouth disease Vesicular lesion on the foot of the same patient.

DIFFERENTIAL DIAGNOSIS

The differential diagnosis for HFMD includes HSV infection, aphthous stomatitis, herpangina, and erythema multiforme major.

COURSE AND PROGNOSIS

Most commonly, HFMD is self-limited, and the viremia is cleared in 7 to 10 days. Prolonged, recurrent cases have been reported and serious sequelae (myocarditis, meningoencephalitis, aseptic meningitis, paralytic disease, fetal demise) can occur.

MANAGEMENT

No treatment for HFMD is needed. Symptomatically, topical application of dyclonine solution or lozenges, lidocaine, or benzocaine may help reduce oral discomfort. Acetaminophen or ibuprofen can be used for symptomatic fever relief. In the event an individual is unable to keep up with oral intake due to oral involvement, hospitalization for IV hydration should be considered.

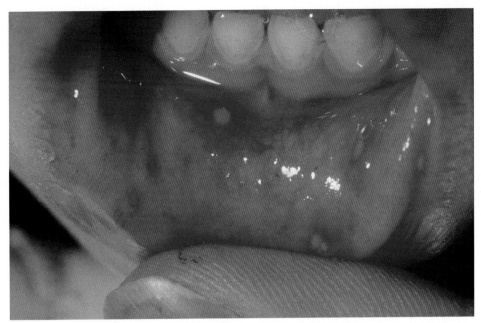

FIGURE 23-31 Hand-foot-and-mouth disease Scattered 3- to 5-mm ulcers on the buccal mucosa of the same patient.

OTHERS

GIANOTTI–CROSTI SYNDROME

Gianotti–Crosti syndrome is a rare, self-limited eruption, characterized by symmetric papules on the face, buttocks, and extremities with mild constitutional symptoms and acute hepatitis.

SYNONYMS Papular acrodermatitis of childhood, papulovesicular acrolocalized syndrome.

EPIDEMIOLOGY

AGE Children: 3 months to 15 years.
GENDER M = F.
INCIDENCE Rare.
SEASON Spring, early summer.
ETIOLOGY Host response to a variety of agents: hepatitis B, EBV >> adenovirus, rotavirus, hepatitis A and C, parainfluenza, Coxsackie, RSV, polio, cytomegalovirus, parvovirus, mumps, HHV-6, human immunodeficiency virus, group A *Streptococcus*, mycoplasma, *Bartonella*, vaccines (polio; diphtheria, pertussis, and tetanus vaccine; mumps–measles–rubella vaccine; hepatitis B, influenza). Rare outbreaks/clustering of cases reported.

HISTORY

Often preceded by an upper respiratory infection, Gianotti–Crosti begins with mild systemic symptoms (malaise, low-grade fever, lymphadenopathy, hepatosplenomegaly, diarrhea) and a rash on the face, buttocks, and extensor surface of the extremities which may be pruritic.

PHYSICAL EXAMINATION

Skin Findings

TYPE Papules, plaques, purpura.
COLOR Flesh-colored, pink, or coppery red.
SIZE 1 to 10 mm.
SHAPE Flat-topped discrete or coalescing lesions (Fig. 23-32).
DISTRIBUTION Face, elbows (Fig. 23-33), knees, buttocks, extremities, palms, soles.

General Findings

FEVER, LAD Cervical, inguinal, and axillary.
OTHER Hepatomegaly, splenomegaly, hepatitis.

DIFFERENTIAL DIAGNOSIS

The differential diagnosis of Gianotti–Crosti includes drug eruption, papular urticaria, viral exanthem, molluscum contagiosum, lichen planus, and lichen nitidus.

LABORATORY EXAMINATIONS

DERMATOPATHOLOGY Epidermal acanthosis, focal spongiosis, exocytosis, mixed dermal infiltrate, dilated dermal capillaries, vascular endothelium swelling.
HEMATOLOGY Leukopenia, monocytosis (approximately 20%), hypochromic anemia.
CHEMISTRY Abnormal liver function tests (aspartate aminotransferase, alanine aminotransferase, alkaline phosphatase). Normal bilirubin.
SEROLOGY May show elevated levels of hepatitis B surface antigen.

COURSE AND PROGNOSIS

Gianotti–Crosti has a self-limited course and the rash resolves spontaneously after 2 to 8 weeks; lymphadenitis lasts for 2 to 3 months; hepatomegaly persists for 3 months.

MANAGEMENT

No treatment for Gianotti–Crosti is necessary because the rash and liver abnormalities resolve spontaneously. Symptomatic relief can be obtained with topical antipruritic agents such as calamine or systemic antihistamines.

The eruption often heals with postinflammatory hypo- or hyperpigmentation in individuals of darker skin types.

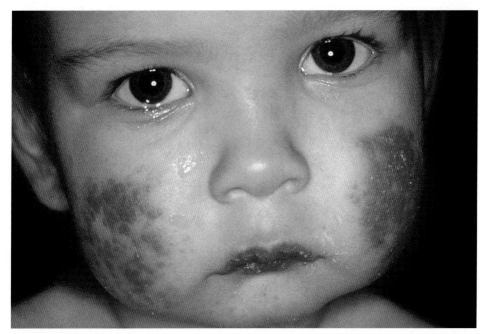

FIGURE 23-32 Gianotti–Crosti syndrome Monomorphous papules coalescing into plaques on the cheeks of a child.

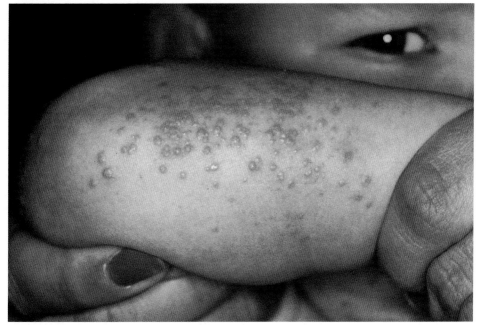

FIGURE 23-33 Gianotti–Crosti syndrome Erythematous papules on the elbow and forearm of the same patient.

ASYMMETRIC PERIFLEXURAL EXANTHEM OF CHILDHOOD

Asymmetric periflexural exanthem of childhood (APEC) is a rare, self-limited eruption, characterized by a unilateral periflexural rash most often of the axilla and trunk presumed to be viral in etiology.

SYNONYM Unilateral laterothoracic exanthem.

EPIDEMIOLOGY

AGE Children: 6 months to 10 years; peak age 1 to 5 years.
GENDER F > M, 2:1.
RACE Caucasians > others.
INCIDENCE Rare.
SEASON Spring.
GEOGRAPHY Europe, northern America.
ETIOLOGY Unclear, thought to be viral.

PATHOPHYSIOLOGY

Seasonal pattern, associated prodrome, familial case reports, and lack of response to antibiotics suggest a viral etiology, but thus far none has been detected.

HISTORY

Often preceded by an upper respiratory or GI prodrome, APEC begins with a unilateral, periflexural (axilla > trunk, arm, thigh), morbilliform, or eczematous rash that spreads to the contralateral side, but maintains a unilateral predominance.

PHYSICAL EXAMINATION

Skin Findings

TYPE Macules, papules (Fig. 23-34).
COLOR Pink, red.
SIZE 1 to 10 mm.
DISTRIBUTION Periflexural: axilla >> trunk, arm, thigh.

General Findings

FEVER, LAD.
OTHER (60%) Diarrhea, rhinitis.

DIFFERENTIAL DIAGNOSIS

The differential diagnosis of APEC includes contact dermatitis, fungal infection, viral exanthema, drug eruption, atypical pityriasis rosea, miliaria, scabies, Gianotti–Crosti syndrome, papular urticaria, and molluscum contagiosum.

LABORATORY EXAMINATIONS

DERMATOPATHOLOGY Superficial perivascular lymphocytic infiltrate, mild spongiosis, exocytosis with dermal inflammation around the eccrine ducts.

COURSE AND PROGNOSIS

APEC has a self-limited course and the rash resolves after 3 to 6 weeks.

MANAGEMENT

No treatment for APEC is necessary because the etiology is unclear and the rash resolves spontaneously. Symptomatic relief can be obtained with antipruritic agents or topical steroids and liberal use of emollients.

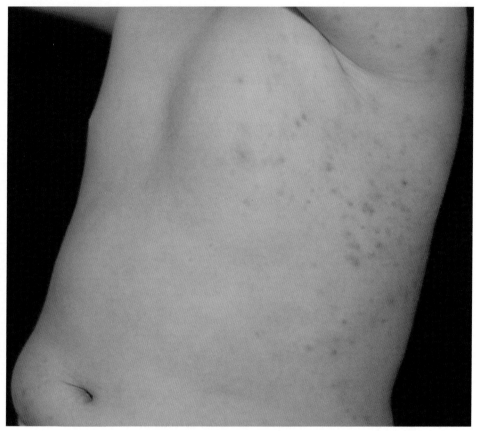

FIGURE 23-34 Asymmetric periflexural exanthem of childhood Unilateral erythematous macules in the axillary area of a child.

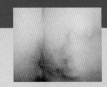

AQUATIC INFESTATIONS

CUTANEOUS LARVA MIGRANS

Cutaneous larva migrans is a skin infestation caused by nematode larvae that penetrate the skin and migrate leaving a characteristic erythematous, serpiginous burrow underneath the skin.

SYNONYM Creeping eruption.

EPIDEMIOLOGY

AGE Children > adults.
GENDER M = F.
INCIDENCE Uncommon; mostly in tropical climates (see **Geography**).
ETIOLOGY Hookworm larvae of cats/dogs (*Ancylostoma braziliense, Uncinaria stenocephala, Ancylostoma caninum*), cattle (*Bunostomum phlebotomum*), or other nematodes.
GEOGRAPHY Common in warm, humid, sandy, coastal areas, central United States, southern United States, central America, South America, and the Caribbean.

PATHOPHYSIOLOGY

In animal hosts (dogs, cats), the hookworm penetrates the skin and spreads through the lymphatic and venous systems to the lungs, breaks through into the alveoli, migrates to the trachea, and is swallowed. The hookworm then matures in the intestine and produces eggs that are excreted by the animal host. Once the animal defecates infested feces, the hookworm ova in the sand or soil hatch into larvae. The larvae penetrates the skin of accidental hosts (humans) when they are stepped on with bare feet or come into contact with other bare skin, but cannot cross the basement membrane and are confined to the epidermis. Thus the larvae wander serpiginously through the epidermis creating visible track patterns, giving the nickname "creeping eruption."

HISTORY

Larvae tend to penetrate the skin and begin to migrate at a rate of 1 to 2 cm/d for 4 weeks to 6 months and may cause pruritus. After aimless wandering, the larvae typically die and the cutaneous tracts self-resolve. Systemic symptoms are absent.

PHYSICAL EXAMINATION

Skin Findings

TYPE Tracks/burrows (Fig. 24-1). Vesicles or bullae can develop in individuals previously sensitized to the invading species.
COLOR Flesh colored to pink.
SIZE Width 2 to 3 mm, extending at 1 to 2 cm/d.
NUMBER One, several, or many tracks.
DISTRIBUTION Exposed sites: feet, lower legs, buttocks >> hands, thighs.

General Findings

Can be associated with peripheral blood eosinophilia and generalized pruritus. Very rare cases of hematogenous dissemination and resultant pulmonary infiltrates have been reported.

DIFFERENTIAL DIAGNOSIS

The differential diagnosis of cutaneous larvae migrans includes phytophotodermatitis, tinea pedis, erythema chronicum migrans, jellyfish sting, contact dermatitis, larva currens, and granuloma annulare.

LABORATORY EXAMINATIONS

DERMATOPATHOLOGY PAS may show larva in a suprabasalar burrow, spongiosis, intraepidermal vesicles, necrotic keratinocytes, and chronic inflammatory infiltrate with many eosinophils.

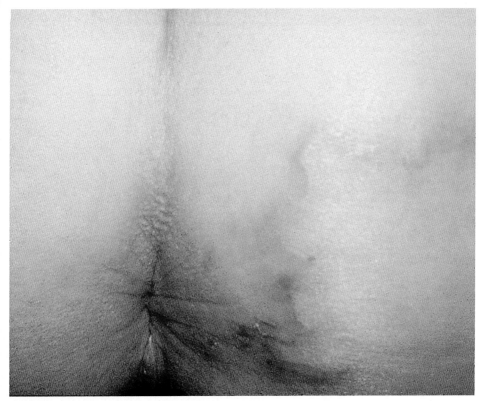

FIGURE 24-1 Cutaneous larva migrans Serpiginous lesion on the buttock of an infant infected with hookworm larvae.

COURSE AND PROGNOSIS

Cutaneous larva migrans is typically self-limited because the human skin is an accidental "dead-end" host. Most larvae die after 2 to 4 weeks of aimless wandering underneath the skin, and the skin rash resolves in approximately 4 to 6 weeks.

MANAGEMENT

Ultimately, the larval eruption will self-resolve in 4 to 6 weeks. Symptomatic relief with topical steroids until the pruritus self-resolves is a safe

treatment of choice. Antihistamines may also offer relief from pruritus.

Severe cases with intense pruritus may be treated with systemic albendazole or ivermectin; side effects include dizziness, nausea, cramps, and vomiting. Systemic albendazole for 3 to 5 days or a single dose of oral ivermectin can achieve rapid cure rates of >90% within 1 week. Topical 10% thiabendazole cream may be better tolerated but must be used thrice daily for 10 days. Historically, attempts at larval destruction modalities including TCA, cryotherapy, or electrocautery aimed at progressing skin burrow were not very effective.

CERCARIAL DERMATITIS

Cercarial dermatitis is an acute allergic pruritic eruption sparing the bathing suit areas of the body that develops following skin infiltration by water-borne *Schistosoma cercariae*.

SYNONYMS Swimmers' itch, collector's itch, schistosome dermatitis, duck itch, duckworms, clam-diggers itch, rice paddy itch.

EPIDEMIOLOGY

AGE Children > adults.
GENDER M = F.
INCIDENCE Common. Often in local episodic outbreaks.
GEOGRAPHY Worldwide; most common in freshwater lakes in north and central United States.
ETIOLOGY Parasitic cercariae of the *Schistosoma* genus have birds, ducks, and cattle as their usual hosts, with snails as the intermediate host. Humans may become an accidental host by contacting either the freshwater or marine form of the parasite.
SWIMMER'S ITCH *Trichobilharzia ocellata* and *T. physellae*, common in swamps.
COLLECTOR'S ITCH *T. stagnicolae*, common in shallow waters.

HISTORY

ONSET Initial exposure causes no symptoms. Subsequent exposures incite an allergic response to a protein residue deposited by the invading parasite. At the time of cercarial penetration, an itching sensation (lasting 1 hour) associated with 1- to 2-mm macules at the sites of penetration may be noted. Cercariae die after penetration into human skin. Initial macules persist a few hours and are followed by a more severe pruritic eruption 10 to 15 hours later. The eruption may progress to a more severe state, peaking in 2 or 3 days and resolving within 7 days. Systemic symptoms are rare.

PHYSICAL EXAMINATION

Skin Findings

TYPE Macules, papules, edema, vesicles, and urticarial wheals.
COLOR Pink to red.
SIZE 3 to 5 mm.
DISTRIBUTION On exposed skin. Spares area covered by clothing (Fig. 24-2).

General Findings

Severe cases may have associated fever, nausea, and malaise.

DIFFERENTIAL DIAGNOSIS

The differential diagnosis of cercarial dermatitis includes seabather's itch, drug eruption, photodermatitis, allergic contact dermatitis, and viral exanthem.

COURSE AND PROGNOSIS

The initial pruritic, macular eruption lasts 1 hour and is followed by a more extensive papular eruption 10 to 15 hours later. This papular eruption generally peaks within 2 to 3 days and self-resolves with no sequelae in 7 to 14 days.

MANAGEMENT

Swimmer's itch is best managed with avoidance of schistosome-infested waters. Attempts have been made to target the snail or waterfowl host as a preventative measure treating the lakes with a mixture of copper sulfate and carbonate, or sodium pentachlorophenate. Since the cercariae do not dwell within the skin, lesions regress spontaneously. Antihistamines, topical calamine, and topical steroids can help relieve symptoms.

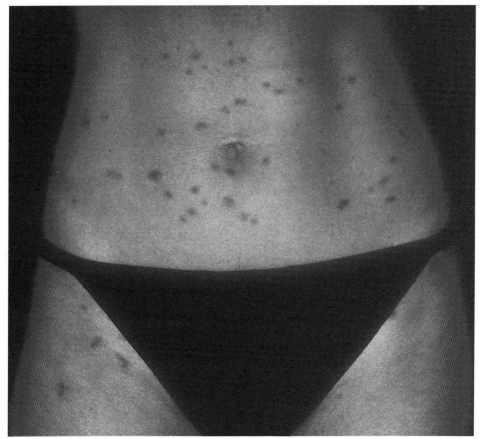

FIGURE 24-2 Cercarial dermatitis: Swimmer's itch Erythematous papules on the exposed areas of a swimmer.

SEABATHER'S ITCH

Seabather's itch is an acute, self-limiting dermatitis, arising shortly after immersion in seawater and characterized by a perifollicular eruption on areas covered by swimsuits.

SYNONYMS Seabather's eruption, marine dermatitis, sea lice.

EPIDEMIOLOGY

AGE Children > adults.
INCIDENCE Common.
GEOGRAPHY Florida, Caribbean, and Cuban salt waters most commonly. Also reported in Asia and Brazil.
ETIOLOGY Planula larvae of sea anemone (*Edwardsiella lineata*) or jellyfish (*Linuche unguiculata*).

HISTORY

The larvae from offending species become trapped between the skin and bathing suits or other garments worn while swimming. Skin lesions develop several hours after bathing in salt water teeming with anemone larvae, as the organisms die and insert their stinging nematocysts into the skin when dry or exposed to fresh water. Skin lesions may itch or burn and persist for 1 to 2 weeks. Systemic symptoms are uncommon but can include headache, malaise, nausea, vomiting, and fever.

PHYSICAL EXAMINATION

Skin Findings

TYPE Macules, papules, wheals, vesiculopapules.
COLOR Erythematous.
SIZE 2 to 3 mm.
DISTRIBUTION Areas covered by bathing suit (Fig. 24-3).

DIFFERENTIAL DIAGNOSIS

The differential diagnosis of seabather's itch includes swimmer's itch, irritant dermatitis, or contact dermatitis.

COURSE AND PROGNOSIS

Seabather's eruption develops several hours after bathing in infested salt water, progresses to a vesiculopapular form, crusts, then spontaneously resolves in 7 to 14 days. It may be intensely pruritic, especially at night. Systemic symptoms are rare, but may include fever, headache, and malaise.

MANAGEMENT

Seabather's eruption may be avoided by washing and drying bathing suit-covered areas of the skin immediately after swimming in infested seawater. Symptomatic treatment includes antipruritic lotions, antihistamines, and limited use of topical or systemic corticosteroids.

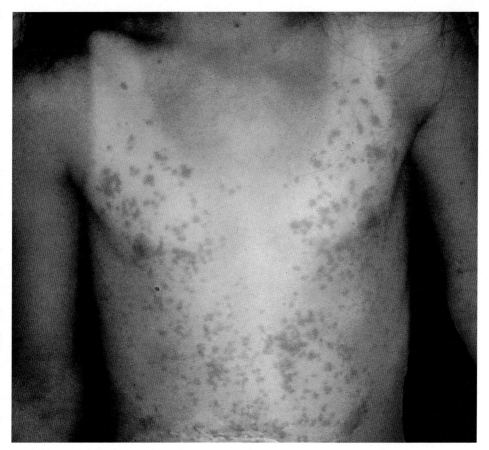

FIGURE 24-3 Seabather's itch Erythematous papules on the unexposed areas of a swimmer.

SEA URCHIN DERMATITIS

Sea urchins are echinoderms with a flat body covered with long, needle-like spines containing venom, which is released once the spine penetrates the skin.

EPIDEMIOLOGY

AGE Any age.
GENDER M = F.
INCIDENCE Uncommon.
GEOGRAPHY Tropical, subtropical climates.
ETIOLOGY Toxins from sea urchin pedicellaria (jaw-like structures that cling to the skin and inject venom) and spines (Fig. 24-4).

HISTORY

Sea urchin dermatitis most commonly occurs when a person accidentally steps on the spines, although handling of the sea urchin can also trigger it to sting. Immediate pain and burning locally is followed by muscle and other systemic symptoms.

PHYSICAL EXAMINATION

Skin Findings

TYPE Puncture site, macule, papule.
COLOR Red–purple.
DISTRIBUTION Exposed areas that brush against the sea urchin: feet (Fig. 24-5).

General Findings

Pedicellaria stings, particularly from the *Toxopneustes pileolus* species common in Japanese waters, can lead to short-lived paralysis, aphonia, neuropathy, or respiratory distress.

DIFFERENTIAL DIAGNOSIS

The differential diagnosis for sea urchin dermatitis includes coral dermatitis, jellyfish stings, insect bites, or snakebites.

COURSE AND PROGNOSIS

Sea urchin dermatitis is typically mild and self-limited. Cases in which larger amounts of spine and pedicellaria are left piercing the skin with larger doses of venom injected can have more severe sequelae (nausea, intense radiating pain, paresthesias, hypotension, respiratory distress, muscular paralysis). More chronic changes can include granuloma formation and hyperpigmentation due to traumatic tattooing from dye contained in sea urchin spines.

MANAGEMENT

All adherent pedicellaria and spines should be removed as quickly as possible to limit the venom infusion. Since no antivenom for any of the venomous echinoderms exists, treatment is supportive and includes hot water immersion (114°F or 45°C) to inactivate heat-labile toxins, ice water immersions for pain relief, prompt analgesia, wound management, and observation for and supportive treatment of systemic symptoms.

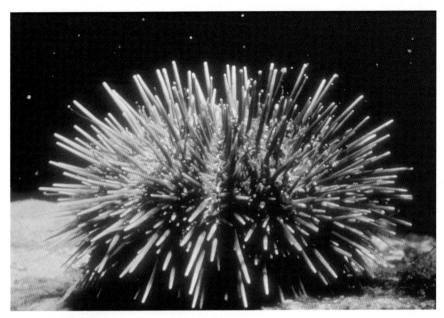

FIGURE 24-4 Sea urchin Spiny projections of sea urchin.

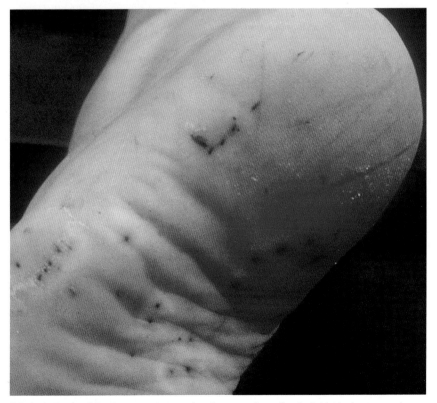

FIGURE 24-5 Sea urchin Puncture sites on the plantar surface of an individual who stepped on a sea urchin.

JELLYFISH DERMATITIS

Jellyfish are radial, symmetric animals with jelly-like bodies and tentacles covered with nematocysts (stinging capsules on tentacles that contain venom).

SYNONYMS *Cnidaria,* Portuguese-man-of-war, hydroids, box jellyfish. Closely related to sea nettles and sea anemones.

EPIDEMIOLOGY

AGE Children > adults.
GENDER M > F.
INCIDENCE Uncommon.
GEOGRAPHY Jellyfish present in temperate, subtropical/tropical waters (Fig. 24-6). Cases commonly reported off coasts of Florida and Australia.
ETIOLOGY Jellyfish venom that contains histamine, prostaglandins, kinin-like factors, and other proteins that may be cardiotoxic or neurotoxic.

PATHOPHYSIOLOGY

Stimulation of the hairs surrounding the jellyfish nematocyte will cause it to eject into the host and express its toxin, which may contain catecholamines, vasoactive amines (e.g., histamine, serotonin), kinins, collagenases, hyaluronidases, proteases, phospholipases, fibrinolysins, dermatoneurotoxins, cardiotoxins, neurotoxins, nephrotoxins, myotoxins, and antigenic proteins.

HISTORY

Immediately after jellyfish contact, intense burning and stinging occur, followed by pruritus and urticaria. Skin necrosis may rarely develop. Residual hyperpigmented streaks may last for months. Depending on the jellyfish species, age of the victim, and amount of venom injected, symptoms can range from mild pruritus to severe systemic shock.

PHYSICAL EXAMINATION

Skin Findings

TYPE Macules, plaques, vesicles, bullae.
COLOR Red, purple, brown.
ARRANGEMENT Linear streaking (Fig. 24-7).
DISTRIBUTION Any exposed site, most common on the legs and arms.

General Findings

Systemic symptoms range from mild malaise, fever, nausea, vomiting, and muscle aches to severe anaphylaxis and cardiac or pulmonary arrest. Stings involving the eye may cause a severe photophobia and keratitis.

DIFFERENTIAL DIAGNOSIS

The differential diagnosis of jellyfish stings includes phytophotodermatitis and contact dermatitis.

LABORATORY EXAMINATIONS

DERMATOPATHOLOGY Nematocysts may be identified; keratinocyte edema, erythrocyte extravasation, and interstitial infiltrate (neutrophils, eosinophils, lymphocytes) may be present.

COURSE AND PROGNOSIS

Eighty-five percent of jellyfish stings are localized with pruritus and burning that gradually self-resolves with mild systemic symptoms. More severe systemic reactions (cardiac arrhythmias, bronchospasm, spastic paralysis, nausea, vomiting, muscle spasms) can be seen in smaller victims injected with more potent jellyfish species venom.

MANAGEMENT

Local skin treatment involves immediate nematocyte inactivation, analgesia, and removal of tentacles or spines. Sterile saline or seawater can be used to wash the area. Warm water immersion or 5% acetic acid (vinegar) left on for 30 minutes will help inactivate the venom. After the inactivation, all adherent tentacles or spines should be removed as quickly as possible (with gloves or tweezers) to reduce venom injections. Vigorous rubbing may trigger firing of nematocysts, and as such should be avoided. Topical anesthetics are helpful once the nematocytes/nematocysts are removed. Cold pack compresses at the sting site for 5 to 10 minutes relieve all but the most severe site pain.

Local or systemic reactions can be treated with antihistamines or corticosteroids. Anaphylactic symptoms can be treated with epinephrine. Antivenoms are available for the most deadly jellyfish (antivenom index published by the American Zoo and Aquarium Association) and, if used promptly, can be lifesaving.

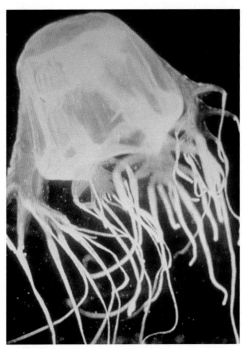

FIGURE 24-6 Jellyfish dermatitis Long tentacles of the jellyfish contain venom and are responsible for the streaky dermatitis.

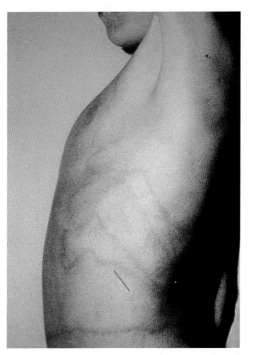

FIGURE 24-7 Jellyfish dermatitis Linear hyperpigmented streaks on the side of a child who brushed against the jellyfish tentacles.

CORAL DERMATITIS

Coral dermatitis is caused by skin accidentally brushing against coral exoskeleton, with resultant laceration, burning, stinging, and foreign body reaction.

SYNONYMS Fire corals, stony corals.

EPIDEMIOLOGY

AGE Children > adults.
GENDER M = F.
INCIDENCE Uncommon.
ETIOLOGY Exoskeleton of the coral.

PATHOPHYSIOLOGY

Exoskeleton of the coral can be spiny and sharp, cutting into exposed skin and resulting in a foreign body reaction.

HISTORY

Corals are located on the floor of the ocean and are accidentally stepped upon or brushed against with a resultant burning, stinging reaction.

PHYSICAL EXAMINATION

Skin Findings

TYPE Papules, pustules.
COLOR Pink, red.
ARRANGEMENT Clustered or linear depending upon exposure pattern.

DISTRIBUTION Exposed sites, commonly legs and feet (Fig. 24-8).

General Findings

May have mild fever, malaise.

DIFFERENTIAL DIAGNOSIS

The differential diagnosis or coral dermatitis includes contact dermatitis, sea jellyfish stings, and sea urchin dermatitis.

COURSE AND PROGNOSIS

Coral dermatitis is self-limited and typically resolves in 2 to 4 weeks. Risk of infection from a coral cut is of greater concern than the toxic effects of the coral. Residual hyperpigmentation can persist for months. Rarely, cutaneous granulomas or a long-standing hypersensitivity reaction may develop at the site of coral dermatitis.

MANAGEMENT

No treatment for coral dermatitis is necessary. Symptomatic relief with analgesics and topical steroids can help.

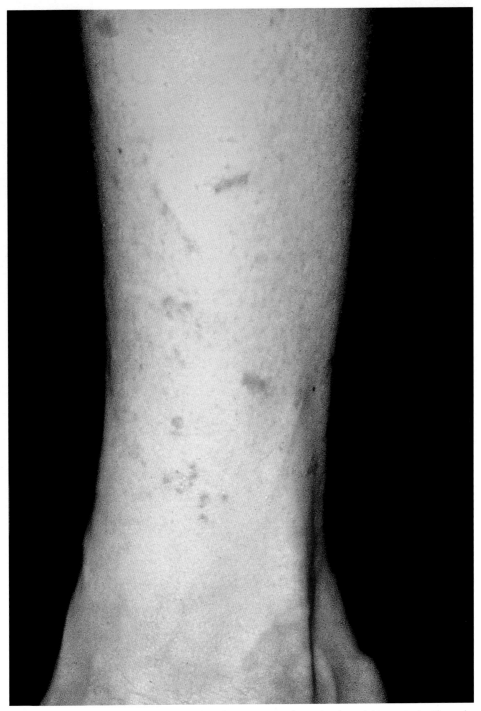

FIGURE 24-8 Coral dermatitis Scattered erythematous papules at the sites of skin contact with coral.

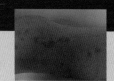

INSECT BITES AND INFESTATIONS

PEDICULOSIS CAPITIS

Pediculosis capitis is an infestation of the scalp by the head louse, which feeds on the human scalp and neck and deposits its eggs on the hair.

SYNONYMS Head lice, louse, nit.

EPIDEMIOLOGY

AGE Children > adults.
GENDER F > M.
PREVALENCE 12 million school children annually in the United States. Ten percent of children worldwide.
INCIDENCE Common.
RACE Caucasian, Asians > blacks.
EPIDEMICS In schools.
SEASON Year-round, but greatest in summer.
ETIOLOGY *Pediculus humanus capitis* (2-mm, six-legged, wingless insect; Fig. 25-1).

PATHOPHYSIOLOGY

Head lice are transmitted from person to person via shared hats, caps, brushes, combs, or head-to-head contact. The *Pediculus humanus capitis* female lays approximately 10 ova per day gluing its eggs to the hair within 1 to 2 mm of the scalp. The ova hatch in 10 days, the louse emerges as a nymph, reaches its adult form 10 days later, and has a life span of 30 days. Lice have anterior mouthparts that attach and feed on blood five times a day. Lice cannot survive for more than 3 days off the human head. Majority of patients have a population of **fewer than 10 head lice.**

HISTORY

Humans contract lice by sharing brushes, hats, close head-to-head contact, etc. The scalp louse deposits nits on the hair next to the scalp, and scalp hair grows 0.5 mm daily (thus, the presence of nits 15 cm from the scalp indicates an infestation that is approximately 9 months old). New viable eggs have a creamy-yellow color; empty eggshells are white. The infestation first manifests as severe pruritus of the back and sides of scalp. Crusts and secondarily impetiginized lesions are common and may extend onto the neck, forehead, face, and ears. In extreme cases, the scalp can become a mass of matted hair, lice, nits, and purulent discharge called plica polonica.

PHYSICAL EXAMINATION

Skin Findings

TYPE Lice, nits (1-mm eggs; Fig. 25-2), macules, papules, excoriations.
SITES OF PREDILECTION Scalp: occipital, postauricular regions.
ASSOCIATED FINDINGS Cervical or posterior auricular lymphadenopathy may be present.

DIFFERENTIAL DIAGNOSIS

The differential diagnosis of pediculosis capitis includes hair casts, dried hairspray or gel, dandruff (epidermal scales), impetigo, seborrheic dermatitis, and tinea capitis.

LABORATORY EXAMINATIONS

DERMATOPATHOLOGY Bite site will show intradermal hemorrhage and a deep, wedge-shaped infiltrate with eosinophils and lymphocytes.
MICROSCOPIC EXAMINATION Shows lice and/or nits adherent to hair.
WOOD'S LIGHT Nits will fluoresce pearly white-blue and are not movable.

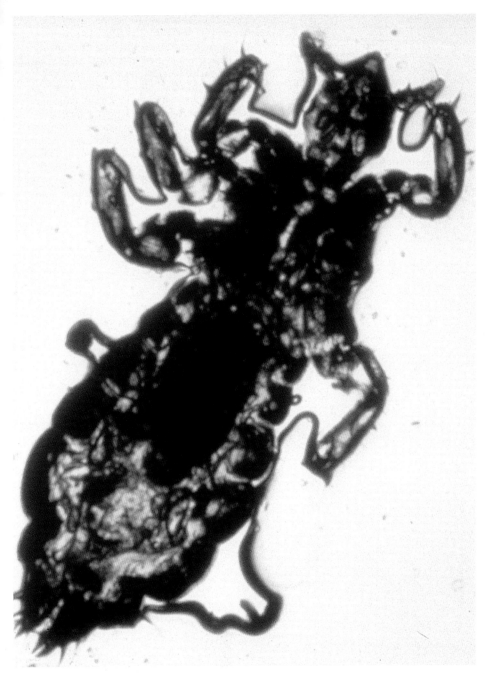

FIGURE 25-1 Pediculus humanus Six-legged wingless insect responsible for head lice.

MANAGEMENT

Head lice are best treated with pediculicides: permethrin, lindane, malathion, or mercuric oxide ointment. The pyrethroids are neurotoxic to lice and current management recommends topical 1% or 5% permethrin applied to scalp and washed off after 10 minutes followed by combing nits out with a fine-toothed comb. The treatment should be repeated 8 to 10 days later. If nits and eggs are still present, pyrethrin/pyrethroid-resistant lice may be present and two applications of 0.5% or 1% malathion should be used combined with fine-toothed combing. Other topical agents that may be first-line treatments for head lice include topical spinosad, topical ivermectin, and topical 5% benzyl alcohol.

Lindane should be avoided in children, because there is potential CNS toxicity associated with overuse or accidental ingestion. Home remedies (such as oils, kerosene, formic acid, and vinegar) are also NOT recommended. All other family members should be checked for asymptomatic lice, because epidemics start in the family, not at school. Floors, play areas, and furniture should be vacuumed. Clothes and bedding should be washed and dried on high heat. Combs and brushes should be soaked in pediculicide for 15 minutes and should not be shared between family members until infection is cleared.

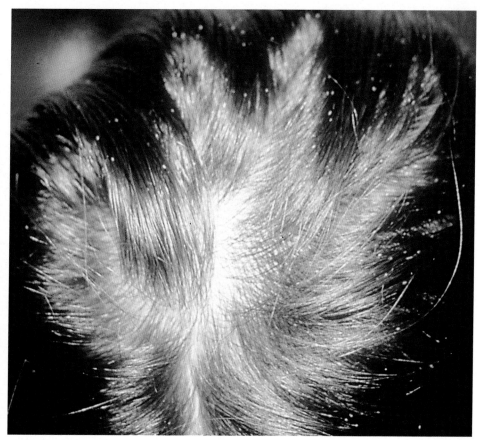

FIGURE 25-2 Head lice Numerous grayish-white lice egg capsules stuck firmly on the hair in a child with head lice.

PEDICULOSIS PUBIS

Pediculosis pubis is an infestation of hairy regions, most commonly the pubic area but at times the hairy parts of the chest, axillae, and upper eyelashes. It is manifested clinically by mild-to-moderate pruritus.

SYNONYMS Crabs, crab lice, pubic lice, phthiriasis.

EPIDEMIOLOGY

AGE 14 to 40 years; most commonly sexually active teenagers and young adults.
GENDER M > F.
INCIDENCE Common.
ETIOLOGY *Phthirus pubis* (1-mm, six-legged insect, crablike in appearance; Fig. 25-3).

PATHOPHYSIOLOGY

The pubic louse lives exclusively on humans and they are transmitted by close physical contact (crowded living conditions, sharing a bed, sharing towels, sexually transmitted). The *P. pubis* female lays 1 to 2 ova per day, has a lifecycle of 35 days and cannot live off the human host for more than 1 day. They remain stationary with their embedded mouth parts in the skin and their claws grasping a coarse hair (pubic, perianal, axillary, eyelashes, eyebrows, facial hair) on either side (Fig. 25-4).

HISTORY

Pediculosis pubis may be asymptomatic or pruritic for months. With excoriation, the lesions may become tender with enlarged regional (inguinal, axillary) lymph nodes. There may also be maculae caeruleae (tâches bleues)—slate-gray, 1-cm macules on the trunk or legs—because of the breakdown product of heme from the louse saliva.

PHYSICAL EXAMINATION

Skin Findings

TYPE Lice, eggs (nits), macules, papules, excoriation, crust.
COLOR Red, blue (maculae caeruleae).
DISTRIBUTION Pubic, axillary areas > trunk. Children: eyelashes, eyebrows.

General Findings

Local lymphadenopathy may be present.

DIFFERENTIAL DIAGNOSIS

The differential diagnosis for pediculosis pubis includes tinea, folliculitis, and scabies.

LABORATORY EXAMINATIONS

DERMATOPATHOLOGY Bite site will show intradermal hemorrhage and a deep, wedge-shaped infiltrate with eosinophils and lymphocytes. The lice themselves do not enter into the skin surface.
MICROSCOPY Lice and nits may be identified with hand lens or microscope.

MANAGEMENT

Pubic lice is best treated with topical pediculicides; permethrin, lindane, or malathion are acceptable treatments. The treatment of choice for pubic lice recommended by the CDC is topical permethrin 1% cream applied for 10 minutes and then washed off. Treatment applied once again 7 to 10 days later may demonstrate the best efficacy. If nits and eggs are still present, resistant lice may be present and 0.5% or 1% malathion should be used. Lindane should be avoided in children, because there is potential CNS toxicity associated with overuse or accidental ingestion.

All sexual contacts should be checked and treated for pubic lice. Clothes and bedding should be washed and dried on high heat to kill ova and parasites. Pediculosis of the eyelashes can be treated with petrolatum bid to eyelashes and mechanical removal. Oral ivermectin can also be used in such patients, or in those who fail topical treatment regimens.

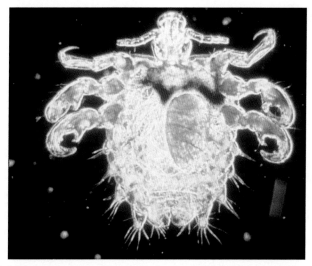

FIGURE 25-3 Phthirus pubis Six-legged crab-like louse responsible for pubic lice.

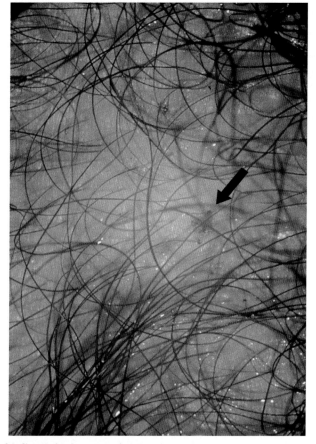

FIGURE 25-4 Pubic lice Pubic louse on a hair in a patient.

PEDICULOSIS CORPORIS

Pediculosis corporis is caused by the body louse that lives on bedding and clothing but intermittently infests humans to feed.

SYNONYM Body lice.

EPIDEMIOLOGY

AGE All ages.
GENDER M = F.
INCIDENCE Common.
ETIOLOGY *Pediculus humanus corporis* (2 to 6 mm, six-legged louse).

PATHOPHYSIOLOGY

Pediculus humanus corporis live on clothing, crawling onto the human host only to feed, predominantly at night. The adult female body louse has a life cycle of 35 days, lays 15 eggs a day on clothing seams and can survive 10 days without a blood meal. On an average, 20 lice can be found on a person with an infestation.

HISTORY

Pediculosis corporis is transmitted via contaminated clothing or bedding. The louse feeds transiently on the skin causing a pruritic eruption, depositing nits on clothes that can remain viable for weeks. Furthermore, the louse can carry rickettsial organisms (epidemic typhus, trench fever, relapsing fever) and transmit them to the human host while feeding.

PHYSICAL EXAMINATION

Skin Findings

TYPE Macule, papule, urticaria, lice, nits (Fig. 25-5).

General Findings

Usually, none present.

DIFFERENTIAL DIAGNOSIS

The differential diagnosis of pediculosis corporis includes eczema and scabies.

LABORATORY EXAMINATIONS

DERMATOPATHOLOGY Bite site will show intradermal hemorrhage and a deep, wedge-shaped infiltrate with eosinophils and lymphocytes. The lice themselves do not enter into the skin surface and will not be seen on histology.
MICROSCOPIC EXAMINATION Lice, nits can be visualized on infested clothes.
WOOD'S LIGHT Nits will fluoresce pearly white-blue.

COURSE AND PROGNOSIS

Undiagnosed pediculosis corporis can lead to worsening pruritus and increased risk of transmission to unaffected individuals.

MANAGEMENT

Because the body louse is rarely on the person's body, treatment is directed more toward patient education. Clothes and bedding should be washed in hot water and then dried on high heat to kill lice and ova. In instances of extensive corporeal lice, a single topical application of permethrin to the entire body can be useful.

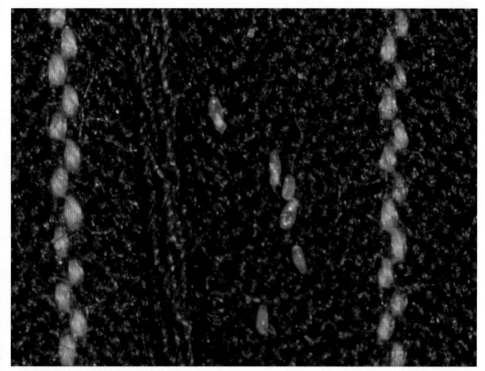

FIGURE 25-5 Body lice Scattered nits seen on the seams of clothing.

SCABIES

Scabies is an infestation by the mite *Sarcoptes scabiei*, characterized by severe pruritus and transmitted by close proximity to an infested person.

 INSIGHT Although resistance to several of the antiparasitics exists and may be growing, many cases of so-called resistant scabies infestation turn out not to be scabies at all.

SYNONYMS 7-year itch, mange.

EPIDEMIOLOGY

AGE In children who are younger than 5 years, young adults (sexually transmitted), bedridden elderly patients.
GENDER M = F.
INCIDENCE Common. Up to 300 million cases annually worldwide.
SEASON Fall, winter.
ETIOLOGY *S. scabiei* var *hominis* (400 μm in size).

PATHOPHYSIOLOGY

The scabies mite can only survive and replicate on human skin and are transmitted by close proximity. Once on the human host, the scabies mite lays eggs under the skin as it burrows. The ova hatch in 5 days, reach maturity in 2 weeks, and then die after 2 months. The mites and eggs can remain alive for 1 to 2 days on clothes or bedding.

HISTORY

One month after exposure, the infested person begins with intractable itching. For pruritus to occur, there must be sensitization to the *S. scabiei* mite. The widespread rash is usually caused by less than 10 mites jumping from site to site on the body. In neonates, immunosuppressed or debilitated patients with more severe infestation, mites can exceed hundreds in number and produce a diffuse scaling eruption (crusted scabies).

PHYSICAL EXAMINATION

Skin Findings

TYPE Burrows, vesicles (Fig. 25-6), excoriations, scale, or crust.
COLOR Gray or flesh-colored, black dot (the mite).
DISTRIBUTION Fingers, wrists, elbows, umbilical area, genital area, feet.

Variants

Nodular scabies: 10-mm, red, nodular lesions on the scrotum, back, feet (Fig. 25-7).

Crusted (formerly Norwegian) scabies: widespread mite infestation causing a crusted generalized rash.

DIFFERENTIAL DIAGNOSIS

The differential diagnosis of scabies includes impetigo, papular urticaria (insect bite), psoriasis, contact dermatitis, atopic dermatitis, or pediculosis.

LABORATORY EXAMINATIONS

DERMATOPATHOLOGY Scabietic burrow, mite, or feces (scybala) in the stratum corneum. Dermis shows a diffuse eosinophilic infiltrate.
SCABIES PREP (Fig. 25-8). A scraping can reveal mites (400-μm round mites with protruding legs), eggs (100-μm oval particles), or feces (10-μm small oval particles).

COURSE AND PROGNOSIS

Scabies pruritus persists for weeks even after adequate treatment, and nodular lesions can take months to years to resolve.

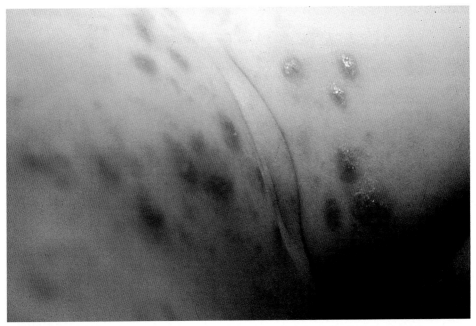

FIGURE 25-6 Scabies Papular and vesicular lesions in the axilla of a child infested with scabies.

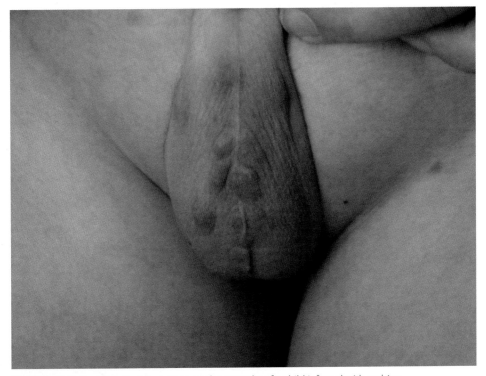

FIGURE 25-7 Scabies Nodular lesions on the genitalia of a child infested with scabies.

MANAGEMENT

A scabicide such as permethrin 5% cream should be applied from neck to toes, left on for 8 hours, and then washed off. Other topical options include lindane, benzyl benzoate, crotamiton, or sulfur. All family members and close contacts should be treated simultaneously and the treatment can be repeated in 1 week to ensure successful eradication. Residual pruritic symptoms and nodules are typical and do not indicate persistent infection. For infants and young children with whole-body involvement, permethrin, 10% crotamiton, or 6% to 10%

sulfur ointment should be applied to all body surface areas. One- or two-dose regimens of oral ivermectin may also be used for the treatment of scabies with similar efficacy. For the management of crusted scabies, both oral and topical treatment in combination are recommended.

Emollients, antihistamines, and topical steroids can be used for symptomatic relief of pruritus. Bedding and clothing should be machine washed in hot water and machine dried on high heat or ironed. Infested articles can also be stored in an airtight garbage bag for more than 72 hours so the mites will die.

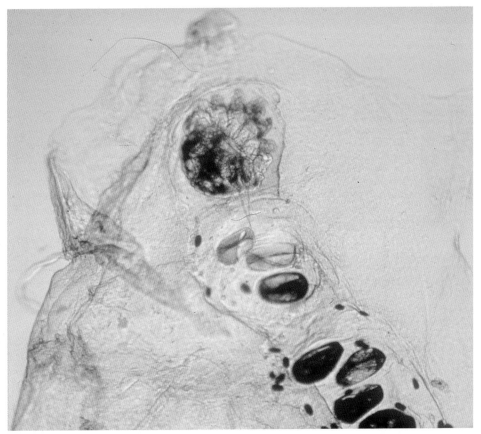

FIGURE 25-8 Sarcoptes scabiei Mite, 400 μm in size, alongside ova (large black ovals), and feces (scattered smaller black dots).

PAPULAR URTICARIA

Papular urticaria is an immunologic-mediated reaction to insect bites, characterized by an intensely pruritic eruption occurring at the bite sites hours to days after the bites. Of note, patients are often unaware of having been bitten.

 INSIGHT Three factors can contribute to the bizarre occurrence of only one child being affected by papular urticaria in a family: (1) Some individuals are more attractive to certain insects; (2) individuals have different levels of reactivity to bites; (3) some patients are very aware of the lesions while others will not notice them unless pointed out.

EPIDEMIOLOGY

AGE Children > adults.
INCIDENCE Extremely common.
RACE Asians > other races.
SEASON Spring, summer.
ETIOLOGY Bites from mosquitoes, gnats, fleas, mites, bedbugs, etc.

PATHOPHYSIOLOGY

Papular urticaria follows an insect bite and is a type I hypersensitivity reaction triggered by injected foreign antigens in a patient who is sensitive.

HISTORY

At the site of a bite, pruritus and erythema occur a few hours after the bite and persist for 1 to 2 weeks or longer. Affected individuals are often not aware of being bitten by insects. Additionally, some family members do not react to bites or are not as highly exposed as the children. Reactions in infants on first exposure may be mild but upon subsequent exposure, young children (aged 1–5 years) have a more severe response. Reactions often subside as the child grows older.

PHYSICAL EXAMINATION

Skin Findings

TYPE Macules, papules (Fig. 25-9), vesicles, excoriations, scars.
COLOR Red.
SHAPE Round, domed.
ARRANGEMENT Usually, in groups of three (representing the "breakfast, lunch, and dinner" of offending insects).
DISTRIBUTION Legs > arms > trunk.

DIFFERENTIAL DIAGNOSIS

The differential diagnosis of papular urticaria includes allergic contact dermatitis, especially to plants such as poison ivy or poison oak.

LABORATORY EXAMINATIONS

DERMATOPATHOLOGY Edema, spongiosis, dermal inflammation with eosinophils.

COURSE AND PROGNOSIS

Papular urticaria is self-limited, but may take weeks to months to clear.

MANAGEMENT

The treatment of papular urticaria is symptomatic with oral antihistamines, antipruritics, or topical steroids. Preventative measures include insect repellents such as DEET (in children or adults) or citronella when outdoors as well as flea/tick control on indoor pets.

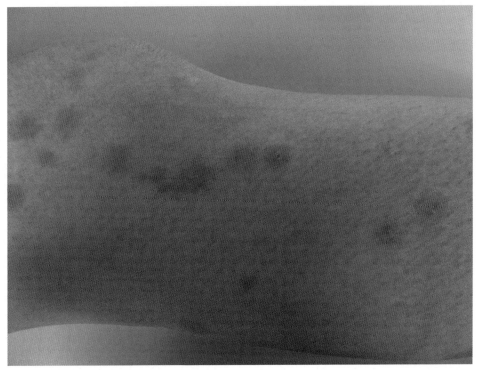

FIGURE 25-9 Papular urticaria Persistent erythematous papules with central vesicles on the leg of a child bitten by insects.

FIRE ANT STING

Fire ant stings are caused by ants of the *Solenopsis* species and are characterized by burning, painful stings that flare immediately and then vesiculate with purulent fluid at the puncture site.

EPIDEMIOLOGY

AGE Children > adults.
GENDER M = F.
INCIDENCE Common, especially in endemic areas.
GEOGRAPHY South America, southern United States.
ETIOLOGY Fire ants (*Solenopsis saevissima*, *Solenopsis richteri*, and *Solenopsis invicta*).

PATHOPHYSIOLOGY

Fire ants grasp the host with their mandibles and then pivot injecting venom with their abdominal stinger in a circular pattern. The venom contains hemolytic factors (triggering mast cells to release histamine) and allergenic proteins.

HISTORY

Fire ants will swarm on a person and bite ferociously, leaving hemorrhage puncta at the site of puncture. The initial reaction is a wheal flaring around the bite site followed by vesiculation. The vesicle becomes cloudy after 10 hours and may last for several days before crusting and potentially leading to scarring. Systemic fever, GI distress, urticaria, and respiratory symptoms are common and become more severe with successive attacks. Rarely anaphylaxis may occur in individuals previously sensitized.

PHYSICAL EXAMINATION

Skin Findings

TYPE Macule, papule, wheal, vesicle (Fig. 25-10).
COLOR Red, pink (Fig. 25-11).
SIZE 1 to 3 cm.
DISTRIBUTION Legs, torso, arms.

DIFFERENTIAL DIAGNOSIS

The differential diagnosis of fire ant bites includes other bites, viral exanthema, or VZV.

LABORATORY EXAMINATIONS

DERMATOPATHOLOGY Perivascular lymphocytic infiltrate with neutrophils and some eosinophils, followed later by vesiculation with neutrophils and epidermal necrosis, dermal edema.

COURSE AND PROGNOSIS

Once bitten, the patient can feel quite ill, and the skin is very itchy and painful at the sites of bites. Systemic reactions can be quite severe (bronchospasm, laryngeal edema, hypotension) and even life-threatening, especially in small children with numerous bites. These reactions tend to increase in severity with subsequent attacks, and fatal anaphylaxis reactions, while rare, are becoming more common.

MANAGEMENT

Local application of cool compresses, topical analgesics, or topical steroids can alleviate the burning, stinging pain. A papain solution of one-fourth meat tenderizer and four parts water, applied topically, can also relieve the itch and burn. Systemic antihistamines, steroids, or epinephrine may be needed in severe cases with signs of respiratory distress. Patients with a known allergy to fire ant bites should carry an epinephrine pen for immediate use in the event of future bites. Fire ants are unable to bite through clothing or shoes, so appropriate cover of feet and legs during outdoor activities can minimize risk of bites.

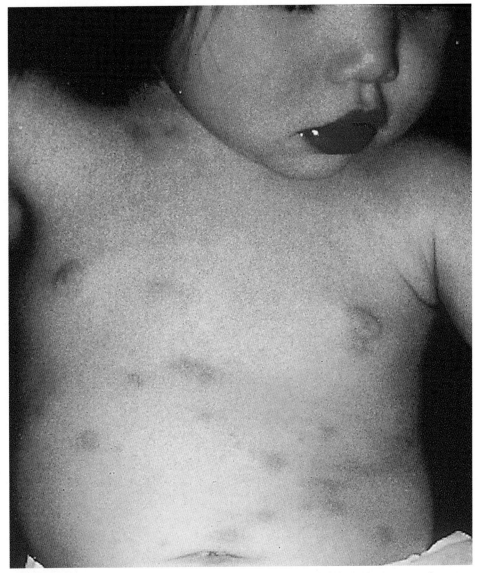

FIGURE 25-10 Fire ant stings Diffuse erythematous papules on a child bitten by numerous fire ants.

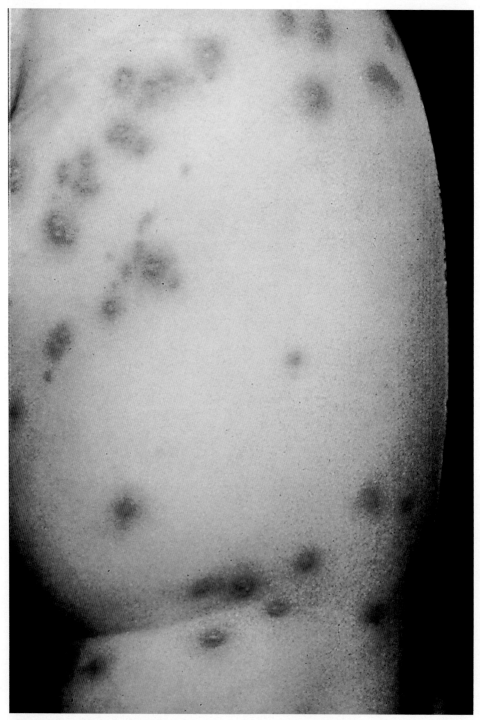

FIGURE 25-11 Fire ant stings Erythematous macules with central pustule formation 24 hours after bites in the same child.

INDEX

Note: Page number followed by f and t indicate figure and table respectively.